Progress in
LIVER DISEASES

VOLUME VI

—————— VOLUME VI ——————

Progress in
LIVER DISEASES

Edited by

HANS POPPER, M.D., Ph.D.

Gustave L. Levy Distinguished Service Professor
Mount Sinai School of Medicine of the
City University of New York

and

FENTON SCHAFFNER, M.D., M.S.

George Baehr Professor of Medicine
and Chief, Division of Liver Diseases
Mount Sinai School of Medicine of the
City University of New York

with 70 contributors

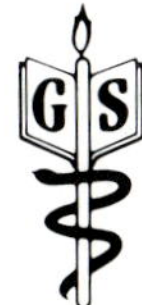

GRUNE & STRATTON
A Subsidiary of Harcourt Brace Jovanovich, Publishers
New York   San Francisco   London

Grune & Stratton, Inc.
111 Fifth Avenue
New York, New York 10003

*Distributed in the United Kingdom by
Academic Press, Inc. (London) Ltd.
24/28 Oval Road, London NW 1*

Library of Congress Catalog Number 61-14102
International Standard Book Number 0-8089-1174-0
Printed in the United States of America

Dedicated to the various national and international associations for
the study of liver diseases around the world.

Contents

CONTENTS

Preface

A progress series in liver diseases, of which this is the sixth volume, contrasts with a textbook. The latter presents comprehensive coverage of the field, whereas the former is devoted to single projections in which areas of particular progress are emphasized. While continuous progress is to be expected, these projections can be compared with the amoeboid movements, where pseudopods form but then disappear with advancement of science, hopefully, by consolidation. Progress in hepatology has been slow since Volume V appeared three years ago, and entailed consolidation and elaboration rather than breakthroughs. Two amoeboid projections listed in Volume V as not yet ready for inclusion, have consolidated and are represented here. One is hepatitis A, now well delineated from hepatitis B, particularly by its lack of chronicity and of a carrier stage. Meanwhile, non-A-non-B hepatitis has been recognized in epidemiologic studies and confirmed in chimpanzee transmissions, and this form, now the most frequent cause of posttransfusion hepatitis, shares these characteristics with hepatitis B, possibly also the association with hepatic cancer. As a matter of fact, chronicity seems to be particularly common, at least with posttransfusion non-A-non-B hepatitis. Environmental liver injury, the second such subject listed in the preface of Volume V, is also now presented in detail, although its frequency as cause of chronic liver disease in man is still in doubt.

The greatest progress since 1961, however, when Volume I appeared, is probably the development of hepatology into an identifiable clinical discipline in the Anglo-American and Germanic countries, as it has been long before in the Latin countries. The ascendency of this discipline is reflected in the bloom and scientific vigor of the associations—international, continental, and national—devoted to the study of the liver and its diseases to which, therefore, this volume is dedicated.

As in previous volumes, the attempt is made to look at hepatic problems from various viewpoints and to present a mixture of theoretical basic-science information, some of which may become clinically useful in the future, and of observations and conclusions applicable today at the bedside. As before, morphology is emphasized primarily by cell and organelle alterations of the hepatocytes and also the various sinusoidal cells, with their role in liver disease just becoming apparent. Chapters devoted to biology and biochemistry represent, as before, the mainstay in the basis of understanding, whether they deal with progress in bilirubin, bile acid or lipoprotein metabolism, or biotransformation. Knowledge of the regulation of hepatocytic maintenance and growth now has practical applications. The role of processes, including transport, in the hepatocytic membranes in liver diseases is still largely based on extrapolation from information about other cells, however, particularly since a clean separation of the various domains of the hepatocytic cell membranes has not yet been accomplished. Such presentation, therefore, had to be postponed, although the knowledge of the receptors and the membrane-supporting cytoskeleton is brought.

In the pathogenesis of liver diseases the greatest progress is the role of the viruses, and a chapter is devoted to hepatitis A and three to hepatitis B. The frequent overlap of information in these chapters was permitted to stand to assist the reader in the appreciation of each chapter. In addition, the effects of drugs and parasites are discussed in detail, as are processes independent of etiology, such as cholestasis and endotoxemia; the first is better understood though not yet fully so, and the latter offers a new approach. As usual, diseases like alcoholic liver injury are looked at again from a new viewpoint as is pediatric liver disease, where progress has been made on the basis of the study of a larger material. Hepatocellular cancer, finally, has been a problem of increasing significance, particularly from a global standpoint. In diagnosis, ''radiologic'' methods have become important tools, often replacing biochemical and histological techniques in overall diagnostic significance. Therapy of liver disease is still symptomatic whether it deals with hepatic coma or vitamin D administration. New surgical procedures, like the jugular-peritoneal shunt of LeVeen, still need controlled trials.

The editors had to weigh the degree of interference with the style of the authors. Franz Ingelfinger, in the preface to the fifth volume, listed various rewards for the authors' efforts, to which we want to add the pleasure in writing their chapters and, most importantly, the opportunity to clarify their thoughts. This reduced editorial license and even such terms as postnecrotic cirrhosis have thus been permitted to stand and, though reluctantly, speculations were not eliminated. The main task of the Editors was to exert pressure for rapid completion to avoid the frequent obsolescence before appearance. The hope is expressed that the volume reflects the labor of love of the authors and Editors who, unfortunately, could not avoid arbitrary decisions in selections.

The Editors

Contributors

DANIEL ALAGILLE, M.D., Professor of Pediatrics, Université Paris-Sud, Head, Department of Pediatrics, Hôpital d'Enfants deBicêtre, and Director, Unité de Recherche d'Hépatologie Infantile de l'Institut National de la Santé et de la Recherche Médicale, Paris, France

WOLFGANG ARNOLD, M.D., Freie Universität Berlin, Universitätskinikum Charlottenburg, Abteilung für Innere Medizin und Poliklinik, Spandauer Damm 130, Berlin, West Germany

D. BERNAERT, Ph.D., Université Libre de Bruxelles, Faculte de Medecine, Laboratoire de Cytologie et de Cancerologie Experimentale, Bruxelles, Belgium

LEONARDO BIANCHI, M.D., Professor of Pathology, University of Basel, Basel, Switzerland

JOHN K. BOITNOTT, M.D., Associate Professor of Pathology, Division of Gastroenterology, The Johns Hopkins University School of Medicine, Baltimore, Maryland

JAMES L. BOYER, M.D., Professor of Medicine, and Director, Liver Study Unit, Department of Medicine, Yale University School of Medicine, New Haven, Connecticut

EUGENE J. BURBIGE, M.D., Assistant Professor in Residence, University of California Davis School of Medicine, and Assistant Chief, G.I. Service, Veterans Administration Medical Center, Martinez, California

PROF. KARL-HERMANN MEYER ZUM BÜSCHENFELDE, M.D., Freie Universität Berlin, Universitätsklinikum Charlottenburg, Abteilung für Innere Medizin und Poliklinik, Spandauer Damm 130, Berlin, West Germany

ARTHUR R. CLEMETT, M.D., Chairman, Department of Radiology, St. Vincent's Hospital and Medical Center, and Clinical Professor of Radiology, New York University School of Medicine, New York, New York

H. DENK, M.D., Professor of Pathology, Division of Gastrointestinal Pathology and Hepatopathology (Hans Popper Laboratory), Department of Pathology, University of Vienna School of Medicine, Vienna, Austria

E. ROLLAND DICKSON, M.D., Associate Professor of Medicine, Mayo Medical School, and Head of a Section in the Division of Gastroenterology and Internal Medicine, Mayo Clinic and Mayo Foundation, Rochester, Minnesota

JULES L. DIENSTAG, M.D., Assistant Professor of Medicine, Harvard Medical School, and Gastrointestinal Unit, Massachusetts General Hospital, Boston, Massachusetts

A.L.W.F. EDDLESTON, D.M., M.R.C.P., Senior Lecturer, and Honorary Consultant Physician, King's College Hospital, London, England

ELWYN ELIAS, B.Sc., M.B., M.R.C.P., Research Associate, Liver Study Unit, Department of Medicine, Yale University School of Medicine, New Haven, Connecticut

GÉRARD FELDMANN, M.D., Associate Professor of Histology, Unité de Recherches de Physiopathologie Hépatique, Hôpital Beaujon, Clichy, and Laboratoire d'Histologie, Embryologie, Cytogénétique, Faculté de Médicine Xavier-Bichat, Paris, France

MURRAY M. FISHER, M.D., Ph.D., Associate Professor of Medicine and Pathology, University of Toronto, and Head, Division of Gastroenterology, Sunnybrook Medical Centre, Toronto, Canada

C. RICHARD FLEMING, M.D., Assistant Professor of Medicine, Mayo Medical School, and Consultant, Division of Gastroenterology and Internal Medicine, Mayo Clinic and Mayo Foundation, Rochester, Minnesota

PETER T. FLUTE, M.D., T.D., M.R.C.P., F.R.C. Path., Professor of Haematology, St. George's Hospital Medical School, London, England

MICHAEL R. FREEMAN, M.D., Research Fellow, Division of Gastroenterology, Department of Medicine, University of Tennessee Center for the Health Sciences, Memphis, Tennessee

SAMUEL W. FRENCH, M.D., Professor of Pathology, University of California Davis School of Medicine, and Chief, Laboratory Service, Veterans Administration Medical Center, Martinez, California

MICHAEL A. GERBER, M.D., Associate Professor of Pathology, Mount Sinai School of Medicine, The City University of New York, New York, New York

MARC A. GOLDMAN, M.D., Former Fellow in Gastroenterology, Medical College of Virginia, Richmond, Virginia, and Gastroenterologist, Springfield, Massachusetts

JOHN L. GOLLAN, M.D., Ph.D., F.R.A.C.P., M.R.C.P., Assistant Professor of Medicine, Gastrointestinal Research Unit, Department of Medicine, and The Liver Center, University of California, San Francisco, California

MARTIN GRÜN, M.D., Medizinische Universitätsklinik Würzburg, West Germany

FRED GUDAT, M.D., Head, Section for Immunology, Department of Pathology, University of Basel, Basel, Switzerland

UWE HOPF, M.D., Freie Universität Berlin, Universitätsklinikum Charlottenburg, Abteilung für Innere Medizin und Poliklinik, Spandauer Damm 130, Berlin, West Germany

THOMAS H. HÜTTEROTH, M.D., Freie Universität Berlin, Universitätsklinikum Charlottenburg, Abteilung für Innere Medizin und Poliklinik, Spandauer Damm 130, Berlin, West Germany

WILLIAM B. JAKOBY, Chief, Section on Enzymes and Cellular Biochemistry, National Institute of Arthritis, Metabolism, and Digestive Diseases, National Institutes of Health, Bethesda, Maryland

E. ANTHONY JONES, M.D., M.R.C.P., Acting Chief, Section on Diseases of the Liver, Digestive Diseases Branch, National Institute of Arthritis, Metabolism, and Digestive Diseases, National Institutes of Health, Bethesda, Maryland

DR. D. L. KNOOK, Deputy Director, Institute for Experimental Gerontology TNO, Rijswijk, The Netherlands

K. S. KOCH, Molecular Biology Laboratory, The Salk Institute, San Diego, California

H. L. LEFFERT, M.D., Cell Biology Laboratory, The Salk Institute, San Diego, California

HEINRICH LIEHR, M.D., Professor of Medicine, Medizinische Universitätsklinik Würzburg, West Germany

RICHARD G. LONG, M.D., M.R.C.P., Honorary Senior Registrar, Royal Postgraduate Medical School, University of London, Hammersmith Hospital, London, England

JURGEN LUDWIG, M.D., Associate Professor of Pathology, Mayo Medical School, and Consultant, Department of Pathology and Anatomy, Mayo Clinic and Mayo Foundation, Rochester, Minnesota

WILLIS C. MADDREY, M.D., Associate Professor of Medicine, Division of Gastroenterology, The Johns Hopkins University School of Medicine, Baltimore, Maryland

C. MAY, Ph.D., Faculté de Medecine, Laboratoire de Cytologie et de Cancerologie Experimentale, Bruxelles, Belgium

TOSHIRO NAKASHIMA, M.D., Professor of Pathology, Kurume University School of Medicine, Kurume, Japan

ADAM NOWOSŁAWSKI, M.D., Professor of Pathology, and Head, Department of Immunopathology, National Institute of Hygiene, Warsaw, Poland

KUNIO OKUDA, M.D., Professor of Medicine, Chiba University School of Medicine, Chiba, Japan

ROBERT L. PETERS, M.D., Professor of Pathology, University of Southern California, and Chief Pathologist, The University of Southern California Liver Unit, Los Angeles, California

M. JAMES PHILLIPS, M.D., Professor and Vice-Chairman, Department of Pathology, University of Toronto, Toronto, Canada

HANS POPPER, M.D., Ph.D., Gustave L. Levy Distinguished Service Professor, Mount Sinai School of Medicine of the City University of New York, New York, New York

JAMES B. RAGLAND, Ph.D., Professor of Biochemistry in Medicine, Division of Gastroenterology, Department of Medicine, University of Tennessee Center for the Health Sciences, Memphis, Tennessee

JUERG REICHEN, M.D., Guest Worker, Section on Diseases of the Liver, Digestive Diseases Branch, National Institute of Arthritis, Metabolism, and Digestive Diseases, National Institutes of Health, Bethesda, Maryland

SEYMOUR M. SABESIN, M.D., Professor of Medicine, and Director, Division of Gastroenterology, Department of Medicine, University of Tennessee Center for the Health Sciences, Memphis, Tennessee

FENTON SCHAFFNER, M.D., George Baehr Professor of Medicine, and Chief, Division of Liver Diseases, Mount Sinai School of Medicine of The City University of New York, New York, New York

BRUCE F. SCHARSCHMIDT M.D., Assistant Professor of Medicine, Gastrointestinal Research Unit, Department of Medicine, and The Liver Center, University of California, San Francisco, California

CHARLES C. SCHWARTZ, M.D., Staff, Gastroenterology Section, Veterans Administration Medical Center, and Assistant Professor of Medicine, Medical College of Virginia, Richmond, Virginia

IRVING J. SELIKOFF, M.D., Professor of Community Medicine and Medicine, Director of Division of Environmental Medicine and Environmental Sciences Laboratory, Mount Sinai School of Medicine, The City University of New York, New York, New York

DAME SHEILA SHERLOCK, M.D., F.R.C.P., Professor of Medicine, Department of Medicine, University of London, and Chairman, Department of Medicine, Royal Free Hospital, Medical School, London, England

DR. DAVID I. H. SIMPSON, Senior Lecturer in Virology, and Honorary Consultant in Virology, Department of Medical Microbiology, The London School of Hygiene and Tropical Medicine, London, England

THOMAS E. STARZL, M.D., Ph.D., Professor and Chairman, Department of Surgery, University of Colorado Medical Center, Denver, Colorado

CLIFFORD J. STEER, M.D., Clinical Associate, Section on Diseases of the Liver, Digestive Diseases Branch, National Institute of Arthritis, Metabolism, and Digestive Diseases, National Institutes of Health, Bethesda, Maryland

ROBERT STERN, M.D., Associate Professor, Department of Pathology, University of California, San Francisco, California

IRMIN STERNLIEB, M.D., Professor of Medicine, Divisions of Genetic Medicine and Gastroenterology, and Associate Director, Liver Research Center, Albert Einstein College of Medicine and Bronx Municipal Hospital Center, Bronx, New York

LEON SWELL, Ph.D., Chief, Lipid Research Laboratory, Veterans Administration Medical Center, and Research Professor of Biochemistry and Medicine, Medical College of Virginia, Richmond, Virginia

JOHN TERBLANCHE, CH.M. (Cape Town), F.R.C.S. (Eng), F.C.S. (S.A.), Professor of Surgery, University of Cape Town and Groote Schuur Hospital, Co-Director of the South African Medical Research Council Liver Research Group, and Head, Department of Surgery, Somerset Hospital, Cape Town, South Africa

JOHN M. VIERLING, M.D., Clinical Associate, Section on Diseases of the Liver, Digestive Diseases Branch, National Institute of Arthritis, Metabolism, and Digestive Diseases, National Institutes of Health, Bethesda, Maryland

Z. RENO VLAHCEVIC, M.D., Chief, Gastroenterology Section, Veterans Administration Medical Center, and Professor of Medicine, Medical College of Virginia, Richmond, Virginia

J. C. WANSON, M.D., Assistant Professor, and Director of the Cytology and Experimental Cancer Laboratories, Université Libre de Bruxelles, Rue Heger Bordet, 1, 1000 Brussells, Belgium

KENNETH S. WARREN, Director for Health Sciences, The Rockefeller Foundation, New York, New York

RICHARD A. WEISIGER, Division of Gastroenterology, Department of Medicine, University of California, San Francisco, California

ROGER WILLIAMS, M.D., F.R.C.P., Director of the Liver Unit, and Consultant Physician, King's College Hospital, London, England

PROF. DR. E. WISSE, Laboratory for Cell Biology and Histology, Free University of Brussels, Brussels, Belgium, and Laboratory for Electron Microscopy, University of Leiden, Leiden, The Netherlands

ALLAN W. WOLKOFF, Assistant Professor, Department of Medicine, Albert Einstein College of Medicine, New York, New York

HSU-CHONG YEH, M.D., Associate Professor of Radiology, Mount Sinai School of Medicine, and Physician-in-charge, Ultrasound Section, Mount Sinai Hospital, New York, New York

LESLIE ZIEVE, M.D., Professor of Medicine, University of Minnesota, Minneapolis, Minnesota

DAVID S. ZIMMON, M.D., Associate Professor of Clinical Medicine, New York University School of Medicine, Chief, Gastroenterology Section, New York Veterans Administration Medical Center, and Gastroenterologist, St. Vincent's Hospital and Medical Center, New York, New York

PROF. ARIE J. ZUCKERMAN, Professor of Microbiology, and Director, Department of Medical Microbiology and WHO Collaborating Centre for Reference and Research on Viral Hepatitis, London School of Hygiene and Tropical Medicine, London

Chapter 1

Morphology and Functional Properties of Isolated and Cultured Hepatocytes

By J. C. WANSON, D. BERNAERT, *and* C. MAY

THE ISOLATION OF HEPATOCYTES in pure fractions devoid of sinusoidal cells, bile duct cells, and fibroblasts provides a useful and interesting experimental model for the study of specific metabolic functions. This model displays numerous advantages when compared to in vivo rat liver perfusion or to incubation of liver slices, namely homogeneity of the cell population and longer cell viability.

Many attempts have been made during the last 25 years to prepare intact hepatic cell suspensions, using either physical or chemical agents (for detailed reviews, see references 1, 2, and 3). The earliest cell preparations were based on mechanical dissociation or the use of divalent metal chelators, such as pyrophosphate, ethylenediamine tetraacetate (EDTA), or citrate,[4] which, by Ca^{2+} removal, release cells from their adhesive forces. An important technical advance was proposed[5] using collagenase as a liver tissue dispersing agent. The yield of isolated intact cells was improved by introducing the continuous recirculating perfusion of the rat liver in situ.[6] A variant of these enzymatic methods was achieved using a two-step procedure that consists of perfusing the rat liver with a Ca^{2+}-free buffered solution followed by enzymatic treatment.[7]

Any successful method for obtaining well-preserved hepatocytes in high yields must involve three critical steps, namely exposure of the tissue to a calcium-free medium, digestion with collagenase, and gentle mechanical action. Cell preservation is estimated by means of dye exclusion tests and morphologic and biochemical criteria.[1,2,6,8,9]

The morphologic analysis of liver tissue reveals hepatocytic cell heterogeneity within the lobule. The use of stereologic techniques has shown that centrolobular cells differ significantly from peripheral ones, taking into account the number and relative volume of mitochondria, lysosomes, and peroxisomes, the proportion of smooth endoplasmic reticulum (SER), and the glycogen content.[10] A gradient in cell size and in hepatocellular fine structure across the entire liver lobule has also been observed.[11] Moreover, hepatocytes display differences in cell ploidy.[12,13] A functional heterogeneity corresponds to this ultrastructural heterogeneity, both of which result from differences in topo-

From the Laboratoire de Cytologie et de Cancérologie Expérimentale, Free University of Brussels, Belgium

This presentation is dedicated to the memory of Professor P. Drochmans graphic metabolic conditions, depending on the quality of the blood supply and the significantly greater volume of bile canalicular space in the portal parenchyma. Numerous authors, using histochemical and biochemical techniques, have detected differences in enzymatic distribution.[14-17] Isolation of intact hepatocytes in suspension provides the opportunity for further separation of different hepatocytic subpopulations according to their size, density, or degree of ploidy. Liver cell subpopulations were separated by isopyknic centrifugation on Ficoll density gradients.[18,19] Two distinct populations of light and heavy hepatocytes are distinguished, which would correspond respectively to centrolobular and peripheral hepatocytes. Furthermore, centrolobular cells can be more efficiently separated from peripheral cells by using drugs or hormones that selectively influence each type of cell.[19-22] A very promising technique, counterflow centrifugation or elutriation, allows the separation of hepatocytes according to cell size and degree of ploidy.[23]

Isolated adult rat parenchymal cells have been used in many laboratories to prepare primary monolayer cultures.[24-32] This experimental model appears suitable for the ultrastructural analysis of cell aggregation [33,34] and for metabolic and pharmacologic studies.[29,30,35] The effects on hepatocytes of drugs, hormones, toxins, and chemical carcinogens can be investigated in vitro, without hormonal or nervous control, and the cells are viable for several days.

The purpose of this presentation is (1) to describe the different steps of the isolation procedure we used to obtain intact adult rat hepatocytes in suspension; (2) to define the morphologic and functional properties of the isolated cells; (3) to analyze the degree of cell heterogeneity in hepatocytic subpopulations separated according to density, cell size, and cell ploidy; and (4) to study their behavior in primary monolayer cultures.

FACTORS INVOLVED IN LIVER TISSUE ADHESION

Hepatic parenchymal cells, or hepatocytes, are arranged in one-cell-thick radiating plates, extending from the periphery to the center of the lobule and separated from each other by sinusoids. Hepatocytes in situ form polyhedral cells, presenting heterogeneous cell surfaces as revealed by scanning electron microscopy of freeze-fractured liver tissue [36,37] and by conventional transmission electron microscopy. Sinusoidal faces, which appear in front of the sinusoids (Fig. 1, Sn), are provided with numerous short (0.5 μ) microvilli (Fig. 1, mv), usually of uniform diameter (0.1 μ), that penetrate into the space of Disse (Fig. 1, Di). At the level of the interhepatocytic faces, three zones of cell contacts can be distinguished: (1) regions of parallel pairs of cell membranes separated by a constant narrow gap of 10–15 nm; (2) regions comprising the bile canaliculus (Fig. 1, BC) endowed with tight junctions (Fig. 1B, ti); and

---

FIG. 1A, B, C—Hepatocytes in situ. Sinusoidal faces display numerous microvilli (mv) penetrating into the space of Disse (Di). Interhepatocytic surfaces present specific cell membrane differentiations, namely bile canaliculi (BC) endowed with tight junctions (Fig. 1B, ti), desmosomes (Fig. 1B, D), and gap junctions (Fig. 1C, G). Notice a Golgi complex (Go) in front of the bile canaliculus (Sn, sinusoid) (1A: ×9,000, 1B: ×21,000; 1C: ×11,000).

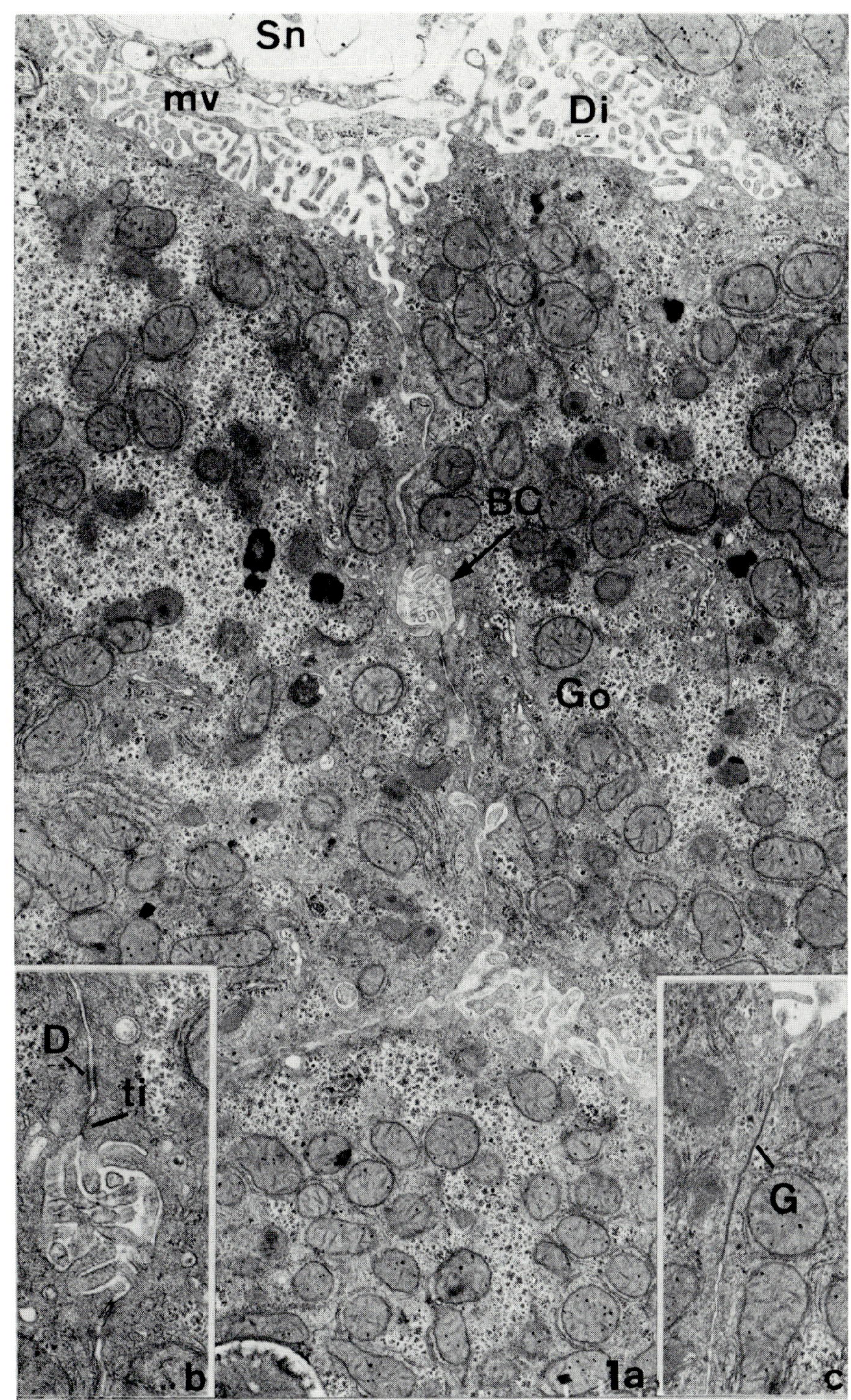

3

(3) regions composed of cell membrane differentiations, such as desmosomes (Fig. 1B, D) and gap junctions (Fig. 1C, G). Although the main specific functions of tight and gap junctions are occlusion of bile compartment and intercellular communication, respectively, these cell membrane differentiations, together with desmosomes, play an important role in liver cohesiveness.

Calcium ions act on plasma membrane adhesiveness.[4,38,39] Preperfusion of the liver with calcium-free Krebs-Ringer solution[2] provokes the dissociation of pairs of adjacent plasma membranes and the cleaving of some membrane domains, namely the desmosomes.[8] Figure 2 illustrates, at high magnification, the effect of a 20-min Ca^{2+} free perfusion. Segments of parallel cell membranes that are normally in close contact (arrows) are dismantled. Some narrow segments remain intimately associated at each side of the bile canaliculus (Fig. 2, BC), where specific membrane differentiations occur, namely tight junctions (arrowheads). Gap junctions also resist the removal of calcium ions.

Finally, the framework of connective tissue, which is composed mainly of numerous collagen fibrils that penetrate deeply inside the liver lobule in the space of Disse, constitutes a well-developed skeleton, which maintains and strengthens the liver architecture. Enzymatic perfusion in the presence of collagenase promotes digestion of this framework and increases the yield of intact isolated cells.[6]

PROCEDURE FOR LIVER CELL PREPARATION

The isolation procedure that we recommend is a multistep process during which cell contacts are weakened, the framework of connective tissue is partly digested, and the final sites of intimate junctions are mechanically broken. The procedure involves the following steps.

Continuous Recirculating Perfusion of the Rat Liver in Situ

The perfusion apparatus consists of a multibulb glass oxygenator that is equipped with a thermometer, a pH meter, and a mixing reservoir, housed in a Plexiglas cabinet, and maintained at constant temperature (37°C).[40] A preperfusion with a Ca^{2+}-free, CO_2-O_2 bubbled Krebs-Ringer solution (300 mOsm; pH 7.4) is performed for 10 min, followed by enzymic perfusion with a Ca^{2+}-free Krebs-Ringer solution containing 0.1% collagenase (200 U/mg) and 0.1% hyaluronidase (460 U/mg) at 37°C for 30 min. Careful control of temperature (37°C), pH (7.0 to 7.4), Po_2 (500 mm Hg), Pco_2 (27 mm Hg), and flow rate (20 ml/min) is maintained during perfusion. This treatment results in a collapsed organ, which is transformed into single hepatocytic cell plates, embedded in a partly digested connective and vascular tissue matrix. After disruption of the surrounding Glisson's capsule, these cell plates can be liberated into the suspension by gentle dissociation with a spatula.

FIG. 2—Partial dislocation of liver tissue after 20 min of perfusion with a Ca^{2+}-free medium. Interhepatocytic surfaces are dismantled (arrows). Adhesion is maintained (arrowheads) at both sides of the bile canaliculus (BC) ($\times$10,000).

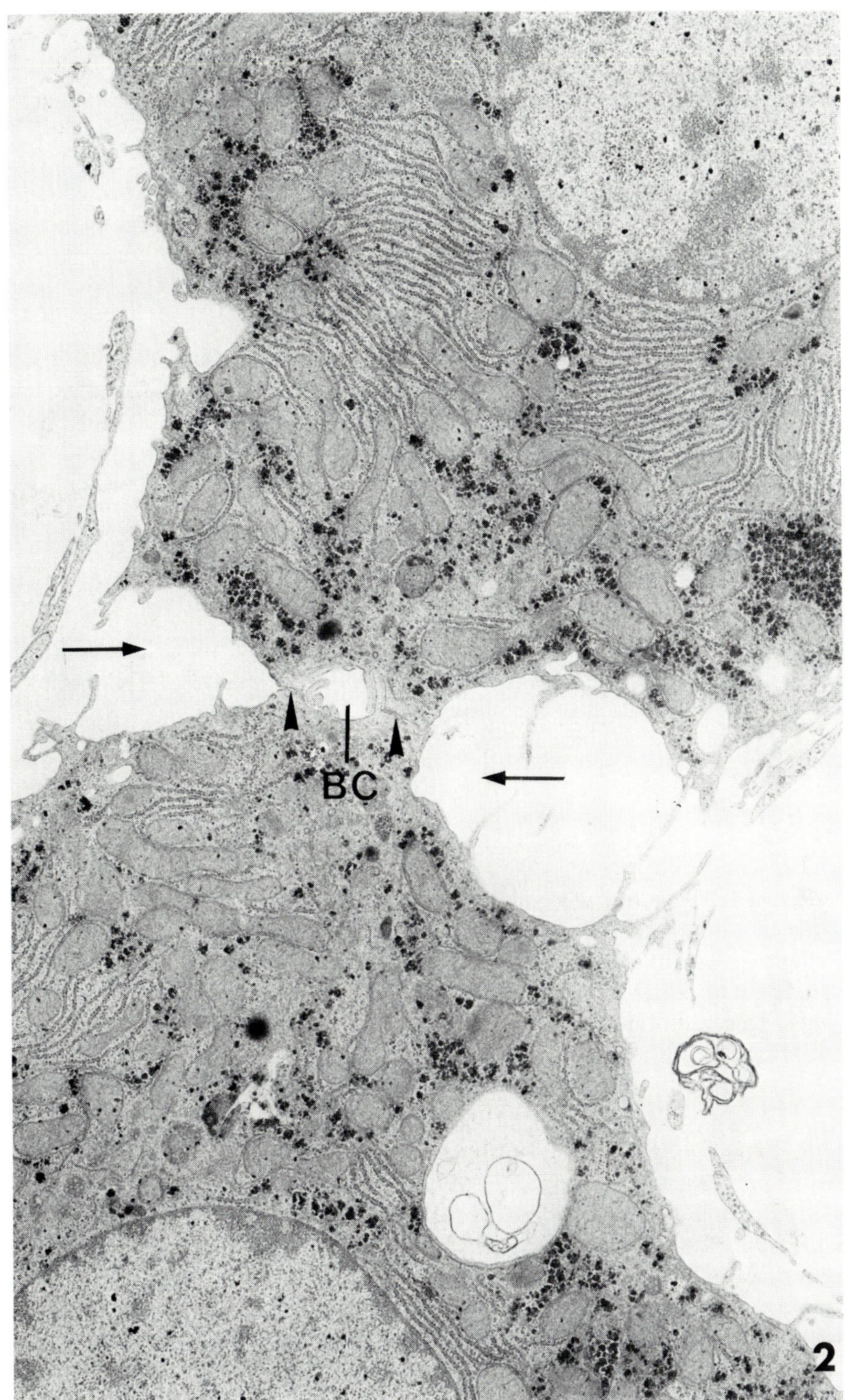

BC
2

Mechanical Dissociation of Hepatic Cell Plates

Mechanical dissociation is accomplished by rolling the cell suspension in a siliconized flask, using a rotary evaporator. This standardized, gentle mechanical treatment is performed at low speed (50 rpm for 5 min) in Ca^{2+}-free, Mg^{2+}-free Krebs-Ringer solution containing 2% dialyzed albumin and 2 mM EDTA (pH 7.2; 37°C). It allows the liberation of a majority of isolated cells, which at this step of the isolation procedure still exhibit their cell surface heterogeneity.[36]

Filtration of the Cell Suspension

The original cell suspension is purified by using Perlon (polyamide PA 6) filters of successively diminishing mesh width, from 100 to 63 μ pore size. Large aggregates are retained on the filters, which account for 10% to 15% of the total material poured on the nylon. Filtration through Perlon of 28-μ pore size is performed when populations of perfectly isolated cells are needed, particularly for the study of cell aggregation in culture.

Washing by a 1-g Sedimentation

A 10–20-ml original cell suspension, diluted into 100 ml of Krebs-Ringer solution, is sedimented at 1 g for 10 min at room temperature. This sedimentation allows purification of the parenchymal cell suspensions by discarding in the supernatant subcellular debris, nonparenchymal cells of small diameter, and damaged hepatocytes.[9]

Preincubation

After sedimentation, the isolated hepatocytes are resuspended in enriched Dulbecco's medium containing 20 mM HEPES (N-2-hydroxyethylpiperazine-N'-2-ethane sulfonic acid) and 40 IU/ml penicillin-streptomycin; the hepatocytes are then incubated for 30 to 60 min at room temperature in a gyratory shaker. During preincubation, hepatocytes become round and acquire homogeneous cell surfaces.

Efficiency and Degree of Purity

Efficiency is evaluated at about 65% to 70% intact isolated cells recovered from the whole liver, i.e. about 50 to 75 $\times$ 10^6 cells per gram of liver tissue, as measured by Coulter counter determinations (Model ZBI, Coulter Electronics Ltd., Dunstable, Bedfordshire, England).

Under the phase contrast microscope, 85% to 90% of the isolated cells appear as well-preserved refringent cells. Few contaminating sinusoidal cells are detected, and few hepatocytes are associated in doublets or triplets.

PROPERTIES OF ISOLATED CELLS

Ultrastructure

Under the transmission electron microscope, isolated hepatocytes present a well-preserved ultrastructure. They display a continuous villous plasma membrane (Fig. 3, mv). Neither cell membrane differentiations, such as desmosomes, tight junctions, or gap junctions, nor remnants of bile canaliculi are detected at the level of the cell surface. The classical biliary polarity, i.e., the presence of Golgi complexes in the peripheral cytoplasm near the bile canaliculi, is also completely lost. Golgi complexes accumulate in the perinuclear area (Fig. 3, Go) intimately associated with lysosomes (Ly). The rough endoplasmic reticulum is composed of parallel running cisternae (RER), and nonswollen

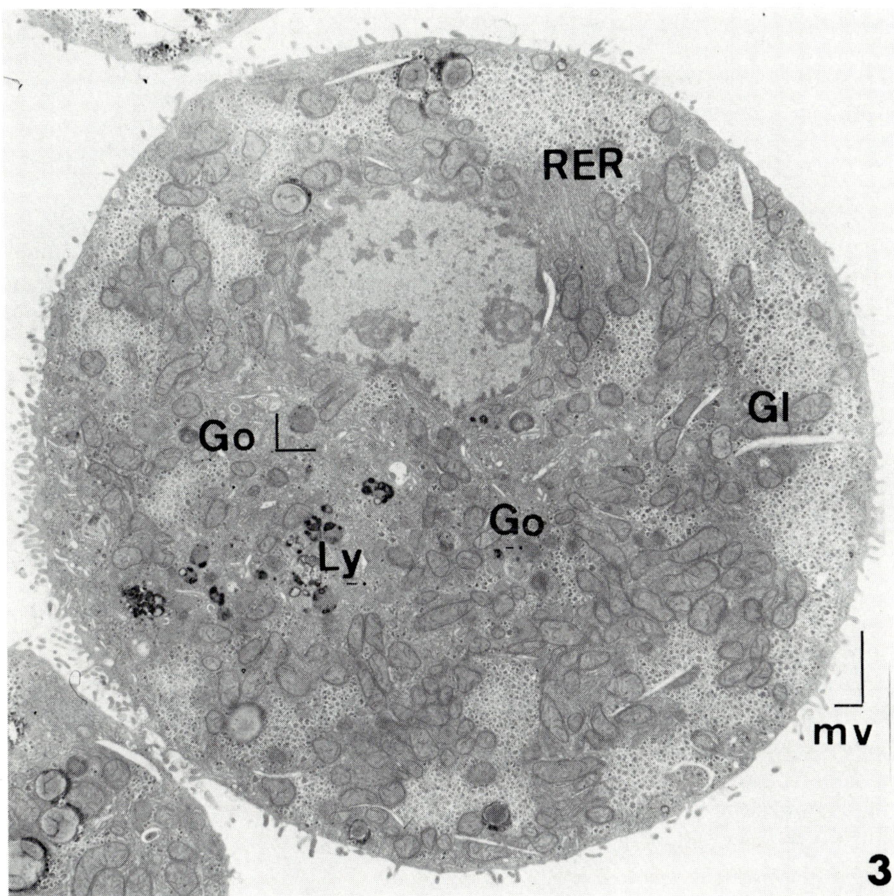

FIG. 3—Isolated hepatocyte, presenting a well-preserved ultrastructure. Notice the numerous microvilli (mv) on the continuous plasma membrane, Golgi complexes (Go) in the perinuclear region, lysosomes (Ly), rough endoplasmic reticulum (RER), and large glycogen areas (Gl) (×6,000).

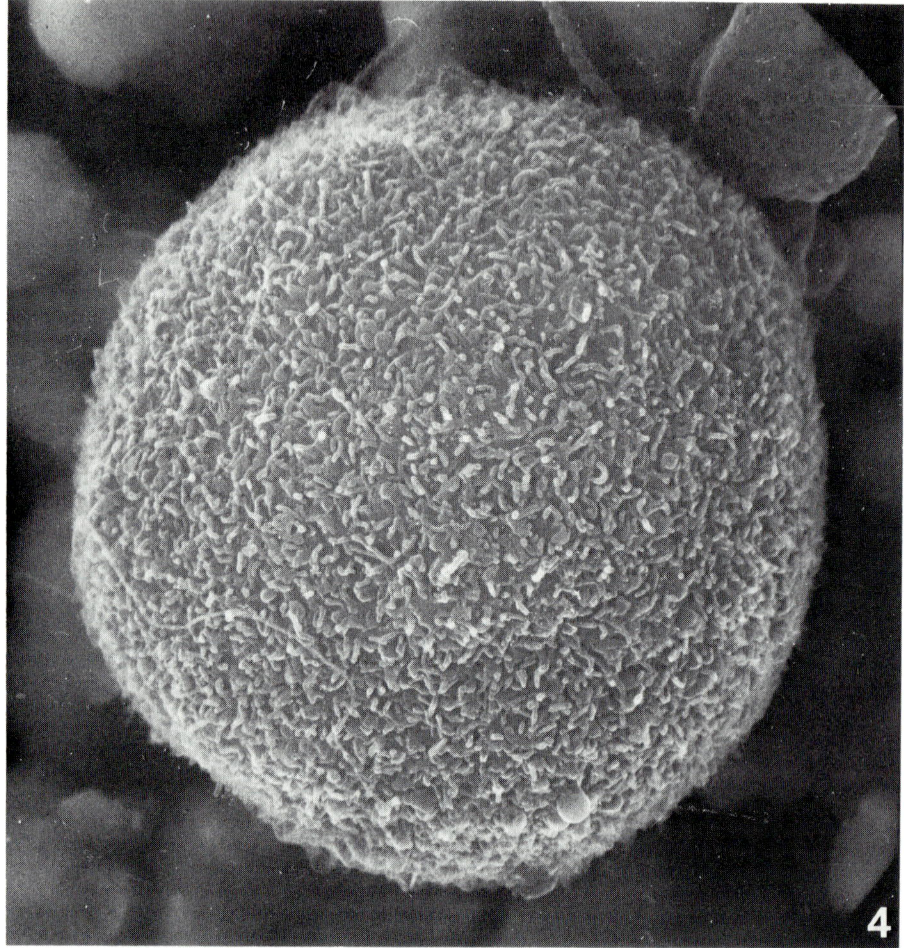

FIG. 4—Scanning electron micrograph of an isolated hepatocyte. The entire cell surface appears covered with numerous microvilli (×6,200).

mitochondria are uniformly distributed inside the cytoplasm. Large glycogen areas mainly composed of α-glycogen particles (Gl) accumulate at the periphery of the cell. Differences in the morphologic properties of isolated hepatocytes are encountered that are reminiscent of the situation in situ (see the next section). Under the scanning electron microscope, the entire cell surface appears covered with numerous microvilli. Hepatocytes are round and form perfectly spherical cells (Fig. 4).

Functional Properties

Glycogen Synthesis in Isolated Hepatocytes

The ability to synthesize glycogen from high concentrations of glucose has been studied in isolated hepatocytes maintained in suspension. The isolated

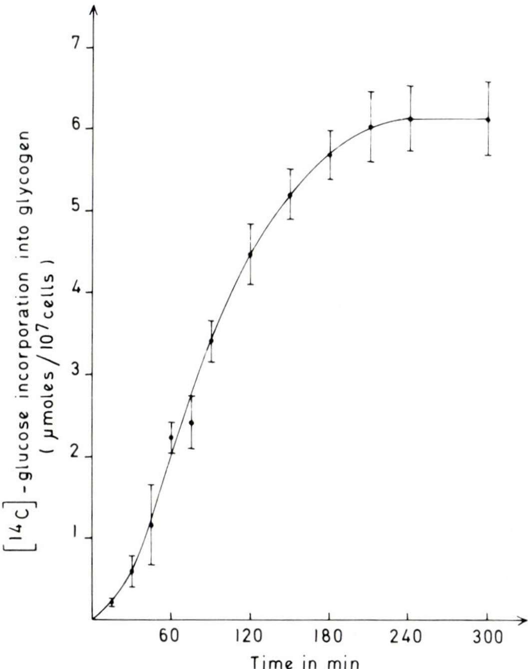

FIG. 5—Kinetics of glucose-^{14}C incorporation into glycogen. Hepatocytes are incubated at 37°C in Dulbecco's medium supplemented with fetal bovine serum, antibiotics, and 40 mM glucose. Mean values are calculated from five experiments. Standard deviations are represented by the vertical lines.

hepatocytes were incubated at 37°C in Dulbecco's medium containing 15% fetal bovine serum, antibiotics, and 40 mM glucose. After a short lag, glycogen synthesis remains linear for 2 to 4 hr and then slows down (Fig. 5). The incorporation rate of glucose into glycogen reaches 2.7 μmole/hr per 10 million incubated cells, or 35 μmol/hr per gram of liver (if 1 g of liver contains about 130 million parenchymal cells). During the first 30 min of incubation, glycogenolysis predominates in the isolated cells. Then, total glycogen content increases and reaches about 137% of the initial value (2.14 mg glycogen per 10^7 cells or 0.106 mg glycogen per milligram of protein) after 4 hr of incubation.

The addition of 20 mU insulin per milliliter of medium does not affect the incorporation rate of glucose during the first 5 hr of incubation. The absence of stimulation of glycogen synthesis by insulin does not result from lack of fixation of the hormone on the receptor sites of the hepatocytes. ^{125}I-insulin is specifically fixed on the isolated hepatocytes, but the fixation is greater at 20°C than at 37°C.[41]

A rapid effect of insulin on glycogenesis in vitro has been argued.[42-45] However, some authors have succeeded in demonstrating stimulation of glycogen synthesis and of the activation of glycogen synthetase by insulin.[46,47]

The glycogen synthetase activity was measured in our cells. Total activity of the enzyme measured in the presence of glucose-6-phosphate (G6P) in the

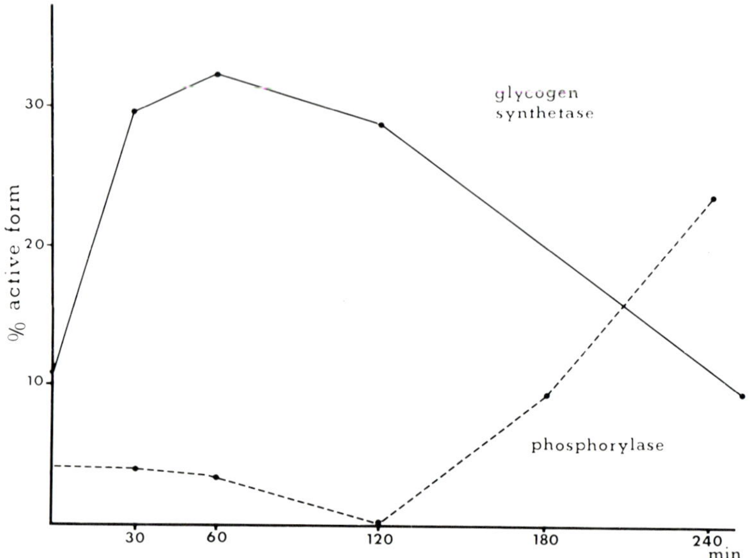

FIG. 6—Effect of glucose on the activities of glycogen synthetase and phosphorylase during incubation at 37°C. This graph presents the percentage of active forms of both enzymes in hepatocytes maintained in suspension.

isolated hepatocytes before incubation reaches 10–15 nmole of glucose incorporated per minute per milligram of protein. At the start of the incubation, the active form represents about 11% of the total synthetase activity; after 1 hr, 32%; and after 2 hr, 29%; in some cases, however, the ratio may increase to 50%. After 4 hr, it is back to its original value of 11% (Fig. 6).

During the activation phase of glycogen synthetase, glycogen phosphorylase is mainly in its inactive form. After 2 hr of incubation, when synthetase becomes inactive, phosphorylase is progressively converted into its active form (Fig. 6).

The ultrastructure of the cells incubated under our conditions was examined after 2 and 4 hr of incubation. After 2 hr of incubation, the homogeneity of the cell population improves. Under close examination, two types of cells may be distinguished: those that contain large accumulations of α-glycogen particles not between the profiles of endoplasmic reticulum, and those that are characterized by hypertrophy of the smooth endoplasmic reticulum. After 4 hr of incubation, the hepatocytes show reproducible structural changes: large accumulations of glycogen, appearance of fat droplets, and the formation of cytolysomes filled with glycogen particles.

In conclusion, the isolated hepatocytes obtained under good ultrastructural conditions are able to synthesize glycogen for at least 4 hr. A high concentration of glucose stimulates glycogenesis and hinders glycogenolysis. The incubation of hepatocytes in the presence of high concentrations of glucose stimulates the conversion of the glycogen synthetase into its active form. Finally, insulin does not stimulate glycogen synthesis in freshly prepared hepatocytes maintained in suspension, although intact receptor sites for insulin have been detected on their plasma membranes (see Chapter 3).

Protein Synthesis in Isolated Hepatocytes

Protein metabolism is well preserved in freshly isolated cells. The kinetics of total protein synthesis may vary, depending on the isolation technique and the incubation medium used. Different experimental conditions were used by many authors for the study of protein synthesis.[1,9,48] When rat hepatocytes are incubated in a culture medium supplemented with serum, which enhances the cell viability, total protein synthesis is maintained for up to 12 hr.[9] The synthesis rate of secreted protein is constant during 20 hr of incubation, whereas the synthesis rate of intracellular protein, which was initially elevated, decreases in the course of time.[48] The incorporation pattern analysis appears complex because of the varying synthesis and degradation rates of the intracellular proteins. Liver cells catabolize 10% to 15% of their own protein during a 20-hr incubation.[48] The various factors influencing the general protein metabolic state of the isolated hepatocytes have also been studied.[49-51]

In our system the rate of leucine incorporation into total protein of the liver cells was determined using Dulbecco's medium. The incorporation rate of leucine is linear for about 4 to 5 hr and reaches 3.5 nmole leucine/hr per milligram of protein (Fig. 7A). With longer incubation periods, the rate of protein synthesis is slightly reduced.

Even in absence of serum the cells remain structurally well preserved after 9 hr of incubation. An interesting morphologic feature is the reconstitution of small cell aggregates in the medium when hepatocytes are incubated in a gyratory shaker for 5 hr.

Specific liver proteins, such as albumin, fibrinogen, transferrin, lipoprotein, and α_1-glycoprotein, are synthesized by isolated liver cells[9,48,52,53] (see Chapter 2). As shown by immunologic methods, albumin is both synthesized and se-

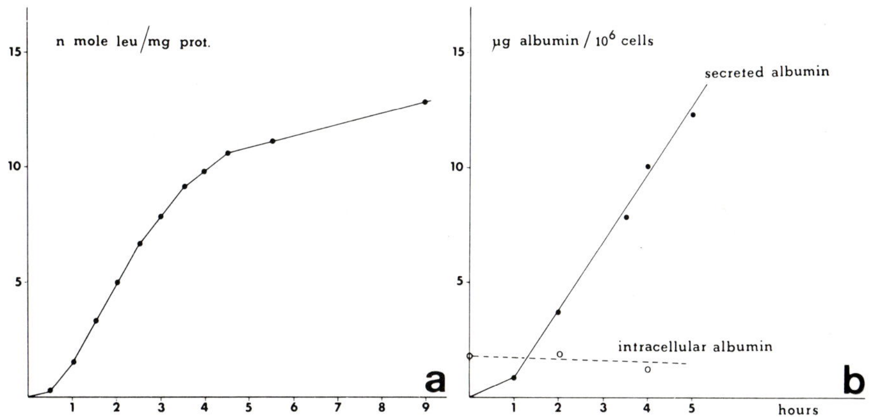

FIG. 7—Kinetics of total protein and albumin synthesis in isolated hepatocytes incubated at 37°C in Dulbecco's medium with antibiotics and without serum. (A) ¹⁴C leucine incorporation into total protein; (B) time course of synthesis of intracellular and secreted albumin.

creted by the cells incubated in Dulbecco's medium at a rate of 3 μg albumin/ hr per 10^6 cells (Fig. 7B). This value, also found by other authors,[9,48] is comparable to the synthesis rate measured in the isolated liver perfused for 12 hr[54] and reaches 40% of the synthesis rate determined in vivo.[55,56] The intracellular albumin concentration remains constant between 1 and 2 μg albumin per 10^6 cells.

SEPARATION OF HEPATOCYTIC SUBPOPULATIONS ACCORDING TO CELL DENSITY OR CELL SIZE

As stated previously, several studies have reported on structural and functional heterogeneity in the liver lobule. The question may be raised whether isolated spherical hepatocytes maintain their specific morphologic, histochemical, morphometric, and biochemical properties after separation and whether it is possible to distinguish several hepatocytic subpopulations, taking into account differences in cell size, cell density, cell ploidy, or amounts and distribution of cell organelles.

Isopyknic Centrifugation

Using 15% to 40% Ficoll density gradients, two types of hepatocytes can be separated.[8] Light hepatocytes, with a mean diameter of 20.5 μ and a mean density of 1.10, present an extended smooth endoplasmic reticulum, numerous small mitochondria, and few glycogen particles. Heavy hepatocytes, with a mean diameter of 19.0 μ and a mean density of 1.14, exhibit a relatively reduced compartment of smooth endoplasmic reticulum but large accumulations of glycogen particles. By stereologic analysis, similar morphologic differences were described between central and peripheral hepatocytes in situ.[10] We therefore suggested that light hepatocytes probably correspond with centrolobular cells and that heavy hepatocytes arise mainly from the peripheral regions.[8] A gradient has been demonstrated in hepatocellular ultrastructure inside the liver lobule, and centrolobular young adult hepatocytes were significantly larger than those in the periportal zone.[11]

A better efficiency in the separation of central and peripheral cells was obtained by enhancing the cell heterogeneity inside the lobule. Two reproducible experimental models were chosen, which increase the lobular heterogeneity by selectively influencing some cells in the lobule. First, intravenous administration of glucose and insulin induces rapid glycogenesis, followed by intense glycogenolysis, preferentially located at the periphery of the lobule.[22] Under these conditions, glycogen permits separation of both cell types. Second, administration of phenobarbital (PB, 100 mg/kg) promotes the proliferation of SER in centrolobular cells, which progressively extends to peripheral cells.[20] The response of hepatocytes to barbiturates showed that the most striking heterogeneity was obtained in the lobule on the third day of PB administration.[21] In this experimental model, centrifugation of isolated cells on Ficoll gradients leads to the separation of light and heavy cells, corresponding respectively to the centrolobular modified hepatocytes and to the peripheral unaffected cells.[19] Morphometric determinations carried out on both cell populations reveal considerable enlargement of centrolobular PB hepatocytes (mean diameter 23.7 μ), while peripheral hepatocytes have a small mean diameter of 19.2 μ.

Elutriation or Counterflow Centrifugation

Counterflow centrifugation separates hepatocytic subpopulations, differing mainly by their cell size and degree of ploidy.[23,57] Fractionation of hepatocytes in different classes with specific properties offers much in the analysis of cell functional heterogeneity and of several liver diseases. For example, preneoplastic liver lesions induced by chemical carcinogens are mainly composed of cells that have a large diameter and are highly polyploid. Selective separation of these hepatocytes in pure fractions would allow detailed analysis of their morphologic and biochemical properties.[58] Hepatocytes in suspension, concentrated in the JE-6 elutriator, adapted to the J-21B Beckmann Centrifuge, were submitted to a counterflow of increasing flow rates from 20 to 25, 30, 35, and 45 ml/min and were separated in five subpopulations (fractions I to V). Fraction I is composed of small diploid cells, presenting a diameter ranging from 15 to 19 μ. Fractions II and III constitute homogeneous populations of well-preserved tetraploid hepatocytes displaying a mean diameter of 20.0 μ. Finally, fractions IV and V are mainly enriched in octoploid cells of large diameter (24 μ) and in doublets and triplets of undissociated cells. Figures 8A and B illustrate the morphologic aspect of the elutriated fractions II (Fig. 8A) and IV (Fig. 8B) under the phase contrast microscope. Figure 8A reveals the high degree of cell size homogeneity of fraction II. The micrograph of Figure 8B shows, at the same final magnification, the presence of hepatocytes of very large size (Fig. 8B, L), contaminated by doublets (D). As confirmed by electron microscopy, elutriated cells maintain good integrity of their organelles, which appear evenly distributed in the different hepatocytic cell classes. Two enzymes, glucose-6-phosphatase, related to the endoplasmic reticulum, and glycogen synthetase, intimately associated to glycogen particles, were tested in the different elutriated fractions: high levels of activity were recorded in the different fractions, which account for the isolation of pure and metabolically active subpopulations.[57]

PRIMARY MONOLAYER CULTURES
OF ADULT RAT HEPATOCYTES

Isolated hepatocytes (3 $\times$ 10^6 cells suspended in 3 ml of medium) were plated in 60-mm plastic Petri dishes in Dulbecco's medium buffered with 20 mM HEPES (pH 7.2) and supplemented with 4 mM glutamine, 5–20 mM glucose, 17% fetal calf serum, and antibiotics (100 μg/ml streptomycin and 100 IU/ml penicillin). Petri dishes were incubated under air and CO_2 (in a ratio of 95:5) at 37°C. The medium was renewed every day.

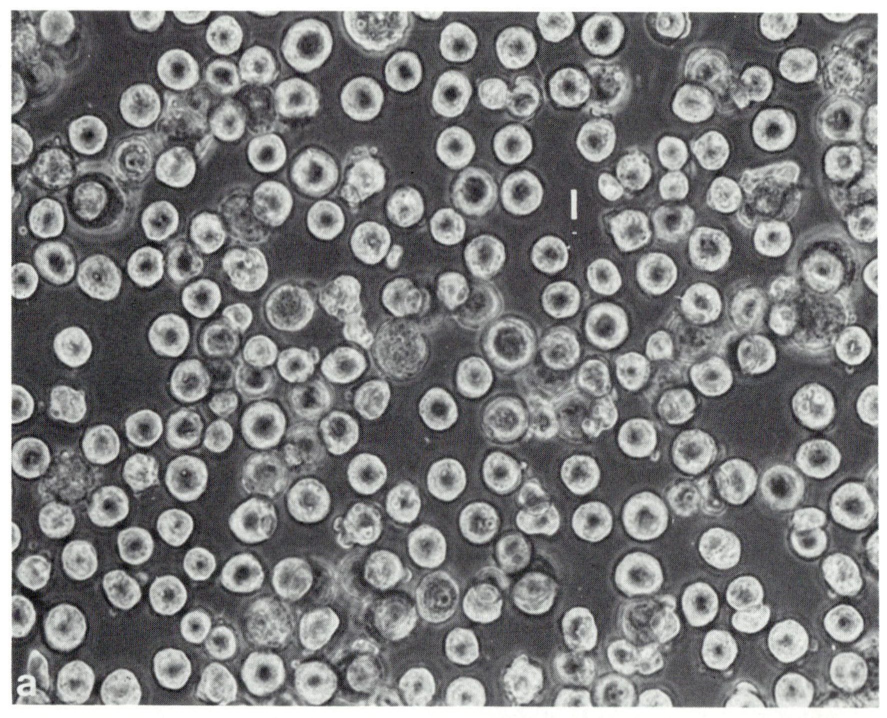
a
I

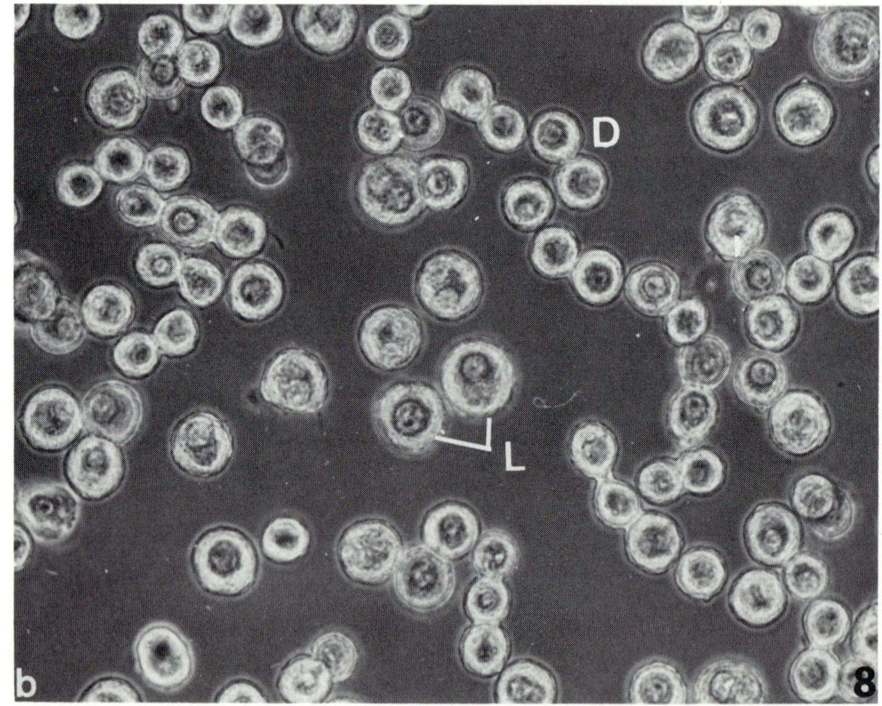
D
L
b
8

Cell Plating

Within 4 hr of incubation, the initially spherical hepatocytes aggregate in groups of two to ten cells and establish their first contacts. These latter consist of closely set, intertwined microvilli of both adjoining cells.[33] Within 24 hr of plating, cell plates of polyhedral hepatocytes are reconstituted. At that time, hepatocytes reveal a high degree of flattening under the scanning electron microscope. Figure 9A illustrates at low magnification the formation of cell trabeculae (T), which are covered by spherical damaged cells in some places. If we assume that these dead cells have a diameter of about 20 μ, each intact flattened hepatocyte displays a diameter of 80–100 μ and extends over a very large surface of the plastic dish. These 24-hr cultured hepatocytes exhibit well-differentiated cell surfaces. Numerous small microvilli are present on their upper surface (Fig. 9B, mv), while interhepatocytic faces (if), which are visualized by artifactual retraction arising during critical point drying, show smooth surfaces and newly formed bile canaliculi (Fig. 9B, arrowheads) containing thin microvilli.

Development of Bile Canaliculi Endowed with Newly Formed Differentiations of the Plasma Membrane

Newly formed bile canaliculi, provided with numerous microvilli, are reconstituted after 24 hr of culture. At both sides of the canaliculi, tight junctions seal the bile compartment and form barriers to the passage of tracers, such as peroxidase or ruthenium red.[33] Figure 10A illustrates the ultrastructural aspect of hepatocytes cultured for 24-hr in a section-plane parallel to the surface of the dish. Ruthenium red, which stains the cell coat intensely, does not penetrate the bile duct (Fig. 10A, BC, arrows). Tight junctions, presenting numerous focal fusions of the external leaflets of both adjacent membranes, are better identified after uranyl acetate staining (Fig. 10B, ti). Moreover, de novo formation of these junctions was studied by the freeze-etching technique. The following sequential stages in their evolution were selected, which are in accordance with those postulated by studies on the in vivo assembly of tight junctions.[59,60] First, 10-nm particles compose a network of linear arrays in the vicinity of the bile canaliculi. In the next step of differentiation, the particles fuse, form short ridge segments, and finally form continuous branched smooth strands, characteristic of the mature tight junction.[33] Desmosomes (Fig. 10B, D) are also reconstituted. They derive from newly formed hemidesmosomes, which are detectable after 4 hr of culture and which induce the differentiation of a duplicate on the corresponding adjacent membrane.

FIG. 8—Phase contrast micrographs of elutriated hepatocytic subpopulations. (A) Homogeneous populations of well-preserved tetraploid cells of intermediate size (I). (B) Hepatocytes of large size (L) and doublets (D) ($\times$300).

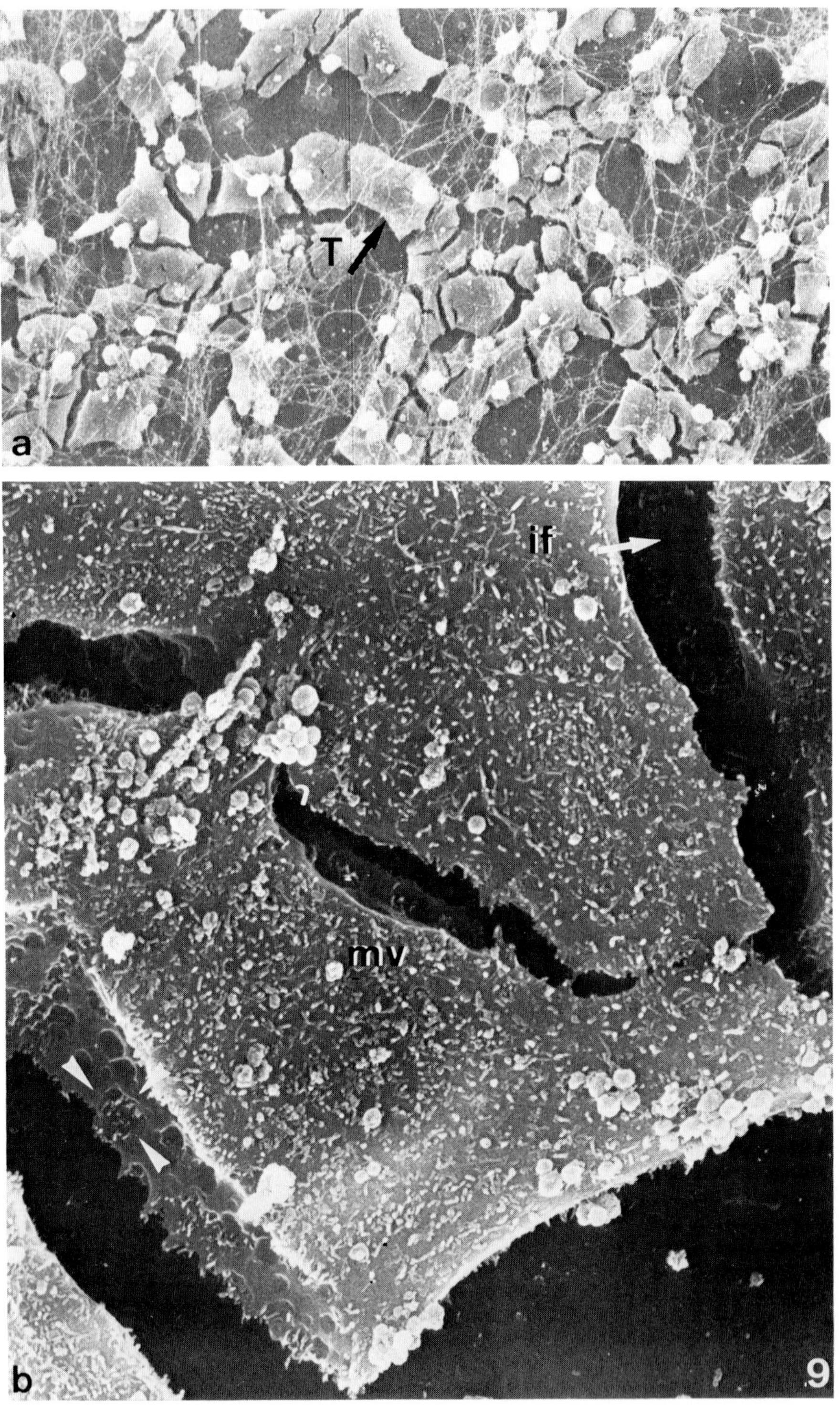

16

Recovery of a Golgi Biliary Polarity

Golgi compexes in situ are polarized with respect to either the bile canaliculi (Fig. 1A) or the cell center. During the isolation procedure, we notice the loss of the classical peripheral location of the Golgi complexes, together with the disappearance of the bile canaliculi. One of the most striking features of these 24-hr hepatocytic cultures is the development of a Golgi biliary polarity, near the newly formed bile canaliculi. Golgi cisternae and vesicles containing lipoprotein particles accumulate near the bile canaliculi, associated with microtubules (Fig. 10B, tu) and microfilaments. The close association of Golgi complexes and bile canaliculi raises the question about the prevailing influence. Is it the Golgi system that induces the differentiation of a biliary segment on a particular site of the plasma membrane, or conversely, is it the local differentiation of a bile canaliculus with its junctional complexes and microtubules that leads to the migration of Golgi elements in their vicinity? Because of the rapidity of the events, it is difficult to determine which has precedence in the process of differentiation to influence or induce subsequent changes. Treatment with antimicrotubular compounds, such as colchicine or nocodazole,[61] which causes the complete disappearance of microtubules (see Chapter 5) and interferes with the intracellular distribution of cell organelles, still allows the reconstitution of bile canaliculi, endowed with tight junctions, in a situation where Golgi elements are randomly distributed. These observations clearly favor the second hypothesis.

Effect of Insulin on Ultrastructure and Glycogenesis
of Rat Liver Cultures

Primary cultures of adult rat hepatocytes carried out in the presence of insulin (20 mU/ml) show increased development and prolongation of their survival time from 3 to about 6 days.[62] After culture with insulin for 48 hr, the cell trabeculae spread considerably more on the surface of the plastic, and after 72 hr, a confluent monolayer of polyhedral cells is formed. The addition of high concentrations of glucose, 20 or 40 mM, to the culture medium, in the absence of insulin, does not influence the morphology of the hepatocytes. By contrast, the addition of insulin in the presence of either glucose concentration induces profound ultrastructural modifications in the hepatocytes. After 24 hr, these changes consist of a significant increase of the SER associated with newly formed glycogen particles. After 48 hr, large amounts of glycogen are stored, lipid droplets are synthesized in the lumen of the SER, and numerous polysomes are present. After 72 hr, cytolysomes filled with glycogen develop in the vicinity of the massed polysaccharide. At the periphery of the cells,

---

FIG. 9—Scanning electron micrographs of hepatocytes in 24-hr culture. (A) Trabeculae (T) are reconstituted, running in all directions. (B) At higher magnification the flattened hepatocytes exhibit numerous microvilli (mv) on their free surfaces and smooth areas and newly formed bile canaliculi (arrowheads) on their interhepatocytic surfaces (if) (9A: ×200; 9B: ×3,100).

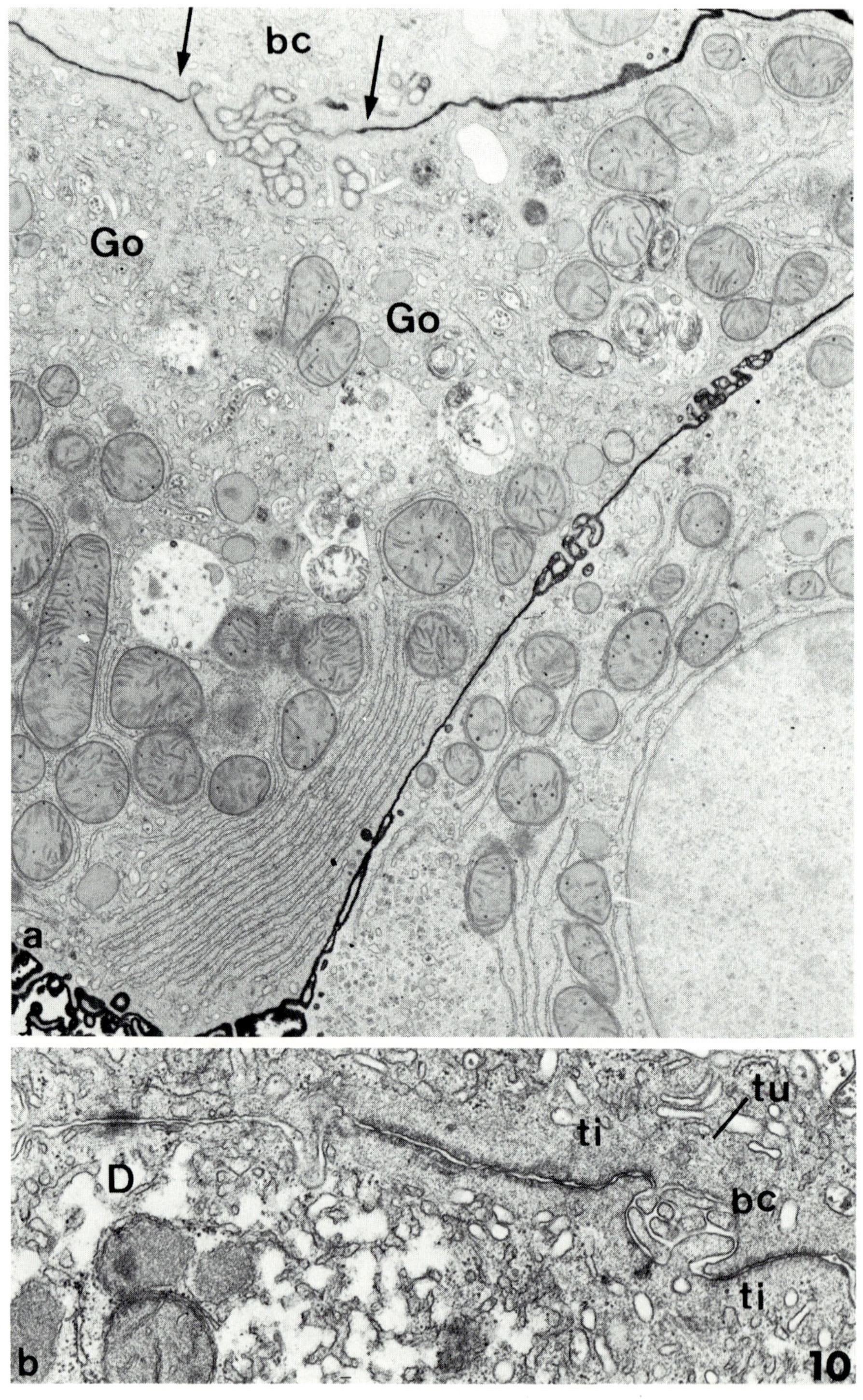

bc
Go
Go
a
tu
ti
D
bc
ti
b
10

flattened lamellae of cytoplasm appear, containing numerous microfilaments and microtubules closely related to accumulated polysomes (see Chapter 5).

Glycogen synthesis has been measured during the first three days of culture in the presence of 20 or 40 mM glucose, with or without insulin. In the absence of the hormone, glycogen synthesis progressively decreases in the hepatocytes with a concomitant loss of total glycogen. The addition of insulin to the cultures only slightly modifies the incorporation of glucose into glycogen after the first 24 hr of culture. By contrast, in the second and third days of culture, insulin induces a threefold to fivefold increase of glycogen synthesis and an accumulation of glycogen in cells which amounts to about three times the control value. This is true for both 20 and 40 mM glucose concentrations.

The glycogen synthetase activity was measured in the cultured cells. Total activity of the enzyme decreases during the culture, except in the culture with insulin after 48 hr. The active form of the enzyme is stimulated after 1 hr of incubation, regresses after 4 hr, and is low after 24 hr. During the second day of culture, after renewal of the medium, the same sequence of events is obtained. The activation rate of the enzyme induced by glucose is increased in presence of insulin.

PERSPECTIVES

Isolation and culture of adult rat hepatocytes constitute experimental models that allow study of the ultrastructural behavior and the specific metabolic properties of parenchymal cells, their degree of differentiation, and their ability to respond to hormonal stimuli, drugs, or toxins. These experimental systems also appear promising in the study of early preneoplastic changes that occur in hepatocytes during chemical carcinogenesis. Isolation of preneoplastic cells in pure fractions[58] and their culture would permit a better analysis of the first alterations that occur and of the sequence of events that lead to the final transformation.

However, numerous problems remain, mainly concerning the degree of viability and the preservation of cell differentiation in long-term cultures. New experimental models, using hormones or growth factors, have to be tested in order to improve these parameters. Similarly, the symbiotic culture of adult rat hepatocytes and sinusoidal cells,[63] which enhances the survival period of hepatocytes in culture, appears to be a useful model for future metabolic studies.

FIG. 10—Electron micrographs of hepatocytes incubated for 24 hr. (A) Bile canaliculi (bc) are formed and are endowed with tight junctions, which do not allow ruthenium red to penetrate inside the bile compartment. (arows). The biliary polarity of the Golgi complex (Go) is restored (×9,300). (B) After uranyl acetate staining, tight junctions (ti) on both sides of the bile canaliculus (bc) and desmosomes (D) are seen. (tu, microtubules) (×19,000).

REFERENCES

1. Schreiber G, Schreiber M: The preparation of single cell suspensions from liver and their use for the study of protein synthesis. Subcell Biochem 2:307–353, 1973
2. Seglen PO: Preparation of isolated rat liver cells. Methods Cell Biol 13:29–83, 1976
3. Jeejeebhoy KN, Phillips MJ: Isolated mammalian hepatocytes in culture. Gastroenterology 71:1086–1096, 1976
4. Anderson NG: The mass isolation of whole cells from rat liver. Science 117:627–628, 1953
5. Howard RB, Christensen AK, Gibbs FA, Pesch LA: The enzymatic preparation of isolated intact parenchymal cells from rat liver. J Cell Biol 35:675–684, 1967
6. Berry MN, Friend DS: High-yield preparation of isolated rat liver parenchymal cells. J Cell Biol 43:506–520, 1969
7. Seglen PO: Preparation of rat liver cells. III. Enzymatic requirements for tissue dispersion. Exp Cell Res 82:391–398, 1973
8. Drochmans P, Wanson JC, Mosselmans R: Isolation and subfractionation on Ficoll gradient of adult rat hepatocytes. Size, morphology and biochemical characteristics of cell fractions. J Cell Biol 66:1–22, 1975
9. Jeejeebhoy KN, Ho J, Greenberg GR, Phillips MJ, Bruce-Robertson A, Sodtke U: Albumin, fibrinogen and transferrin synthesis in isolated rat hepatocytes suspensions. A model for the study of plasma protein synthesis. Biochem J 146:141–155, 1975
10. Loud AV: A quantitative stereological description of the ultrastructure of normal rat liver parenchymal cells. J Cell Biol 37:27–46, 1968
11. Schmucker DL, Mooney JS, Jones AL: Stereological analysis of hepatic fine structure in the Fisher 344 rat. Influence of sublobular location and animal age. J Cell Biol 78:319–337, 1978
12. Nadal C, Zajdela F: Polyploïdie somatique dans le foie de rat. I. Le rôle des cellules binucléées dans la genèse des cellules polyploïdes. Exp Cell Res 42:99–116, 1966
13. James J: The genesis of polyploidy in rat liver parenchymal cells. Cytobiologie 15:410–419, 1977
14. Novikoff A: Cell heterogeneity within the hepatic lobule of the rat. J Histochem Cytochem 7:240–244, 1959
15. Chiquoine D: The distribution of glucose-6-phosphatase in the liver and kidney of the mouse. J Histochem Cytochem 1:429–437, 1953
16. Sasse D, Katz N, Jungermann K: Functional heterogeneity of rat liver parenchyma and of isolated hepatocytes. FEBS Lett 57:83–88, 1975
17. Guder WG, Schmidt U, Funk B, Weiss J, Purschel S: Liver cell heterogeneity. The distribution of pyruvate kinase and phosphoenolpyruvate carboxykinase (GTP) in the liver lobule of fed and starved rats. Hoppe Seylers Z Physiol Chem 357:1793–1800, 1976
18. Castagna M, Chauveau J: Séparation des hépatocytes isolés de rat en fractions cellulaires métaboliquement distinctes. Exp Cell Res 57:211–222, 1969
19. Wanson JC, Drochmans P, May C, Penasse W, Popowski A: Isolation of centrolobular and perilobular hepatocytes after phenobarbital treatment. J Cell Biol 66:23–41, 1975
20. Burger P, Herdson PB: Phenobarbital-induced fine structural changes in rat liver. Am J Pathol 48:793–803, 1966
21. Menard D, Penasse W, Drochmans P, Hugon JS: Glucose-6-phosphatase heterogeneity within the hepatic lobule of the phenobarbital-treated rat. Histochem 38:229–239, 1974
22. Russo E, Drochmans P, Penasse W, Wanson JC: Heterogeneous distribution of glycogen within the rat liver lobule, induced experimentally. J Submicrosc Cytol 7:31–45, 1975
23. Bernaert D, Wanson JC, Mosselmans R, De Paermentier F, Drochmans P: Caractérisation morphologique, morphométrique et biochimique de sous-populations d'hépatocytes de rat adulte, séparées par élutriation. Arch Intern Physiol Bioch 86:408–409, 1978
24. Iype Pt: Cultures from adult rat liver cells I. Establishment of monolayer cell culture from normal liver. J Cell Physiol 78:281–288, 1971
25. Alwen J. Gallhai-Atchard J: A method of maintaining parenchymal cells from adult rat liver in vitro. J Cell Sci 2:249–260, 1972
26. Chapman GS, Jones AL, Meyer UA, Bissell DM: Parenchymal cells from adult rat

liver in nonproliferating monolayer culture. II. Ultrastructural studies. J Cell Biol 59:735–747, 1973

27. Bissell DM, Hammaker LE, Meyer UA: Parenchymal cells from adult rat liver in nonproliferating monolayer culture. I. Functional studies. J Cell Biol 59: 722–734, 1973

28. Alwen J, Lawn AM: The reaggregation of adult rat liver cells maintained in vitro. Exp Cell Res 89:197–205, 1974

29. Bonney RJ, Becker JE, Walker PR, Potter VR: Primary monolayer cultures of adult rat liver parenchymal cells suitable for study of the regulation of enzyme synthesis. In Vitro 9:399–413, 1974

30. Pariza MW, Yager JD, Goldfarb J, Gurr A, Yanagi S, Grossman SH, Becker JE, Barber TA, Potter VR: Biochemical, autoradiographic, and electron microscopic studies of adult rat liver parenchymal cells in primary culture. Edited by LE Gerschenson and EB Thompson: Gene Expression and Carcinogenesis in Cultured Liver. New York, Academic Press, 1975, pp 137–167

31. Michalopoulos G, Pitot HC: Primary culture of parenchymal liver cells on collagen membranes. Exp Cell Res 94:70–78, 1975

32. Michalopoulos G, Sattler GL, Pitot HC: Hormonal regulation and the effects of glucose on tyrosine aminotransferase activity in adult rat hepatocytes cultured on floating collagen membranes. Cancer Res 38:1550–1555, 1978

33. Wanson JC, Drochmans P, Mosselmans R, Ronveaux MF: Adult rat hepatocytes in primary monolayer culture. Ultrastructural characteristics of intercellular contacts and cell membrane differentiations. J Cell Biol 74:858–877, 1977

34. Moscona AA: Cell aggregation: properties of specific cell-ligands and their role in the formation of multicellular systems. Dev Biol 18:250–277, 1968

35. Bissell DM, Guzellian PS: Microsomal functions and phenotypic change in adult rat hepatocytes in primary monolayer culture. Edited by LE Gerschenson and EB Thompson: Gene Expression and Carcinogenesis in Cultured Liver. New York, Academic press, 1975, pp 119–136

36. Drochmans P, Wanson JC, May C, Bernaert D: Ultrastructural and metabolic studies of isolated and cultured hepatocytes. Edited by Elsevier/Excerpta Medica/North-Holland and Elsevier/North-Holland: Hepatotrophic Factors (Ciba Foundation Symposium 55), Amsterdam, 1978, pp 7–29

37. Motta PM: The three-dimensional fine structure of the liver as revealed by scanning electron microscopy. Int Rev Cytol, Suppl 6:347–399, 1977

38. Curtis A: Cell contact and adhesion. Biol Rev (Camb) 37:82–129, 1962

39. Hays RM, Singer B, Malamed S: The effect of calcium withdrawal on the structure and function of the toad bladder. J Cell Biol 25:195–208, 1965

40. Hems R, Ross BD, Berry MN, Krebs HA: Gluconeogenesis in the perfused rat liver. Biochem J 101:284–292, 1966

41. Bernaert D, Wanson JC, Remion C, Ooms H, Popowski A: Culture of hepatocytes isolated from adult rats. Effect of insulin on the ultrastructure and on the glycogenesis. J Cell Biol 70:160a, 1976

42. Glinsmann WH, Pauk G, Hern E: Control of rat liver glycogen synthetase and phosphorylase activities by glucose. Biochem Biophys Res Commun 39:774–782, 1970

43. Hers HG, De Wulf H, Stalmans W: The control of glycogen metabolism in the liver. FEBS Lett 12:73–82, 1970

44. Miller TB Jr, Larner J: Mechanism of control of hepatic glycogenesis by insulin. J Biol Chem 248:3483–3488, 1973

45. Seglen PO: Effects of anaerobiosis, glucose, insulin and glucagon on glycogen metabolism in isolated parenchymal rat liver cells. FEBS Lett 36:309–312, 1973

46. Akpan JO, Gardner R, Wagle SR: Studies on the effects of insulin and acetylcholine on activation of glycogen synthase and on glycogenesis in hepatocytes isolated from normal fed rats. Biochem Biophys Res Commun 61: 222–229, 1974

47. Witters LA, Alberico L, Avruch J: Insulin regulation of glycogen synthase in the isolated rat hepatocyte. Biochem Biophys Res Commun 69:997–1003, 1976

48. Crane LJ, Miller DL: Plasma protein synthesis by isolated rat hepatocytes. J Cell Biol 72:11–25, 1977

49. Seglen PO: Incorporation of radioactive amino acids into protein in isolated rat hepatocytes. Biochim Biophys Acta 442:391–404, 1976

50. Seglen PO: Protein-catabolic state of isolated rat hepatocytes. Biochim Biophys Acta 496:182–191, 1977

51. Seglen PO: Inhibitor of protein degradation

formed during incubation of isolated rat hepatocytes in a cell culture medium. Exp Cell Res 107:207–217, 1977

52. Jeejeebhoy KN, Ho J, Breckenridge C, Bruce-Robertson A, Steiner G, Jeejeebhoy J: Synthesis of VLDL by isolated rat hepatocytes in suspension. Biochem Biophys Res Commun 66:1147–1159, 1975

53. Jeejeebhoy KN, Ho J, Mehra R, Jeejeebhoy J, Bruce-Robertson A: Effects of hormones on the synthesis of α_1 (acute-phase) glycoprotein in isolated rat hepatocytes. Biochem J 168:347–352, 1977

54. John DW, Miller LL: Regulation of net biosynthesis of serum albumin and acute phase plasma proteins. Induction of enhanced net synthesis of fibrinogen, α_1-acid glycoprotein, α_2 (acute phase)-globulin, and haptoglobin by amino acids and hormones during perfusion of the isolated normal rat liver. J Biol Chem 244:6134–6142, 1969

55. Kirsch R, Frith L, Black E, Hoffenberg R: Regulation of albumin synthesis and catabolism by alteration of dietary protein. Nature 217:578–579, 1968

56. Jeejeebhoy KN, Phillips MJ, Bruce-Robertson A, Ho H, Sodtke U: The acute effect of ethanol on albumin, fibrinogen and transferrin synthesis in the rat. Biochem J 126:1111–1126, 1972

57. Bernaert D, Wanson JC, Mosselmans R, De Paermentier F, Drochmans P: Separation of adult rat hepatocytes in distinct subpopulations by centrifugal elutriation. J Biol Cell (in press)

58. Wanson JC, Bernaert D, Penasse W, Drochmans P, Bannash P: Elutriated hepatocytic subpopulations isolated from N-nitrosomorpholine treated rats. Arch Intern Physiol Bioch 86:470–471, 1978

59. Montesano R, Friend DS, Perrelet A, Orci L: In vivo assembly of tight junctions in foetal rat liver. J Cell Biol 67:310–319, 1975

60. Elias PM, Friend DS: Vitamin-A-induced mucous metaplasia. An in vitro system for modulating tight and gap junction differentiation. J Cell Biol 68:173–188, 1976

61. De Brabander M, Wanson JC, Mosselmans R, Geuens G, Drochmans P: Effects of antimicrotubular compounds on monolayer cultures of adult rat hepatocytes. J Biol Cell 31:127–140, 1978

62. Bernaert D, Wanson JC, Drochmans P, Popowski A: Effect of insulin on ultrastructure and glycogenesis in primary cultures of adult rat hepatocytes. J Cell Biol 74:878–900, 1977

63. Wanson JC, Drochmans P, Mosselmans R, Knook DL: Symbiotic culture of adult hepatocytes and sinus-lining cells. Edited by E Wisse and DL Knook: Kupffer Cells and Other Liver Sinusöidal Cells. Amsterdam, Elsevier/North-Holland Biomedical Press, 1977, pp 141–150

Chapter 2

Morphologic Aspects of Hepatic Synthesis and Secretion of Plasma Proteins

By GÉRARD FELDMANN, M.D.

AS SHOWN BY different biochemical approaches to various experimental procedures, such as perfused isolated liver,[1] total hepatectomy,[2] incubation of liver slices,[3] or hepatic subcellular fractions[4,5] in suitable conditions, the liver produces most of the plasma proteins except for the immunoglobulins.[6] Although a great deal of information is available on the biosynthesis of plasma proteins by the whole liver, our knowledge about the type, number, and distribution of the hepatic cells that produce these proteins is still rather limited.

The liver does not form a homogeneous cellular mass. In addition to the cells of the portal spaces, several types of cells are represented in the hepatic lobule.[7] The most abundant, the hepatocytes, form about 78% of the parenchymal volume;[8] in the sinusoids, three additional kinds of cells are present: endothelial cells, Kupffer cells, and fat-storing cells.[7] Moreover, within the lobule, these cells are arranged according to a definite order, and it is usual to describe several zones that are functionally different within the lobule. At first glance, each of the four types of cells present in the lobule would be able to produce plasma proteins, since the organelles in which the synthesis and the secretion of these proteins take place are present in their cytoplasm. For reasons that will be developed later, however, the hepatocytes are likely to represent the cells mainly responsible for this synthesis. Theoretically, we can imagine that every hepatocyte is able to produce every protein; indeed, on light or electron microscopy, it is impossible to distinguish one hepatocyte from another. Hepatocytes located in different parts of the hepatic lobule do not function identically, however. As far back as 1923, Noel, using histochemical techniques,[9] demonstrated a different activity of the periportal zone than that of the centrolobular zone, while the middle zone was in an intermediate state. More recently, with histoenzymatic methods, it has been shown that the distribution of several hepatocyte enzymes varies from one part of the hepatic lobule to another.[10] Ultrastructural stereologic methods demonstrated significant differences in the size and number of several cytoplasmic organelles in the different zones of the same lobule.[11] The distribution of some of the enzymes responsible for glucogenesis is not similar in microdissected periportal

From the Unité de Recherches de Physiopathologie Hépatique, INSERM, Hôpital Beaujon, 92118 Clichy Cedex, and the Laboratoire d'Histologie, Embryologie, Cytogénétique, Faculté de Médècine Xavier Bichat, 75018, Paris, France.

Supported by grant 7650817 from INSERM.

or perivenous rat tissue.[12] A similar situation could exist for the hepatocytes engaged in the production of plasma proteins. However, in contrast to enzymes, for which histochemical techniques are available, the localization of plasma proteins in the hepatocytes entails technical difficulties. The histochemical methods currently available to demonstrate a protein in a cell are, for the most part, difficult and not entirely specific;[13] they are only able, at best, to indicate the presence of biochemically comparable proteins, but they are unable to ascertain the nature of these proteins. The only easy procedure for detecting a protein in a cell is immunofluorescence. This technique, proposed about 25 years ago,[14] is based on the use of specific antibodies against a given protein and labeled with fluorochromes. The first results provided by immunofluorescence of the human liver were obtained in 1964, when albumin and fibrinogen were located in the normal liver;[15] about 10% and 1% of the hepatocytes contained albumin and fibrinogen, respectively, and the protein-containing cells were scattered throughout the hepatic lobule. Comparable results were obtained in humans for prothrombin[16] and for transferrin.[17] These patterns, a small percentage of protein-containing cells with an irregular lobular distribution, were also observed in animals; for instance, in the dog, prothrombin was found in 10% to 20% of hepatocytes,[16] whereas haptoglobin was seen in only about 2% of these cells[18] and fibrinogen in a small number of cells.[19] Despite their interest, the importance of these findings remain limited, since among the protein-containing hepatocytes, those cells synthesizing the protein cannot be distinguished by immunofluorescence from those accumulating it passively. Indeed, immunofluorescence cannot be applied to electron microscopy, which appears to be the only morphologic procedure that can demonstrate which organelles in a cell are responsible for the synthesis and the secretion of protein.

Immunocytochemical techniques were greatly improved in 1966 when antibodies were labeled not by fluorochrome but by an enzyme.[20,21] The principles of the immunoenzymatic techniques are similar to those of the immunofluorescent techniques and have been reviewed in a recent symposium.[22] Instead of demonstrating the protein by means of an ultraviolet examination of the tissue section, it is demonstrated by a specific histochemical method that is usable both on light and electron microscopy. Of the numerous enzymes proposed, the most popular is horseradish peroxidase, and the term "immunoperoxidase" is used just as currently as the word "immunofluorescence." The histochemical reaction,[23] determined by peroxidase, gives dark brown deposits on light microscopy and electron-dense precipitates on electron microscopy. One advantage of the immunoenzymatic techniques is that they allow reinvestigation of the cells already examined on light microscopy, using ultrastructural techniques to check the results obtained in the first instance. Their sensitivity and specificity make these techniques a good tool to investigate the subcellular mechanisms of protein synthesis and secretion.[24]

This review surveys the information brought by the immunoperoxidase method to the morphologic knowledge of hepatic synthesis and secretion of plasma proteins. The results obtained with immunoperoxidase will be compared with those obtained with immunofluorescence, since, at least on light microscopy, these two techniques give similar results.

LOCALIZATION OF PLASMA PROTEINS
IN THE NORMAL LIVER

Several proteins produced by the liver, such as albumin, fibrinogen, ceruloplasmin, α_1-antitrypsin (α_1-AT), α_1-fetoprotein, and C-reactive protein (CRP), were investigated in the normal liver using immunoperoxidase.[25–31] For five of these proteins—albumin, fibrinogen, ceruloplasmin, α_1-AT, and α-fetoprotein—the results obtained were quite similar. CRP was not detectable in the normal rabbit liver;[31] the probable reason for this will be discussed later.

Using light microscopy, in either humans or rats (Figs. 1 and 2), the plasma protein being investigated, regardless of type, was always detected in only some hepatocytes and never in the Kupffer cells, the endothelial cells, or the fat-storing cells. In the hepatocytes, the protein was visible only in the cytoplasm and never in the nucleus. The intensity of the reaction varied from one cell to another. Some cells contained a large amount of the plasma protein being investigated, while in others the staining was moderate or weak. Generally, the reaction was diffuse throughout the cytoplasm. In some hepatocytes, however, dark brown deposits were visible in only a part of the cytoplasm. The protein-containing cells were randomly distributed within the hepatic lobule between the portal space and the central vein. These protein-containing cells, in some areas in the lobule, were clustered in small groups of 5 to 20 hepatocytes. In other places, one isolated hepatocyte containing the protein was visible, while the cells around it did not demonstrate any protein. Some protein-containing hepatocytes were clustered in the vicinity of the portal space or the central vein, but this aspect was not constant, and it was impossible to describe a diffuse lobular distribution for any protein. Within the sinusoidal spaces a small quantity of protein was sometimes visible close to the plasma membrane of the hepatocytes. Except for the lumens of the vessels, no protein was visible in the portal space; in particular, no protein was detectable in the biliary epithelial cells.

The number of hepatocytes containing the protein varied greatly from one hepatic lobule to another. Some lobules did not contain any cell with detectable protein. In the rat, striking differences in the number of hepatocytes containing the protein were observed between two specimens taken from different hepatic lobes. As a consequence of this irregular distribution, it was difficult to accurately assess the percentage of protein-containing cells. A rough estimate can be made, however. In normal humans, a mean of 36% hepatocytes contained albumin.[25] In the rat, the mean was between 10% and 15%.[30] The percentage was lower during the postnatal period; 24 hr after birth, albumin was present in only about 5% of the hepatocytes, while 5 days later the protein was recognizable in about 15% of the cells.[30] For fibrinogen, comparable results

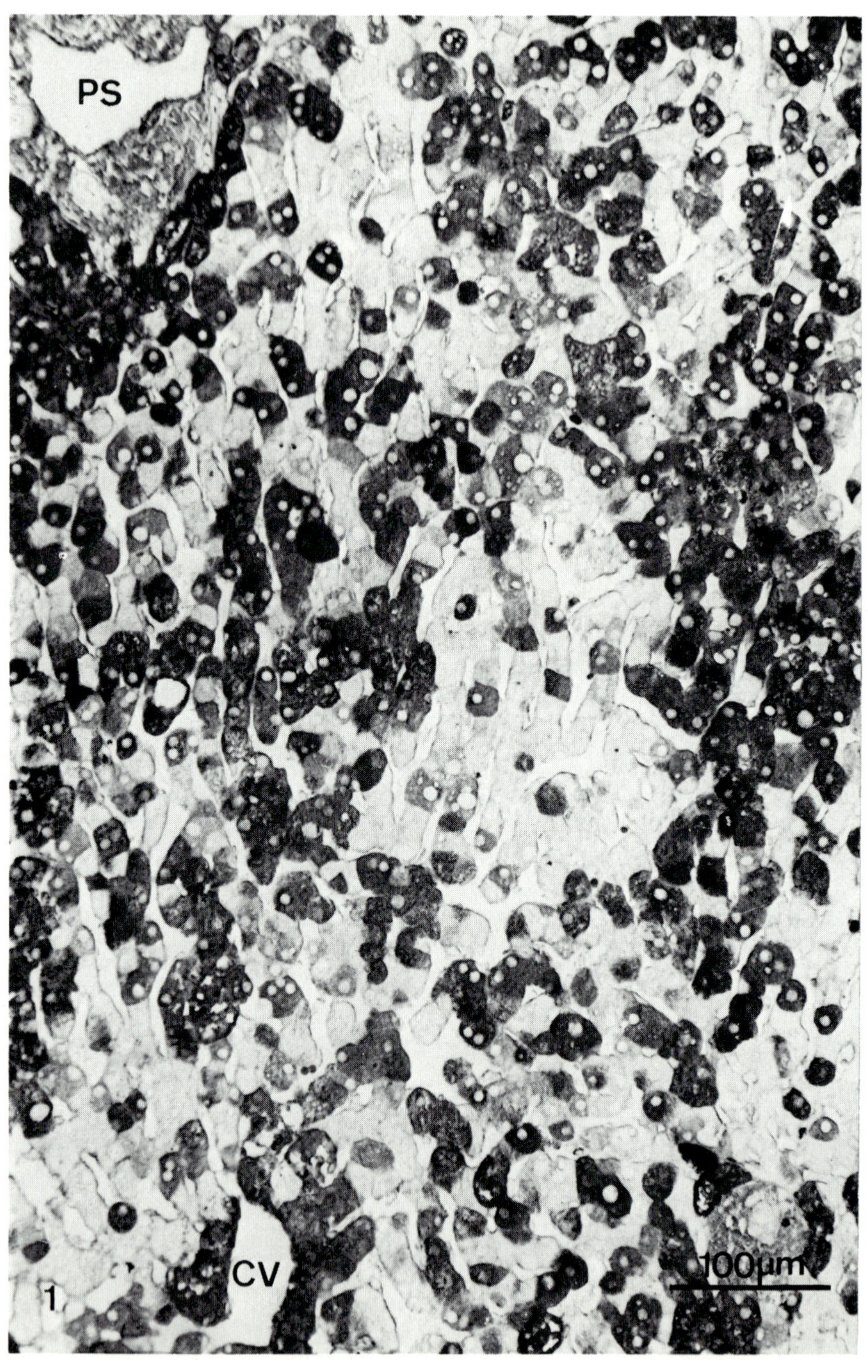

FIG. 1—Light-microscopic appearance of normal human liver. Localization of albumin. The dark brown deposits indicating the presence of the protein are visible in some hepatocytes only randomly distributed in the hepatic lobule (PS, portal space; CV, central vein) (× 220).

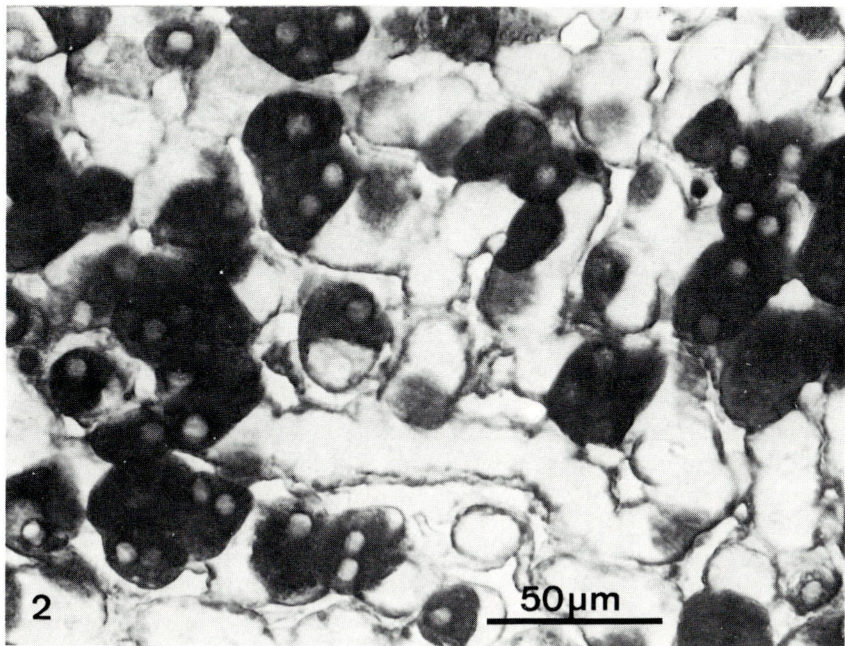

FIG. 2—Light-microscopic appearance of normal human liver, showing albumin confined to cytoplasm of hepatocytes. Some cells contain a large amount of albumin, while in others the staining is moderate or weak. A small quantity of albumin is visible along the plasma membrane of the hepatocytes ($\times$ 475).

were obtained in adult human[32] and in the adult rat;[27] very few hepatocytes (not more than 1%) contained this protein. In humans, α_1-AT was found in only 1% to 5% of the hepatocytes,[28] while ceruloplasmin was present in about 10% of the hepatocytes.[26] No α_1-fetoprotein-containing hepatocytes were seen in the liver of the adult rat, but some cells with this protein were visible during the postnatal period.[29]

These results suggest that the hepatocytic localization is very general for the plasma proteins produced by the liver. They confirm the results obtained with immunofluorescence for albumin,[15,33] fibrinogen,[19] prothrombin,[16] haptoglobin,[18] transferrin,[17,34] and α-fetoprotein. This last protein was investigated on several occasions in humans as well as in the experimental animal, by immunofluorescence[35,36] and by immunoperoxidase,[37] and a similar hepatocyte localization was found with both techniques. Similarly, the results with immunofluorescence for transferrin[17] were confirmed with immunoperoxidase.[38] The β-apoprotein of lipoproteins was also located in the cytoplasm of the hepatocytes.[39] Plasma proteins (albumin,[15] fibrinogen,[15] or transferrin[17]) were reported to be present in Kupffer cells and in hepatocytes in studies based on immunofluorescence. Theoretically, the Kupffer cells, as already stated, are able to produce plasma proteins because they contain all the organelles necessary for this production. Several findings suggest, however, that their contribution to the production of plasma proteins is unlikely or at least very limited. First, plasma proteins have not been detected within Kupffer cells for all the proteins investigated. Moreover, for the same protein, conflicting results have been published. For instance, albumin in the Kupffer cells was reported[15] but not confirmed.[25,30,33] The discrepancy could be explained by technical differences in the preparation of the liver specimens or of the antibodies. Second, the localization observed by immunofluorescence could result from pinocytosis of plasma proteins and not from active synthesis. Many more Kupffer cells containing haptoglobin were observed during the catabolic phase of experimental inflammation than during the anabolic phase.[18] Third, direct evidence regarding the role of the Kupffer cells in the synthesis of plasma proteins is lacking. Several proteins, such as one of the components of complement or proaccelerin, could be produced by these cells.[40] The production of these plasma proteins has, in fact, been demonstrated for macrophages in general but not specifically for Kupffer cells.[41] No satisfactory biochemical or morphologic data regarding the endothelial cells or the fat-storing cells support the view that these cells contribute significantly to the synthesis of plasma proteins.

In all the studies conducted with light microscopy, either with immunofluorescence or with immunoperoxidase, the protein investigated was detectable in only a part, sometimes a very small part, of the hepatocytes, and comparable percentages of protein-containing hepatocytes have been reported for the different proteins studied. The only exception was the localization of the β-apoprotein of lipoproteins, which was present in all the hepatocytes.[39] The difference between these results and others was not discussed by the authors.

The random distribution of hepatocytes containing plasma proteins was also observed by most authors.[15-19,25-30,32-34,37,38] By contrast, with some enzymes, it seems impossible to ascribe for any given protein a preferential lobular localization. We sometimes observed some protein-containing hepatocytes around the portal space or the central vein; this was also pointed out by others,[15] but the localization is not constant and does not constitute an argument favoring a diffuse lobular localization.

The absence of detectable CRP[31] or α-fetoprotein[29] in the normal adult liver is probably related to the very low amount of protein produced. Consequently, it is difficult to locate the hepatocytes that are responsible for this synthesis. One illustration of this situation was given in two inherited diseases characterized by the absence of a plasma protein. One of these diseases was observed in a girl with α_1-antitrypsin deficiency with a very rare genotype, the genotype Pi___, in which plasma α_1-AT was absent;[42] the other was observed in 3 patients with little or no plasma ceruloplasmin.[43] No hepatocyte with α_1-AT or ceruloplasmin could be found in these patients even using electron microscopy.[42,43]

Similar results were obtained, by electron microscopy, in the hepatocytes in which albumin, fibrinogen, α_1-AT, and ceruloplasmin were visible by light microscopy. Each protein was located on the same cytoplasmic organelles, the rough endoplasmic reticulum (RER), the smooth endoplasmic reticulum (SER), and the Golgi apparatus (GA) (Fig. 3). These findings suggest, therefore, that

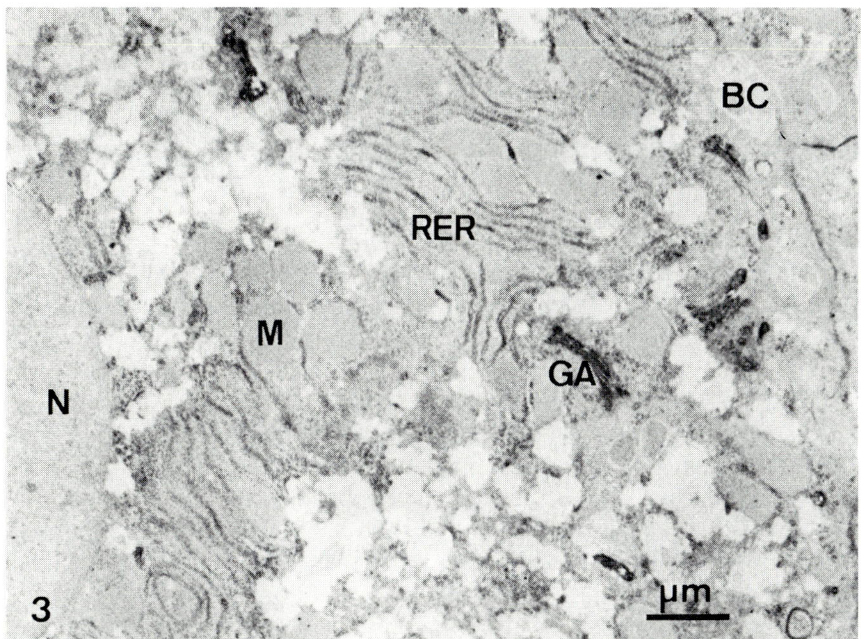

FIG. 3—Electron-microscopic appearance of a part of a normal rat hepatocyte. The electron-dense precipitates indicating the presence of albumin are located in the rough endoplasmic reticulum (RER) and the Golgi apparatus (GA); smooth endoplasmic reticulum is not visible in this figure. The electron-transparent spots correspond to glycogen that is unstained (N, nucleus; M, mitochondria; BC, bile canaliculus) ($\times$ 11,050).

the hepatocyte in which a protein is detectable is a cell engaged in the synthesis and the secretion of this protein, since, according to a current concept,[44] these three organelles form an intracytoplasmic network in which the protein is synthesized on the RER and then passes through the SER and the GA before being secreted into the plasma. With immunoperoxidase, the electron-dense precipitates indicating the protein were generally visible on the membranes of these organelles with only a small amount in their lumens. In the RER, the protein was present in only some of the cisternae forming this organelle and sometimes on the nuclear external membrane. Some ribosomes bound to the membranes of the RER displayed some protein. In the SER, a discrete localization was found on the membranes of the smooth vesicles. In the GA, in addition to the saccular localization, the protein was present in vesicles located around this organelle. Some variations were observed from one hepatocyte to another. In some cells the protein was only detectable in the RER, while in others, it was present in the GA and not in the RER or the SER. The plasma proteins were not found in any other cytoplasmic organelle, and no protein was detectable on free ribosomes. Near the plasma membrane, no observation suggested exocytosis of the protein toward the plasma, with one possible exception reported for the lipoproteins.[39] A small quantity of protein was found in areas in the space of Disse. The absence of proteins in the sinusoidal cells was confirmed by electron microscopy. The location of plasma proteins on the RER, SER, and GA was also observed by electron microscopy for two other proteins produced by the liver, α-fetoprotein[45] and the β-apoprotein of lipoproteins.[39] The localization on the GA was not always found, however.[45,46] Localization of albumin in the cytosol has been reported.[46] The discrepancies between these findings and our results may be explained by technical differences in the preparation of liver tissue.

The finding of protein on the RER, the SER, and the GA agrees with the results of biochemical studies performed in the rat on hepatic subcellular fractions obtained after homogenization of the liver. For albumin, the three subcellular steps are well documented. It is now well established with radioactive amino acids that albumin is synthesized by the RER[47] and then passes into the SER[48] and the GA[49] before reaching the plasma. Biochemical information on the other proteins is not so abundant, but the synthesis of fibrinogen[50,51] and other glycoproteins by microsomes has been demonstrated.[52,53]

Thus the findings obtained by immunoperoxidase techniques agree with those obtained from biochemical studies. In addition, the morphologic technique provides information on synthesis and secretion that cannot be obtained with other techniques.

First, the use of electron microscopy now allows us to distinguish between cells that are actively engaged in protein synthesis and those that merely accumulate a protein.

Second, whereas biochemical studies give only an overall view of synthesis and secretion, this technique demonstrates that only some hepatocytes are working at a given time.

Third, whatever the protein investigated, the subcellular pathways seem to be identical. Proteins produced by the liver are biochemically very different. Some are composed only of amino acids; others, such as the glycoproteins, are made of amino acids and carbohydrates; and still others, such as the lipoproteins, contain lipids. Carbohydrates[54,55] or lipids[56] are added to the polypeptide chains in the SER and/or the GA. Apparently, this addition does not greatly modify the protein, at least immunologically, since it is detected on every organelle. Moreover, the location of the protein on some of the ribosomes bound to the membranes of the RER suggests that the protein acquires its antigenic conformation early, a suggestion that agrees with several biochemical studies performed on ribosomes showing that albumin was detectable immunologically in albumin-synthesizing ribosomes.[57,58] The absence of protein on cytoplasmic free ribosomes also agrees with several observations regarding the manufacture of the proteins exported into the plasma by the ribosomes bound to the RER, while the proteins remaining inside the hepatocytes are made by the free ribosomes.[59,60]

Fourth, the small amount of protein in the lumens of the RER, SER, and GA indicates that each hepatocyte produces only a little protein or that the protein is quickly exported into the plasma. By contrast with numerous exocrine or endocrine cells, the protein does not seem to be stored in the hepatocyte before its secretion.

Fifth, the fact that the protein is present in some cells either in the RER or in the GA suggests either cyclic activity or that the transit time of the protein is not identical in the two organelles. Kinetic studies have shown that albumin remains longer in the GA[49] than in other organelles.

The immunoperoxidase technique did not provide morphologic data on the protein pathway between the GA and the plasma membrane, however. After the GA, at least in the pancreatic exocrine cells, the protein is taken up by vacuoles that go to the cellular membrane.[44] This step was not elucidated in the liver by immunoperoxidase.

HEPATIC LOCALIZATION OF PLASMA PROTEINS AFTER EXPERIMENTAL MODIFICATION OF THEIR SYNTHESIS OR SECRETION

One of the main questions raised by the small percentage of protein-producing hepatocytes in the normal liver is whether or not these cells are specialized for the synthesis of a given protein. To obtain more information on this point, several animal experiments were performed in an attempt to increase the hepatic synthesis of a given protein. In this manner, when such a protein is investigated in the liver with peroxidase-labeled antibodies, several results are possible using light microscopy: (1) the percentage of protein-containing hepatocytes could be similar to that observed in the normal state; or (2) the percentage of protein-containing hepatocytes could be greater than that observed in the normal state. Using electron microscopy, in the second case, protein could be detectable in large amounts in the RER, SER, and GA of the hepatocytes. The first result would constitute an argument for specialization, while the second would argue against this specialization.

Hepatic synthesis of albumin, fibrinogen, and CRP was increased in the following experiments. For albumin, a nephrotic syndrome was induced in the rat with puromycin[61] or with autologous immune complexes.[62] The rats were studied when plasma albumin concentration was very low and when proteinuria was at its maximum. Under such conditions, albumin hepatic synthesis is at least doubled.[63] Albumin was present in almost all the hepatocytes in a nephrotic rat,[64] whereas in the normal rat it was visible in only 15% of the hepatocytes. Using electron microscopy, the protein was mainly located in the dictyosomes of the GA, which were hypertrophied, very numerous, and filled with albumin (Fig. 4).

For fibrinogen and CRP, comparable experiments were performed in the rat and in the rabbit, respectively. These two proteins belong to the group of plasma proteins, the plasma concentration of which increases strikingly in the initial stage of any inflammatory reaction.[65] This increase is caused by an increase of hepatic synthesis of these proteins.[65] In the experimental animal, an inflammatory reaction can be induced by administering turpentine. Turpentine was injected subcutaneously to rats, and the animals were sacrificed 8, 16, 24, 32, and 72 hr after its administration.[66] The percentage of fibrinogen-containing hepatocytes did not vary at 8 hr. At 16 hr, when fibrinogen plasma

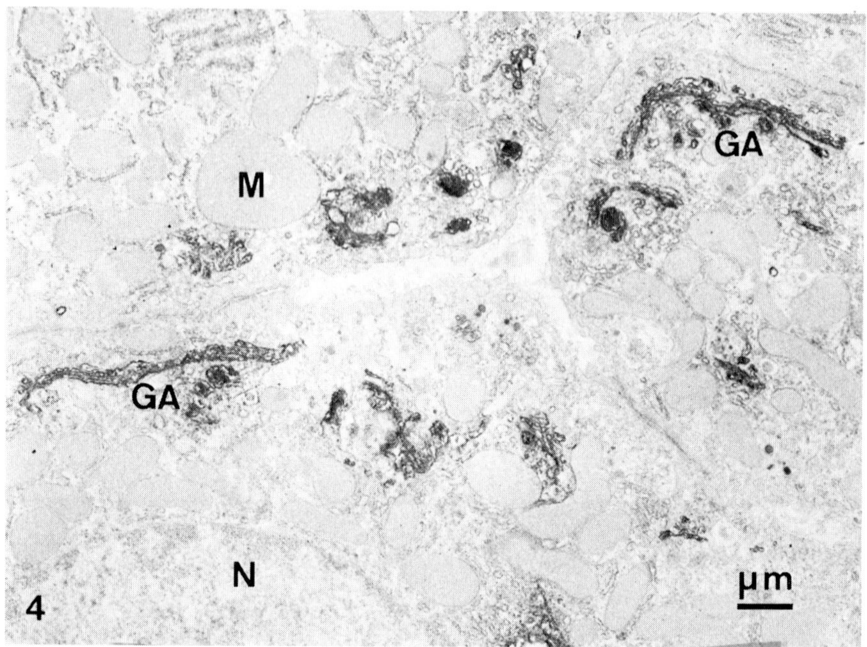

FIG. 4—Electron-microscopic appearance of three hepatocytes in a nephrotic rat. Numerous Golgi apparatus (GA) cysternae filled with albumin are visible (N, nucleus; M, mitochondria) (× 7,480).

concentration was about 800 mg/dl, numerous fibrinogen-containing hepatocytes were visible around the portal spaces. At 24 and 32 hr, when fibrinogen plasma concentration was 1000 and 1200 mg/dl, almost all the hepatocytes contained fibrinogen (Fig. 5). By electron microscopy, much of this protein was visible in the lumens of the RER (Fig. 6), the SER, and the GA. At 72 hr when the plasma concentration of fibrinogen decreased, only a few hepatocytes with fibrinogen were visible in the liver, and the ultrastructural appearance of the organelles engaged in synthesis and secretion of this protein was similar to that observed in the normal liver.

Turpentine was also injected into rabbits for the study of CRP. Although no CRP-containing hepatocytes were demonstrated in the normal rabbit,[31] hepatocytes with CRP were visible as early as 8 hr after turpentine administration, mainly around the portal spaces; this percentage then increased to a maximum at 24 hr, decreasing at 38 hr after turpentine administration.[31] By electron microscopy, large amounts of the protein were visible in the RER, the SER, and the GA at 24 hr.[31]

A common interpretation can be given for these three experiments. When the hepatic synthesis of a protein is increased, all or almost all the hepatocytes work together to produce the protein. Consequently, this finding represents an indirect but strong argument in favor of the view that the hepatocytes are not specialized in the synthesis of a single protein. The results for albumin, fibrinogen, and CRP agree with those obtained with immunofluorescence by several researchers for prothrombin[16] or transferrin.[34] For instance, when hepatic syn-

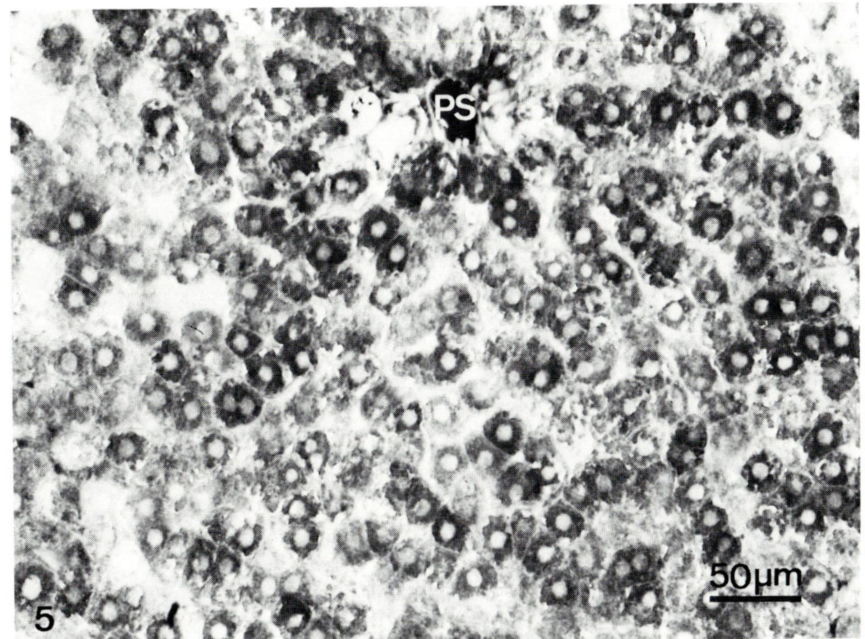

FIG. 5—Light-microscopic appearance of a rat liver during an inflammatory reaction. Numerous hepatocytes with fibrinogen are visible (PS, portal space) (× 250).

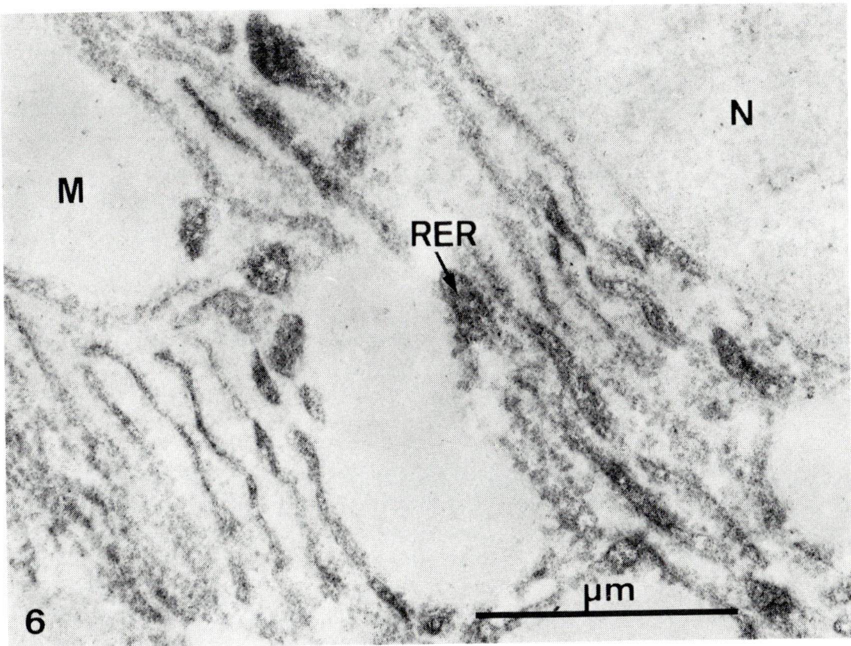

FIG. 6—Electron-microscopic appearance of a part of a rat hepatocyte during an inflammatory reaction. Fibrinogen is visible in large amounts in the lumens of the rough endoplasmic reticulum (RER) (N, nucleus; M, mitochondria) (× 35,700).

thesis of prothrombin was stimulated by vitamin K_1, the protein was demonstrated in all the hepatocytes,[16] whereas in the normal state, it was present in only about 20% of these cells.[16] Similarly, 3 to 4 days after acute blood loss in the rat, transferrin was present in 60% to 70% of the hepatocytes, while in the normal state, the amount of transferrin did not exceed 20%.[34] Only with the immunoperoxidase technique, however, can we ascertain that the changes in plasma protein concentration are due to an increase in synthesis and secretion, since the protein is detectable in large amounts in the lumens of the organelles responsible for these functions in the hepatocyte.

Another experimental result reinforces the view that the hepatocytes are not specialized in the synthesis of a single protein. When the secretion of a protein is inhibited, the protein is found in almost all the hepatocytes. Colchicine inhibits the secretion of plasma proteins by the liver. Under suitable conditions, this drug does not change the synthesis but inhibits the secretion by acting on the microtubules of the hepatocyte,[67,68] the organelles of which are probably involved in the secretion of plasma proteins. Eight hours after a single dose of colchicine, fibrinogen was present in numerous hepatocytes located around the portal space.[27] By electron microscopy, at this time the protein accumulated in the lumens of the RER, suggesting that its secretion was inhibited immediately after synthesis.[27]

The reasons why only some hepatocytes are at work normally for a given protein are not obvious. Cyclic activity is likely. Biochemical studies have demonstrated that for two proteins, albumin and fibrinogen, only one-third[69] and one-tenth[70] of the liver, respectively, are sufficient to maintain a normal plasma concentration of these two proteins. However, the influence of various physiologic factors[71] that interfere with hepatic synthesis of plasma proteins has not been investigated by morphologic techniques. As observed by immunofluorescence, the number of albumin-containing hepatocytes in the rat was very low when the animals received a diet devoid of protein.[72]

Finally, it is not known whether a single hepatocyte is able to produce more than one protein at the same time. Using antihuman albumin and antihuman fibrinogen antibodies labeled with two different fluorochromes, it has been shown that these two proteins are present in the same cells,[15] but this work has not been confirmed. Several preliminary results suggest, however, that during an inflammatory state the hepatocytes located around the portal space could produce fibrinogen, haptoglobin, orosomucoid, and α_2-macroglobulin simultaneously.[73]

HEPATIC LOCALIZATION OF PLASMA PROTEINS IN VARIOUS LIVER DISEASES

Although few results are available, some information has been obtained in some liver diseases.

In Pi ZZ α_1-AT deficiency, both immunofluorescence[74–76] and immunoperoxidase[77,78] techniques have indicated that the diastase-resistant periodic acid-Schiff (PAS)-positive globules observed in the hepatocytes by light mi-

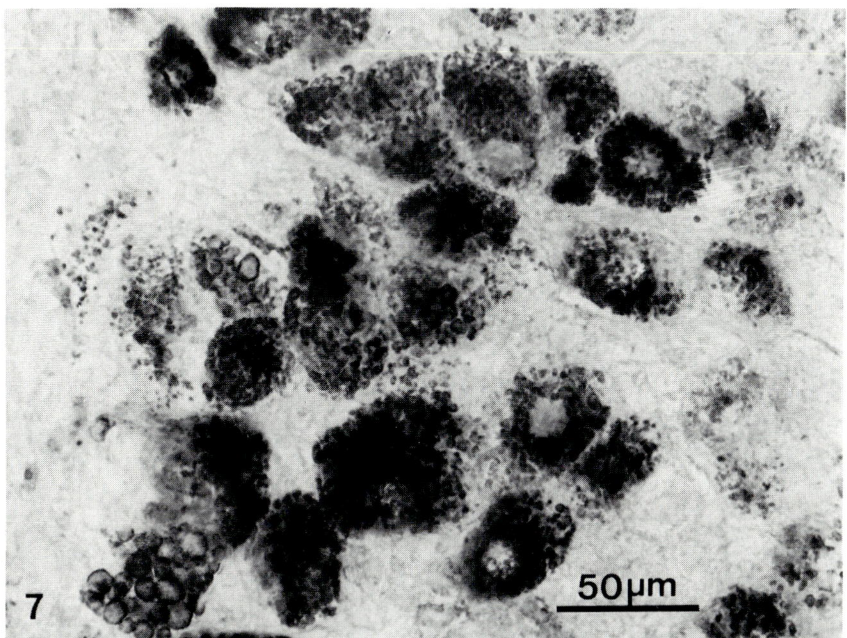

FIG. 7—Light-mciroscopic appearance of a liver from a patient with α_1-antitrypsin deficiency. Numerous globules with α_1-antitrypsin are visible in some hepatocytes ($\times$ 382).

croscopy were composed of α_1-AT (Fig. 7). α_1-Antitrypsin was not demonstrated in every hepatocyte.[74–78] The percentage of α_1-AT-containing hepatocytes varied greatly from one patient to another. This percentage could be related to the genotype.[76] It could be larger in homozygous patients with the genotype Pi ZZ than in heterozygous patients with the genotype Pi MZ. Using immunoperoxidase with electron microscopy[78] (Fig. 8), it has been shown that α_1-AT accumulated in large amounts in the RER and the SER of the hepatocytes, while no protein was detectable on the GA.[28] These findings suggest that the biochemical defect(s) responsible for the abnormality of the protein could be, at least in part, in the SER. In vitro studies have demonstrated that the Z α_1-AT is deficient in sialic acids.[79] Glycosidation of proteins takes places in the SER and/or in the GA.[54,55] The last carbohydrate to be added is sialic acid, which could be essential for the secretion of a glycoprotein;[54,55] without it, the protein would not be secreted and would accumulate in the SER and the RER.

Preliminary results have been obtained for albumin in human alcoholic cirrhosis. As in the normal liver, albumin was located in the cytoplasm of some of the hepatocytes. One finding was striking, however. Albumin-containing hepatocytes were visible only in some cirrhotic nodules (Fig. 9). By electron microscopy, large amounts of albumin were found in the RER and the GA of some patients,[43] while no or almost no albumin was observed in these organelles in the normal liver. These findings are difficult to interpret. Albumin

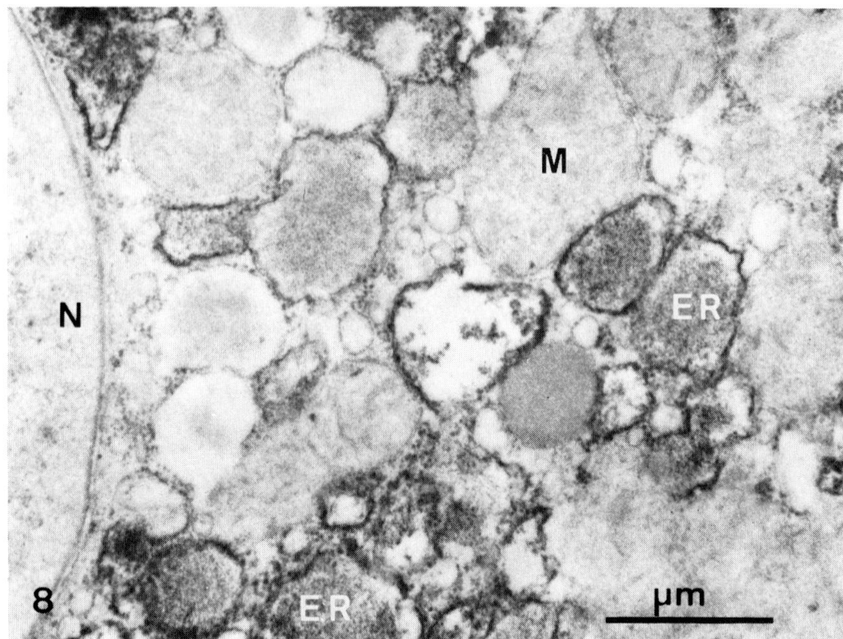

FIG. 8—Electron-microscopic appearance of part of a hepatocyte in a patient with α_1-antitrypsin deficiency. Electron-dense precipitates demonstrating the presence of the protein are visible in the dilated endoplasmic reticulum (ER) (N, nucleus; M, mitochondria) ($\times$ 23,000).

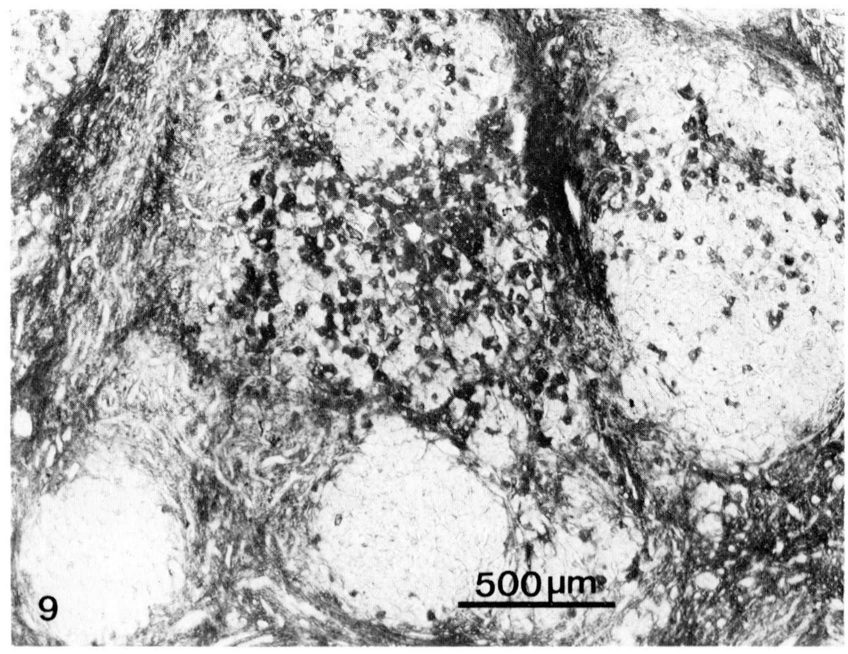

FIG. 9—Light-microscopic appearance of the liver of a patient with alcoholic cirrhosis. Hepatocytes with albumin are visible only in some nodules ($\times$ 382).

hepatic synthesis could be increased in some patients with alcoholic cirrhosis,[80] but possibly the accumulation of albumin could also reflect altered secretion of this protein.[43] Alcohol feeding to rats produced accumulation in the liver of export proteins, particularly albumin; this accumulation was associated with a decrease of polymerized tubulin [81] (see Chapter 5).

α-Fetoprotein was investigated on several occasions in hepatocellular carcinomas in humans[35,36] and during experimental carcinogenesis.[82] In human hepatocellular carcinomas, α-fetoprotein was located by immunofluorescence in only some tumor cells randomly distributed in the tumor mass, and not in all the cases examined with this technique.[35,36] Conflicting results have been reported in experimental carcinogenesis.[82] α-Fetoprotein-containing hepatic cells were present with no special morphologic features in some cases, while in others, the protein was located in "transitional" cells, different from the normal hepatocytes. This last feature has been emphasized using the affinity of radio-labeled estrogens for α-fetoprotein.[83] The presence of transitional cells has not been intensively studied by electron microscopy with immunoperoxidase, however, and the ultrastructural demonstration of these cells is still lacking, as is information on the fine structure of α-fetoprotein-containing tumor cells in human primary hepatocellular carcinomas.

Immunoperoxidase was used to study the liver in tyrosinosis,[29] a hereditary disease characterized by a defect in tyrosine metabolism associated with chronic liver disease and with a very high concentration of α-fetoprotein in the plasma. Numerous α-fetoprotein-containing hepatocytes were observed in these patients. Whether the α-fetoprotein-containing cells indicate a premalignant disorder is unclear, since no ultrastructural studies were performed. However, primary hepatocellular carcinomas do arise in tyrosinosis.

Finally, an interesting observation was made on patients with alcoholic hepatitis.[84] The liver of 9 of 18 patients studied with immunofluorescence showed numerous α-fetoprotein-containing hepatocytes, whereas the plasma concentration of this protein was normal in most of these patients. The explanation for this observation remains unclear, but some of the cells were located near areas of hepatocytic regeneration. α-Fetoprotein increases in the plasma during hepatic regeneration, and conceivably α-fetoprotein could be detected with morphologic methods in the hepatocytes even with unaltered plasma concentration.

REFERENCES

1. Miller LL, Bale WF: Synthesis of all plasma protein fractions except gamma globulins by the liver. The use of zone electrophoresis and lysine-ϵ-C[14] to define the plasma proteins synthesized by the isolated perfused liver. J Exp Med 99:125–132, 1954

2. Kukral JC, Kerth JD, Pancner RJ, Cromer DN, Henagar GC: Plasma protein synthesis in the normal dog and after total hepatectomy. Surg Gynecol Obstet 113:360–372, 1961

3. Peters T Jr, Anfinsen CB: Production of radioactive serum albumin by liver slices. J Biol Chem 182:171–179, 1950

4. Campbell PN, Greengard O, Kernot BA: Studies on the synthesis of serum albumin by isolated microsome fraction from rat liver. Biochem J 74:107–117, 1960

5. Sarcione EJ: The initial subcellular site of incorporation of hexoses into liver protein. J Biol Chem 239:1686–1689, 1964

6. Schultze HE, Heremans JF: Molecular Bi-

ology of Human Proteins with Special Reference to Plasma Proteins. Amsterdam, Elsevier, 1966, pp 354–355

7. Bloom W, Fawcett DW: A Textbook of Histology (ed 10). Philadelphia, WB Saunders, 1975, pp 688–725

8. Blouin A, Bolender RP, Weibel ER: Distribution of organelles and membranes between hepatocytes and nonhepatocytes in the rat liver parenchyma. A stereological study. J Cell Biol 72:441–455, 1977

9. Noël R: Recherches histo-physiologiques sur la cellule hépatique des mamifères. Arch Anat Microsc Morphol Exp 19:1–159, 1923

10. Wachstein M: Cyto- and histochemistry of the liver. Edited by C Rouiller: The Liver. Morphology, Biochemistry, Physiology. Vol. I New York, Academic Press, 1963, pp 137–194

11. Loud AV: A quantitative stereological description of the ultrastructure of normal rat liver parenchymal cells. J Cell Biol 37:27–46, 1968

12. Katz N, Teutsch HF, Jungermann K, Sasse D: Heterogeneous reciprocal localization of fructose-1,6 bis-phosphatase and of glucokinase in microdissected periportal perivenous rat liver tissue. FEBS Lett 83:272–276, 1977

13. Pearse AGE: Histochemistry. Theoretical and Applied (ed 3). Vol. I. London, Churchill, 1968, pp 106–179

14. Coons MH, Kaplan HH: Localization of antigen in tissue cells. II. Improvements in a method for the detection of antigen by means of fluorescent antibody. J Exp Med 91:1–13, 1950

15. Hamashima Y, Harter JG, Coons HH: The localization of albumin and fibrinogen in human liver cells. J Cell Biol 20:271–279, 1964

16. Barnhart MI: Prothrombin synthesis: an example of hepatic function. J Histochem Cytochem 8:740–751, 1965

17. Lane RS: Localization of transferrin in human and rat liver by fluorescent antibody technique. Nature 215:161–162, 1967

18. Peters JH, Alper CA: Haptoglobin synthesis. II. Cellular localization studies. J Clin Invest 45:314–320, 1966

19. Barnhart MI, Forman WB: The cellular localization of fibrinogen as revealed by the fluorescent antibody technique. Vox Sang 8:461–473, 1963

20. Avrameas S, Uriel J: Méthode de marquage d'antigènes et d'anticorps avec des enzymes et son application en immunodiffusion. CR Acad Sci (Paris) 262:2543–2545, 1966

21. Nakane PK, Pierce GB: Enzyme-labeled antibodies: Preparation and application for the localization of antigens. J Histochem Cytochem 14:929–931, 1966

22. Feldmann G, Druet P, Bignon J, Avrameas S: Immunoenzymatic Techniques. Amsterdam, North-Holland, 1976

23. Graham RC Jr, Karnovsky MJ: The early stages of absorption of injected horseradish peroxidase in the proximal tubules of mouse kidney: Ultrastructural cytochemistry by a new technique. J Histochem Cytochem 14:291–302, 1966

24. Avrameas S: Enzyme markers: Their linkage with proteins and use in immuno-histochemistry. Edited by P Stoward: Fixation in Histochemistry. London, Chapman and Hall, 1973, pp 183–192

25. Feldmann G, Penaud-Laurencin J, Crassous J, Benhamou JP: Albumin synthesis by human liver cells: Its morphological demonstration. Gastroenterology 63: 1036–1048, 1972

26. Feldmann G: Plasma protein synthesis by human liver cells: Its morphological demonstration with antibodies labelled with peroxidase. Edited by E Wisse, WTh Daems, I Molenaar, and P Van Duijn: Electron Microscopy and Cytochemistry. Amsterdam, North-Holland, 1974, pp 145–149

27. Feldmann G, Maurice M, Sapin C, Benhamou JP: Inhibition by colchicine of fibrinogen translocation in hepatocytes. J Cell Biol 67:237–243, 1975

28. Feldmann G, Guillouzo A, Maurice M, Guesnon J: Depressed secretion of plasma proteins synthesized by the liver: An ultrastructural investigation based on immunoperoxidase. Edited by G Feldmann, P Druet, J Bignon and S Avrameas: Immunoenzymatic Techniques. Amsterdam, North-Holland, 1976, pp 379–394

29. Guillouzo A, Feldmann G, Belanger L: Localization of alpha-fetoprotein-containing liver cells in tyrosinosis and in newborn rat. Edited by WH Fishman and S Sell: Oncodevelopmental Gene Expression. New York, Academic Press, 1976, pp 647–654

30. Guillouzo A, Feldmann G, Maurice M, Sapin C, Benhamou JP: Ultrastructural dis-

tribution of albumin in rat hepatocytes during post-natal development. J Microsc Biol Cell 26:35–41, 1976

31. Kushner I, Feldmann G: Control of the acute phase response. Demonstration of C-reactive protein synthesis and secretion by hepatocytes during acute inflammation in the rabbit. J Exp Med 148:466-477, 1978

32. Feldmann G: unpublished results

33. Lane RS: The cellular distribution of albumin in normal rat liver demonstrated by immunofluorescent staining. Clin Sci 36:157–159, 1969

34. Lane RS: Transferrin synthesis in the rat: A study using the fluorescent antibody technique. Br J Haematol 15:355–364, 1968

35. Goussev AI, Engelhardt NV, Masseyeff R, Camain R, Basteris B: Immunofluorescent study of alpha-foetoprotein (αfp) in liver and liver tumors. II. Localization of αfp in the tissues of patients with primary liver cancer (PLC). Int J Cancer 7:207–217, 1971

36. Purtillo DT, Yunis EF: α-Fetoprotein. Immunofluorescent localization in human fetal liver and hepatoma. Lab Invest 25:291–294, 1971

37. Nayak NC, Mital I: The dynamics of α-fetoprotein and albumin synthesis in human and rat liver during normal ontogeny. Am J Pathol 86:359–374, 1977

38. Kraemer M, Foucrier J: Mise en évidence immunoenzymatique de la transferrine dans le foie de rat. Résultats préliminaires. CR Acad Sci (Paris) 283:83–85, 1976

39. Alexander CA, Hamilton RL, Havel RJ: Subcellular localization of B apoprotein of plasma lipoproteins in rat liver. J Cell Biol 69:241–263, 1976

40. Vernon-Roberts B: The Macrophage. Cambridge, Cambridge University Press, 1972, pp 144–145

41. Stecher VJ, Thorbecke GJ: Sites of synthesis of serum proteins. I. Serum proteins produced by macrophages in vitro. J Immunol 99:643–652, 1967

42. Feldmann G, Martin JP, Sesboue R, Ropartz C, Perelman R, Nathanson M, Seringe P, Benhamou JP: The ultrastructure of hepatocytes in alpha-1-antitrypsin deficiency with the genotype Pi___. Gut 16:796–799, 1975

43. Feldmann G, Maurice M: Morphological findings of liver protein synthesis and secretion. Edited by H Popper, L Bianchi, and W Reuter. Membrane Alterations as Basis of Liver Injury. Lancaster, England, MTP Press, 1977, pp 61–76

44. Palade G: Intracellular aspects of the process of protein synthesis. Science 189:347–358, 1975

45. Peyrol S, Grimaud JA, Pirson Y, Chayvialle JA, Touillon C, Lambert R: Ultrastructural immunoenzymatic study of α-fetoprotein producing cells in the human fetal liver. J Histochem Cytochem 25:432–438, 1977

46. Lin CT, Chang JP: Electron microscopy of albumin synthesis. Science 190:465–467, 1975

47. Peters T Jr: The biosynthesis of rat serum albumin. I. Properties of rat albumin and its occurence in liver cell fractions. J Biol Chem 237:1181–1185, 1962

48. Peters T Jr: The biosynthesis of rat serum albumin. II. Intracellular phenomena in the secretion of newly formed albumin. J Biol Chem 237:1186–1189, 1962

49. Glaumann H, Ericsson JLE: Evidence for the participation of the Golgi apparatus in the intracellular transport of nascent albumin in the liver cell. J Cell Biol 47:555–567, 1970

50. Barnhart ML, Anderson GF: Intracellular localization of fibrinogen. Proc Soc Exp Biol Med 110:734–737, 1962

51. Williams CA: Analysis of "acute phase" protein synthesis in the mouse by immunoelectrophoresis. Edited by MA Rothschild and T Waldmann: Plasma Protein Metabolism. Regulation of Synthesis, Distribution, and Degradation. New York, Academic Press, 1970, pp 383–392

52. Jamieson JC, Ashton FE: Studies on acute phase proteins of rat serum. III. Site of synthesis of albumin and α_1-acid glycoprotein and the contents of these proteins in liver microsome fractions from rats suffering from induced inflammation. Can J Biochem 51:1034–1045, 1973

53. Redman CM, Cherian MG: The secretory pathways of rat serum glycoproteins and albumin. Localization of newly formed proteins within the endoplasmic reticulum. J Cell Biol 52:231–245, 1972

54. Spiro RG: Glycoproteins: their biochemistry, biology and role in human disease. N Engl J Med 281:991–1001; 1043–1056, 1969

55. Clauser H, Herman G, Rossignol B, Harbon S: Biosynthesis of glycoproteins. Biosynthesis at the cellular and subcellular

level. Edited by A Gottschalk: Glycoproteins. Their Composition, Structure and Function (ed 2). Part B. Amsterdam, Elsevier, 1972, pp 1151–1169

56. Claude A: Growth and differentiation of cytoplasmic membranes in the course of lipoprotein granule synthesis in the hepatic cell. I. Elaboration of elements of the Golgi complex. J Cell Biol 47:745–766, 1970

57. Warren WA, Peters T Jr: Binding of purified antialbumin by rat liver ribosomes. J Biol Chem 240:3009–3015, 1965

58. Taylor JM, Schimke RT: Specific binding of albumin antibody to rat liver polysomes. J Biol Chem 249:3597–3601, 1974

59. Campbell PN, Serck-Hanssen G, Lowe E: Studies on the protein-synthesizing activity of the ribosomes of rat liver. The activity of free polysomes. Biochem J 97:422–431, 1965

60. Redman CM: Biosynthesis of serum proteins and ferritin by free and attached ribosomes of rat liver. J Biol Chem 244:4308–4315, 1969

61. Frenk S, Antonowicz I, Craig JM, Metcoff J: Experimental nephrotic syndrome induced in rats by aminonucleoside. Renal lesions and body electrolyte composition. Proc Soc Exp Biol Med 89:424–427, 1955

62. Heymann W, Hackel DB, Harwood S, Wilson SGF, Hunter JLP: Production of nephrotic syndrome in rats by Freund's adjuvants and rat kidney suspension. Proc Soc Exp Biol Med 100:660–664, 1959

63. Katz J, Bonorris G, Okuyama S, Sellers AL: Albumin synthesis in perfused liver of normal and nephrotic rats. Am J Physiol 212:1255–1260, 1967

64. Maurice M, Feldmann G, Druet P, Laliberté F, Bouige D: Immunoperoxidase localization of albumin in hepatocytes of nephrotic rats with special reference to changes in the Golgi apparatus. Lab Invest 40:39–45, 1979.

65. Koj A: Acute-phase reactants. Their synthesis, turnover and biological significance. Edited by AC Allison: Structure and Function of Plasma Proteins. Vol. I. London, Plenum Press, 1974, pp 73–131

66. Damianov B, Rogier E, Maurice M, Druet P, Feldmann G: Localisation hépatique du fibrinogène au cours de la phase aiguë de la réaction inflammatoire. Biol Cell 29:12a, 1977

67. Le Marchand Y, Singh A, Assimacopoulos-Jeannet F, Orci L, Rouiller C, Jeanrenaud B: A role for the microtubular system in the release of very low density lipoproteins by perfused mouse livers. J Biol Chem 248:6862–6870, 1973

68. Redman CM, Banerjee D, Howell K, Palade GE: Colchicine inhibition of plasma protein release from rat hepatocytes. J Cell Biol 66:42–59, 1975

69. Rothschild MA, Oratz M: Albumin synthesis and degradation. Edited by AC Allison: Structure and Function of Plasma Proteins. Vol. II. London, Plenum Press, 1976, pp 79–105

70. Regoeczi E: Fibrinogen. Edited by AC Allison: Structure and Function of Plasma Proteins. Vol. I. London, Plenum Press, 1974, pp 133–167

71. Sidransky H: Regulatory effect of aminoacids on polyribosomes and protein synthesis of liver. Edited by H Popper and F Schaffner: Progress in Liver Diseases. Vol. IV. New York, Grune & Stratton, 1972, pp 31–43

72. Chandrasakharam N, Fleck A, Munro HN: Albumin content of rat hepatic cells at different levels of protein intake. J Nutr 92:497–502, 1967

73. Courtoy PJ, Lombart C, Feldmann G, Moguilevsky N, Rogier E: Etude de la synthèse hépatique des glycoproteines de la réaction inflammatoire: cinétique et localisation chez le rat. Biol Cell 33:28a, 1978

74. Sharp HL: Alpha-1-antitrypsin deficiency. Hosp Pract 6:83–96, 1971

75. Gordon HW, Dixon J, Rogers JC, Mittman C, Lieberman J: Alpha-1-antitrypsin (A_1-AT) accumulation in livers of emphysematous patients with A_1-AT deficiency. Hum Pathol 3:361–370, 1972

76. Aagenaes Ø, Matlary A, Elgjo K, Munthe E, Fargerhol M: Neonatal cholestasis in alpha-1-antitrypsin deficient children. Acta Paediatr Scand 61:632–642, 1972

77. Palmer PE, Delellis RA, Wolfe HJ: Immunohistochemistry of liver in alpha-1-antitrypsin deficiency. A comparative study. Am J Clin Pathol 62:350–354, 1974

78. Feldmann G, Bignon J, Chahinian P, Degott C, Benhamou JP: Hepatocyte ultrastructural changes in α_1-antitrypsin deficiency. Gastroenterology 67:1214–1224, 1974

79. Sharp HL: The current status of α_1-antitrypsin, a protease inhibitor, in gastrointes-

tinal disease. Gastroenterology 70:611–621, 1976

80. Rothschild MA, Oratz M, Zimmon D, Schreiber SS, Weiner I, Van Caneghem A: Albumin synthesis in cirrhotic subjects with ascites studied with carbonate-^{14}C. J Clin Invest 48:344–350, 1969

81. Baraona E, Leo MA, Borowsky SA, Lieber CS: Pathogenesis of alcohol-induced accumulation of protein in the liver. J Clin Invest 60:546–554, 1977

82. Abelev GI: Cellular aspects of alpha-fetoprotein synthesis. Edited by WH Fishman and S Sell: Onco-developmental Gene Expression. New York, Academic Press, 1976, pp 191–202

83. Uriel J, Aussel C, Bouillon D, Loisillier F, de Nechaud B: Liver differentiation and the oestrogen-binding properties of α-fetoprotein. Ann NY Acad Sci 259:119–130, 1975

84. Husby G, Strickland RG, Caldwell JL, Williams RC Jr: Localization of T and B cells and alpha fetoprotein in hepatic biopsies from patients with liver disease. J Clin Invest 56:1198–1209, 1975

Chapter 3

Cell Surface Receptors in the Liver

By E. ANTHONY JONES, M.D., M.R.C.P., JOHN M. VIERLING, M.D., CLIFFORD J. STEER, M.D., *and* JUERG REICHEN, M.D.

A variety of hepatic cell surface receptors have been tentatively identified and appear to play important roles in hepatic physiology. Hepatic cell surface receptors are involved in (1) the mediation of the metabolic effects of some polypeptide hormones, (2) the transport of a variety of inorganic and organic solutes, (3) the uptake of certain hematinics, (4) the uptake of modified glycoproteins and lipoproteins, (5) the clearance of particles coated with specific immunologically active molecules, and (6) the interaction of the liver with certain exogenous agents. This chapter is concerned primarily with the first five phenomena. With only a few exceptions, the interaction of the cell surface of hepatic cells with exogenous agents such as drugs, viruses, and bacterial toxins is not discussed in this review.

Appropriate definitions of cell surface receptors should take into account current concepts of the structure and properties of cell membranes. In this context, the fluid mosaic membrane model[1] appears to be particularly germane. The cell membrane is regarded as a fluid lipid bilayer interdispersed with integral or intrinsic and surface or extrinsic membrane proteins. The former proteins extend through both layers of lipid. Hydrophobic areas are embedded in the bilayer, while hydrophilic areas are exposed to either aqueous surface of the membrane. By contrast, extrinsic proteins do not traverse the membrane and are embedded to a lesser extent in the bilayer. The model allows for considerable lateral mobility of membrane proteins. Such mobility could occur as a result of random Brownian movement or be governed by specific structures such as the microfilament system.[2] Cell surface receptors appear to be integral membrane proteins.[1,3]

A useful, operative definition of cell surface receptors has been proposed.[4] They can be defined as molecules in the cell membrane that are "uniquely capable of recognizing and interacting with" a ligand "with a high degree of selectivity and affinity and which, in addition, possess the capability of conveying the occurrence of the interaction to biochemical processes resulting in metabolically significant events." Thus the receptor is considered to have two distinct functions: the recognition of the ligand and, when ligand and receptor have interacted, the activation of other molecules in order to generate the specific biologic response. A cell surface receptor can also be defined as a cell membrane component "which has the ability to selectively recognize and

From the Section on Diseases of the Liver, Digestive Diseases Branch, National Institute of Arthritis, Metabolism and Digestive Diseases, National Institutes of Health, Bethesda, Maryland.

43

bind'' a ligand ''and which has binding characteristics consistent with a potential for signal generation.''[3] This definition implies that the binding of analogs of the ligand to the receptor should exhibit specificities that parallel the
biologic effects of the analogs and that the kinetics of ligand-receptor interaction should be consistent with the kinetics and dose response of the biologic
effects induced by the ligand. The concept of biologic response to receptor-
ligand interaction, depending on the conveyance of this occurrence over a
finite distance (i.e., signal generation), includes the possibility that the molecular structures responsible for recognizing and binding a ligand are separate
from those responsible for effecting the biologic response. Receptor and effector functions may reside in different regions of a single molecule, or they
may reside in separate molecules that interact directly or indirectly in the fluid
mosaic membrane. Different possibilities of such an arrangement have been
discussed by Singer and Nicholson[1] (Fig. 1). It is evident from the above

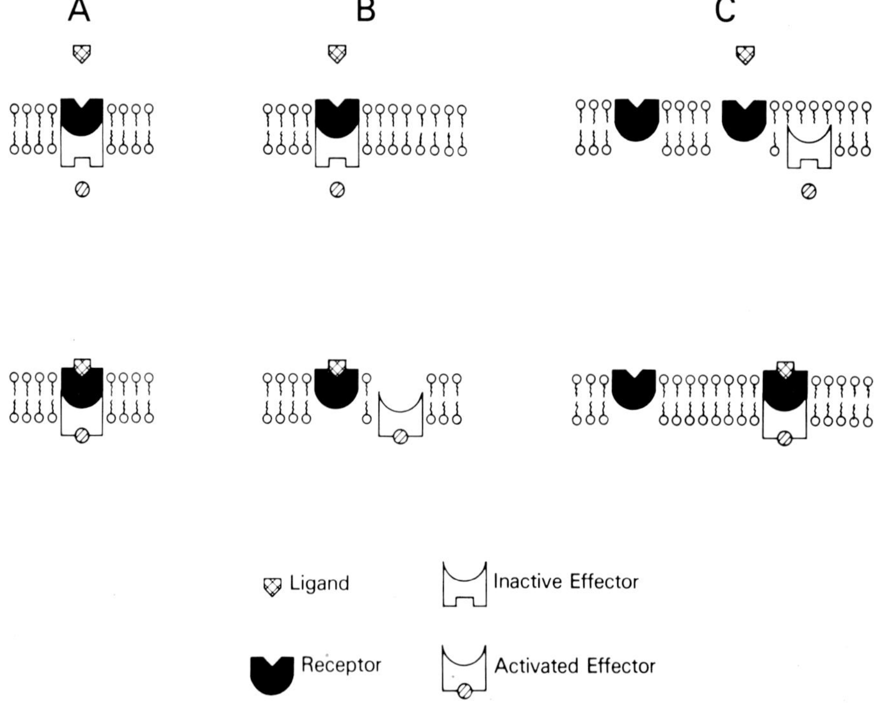

FIG. 1—Models of ligand-receptor interaction. Receptor and effector molecules are depicted in
a lipid bilayer. The upper part of the figure shows receptors unoccupied by ligand and nonactivated
effectors. The lower part shows effectors that have become activated as a result of ligand-receptor
binding. Note the conformational change in the effector associated with its activation. In model
A the receptor and effector site are on the same molecule. In model B the conformational change
induced by ligand-receptor interaction results in the separation of the activated effector from the
ligand-receptor complex. In model C, receptors and effectors are separate units that are both
considered to be capable of lateral movement within the bilayer. In this model, based on the
concepts proposed by Singer and Nicholson,[1] ligand-receptor binding increases the probability of
receptor-effector interaction.

definitions that the demonstration of binding of a ligand to a cell membrane per se does not imply that the binding is to a receptor.

These concepts have been developed primarily to account for the action of polypeptide hormones. They may, however, also apply to completely unrelated biologic phenomena, such as solute transport or the interaction of immunologically active molecules with hepatic cells. The finding that a variety of ionic solutes cross cell membranes at much faster rates than those predicted from their physicochemical properties has led to the concept of carrier-mediated transport.[5] The formation of a complex between a carrier, presumably the hydrophylic region of a membrane protein, and a solute undergoing selective transport can be described by kinetics similar to those of receptor-ligand interactions. In the case of carrier-mediated transport, the biologic response can be regarded as the transfer of the solute across the membrane. In the case of the binding of immunologically active molecules to cell surface membranes, the molecular structures involved are probably much larger than those involved in polypeptide hormone binding or solute transport.

Processes in the liver that are mediated by parenchymal cell surface receptors must be differentiated from those mediated by nonparenchymal cell surface receptors. The action of polypeptide hormones, the uptake and transport of inorganic and organic solutes, and the uptake of hematinics and lipoproteins are examples of processes mediated by cell surface receptors on hepatocytes. By contrast, the immunospecific clearance of particles in the circulation is a process mediated specifically by cell surface receptors on nonparenchymal cells. Some processes, such as the hepatic uptake of certain specifically modified glycoproteins, appear to be mediated by cell surface receptors on either parenchymal or nonparenchymal cells.

METHODOLOGIC CONSIDERATIONS

Many direct studies of ligand-receptor interaction and carrier-mediated transport have involved the standard methods applied to competitive protein-binding assays.[6] Typically, an isotopically labeled purified ligand is incubated with a suitable receptor preparation. The labeled ligand-receptor complex is then separated from free labeled ligand by centrifugation, filtration, adsorption, or precipitation; thereafter, receptor-bound radioactivity is determined. By repeating the incubation over different time periods with varying amounts of unlabeled ligand or related compounds, the kinetics of ligand-receptor interaction, as well as the specificity, stoichiometry, and saturability of the binding reaction, can be determined.

Preparations of liver used as a source of receptor include intact cells, particulate fractions of cells, and solubilized mixtures of proteins obtained from solubilization of cell suspensions or particulate fractions. Each type of preparation has its own advantages and disadvantages. Isolated intact cells can be obtained from tissue culture or by enzymatic and/or mechanical disruption of the liver. Appropriate methods of isolation have been discussed elsewhere.[7,8] Suitable long-term cultures of hepatic cells have not yet been established.

Furthermore, if they are, it will be necessary to determine whether transformation or adaptation of cells in culture has affected their populations of cell surface receptors. The viability of freshly prepared cell suspensions needs to be assessed, since the duration of viability of cells in such suspensions is limited (see Chapter 1). Criteria used to assess viability include measurements of the exclusion of dyes such as trypan blue, enzyme leakage, membrane potential, gluconeogenesis, synthesis of export proteins, and metabolic responses to hormones.[7-9] Since most suspensions of dispersed cells are metabolically active, ligand binding and biologic response may be studied simultaneously and correlated.[10,11] Studies with intact cells may be hampered by ligand degradation, however. Furthermore, the use of enzymes such as collagenase or pronase in the isolation of the cells may alter the number or structure of their cell surface receptors.[6] A potentially important advantage of working with dispersed cells is the possibility of conducting separate studies with purified preparations of parenchymal and nonparenchymal cells.[12]

Particulate cell fractions have the advantage of being more stable on storage and unaffected by ligand-degrading enzymes in some instances. Relevant to this review are studies conducted with purified liver plasma membrane fractions. These can be obtained by homogenization of whole liver or of isolated hepatocytes, followed by several steps of differential and/or isopyknic centrifugation.[13-17] In work with plasma membrane fractions, every preparation must be assessed for yield and purity by measurement of appropriate marker enzymes, phase and transmission electron microscopy, and acrylamide gel electrophoresis.[13-17] If the preparations are obtained from a whole liver homogenate, membranes from nonparenchymal cells may contribute significantly to the final preparation.[18]

Solubilized cell fractions have been valuable in attempts to purify and characterize hepatic cell surface receptors. Solubilizing agents include neutral, anionic, and cationic amphipaths. In addition to solubilizing agents, hydrophobic bonds that anchor protein receptors in the lipid bilayer may be broken by the use of chaotropics, limited proteolytic digestion, or other enzymatic treatments.[19,20] Like original intact membrane preparations, solubilized surface membranes may be contaminated by material from intracellular organelles. Rigorous criteria are required to follow the extent of solubilization, since different agents may have different capacities to solubilize proteins from the lipid bilayer. Furthermore, detergent-receptor interactions have to be taken into account. Solubilization of receptors with strong anionic detergents usually results in the entire surface of the receptor becoming coated with negative charges, with concomitant loss of binding activity. Nonionic detergents are thought to coat only the hydrophobic areas of protein molecules, leaving their biologically active hydrophilic sites exposed. Some integral membrane proteins show varying degrees of phospholipid dependence, addition of phospholipids after solubilization being necessary to restore their full biologic activity. Solubilized membrane proteins have been most widely used in the partial purification of receptor proteins by affinity chromatography.[21,22] The limitations and possible pitfalls of this method have been discussed elsewhere.[21] A promising approach to the understanding of receptor function may be the reconstitution of biologically active systems by incorporation of pure receptor proteins into liposomes.[23]

CURRENT CONCEPTS OF LIGAND-RECEPTOR INTERACTIONS

The binding of a ligand to its receptor is generally a rapid process that is usually reversible. The time course and extent of binding depend on temperature, physicochemical environment, ligand concentration, and concentration and spatial arrangement of the receptors. After dissociation from its receptor, a ligand is usually identical to the native ligand in terms of physical properties, biologic activity, and the capacity to interact with antibodies and other membrane receptors.[24,25]

A finite number of receptor sites for a ligand exist on a particular cell surface. The interaction of ligand (L) with unoccupied receptor (R) on the cell surface can be analyzed mathematically in terms of the law of mass action.[6,26-28] Thus,

$$[L] + [R] \underset{k_{-1}}{\overset{k_1}{\rightleftharpoons}} [LR] \tag{1}$$

In equation (1), k_1 and k_{-1} are the association and dissociation rate constants, respectively, while $[L]$, $[R]$, and $[LR]$ are the concentrations of free ligand, unoccupied receptor, and ligand-receptor complex, respectively. It follows that

$$\frac{k_1}{k_{-1}} = \frac{[LR]}{[L][R]} = K_a \tag{2}$$

where K_a is the association constant with the dimensions M^{-1}. The reciprocal of the association constant yields the dissociation constant with the dimensions M. According to this equation, the concentration of ligand bound (c_b) at any given concentration of free ligand (c_f) can be described by the general binding isotherm[28] as follows:

$$c_b = P\left(\frac{K_a c_f}{1 + K_a c_f}\right) \tag{3}$$

where P is the maximal binding capacity or the maximal number of binding sites, if the receptor can be identified. Deviations from this behavior are frequently encountered. For instance, deviations may be caused by nonsaturable binding, which is often referred to as nonspecific binding[3] (Fig. 2). This can be taken into account by adding a linear term to equation (3):

$$c_b = P\left(\frac{K_a c_f}{1 + K_a c_f}\right) + q c_f \tag{4}$$

where q is a coefficient, describing the fraction nonspecifically bound. Another cause of deviation from the general binding isotherm described by equation (3) would be the presence of several distinct classes of binding sites. The net

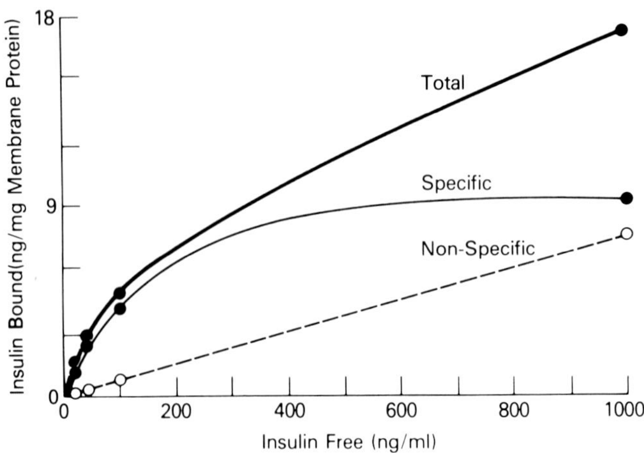

FIG. 2—Binding of insulin to rat liver plasma membranes. Total, specific, and nonspecific insulin bound are plotted against the concentration of free insulin. Note that the specific binding, which presumably reflects the interaction of insulin with its receptor, shows saturability. By contrast, nonspecific binding is directly proprotional to the concentration of free insulin. Total observed binding is the sum of specific and nonspecific binding (see equation 4). Nonspecific binding must be taken into account in analyzing data on the binding of ligands. (From reviews by Kahn.[3,6] Reproduced by permission from the Plenum Publishing Company, New York and the *Journal of Cell Biology*.)

concentration bound can then be expressed by summation of the amount bound to each class:

$$c_b = \sum_{i=1}^{n} P_i \left(\frac{K_{ai}c_f}{1 + K_{ai}c_f} \right) \tag{5}$$

In equation (5), i describes the ith of n classes of different binding sites, each of which is characterized by its maximal binding capacity and association constant. Deviation from the general binding isotherm described in equation (3) can also occur in the presence of heterogeneous binding sites and/or the occurrence of site-site interactions (cooperativity). These phenomena can be expressed mathematically by incorporating the Hill coefficient[29,30] into equation (3) as follows:

$$c_b = P \left[\frac{(K_a c_f)^h}{1 + (K_a c_f)^h} \right] \tag{6}$$

where h is the Hill coefficient, which is dimensionless. $h < 1$ can result from heterogeneity of the binding sites or negative cooperativity. The latter is thought to be caused by site-site interactions that decrease the probability of binding at high ligand concentrations. By contrast, $h > 1$ may be caused by positive cooperativity, which can result from site-site interactions increasing the probability of binding at high ligand concentrations. The influence of h on the binding isotherm is illustrated schematically in Figure 3. Negative cooperativity may augment sensitivity of the cell to receptor-ligand interactions at

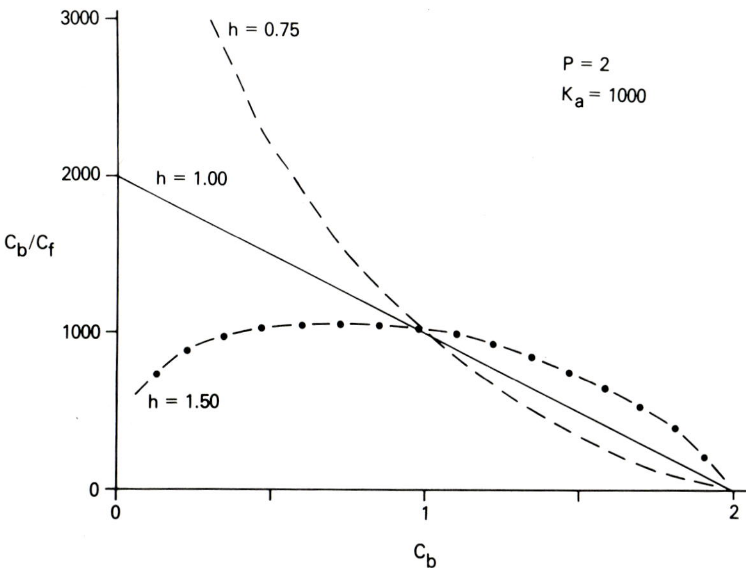

FIG. 3—Scatchard plots[6] of ligand-receptor interaction. The ratio of the concentrations of bound to free ligand (c_b/c_f) is plotted against the concentration of bound ligand (c_b). In this hypothetical example, a maximum binding capacity (P) of 2 (e.g., sites per receptor molecule) and an association constant (K_a) of 1000 M^{-1} are assumed. If the Hill coefficient (see equation 6) is 1.0, the plot is linear (solid line). This relationship is typical of that predicted for a single class of homogeneous binding sites according to the general binding isotherm (see equation 3). Note that K_a can be derived by dividing the intercept with the ordinate by P. When h is less than 1.0 (dashed line), a larger fraction of ligand is bound at low ligand concentrations than would be predicted from equation 3 (negative cooperativity). The reverse holds true when h is greater than 1.0 (alternate dashes and dots) (positive cooperativity). The effect of h on the binding isotherm can be predicted from equation 6.

low concentrations of ligand while buffering the cell against acutely elevated levels of ligand.[31]

Expansions of the simple model outlined above, which are all concerned with the analysis of steady-state data, have been discussed in detail elsewhere.[32–34] By contrast, the model proposed by Frieden[35] permits analysis of kinetic data. This possibility is of importance in studies of ligand-receptor interactions, since it is often difficult, if not impossible, to differentiate between heterogeneity and negative cooperativity ($h < 1$) of binding sites from steady-state binding data.[30] The phenomenon of negative cooperativity is of particular importance in the interaction of insulin with its receptor[31,36] (see Insulin).

All the models cited are based on the assumption that the biologic response to ligand-receptor interaction is a function of the fraction of binding sites which are occupied (occupancy theory). Certain deviations from this expected behavior have led to the formulation of the rate theory[37] in which the biologic response is regarded as a function of the "forward reaction velocity" (v_f):

$$v_f = k_1[L][R] - \left(\frac{k_1^2[L][R]}{k_1[L] + k_{-1}}\right)(1 - e^{-(k_1[L] + k_{-1})t}) \tag{7}$$

The main difference between the occupancy theory and the rate theory is that the former predicts the elicited response in terms of a continuous process, whereas the latter predicts it in terms of a series of discrete quanta.

Different possibilities for the coupling of ligand-receptor binding and elicitation of the biologic response have been considered.[1] A poor correlation between biologic response and ligand binding seems difficult to explain in terms of a single molecule with both receptor and effector functions (model A in Fig. 1). A more complex model is necessary to account for cooperative interactions between receptors[31,36,38] and the effect of regulatory factors on ligand binding.[39,40] The most comprehensive model is the one based on the concepts proposed by Singer and Nicholson[1] (model C in Fig. 1). This model includes separate receptor and effector molecules embedded in the lipid membrane and allows for their lateral mobility. The binding of ligand to receptor increases the probability of interaction between receptor and effector. This model explains several phenomena. For instance, the model can account for a maximal biologic response to insulin being observed when only a certain fraction of the total number of insulin receptor sites are occupied by insulin molecules, an example of the phenomenon of spare receptors.[6] It can also account for nonlinear coupling between receptor occupancy and biologic response. In addition, the biologic response may not be proportional to a given receptor occupancy for different ligands. This can be explained by the different intrinsic capacities of individual ligands to initiate the biologic response.[3] Several combinations of the phenomena discussed have been described. Thus, different ligands can induce the same biologic response if their occupied receptors converge on the same effector.[41] If a single effector can be stimulated by the binding of different ligands with their respective receptors, nonadditive activation of a biologic response may occur when more than one of the ligands is present at maximal concentration.[41] Furthermore, multiple biologic responses can be initiated by a single ligand if its receptor-ligand complex interacts with more than one effector.[42]

It is evident from the comprehensive model (Fig. 1) that an important determinant of coupling is the fluidity of the membrane, since this property allows for the lateral movement of both receptor and effector.[1,43-45] The demonstration of cooperative phenomena[31,36,38] is consistent which such lateral movement.

An important determinant of the magnitude of the biologic response is the number of receptors present on the cell surface. There is a constant turnover of cell proteins, the reported half-lives for specific glycoprotein enzymes ranging from 2 hr to 16 days.[46] Clearly the concentration of a cell surface receptor is related to its prevailing rates of synthesis and degradation. Certain hormones exert a negative feedback control of the concentration of their receptors on cell surfaces.[47] This can occur if binding of ligand promotes receptor degradation by membrane-bound proteases, endocytosis, or shedding of the ligand-receptor complex into extracellular fluid.[3] By contrast, prolactin induces its own receptor.[48] No studies have established the synthesis of structurally abnormal, mutant receptors.

HEPATIC CELL SURFACE RECEPTORS FOR HORMONES

Insulin

A receptor for insulin on the plasma membrane of hepatocytes has been identified, extensively characterized, and partially purified.[6,22,44,49,50] The two classical functions incorporated into the definition of a receptor are exhibited by the insulin receptor. Thus the binding of insulin to its receptor on the hepatocyte is followed by changes in the intermediary metabolism of the hepatocyte characteristic of the action of insulin. This receptor appears to possess the same properties as insulin receptors in other tissues and species with respect to the characteristics of insulin binding and the inhibition of such binding by anti-insulin receptor antibodies.[49,51]

The insulin receptor characterized in rat liver plasma membranes is a glycoprotein, the molecular weight of which is estimated to vary between 135,000 and 300,000. The receptor molecule possesses subunits, which have a molecular weight estimated to be about 75,000.[22,44,50] Steady-state binding of insulin to its receptor occurs within a few minutes at 37°C but takes several hours at lower temperatures.[10,27,52,53] There is a gradual decline in binding on prolonged incubation, probably as a result of insulin and receptor degradation.[52,53] Binding of insulin to its receptor appears to be fully reversible at lower temperatures, but dissociation is not a simple first-order reaction[52] (Table 1). When insulin dissociates from its receptor under these conditions it is identical to native insulin, suggesting that the site of binding of insulin to its receptor is distinct from its major site of catabolism.[24] The insulin-degrading enzymes found in most liver plasma membrane preparations are probably intracellular contaminants.[54] Insulin binding to surface receptors may facilitate insulin degradation, however, possibly by promoting its entry into the cell and exposure to proteolytic enzymes.[54–58] Some binding of insulin to liver plasma membranes is saturable, while another component of binding is nonsaturable and represents nonspecific binding[3,6] (Fig. 2). The saturable binding is characterized by a high affinity for insulin and presumably represents the physiologically important binding of insulin to its receptor.[3,52]

Trypsin reduces the senitivity of adipocytes to insulin apparently by decreasing the total amount of receptor available for binding. Although insulin-receptor binding is not affected by incubating cell membranes with neuraminidase alone, the binding is lost after exposure to a combination of neuraminidase and β-galactosidase.[44] This suggests that galactosyl groups, but not sialic acid residues, are involved in insulin recognition and are probably a chemical constituent of the receptor.

A close correlation has been found between the affinity of a variety of insulins from different species, insulin analogs, and insulin derivatives for insulin receptors on hepatocytes and adipocytes and their capacity to induce insulin-like biologic responses.[10,59-61] Such specificities have permitted the mapping of structure-function relationships for the insulin molecule.[62] A competitive antagonist of insulin has not yet been found among the insulin analogs tested.

TABLE 1.—*Binding Properties of Some Ligands to Hepatic Plasma Membranes*.

Ligand	Animal	Number of Sites/Cell	Association Constant (K_a)	Rate Constants*		References
				Association (k_1)	Dissociation (k_{-1})	
		(10^5)	(10^9M^{-1})	$(10^6s^{-1}M^{-1})$	$(10^{-3}s^{-1})$	
Insulin	Rat, mouse	1.0–2.5	0.12	0.13–1	0.7	3
Glucagon	Rat	1.1	~1.5	1	4	3
Vasoactive intestinal polypeptide	Rat	—	5.9–6.3	13	2.3	115
Human growth hormone	Pregnant rabbit	—	0.05	—	—	116
Human growth hormone	Male rat	0.06–0.22	1.14–1.16	—	—	117,118
Human growth hormone	Female rat	0.16–0.21[+]	0.96–1.24[+]	—	—	117–119
Bovine growth hormone	Male rat	0.39	0.30	—	—	118
Bovine growth hormone	Female rat	0.59	0.36	—	—	118
Ovine prolactin	Male rat	0	—		—	118
Ovine prolactin	Female rat	0.42	0.82	—	—	118
L-triiodothyronine	Rat	—	0.31	—	—	125
Prostaglandin E_1	Rat	—	0.83	—	—	126
Sulfobromophthalein	Rat	—	0.035	—	—	170
Vitamin B_{12}-rat transcobalamin II complex	Rat	—	5.5	—	—	189

*Rate constants are temperature dependent.

[+]In one study,[118] nonlinear Scatchard plots were obtained and were attributed to binding to both somatogenic and lactogenic binding sites.

Direct studies of the binding of labeled insulin to intact hepatocytes[10] and the finding that the concentration of insulin receptors is enriched 30- to 100-fold during purification of plasma membranes of hepatocytes[6,16,59] indicate that insulin receptors are present in the highest concentration on plasma membranes. Furthermore, electron-microscopic radioautography revealed that the plasma membrane of hepatocytes is the initial site of localication of labeled insulin in vivo.[63] Using ferritin-labeled insulin, the density of insulin receptors on hepatocytes was about $90/\mu^2$. The receptors were not uniformly distributed on these membranes. They appeared to be diffusely distributed in some areas, whereas in others, clusters containing 3 to 12 ferritin-insulin molecules were observed. Binding sites in freeze-etched preparations of liver membranes corresponded to intramembrane particles that could be seen embedded in the phospholipid bilayer. No receptors were found on the inside of membranes by this technique, suggesting that the binding site of the receptors faces only the external surface of the plasma membrane.[64] The half-life of the receptor in rat liver plasma membrane preparations at 30° to 37°C is approximately 4 hr.[52,53] Digestion of liver cell membranes with phospholipases A and C results in augmented insulin binding owing to an increased binding capacity of the membranes, persumably as a result of the unmasking of additional binding sites that are normally hidden within the phospholipid bilayer. Extraction of membranes with organic solvents has a similar effect.[65]

Although close correlations between the time course of receptor occupancy and the onset of insulin-induced biologic effects have been found, the interaction of insulin with its receptor on fat cells exhibits the phenomena of spare receptors and nonlinear coupling.[66] Of particular interest is the observation of negatively cooperative site-site interactions by the insulin receptor on hepatocytes of several species.[31,36,67,68] Negative cooperativity is retained by solubilized insulin receptors, suggesting that complete membrane integrity is not required for site-site interactions. The phenomenon of negative cooperativity is associated with a fourfold decrease in the size of the solubilized receptor, possibly owing to the dissociation of subunits, and results in an appreciable decrease in receptor affinity.[49,67] The structural requirements for binding of insulin probably include all the submolecular regions of the insulin receptor necessary for the induction of bioactivity. By contrast, the structural requirements for the induction of negative cooperativity are probably distinct from the bioactive sites of the receptor molecule.[3,68] Insulin receptors undergo a change from a slow dissociating state to a fast dissociating state as occupancy increases, and the proportion of sites in each state may be a function of both the occupancy of receptor sites by insulin monomer and the physiochemical environment. Lateral mobility of insulin receptors is suggested by the finding that negative cooperativity exhibited by these receptors shows a sharp inflection point in the Arrhenius plot at about 21°C.[36] A sharp transition at about this temperature has also been associated with the formation of clusters in artificial lipid layers[69] and a phase transition of membrane phospholipids.[70] Furthermore, concanavallin A, which inhibits the migration of a variety of receptors and surface antigens, also inhibits site-site interactions among insulin receptors.[31]

The concentration of insulin receptors on hepatocytes may be altered by metabolic, hormonal, and possibly genetic factors and may be of importance in the pathogenesis of human disease states characterized by insulin resistance or sensitivity. Liver membranes from the hyperinsulinemic and insulin-resistant obese hyperglycemic mouse (ob/ob) bind only 20% to 25% as much insulin per milligram of membrane protein as those of thin littermates,[53,71] and the perfused liver of ob/ob mice is less efficient in removing insulin from the perfusate than that of normal mice.[72] The properties of the hepatic insulin receptor of the ob/ob mouse appear to be the same as those of normal control mice.[53,71] These findings indicate that the number of insulin receptors is selectively reduced in the ob/ob mouse. Reduced numbers of insulin receptors on hepatocytes have also been found in other genetically obese insulin-resistant mice[73,74] and in mice and rats with artificially induced insulin resistance.[74–77] Chickens have one-fifth fewer insulin binding sites on their hepatocytes than do rats, an observation that may explain the relatively greater degree of physiologic insulin resistance in the chicken.[78] Conversely, insulin-deficient states in animals are associated with an increased concentration of insulin receptors on plasma membranes of hepatocytes[79,80] When the cause of the abnormal insulin concentration is removed or corrected, the concentration of insulin receptors tends to return to normal.[6,80] This can occur, for instance, in obesity as a result of diet restriction.[6] Diet alone appears to modify the insulin receptor, as the livers of rats fed a high-glucose diet bind 50% more insulin than do those rats fed a high-lipid diet.[81] An inverse relationship appears to exist between the degree of insulin resistance and the number of insulin receptors on hepatocytes,[6,80] suggesting that insulin exerts a negative feedback control of its receptors.

Polyclonal IgG antibodies directed at insulin receptors have been found in some disease states characterized by insulin resistance. Individual antireceptor antibodies appear to interact with different regions of the insulin receptor and consequently produce different effects on receptor affinity and capacity, site-site interactions among receptors, and biologic responses.[82]

Insulin has an overlapping spectrum of activities with several serum growth factors, in particular nonsuppressible insulinlike activity soluble in acid ethanol (NSILA-s), multiplication-stimulating activity, and the somatomedins.[83] NSILA-s and insulin compete for binding to the insulin receptor in proportion to their relative insulinlike potencies.[84] NSILA-s can competitively inhibit insulin degradation by rat liver plasma membranes.[85]

Glucagon

Receptors for glucagon have been identified on hepatocytes. They are present in highest concentration on the plasma membranes.[6,10,16] The receptor is probably a lipoprotein with an estimated molecular weight of about 190,000 and there is evidence of subunits with estimated molecular weights in the range of 23,000–90,000.[86,87] Binding of glucagon to hepatic plasma membranes is decreased after the membranes have been exposed to trypsin and phospholipases.[11,25,88,89]

Native glucagon competes with labeled glucagon for soluble binding sites and displaces labeled glucagon from complexes with the receptor. Binding of glucagon to its receptor is complete within 20 min at 30°C and is readily reversible.[86] Rat liver plasma membranes bind approximately 2.6 pmole glucagon per milligram of membrane protein, the glucagon receptors being saturated by concentrations of glucagon in the range of 4–8×10^{-8} M [25] (Table 1). After glucagon dissociates from its receptor, it is identical to native glucagon.[25] As is the case for insulin, the site of binding of glucagon to its receptor is probably not the same as its site of catabolism.[90,91]

The binding of glucagon to its receptor is specific. Secretin and other peptides do not interfere with glucagon binding.[25] Enteroglucagon can bind to some but not all of the hepatic receptors for pancreatic glucagon.[92] Des-l-histidine glucagon (DHG) is an effective competitive inhibitor of glucagon, although it causes structural coupling between the glucagon receptor and the effector unit.[93] It has about one-tenth of the affinity of glucagon for its receptor, but mediates no glucagonlike biologic activity.[94] This observation suggests that different regions of the glucagon molecule are important for binding to the receptor and for mediating the biologic response. Hydrophilic residues at the carboxy terminal region of glucagon are involved in the process of recognition at the glucagon receptor but do not participate in the sequence of events leading to the mediation of the biologic response. The amino-terminal histidyl residue in glucagon plays an important role in the expression of hormone action and contributes to the recognition process.[95] DHG apparently interacts reversibly with the glucagon receptor, since its effect can be reversed by the addition of excess native glucagon.[96]

The affinity of glucagon for its hepatic receptor can be altered by the binding of a different ligand to hepatic membranes.[39,40,97,98] For instance, the guanyl nucleotide GTP stimulates the dissociation of glucagon from its receptor. The binding isotherm is complex, 90% of the binding sites having a lower apparent dissociation constant and a small proportion of sites having a higher affinity for the hormone.[99] The hormone and nucleotide may act in concert with the glucagon receptor as an allosteric regulator of the biologic response to glucagon.[39,40,97-99]

The interaction of glucagon with isolated plasma membranes from homogenized liver was the first hormone-responsive adenylate cyclase system extensively studied.[100] Binding of glucagon to liver plasma membranes correlates with the activity of the hepatic adenylate cyclase system. This system is responsible for mediating some of the biologic responses to glucagon.[25] Either GTP or ATP is required for the activation of rat liver adenylate cyclase by glucagon.[101] In the rat, enteroglucagon-induced maximal stimulation of hepatic plasma membrane adenylate cyclase is only 70% of that generated by pancreatic glucagon.[102] In the dog, however, immunoreactive glucagon derived from the gastric fundus is more active than immunoreactive glucagon derived from the pancreas in stimulating hepatic adenylate cyclase activity, an observation not attributable to differences in the binding of the two glucagons to liver plasma membranes.[103] According to the assay conditions, half-maximal activation of adenylate cyclase in rat liver plasma membranes occurs at glucagon concentrations in the range of 4×10^{-9} to 5×10^{-10} M.[98,104] At both maximally and half-maximally stimulating glucagon concentrations, adenylate cyclase is activated within seconds of the addition of glucagon, and the activation is reversible, the system apparently following the law of mass action.[101] The concentration ranges over which glucagon-dependent adenylate cyclase activity is stimulated and over which glucagon binds to liver membranes are the same.[25] Steady-state activation is established before steady-state binding, however.[96] Furthermore, the glucagon receptor of rat liver plasma membranes can couple to adenylate cyclase without activating it.[93] Observed discrepancies between glucagon binding and adenylate cyclase activation, such as nonlinear coupling and spare receptors,[39,96,105] cannot be adequately accounted for either by the occupancy theory or by the rate theory of hormone action. Observations on the dissociation of glucagon from its hepatic receptor[96] and the finding of an abrupt increase in the energy of activation for glucagon-stimulated hepatic adenylate cyclase at temperatures above $32°C$[106] suggest that the glucagon receptor undergoes allosteric changes. This phenomenon could account for the apparent heterogeneity of binding of glucagon to hepatocytic plasma membranes[107] and partially purified glucagon receptors.[86] Changes in the energy of activation do not correlate with changes in the binding of the hormone to its receptor, however. The concerted interdependent mechanisms of the activation of hepatic adenylate cyclase by glucagon and GTP might be explained by cooperative interactions between multiple glucagon binding sites and GTP-binding sites in response to ligand binding that result in conformational changes in the enzyme system.[98] Indeed, in one study, glucagon induced conformational changes in plasma membranes of rat liver, and these changes correlated with the activity of the adenylate cyclase system.[108] The lipid environment of the glucagon receptor in the hepatocytic plasma membrane apparently plays a role in the regulation of adenylate cyclase.[109]

The sensitivity of the rat heaptic adenylate cyclase system to glucagon is low during fetal life,[110] hepatic regeneration provoked by partial hepatectomy,[111] and sustained glucagon stimulation.[112] By contrast, it is increased by feeding,[113] diabetes,[114] and uremia.[77] These phenomena can be attributed to changes in the binding affinity or capacity of the plasma membranes for glucagon.

Vasoactive Intestinal Polypetide and Secretin

Vasoactive intestinal polypeptide (VIP) and secretin appear to bind to rat liver plasma membranes at common saturable binding sites that are distinct from those for glucagon. Binding of labeled VIP and secretin to these binding sites can be inhibited by enteroglucagon, however. VIP stimulates plasma membrane adenylate cyclase, but the maximal response is appreciably less than that generated by pancreatic glucagon. VIP and secretin inhibit the binding of labeled VIP in proportion to their respective abilities to activate adenylate cyclase. Binding of VIP is decreased and its dissociation rate increased by guanyl nucleotides[102,115] (Table 1).

Growth-Promoting and Lactogenic Hormones

Human growth hormone binds to rabbit[116] and mouse[71] liver plasma membranes. Binding studies employing intact rat hepatocytes suggest that these cells possess separate binding sites for hormones with somatogenic and lactogenic properties. Growth hormones with both somatogenic and lactogenic properties, such as human growth hormone, bind to both types of binding sites. The numbers of these binding sites on hepatocytes vary with species and exposure to sex hormones[117–119] (Table 1). Prolactin induces the lactogenic hormone binding site on hepatocytes.[48] It has not been established that the hepatocellular binding sites for hormones with growth-stimulating and prolactin actions are true receptors involved in mediating the biologic effects of these hormones. NSILA-s, multiplication-stimulating factor, and somatomedin A, all of which have growth-promoting properties, compete with growth hormone for binding sites on rat liver plasma membranes in proportion to their relative growth-promoting potencies. In addition, these substances have weak insulin-like activities and compete for the hepatic insulin receptor in proportion to their relative potencies in inducing insulin-like effects[84] (see Insulin).

Catecholamines

Although the distinction between α- and β-adrenergic functions is less clear than in other systems these adrenergic effects have been demonstrated in hepatocytes.[120] Such effects may be mediated by cell surface receptors,[121,122] and binding data consistent with the existence of such receptors have been generated in rats.[123]

L-triiodothyronine and L-thyroxine

Saturable binding sites for L-triiodothyronine (T_3) have been demonstrated on rat liver plasma membranes. The corresponding D isomer and L-thyroxine are less potent than L-T_3 in competing for these binding sites. These findings suggest that the transport of L-T_3 and other thyroid hormones into hepatocytes involves their binding to proteins on the plasma membrane[124,125] (Table 1) (see Hepatocellular Carrier-mediated Transport).

Prostaglandins

Specific binding of prostaglandin E_1 to liver plasma membranes has been convincingly demonstrated[126] (Table 1). The receptor has been isolated and characterized as a protein with molecular weight of 105,000.[127] The effects of prostaglandins on hepatocellular metabolism have not yet been fully elucidated, but these substances may be responsible for the fine regulation of the adenylate cyclase system[128,129] in which the prostaglandins could act as local intercellular hormones.[128]

Binding sites for prostaglandin F_{2a} on liver plasma membranes have also been reported.[129] These binding sites are distinct from the receptors for prostaglandin E_1 and are unrelaled to the prostaglandin receptor-adenylate cyclase complex.[128] Their biologic significance is unknown.

While receptors for other hormones undoubtedly exist in the liver (e.g., receptors for glucocorticoids), it has not been established that any of them are located in cell surface membranes.

HEPATOCELLULAR CARRIER-MEDIATED TRANSPORT

As stated in the introduction, carrier-mediated transport shares similar kinetic features with ligand-receptor interactions, and in some nonhepatic systems, such carrier molecules have been isolated and characterized. This section discusses some transport systems that fulfill the criteria of carrier-mediated transport even though the responsible carrier has not yet been isolated.

Na^+, K^+-Stimulated Adenosine Triphosphatase

The exchange transport of Na^+ and K^+ is an essential feature of a wide variety of animal cells. This transport system contributes to the maintenance of the osmolarity of the cell, and influences fluid transport in some glands.[130,131] The association of this Na^+ pump with the enzyme Na^+, K^+-stimulated adenosine triphosphatase is well established,[130,131] and the presence of this enzyme on rat liver plasma membrane has been demonstrated.[132] The activity of this enzyme can be manipulated by a variety of hormones[133,134] and drugs,[134–136] as well as by bile salts.[137] In several instances, changes in the activity of the enzyme have been paralleled by changes in bile-salt-independent bile flow,[133–135] a finding that has lent support to the hypothesis that this fraction of hepatocellular bile may be dependent upon the activity of this enzyme in the canalicular membrane. The recent demonstration that the enzyme is localized mainly on the lateral part of the hepatocellular surface membrane[138] sheds doubt on this assumption, however. Alternative models for isotonic water transport have been proposed for the liver[139] or may be inferred from appropriate studies in other organs.[140,141]

Hexoses and Amino Acids

The hepatocyte, like many other metabolically active cells, possesses a variety of transport systems for the uptake of substrates of cellular metabolism such as amino acids and hexoses. Although there is good evidence for carrier-mediated transport for many substrates of this type, none of the hypothetical carriers has been identified or isolated from the hepatocyte.

Facilitated diffusion for hexoses has been demonstrated in the perfused liver of the rat,[142] in the dog,[143,144] and in sheep,[145] and specific binding of D-glucose to rat liver plasma membranes has been shown.[146] Whether the hexose transport system in the liver is coupled to Na^+ flux, as it appears to be in other organs,[147] remains to be established. Uptake of glucose into plasma membrane vesicles is stimulated to a slight degree by insulin,[146] although it is generally thought that insulin does not affect the transmembrane movement of the postulated carrier-sugar complex.[137,147]

The amino acid transport systems have been studied mainly in isolated rat hepatocytes, either freshly prepared or maintained in primary culture. The classification and general features of animal amino acid transport systems have been reviewed elsewhere.[148,149] The hepatocyte, in common with many other cells derived from mammals, exhibits three different systems for the transport of neutral amino acids, designated as the A, L, and ACS systems.[149,150] While the A and ACS systems apparently involve a Na^+ flux coupled active process,[151–155] the L system predominantly exhibits features of facilitated diffusion,[151,155] with only a small component of transport appearing to depend on an active process.[150] The characteristics of the binding of different amino acids to liver plasma membranes or components of liver plasma membranes remain to be established. In cultured hepatocytes, insulin increases the transport of α-aminoisobutyric acid, a nonmetabolized amino acid, via a cycloheximide sensitive step.[154]

Organic Anions and Other Cationic and Neutral Compounds

The liver is the major organ in mammals responsible for inactivating biologically active molecules, neutralizing toxic substances, and chemically modifying a variety of endogenous and exogenous compounds to facilitate their excretion. Related to these functions the liver possesses distinct and highly specialized transport systems. Characteristics of the binding of appropriate solutes to liver plasma membranes have been determined only for a few of these. In view of their prominent role in bile formation, a transport system for organic anions has long been postulated.[156]

The hepatocyte apparently possesses two distinct systems for the transport of organic anions, one responsible for the transport of bile salts[157–159] and the other for the transport of organic anionic dyes such as bilirubin, sulfobromophthalein, and indocyanine green.[160–164] The bile salt transport system has been found to be saturable in the dog,[157] in the perfused rat liver,[158] and in isolated hepatocytes.[159] In the perfused rat liver and in isolated hepatocytes this transport system has been shown to be Na^+-flux-coupled[158–160] and probably concentrative.[159] Specific binding of bile salts to rat liver plasma membranes has been described,[165] although the relevance of the observed binding to bile salt transport remains to be established.

The transport system for organic anionic dyes has been less well defined than that for bile salts. Saturable uptake of sulfobromophthalein and/or bilirubin has been described in the dog[166] and the rat,[162,163] and for indocyanine green, in the rat[161] and in man.[167] These findings could be explained by simple diffusion and subsequent binding to intracellular acceptor proteins[168,169] (see Chapter 11). Indeed in one study, sulfobromophthalein transport into isolated rat hepatocytes did not fulfill the criteria for carrier-mediated transport.[164] Saturable binding sites for sulfobromophthalein on liver plasma membranes (Table 1) with specificity comparable to organic anionic dye transport in vivo have been described.[170] Furthermore, discrete proteins with high affinities for sulfobromophthalein[171,172] and bilirubin[171] have been extracted from liver plasma membrane fractions. These findings favor the existence of membrane carriers for organic anionic dyes.

TABLE 2.—*Receptors for Glycoproteins in the Mammalian Liver*

Glycoprotein	Enzyme Used in Preparation	Sugar Residue Cleaved	Terminal Sugar Residue	Hepatic Receptor	
				Hepatocytes	Nonparenchymal Cells
Intact	—	—	Sialic acid	−	−
Asialo-derivative	Neuraminidase	Sialic acid	Galactose	+++	−
Agalacto-derivative	β-galactosidase	Galactose	N-acetylglucosamine	−	++
Ahexosamino-derivative	N-acetylglucosaminidase	N-acetylglucosamine	Mannose	−	+++

is located on the plasma membrane of hepatocytes but not of nonparenchymal cells[12] (Table 2).

The rapid removal of desialylated α_1-antitrypsin but not intact α_1-antitrypsin from the human circulation has been ascribed to the action of HBP.[197] Furthermore, HBP has recently been isolated from the human liver.[198]

Neuraminidase is widely distributed in vivo and occurs as a constituent of certain infectious agents such as the influenza virus.[199] Direct proof that desialylation of glycoproteins occurs in vivo is lacking, however. Although the precise physiologic role of HBP has not been established, it may play a role in the catabolism of glycoproteins. After binding to hepatocytes, desialylated glycoproteins are taken up by endocytosis and then undergo proteolytic degradation in lysosomes.[200] Small but detectable quantities of asialoglycoproteins exist in the plasma of normal subjects. In patients with chronic hepatocellular diseases the plasma concentrations of asialoglycoproteins are appreciably greater than in normal subjects.[201] Accumulation of asialoglycoproteins in the circulation of patients with liver diseases could arise from defective synthesis of the carbohydrate moiety of glycoproteins, decreased perfusion of hepatocytes, or suboptimal amounts of HBP on the surface membrane of hepatocytes.

A hepatic glycoprotein recognition system distinct from HBP has been defined in the rat.[202] After intravenous infusion, many glycoprotein lysosomal hydrolases are rapidly cleared from the circulation by the liver in mammals.[203–205] Hepatic clearance of these enzymes is saturable.[204] Uptake of these enzymes by the liver can be abolished by pretreating them with sodium periodate, which oxidizes sugar residues, but not by administration of an excess of a desialylated glycoprotein.[203,205] These findings suggest that the hepatic clearance of lysosomal hydrolases is mediated by sugar residues other than galactosyl groups and point to the existence of receptor specific hepatic recognition systems other than that for desialylated glycoproteins in the mammal. Recently, recognition sites for both N-acetylglucosamine and mannose terminated glycoproteins have been identified on the surface membrane of nonparenchymal cells[12] (Table 2). Of potential relevance to these findings is the isolation from homogenates of mammalian liver of a binding protein for mannan, a polysaccharide of mannose. This protein has the property of binding both N-acetylglucosamine and mannose-terminated glycoproteins.[206] Neither the cellular nor the organelle distribution of this protein has been determined.

The distribution of cellular uptake of glycoproteins possibly may be influenced by specifically modifying their carbohydrate moieties,[207,208] since the different glycoprotein receptors vary in their relative distribution on hepatocytes versus nonparenchymal cells[12] (Table 2).

LIPOPROTEINS

High-affinity saturable binding sites for homologous low-density lipoproteins have been found in liver membranes of the pig. Binding of low-density lipoproteins to these sites is inhibited by very low density lipoproteins and by high-density lipoproteins.[209] Specific binding of chylomicron remnants to rat liver plasma membranes has also been demonstrated. The inhibition of this binding by exposure of the membranes to trypsin led to the suggestion of a hepatic protein receptor for chylomicron remnants[210] (see Chapter 13).

IMMUNOLOGIC PHENOMENA AND HEPATIC CELL SURFACE RECEPTORS

In Vivo Studies of Receptors for Immunoglobulin and Complement on Nonparenchymal Cells

Recognition of the existence of receptors for immunologically active molecules on Kupffer cells has emerged from a series of investigations into the pathogenesis of the acquired autoimmune hemolytic anemias.[211] In a guinea pig model of immune hemolytic anemia, autologous ^{51}Cr-labeled erythrocytes, sensitized with purified IgM anti-guinea pig erythrocyte antibody, were infused intravenously.[212,213] Following the infusion, the curve of peripheral venous blood radioactivity was complex, being characterized by an initial rapid clearance of labeled cells from the circulation, followed by a slower reaccumulation of a proportion of the cleared labeled cells in the circulation. Analogous studies in humans yielded similar results and organ localization studies in both animals and humans showed that the liver was the primary site of sequestration of the labeled cells.[212-215] The rate limiting factor in the hepatic sequestration of IgM-sensitized cells is the rate of liver blood flow.[215] This sequestration was mediated by complement-specific receptors, as the clearance process did not occur in guinea pigs with congenital C4 deficiency or in guinea pigs depleted of the terminal complement components, including C3, by the administration of protein extracts of cobra venom.[212,213] IgM agglutinin-induced hepatic sequestration of erythrocytes depends on the binding of C3 or a conversion product of C3 to the surface of erythrocytes in the rabbit. It has been directly demonstrated in this species that the hepatic sequestration of such cells resulted from their binding to the surface membrane of Kupffer cells.[216] Studies in humans following the intravenous administration of IgM-sensitized erythrocytes showed that C3b rapidly binds to the erythrocyte surface as a result of local activation of the classical complement pathway.[214] Based on these findings, it can be concluded that the hepatic sequestration of IgM-sensitized erythrocytes is mediated by a receptor for C3b on the surface membrane of Kupffer cells. Such a receptor specific for the C3b fragment of C3 has been demonstrated on human alveolar macrophages.[217] Cells bound to Kupffer-cell receptors undergo one of two fates: permanent removal from the circulation by phagocytosis[216] or release back into the circulation.The latter process occurs as a consequence of the action of the plasma enzyme C3b inactivator, which cleaves C3b into two fragments: C3d, which remains erythrocyte-bound, and C3c, which is released into the plasma. Since C3d-coated erythrocytes have a lower affinity for the surface of Kupffer cells, they are released back into the circulation, where they have an almost normal survival.[214,215] The magnitude of the clearance of IgM-sensitized cells and of their phagocytosis by Kupffer cells varies directly with the number of C1-fixing sites on the surface of each erythocyte. A minimum number of 20 such sites per cell is required to initiate clearance[214] (Fig. 4).

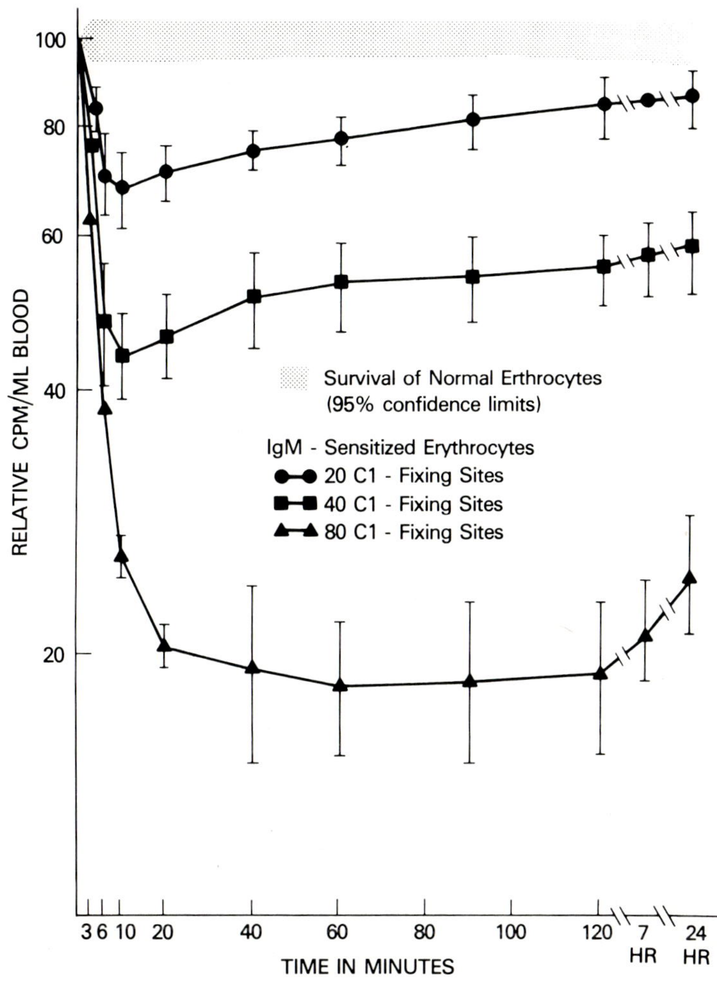

FIG. 4—Hepatic C3b-receptor-mediated clearance in normal human subjects. Blood radioactiv-ity-time curves after the intravenous injection of IgM isoagglutinin-sensitized ^{51}Cr-labeled autolo-gous erythrocytes are shown. The injected cells rapidly become coated with C3b in vivo. The three curves depict data obtained employing levels of sensitization of 20 (3 individuals), 40 (5 individuals), and 80 (3 individuals) C1-fixing sites per erythrocyte, respectively. Vertical lines represent ± 1 SEM. Each subject received a total dose of 5 μCi of ^{51}Cr. All counts per milliliter of blood are expressed relative to a hypothetical zero time value of 100. The nadir of the curves, which reflect the magnitude of clearance, are lower the larger the number of C1-fixing sites per erythrocyte. Reaccumulation of blood radioactivity after the nadir reflects the delivery of C3d-coated labeled erythrocytes into the circulation as a consequence of the cleavage by C3b inacti-vator of C3b on labeled erythrocytes bound to Kupffer cells. The extent to which the blood radioactivity curves fail to regain their zero time values is an index of the magnitude of phago-cytosis of Kupffer cell-bound labeled erythrocytes. (From the study of Atkinson and Frank.[214] Reproduced by permission of the *Journal of Clinical Investigation*.)

C3b-Receptor-Specific Defect in Primary Biliary Cirrhosis

The hepatic C3b-receptor-mediated clearance of IgM-sensitized ^{51}Cr-labeled autologous erythrocytes has been studied in patients with chronic liver diseases.[218] Each of 6 patients with primary biliary cirrhosis exhibited an unequivocal defect in C3b-receptor-mediated clearance function of Kupffer cells (Fig. 5), whereas this function was entirely normal in patients with chronic active hepatitis and compensated alcoholic cirrhosis. The defect in C3b-receptor function in primary biliary cirrhosis was specific, since the clearance of IgG-sensitized ^{51}Cr-labeled autologous erythrocytes from the circulation of the same patients, a process predominantly mediated by receptors for the Fc region of IgG on the surface of fixed macrophages in the spleen,[211] was either normal or accelerated.[218] The defect could not be explained by reduced hepatic blood flow or a generalized defect in hepatic reticuloendothelial phagocytic function, since the clearance from the plasma of both tracer and test doses of microaggregated albumin was normal in the patients with primary biliary cirrhosis. The defect in C3b-receptor-mediated clearance did not correlate with the duration of symptoms attributable to the disease, with the hepatic histologic

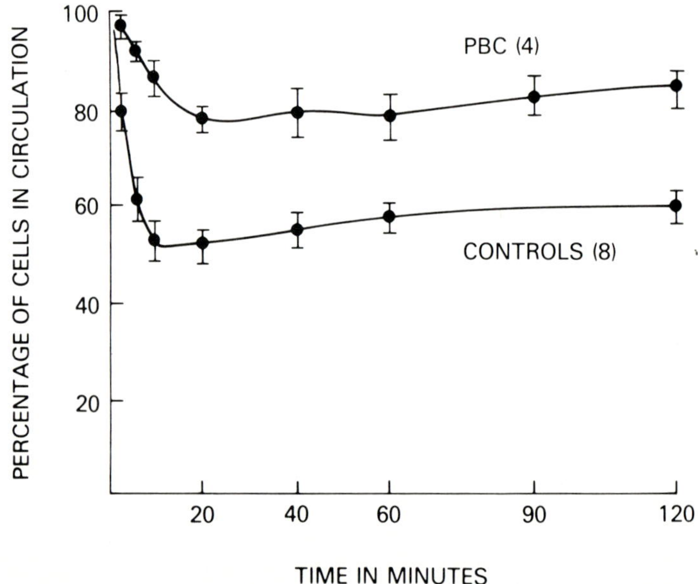

FIG. 5—Hepatic C3b-receptor-mediated clearance defect in primary biliary cirrhosis (PBC). Data on blood radioactivity after the intravenous administration of IgM isoagglutinin-sensitized radiochromated erythrocytes in 8 normal subjects and 4 patients with PBC are shown. Not included in this figure are corresponding data on 2 patients with PBC who were studied using an IgM-cold agglutinin. Presentation of the data is analogous to that in Figure 4. In each of the 12 studies the level of sensitization employed was 40 C1-fixing sites per erythrocyte. The initial mean disappearance rate of radioactivity from the circulation is much slower and the mean nadir of the blood radioactivity curve much higher ($p < 0.001$) for the group with PBC than are corresponding values for the group of normal subjects. (From the study of Jaffe et al.[218] Reproduced by permission of the *Journal of Clinical Investigation*.)

stage of the disease, or with biochemical indices of cholestasis in serum. Indeed, in a patient with severe cholestasis caused by large duct biliary obstruction, C3b-receptor-specific clearance was entirely normal. Furthermore, measurements of serum complement indicated that the defect was not caused by a deficiency of components of the classical pathway or by increased activity of C3b inactivator.[218]

Compartmental analysis of the experimental data indicated that the defect in C3b-receptor-mediated clearance in primary biliary cirrhosis could be explained solely on the basis of a decreased rate of deposition of C3b-coated cells onto Kupffer cell receptors.[219] One possible explanation for this finding would be decreased availability of these receptors in primary biliary cirrhosis. This could occur if a large proportion of them are occupied by either excess free C3b or immune complexes containing C3b.[220]

In Vitro Studies of Receptors for Immunoglobulin and Complement on Nonparenchymal Cells

Studies of immunospecific receptor-mediated clearance in vivo have been complemented by in vitro studies of surface receptors for immunologically active molecules on hepatic sinusoidal cells. Specific binding of sheep erythrocytes coated with IgG (EA) or IgM and C3 (EAC) to cultured rat hepatic sinusoidal cells has been demonstrated, indicating receptors for Fc and C3 on the surface membrane of these cells.[221,222] Binding of EA was independent of phagocytosis. The latter, but not the former, was inhibited by mild treatment with trypsin, was energy-dependent, and possibly involved the microfilament system.[222,223] Following exposure to EA, subsequent Fc- receptor-mediated phagocytosis was inhibited and returned to control values only after prolonged culture. Incubation of sinusoidal cells with neuraminidase increased both binding and phagocytosis of EA, presumably by exposing additional Fc receptors in the surface membrane. Although binding of EAC appeared to be efficient, less than 20% of the bound EAC underwent phagocytosis,[222] an observation in accord with the results of C3b-receptor-mediated clearance in vivo that indicate that binding of EAC to C3b receptors is a poor stimulus for phagocytosis.[214,215] By contrast to the binding of EA, binding of EAC was readily inhibited by trypsin. Newborn calf serum stimulates the phagocytosis of bound EAC by an unknown mechanism. The limiting factor in phagocytosis of both EA and EAC may be cellular volume rather than the availability of surface receptors.[222] The mechanism of phagocytosis of bound EA is different from that of bound EAC in that the former process involves appreciably more membrane activity than does the latter.[223] Analogous studies employing monocytes and macrophages from extrahepatic tissues [217,224-226] emphasize the similarities in both the types and functions of receptors for immunologically active molecules on the cell surface of sinusoidal cells in the liver and other circulating and extrahepatic fixed macrophages. Although fixed macrophages of the liver have not been specifically evaluated for cell surface receptors for C4b and C3d, receptors for these complement components have been identified on other cells derived from the reticuloendothelial system.[227]

Receptors for Immunoglobulin and Complement on Hepatocytes

Only relatively limited information exists regarding receptors for immunologically active molecules on the surface membrane of hepatocytes. One study, however, on the capacity of hepatocytes isolated from rabbits and humans to bind immunoglobulin and complement has been reported.[228] The presence of Fc receptors on parenchymal cells was suggested by the binding of aggregated IgG and, to a lesser extent, native IgG as detected by immunofluorescence. Binding of preformed antigen-antibody complexes prepared in antibody excess appeared to be mediated by Fc receptors, since complexes of antigen-F(ab)$_2$ did not bind. Isolated human hepatocytes did not react with fluorescinated anti-C1q, C4, or C3 spontaneously. Direct binding of purified human and guinea pig C3 was demonstrated, however, suggesting a cell surface receptor for C3 on hepatocytes. In contrast to corresponding results obtained with isolated rat sinusoidal cells,[222] neuraminidase treatment of hepatocytes had no effect on the binding of aggregated immunoglobulin. The binding of C3 to hepatocytes was increased by neuraminidase, however. Trypsin treatment had little effect on the binding of aggregated immunoglobulin but readily inhibited binding of C3. Attempts to form rosettes with hepatocytes exposed to EA (IgG) or EAC were unsuccessful.[228] This lack of correlation between apparent receptor-mediated binding observed by immunofluorescence and with particulate reagents requires further investigation.

Immunologic Properties of the Hepatic Receptor for Asialoglycoproteins

A possible role for hepatic cell surface receptors in the modulation or modification of cellular immune responses has been suggested by the demonstration that the hepatocyte-specific receptor for asialoglycoproteins (HBP) (see Glycoproteins) can selectively induce desialylated human lymphocytes to exhibit both mitogenesis[229] and cytotoxicity.[230] Observations that HBP possesses several lectinlike properties prompted an evaluation of HBP as a potential mitogen.[229] Purified HBP can indeed induce mitogenesis in desialylated, but not in intact lymphocytes, probably as a result of the interaction of HBP with exposed galactosyl residues on the surface of the desialylated cells (see Glycoproteins). Prior treatment of HBP with neuraminidase greatly decreased its ability to induce mitogenesis in desialylated lymphocytes, suggesting that the mitogenic effect of HBP depends on its content of sialic acid. Studies employing enriched subpopulations of lymphocytes indicated that HBP induced transformation predominantly in a subpopulation containing T and K cells.[229] These findings, as well as the previous observation that desialylated lymphocytes, after their intravenous administration to animals, are selectively taken up by the liver rather than by the spleen and lymph nodes,[231-233] prompted the idea that HBP might also induce desialylated lymphocytes to exhibit increased cytotoxicity and that this hepatic cell surface receptor may play a role in a mechanism of hepatocellular injury.

That HBP can specifically induce desialylated lymphocytes to mediate increased cytotoxicity was subsequently demonstrated[230] (Fig. 6). Cytotoxicity

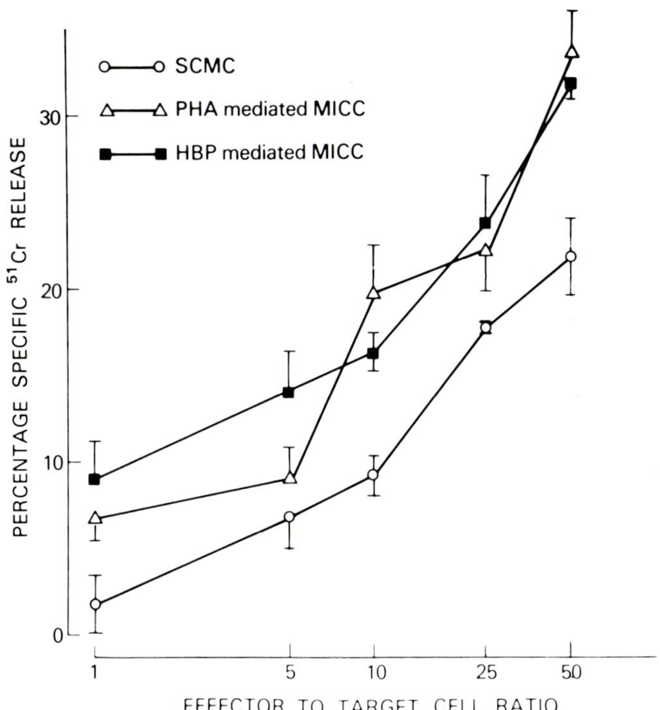

FIG. 6—Mitogen-induced cellular cytotoxicity (MICC) mediated by the hepatic cell surface receptor that specifically binds desialylated glycoproteins (HBP). Values for cytotoxicity mediated by desialylated macrophage-depleted human lymphocytes against Chang target cells are shown in the presence of medium alone (spontaneous cell-mediated cytoxicity, SCMC), medium containing 1 μg phytohemagglutinin (PHA) per milliliter and medium containing 1.56 μg HBP per milliliter. The index of cytotoxicity is radioactivity released from ^{51}Cr-labeled target cells. Each point represents the mean of three experimental values. Vertical lines represent ± 1 SEM. HBP is as potent as the powerful lectin PHA in inducing cytotoxicity in this system. (From the study of Vierling et al.[230] Reproduced by permission of *Gastroenterology*.)

was induced when desialylated but not intact lymphocytes were exposed to either purified HBP or HBP present as a normal constituent of the surface membrane of isolated rabbit hepatocytes. The cytotoxicity mediated by desialylated lymphocytes against isolated rabbit hepatocytes was blocked by a desialylated glycoprotein but not by a native glycoprotein, suggesting that cytotoxocity resulted from the specific interaction of HBP with the desialylated lymphocytes. These observations demonstrated the capacity of HBP, as a normal constituent of the plasma membrane of mammalian hepatocytes, to induce cytotoxicity. They are insufficient to prove a role for HBP in hepatic injury in vivo, however. The hypothesis that this might occur was strengthened by the assumption that the selective accumulation of desialylated lymphocytes in the liver[231−233] was mediated by their specific binding to HBP on hepatocytes. This assumption, however, should be tentative, since cellular elements of the blood during their passage through the liver may be restricted to the sinusoids and hence would not come into intimate and immediate contact with the plasma membrane of hepatocytes. Since HBP has not been demonstrated on the surface of sinusoidal cells[12] (see Glycoproteins), it is possible that hepatic sequestration of desialylated lymphocytes may not be mediated by their interaction with HBP. The observation that sera of rodents and humans contain a natural antibody that rapidly adheres to desialylated lymphocytes[234] suggests that desialylated cells in vivo may become coated with immunologically active molecules on their surface membranes and that these cells could, therefore, bind to Fc or C3 receptors present on sinusoidal lining cells. Although the precise role of HBP as a stimulus of cytotoxicity in vivo remains unclear, the finding that a small change in the structure of the carbohydrate moiety of glycoproteins in the surface membrane of lymphocytes can result in augmented cytotoxicity as a result of their specific interaction with a normal constituent of the surface membrane of another cell raises the possibility that this may be a mechanism of cellular injury in vivo.

BASES FOR FUTURE STUDIES

Our understanding of cell surface receptors in the liver is currently far from complete. Only one receptor has been isolated in a pure form: the mammalian receptor that specifically binds desialylated glycoproteins.[195,196] For only two receptors are there adequate data correlating ligand-receptor binding with biologic response: the insulin[66] and glucagon[96] receptors. These two receptors, although extensively studied, have only been partially purified.[22,86] In most instances, data cited for the existence of other cell surface receptors are limited to the demonstration of specific binding sites on hepatic plasma membranes without any correlations of ligand-receptor interaction with biologic response. The concept that receptors may be involved in carrier-mediated transport is largely hypothetical in spite of some encouraging studies. At least some cell surface receptors play important roles in the regulation of metabolic processes in the liver, however. Also changes in the surface membrane concentration of at least one of these receptors, the insulin receptor, are of importance in the pathogenesis of disease states.[6] Finally, the dynamic state of the plasma membrane of liver cells may be relevant to mechanisms of hepatocellular injury that might involve altered receptor activity.[235] The mediation of mitogen-induced cellular cytotoxicity by the receptor for desialylated glycoproteins may provide a model for the specific participation of a cell surface receptor in a process leading to the hepatocellular injury.[230] Future investigations of hepatic cell surface receptors will provide valuable new insights into hepatic physiology and pathophysiology as well as mechanisms of liver injury.

ACKNOWLEDGMENTS

The authors are most grateful to Drs. Jeffrey S. Flier and Jerry D. Gardner for their constructive criticisms of this review and to Mrs. Phyllis Kline for her secretarial proficiency.

REFERENCES

1. Singer SJ, Nicolson GL: The fluid mosaic model of the structure of cell membranes. Science 175:720–731, 1972
2. Ash JF, Louvard D, Singer SJ: Antibody-induced linkages of plasma membrane proteins to intracellular actomyosin-containing filaments in cultured fibroblasts. Proc Natl Acad Sci USA 74:5584–5588, 1977
3. Kahn CR: Membrane receptors for hormones and neurotransmitters. J Cell Biol 70:261–286, 1976
4. Cuatrecasas P: The insulin receptor. Diabetes 21 (Suppl 2):396–402, 1972
5. Wilbrandt W and Rosenberg T: The concept of carrier transport and its corollaries in pharmacology. Pharmacol Rev 13:109–183, 1961
6. Kahn CR: Membrane receptors for polypeptide hormones. Edited by ED Korn: Methods in Membrane Biology. Vol. 3. New York, Plenum, 1975, pp 81–146
7. Berry MN, Friend DS: High yield preparation of isolated rat liver parenchymal cells. J Cell Biol 43:506–520, 1969
8. Jeejeebhoy KN, Ho J, Greenberg GR, Phillips MJ, Bruce-Robertson A, Sodke V: Albumin, fibrinogen and transferrin synthesis in isolated rat hepatocyte suspensions. Biochem J 146:141–155, 1975
9. Baur H, Kasperek S, Pfaff E: Criteria of viability of isolated liver cells. Hoppe Seylers Z Physiol Chem 356:827–838, 1975
10. Freychet P, Rosselin G, Rancon F, Fouchereau M, Broer Y: Interactions of insulin and glucagon with isolated rat liver cells. I. Binding of hormones to specific receptors. Horm Metab Res Suppl 5:72–78, 1974
11. Rosselin G, Freychet P, Fouchereau M, Rancon F, Broer Y: Interactions of insulin and glucagon with isolated rat liver cells. II. Dynamic changes in the cyclic AMP induced by hormones. Horm Metab Res Suppl 5:78–86, 1974
12. Steer CJ, Jones EA, Hickman JW: Indentification and localization of specific glycoprotein receptors on parenchymal and nonparenchymal rat liver cells. Clin Res 26:499A, 1978
13. Neville DM Jr: Isolation of an organ specific protein antigen from cell-surface membrane of rat liver. Biochim Biophys Acta 154:540–552, 1968
14. Song CS, Rubin W, Rifkind AB, Kappas A: Plasma membranes of the rat liver. Isolation and enzymatic characterization of a fraction rich in bile canaliculi. J Cell Biol 41:124–132, 1969
15. Touster O, Aronson NN Jr, Dulaney JT, Hendrickson H: Isolation of rat liver plasma membranes. Use of nucleotide pyrophosphatase and phosphodiesterase I as marker enzymes. J Cell Biol 47:604–618, 1970
16. Neville DM Jr, Kahn CR: Isolation of plasma membranes for cell surface membrane receptor studies. Edited by AI Laskin, JA Last: Methods in Molecular Biology. Vol. 5. New York, Marcel Dekker, 1974, pp 57–85
17. Wisher MH, Evans WH: Functional polarity of the rat hepatocyte surface membrane. Isolation and characterization of plasma-membrane subfractions from the blood-sinusoidal, bile-canalicular and contiguous surfaces of the hepatocyte. Biochem J 146:375–388, 1975
18. Blouin A, Bolender RP, Weibel ER: Distribution of organelles and membranes between hepatocytes and nonhepatocytes in the rat liver parenchyma. J Cell Biol 72:441–455, 1977
19. Helenius A, Simons K: Solubilization of membranes by detergents. Biochim Biophys Acta 415:29–79, 1975
20. Tanford C, Reynolds JA: Characterization of membrane proteins in detergent solutions. Biochim Biophys Acta 457:133–170, 1976
21. Cuatrecasas P, Anfinsen CB: Affinity chromatography. Ann Rev Biochem 40:259–278, 1971
22. Cuatrecasas P: Affinity chromatography and purification of the insulin receptor of liver cell membranes. Proc Natl Acad Sci USA 69:1277–1281
23. Korenbrot JT: Ion transport in membranes. Incorporation of biological ion-translocating proteins in model membrane systems. Annu Rev Physiol 39:19–49, 1977
24. Freychet P, Kahn CR, Roth J, Neville DM Jr: Insulin interactions with liver plasma membranes: Independence of binding of the hormone and its degradation. J Biol Chem 247:3953–3961, 1972
25. Rodbell M, Kraus HMJ, Pohl SL, Birnbaumer L: The glucagon-sensitive adenyl cyclase system in plasma membranes of rat

liver. III. Binding of glucagon: method of assay and specificity. J Biol Chem 246:1861–1871, 1971

26. Rodbard D: Mathematics of hormone-receptor interaction. I. Basic principles. Edited by BW O'Malley and AR Means: Receptors for Reproductive Hormones. New York, Plenum, 1973, pp 289–326

27. Birnbaumer L, Pohl SL, Kaumann AJ: Receptors and acceptors: A necessary distinction in hormone binding studies. Edited by P Greengard and GA Robinson: Advances in Cyclic Nucleotide Research. Vol. 4. New York, Raven Press, 1974, pp 239–281

28. Klotz IM: Protein interactions with small molecules. Acc Chem Res 7:162–168, 1974

29. Hill AR: The combinations of haemoglobin with oxygen and with carbon monoxide. Biochem J 7:471–480, 1913

30. Pliska V: Heterogeneous binding sites in neurophysin-like macromolecules: Some theoretical and computational considerations. Ann NY Acad Sci 248:480–493, 1975

31. De Meyts P: Cooperative properties of hormone receptors in cell membranes. J Supramol Struct 4:241–258, 1976

32. Monod J, Wyman J, Changeux JP: On the nature of allosteric transitions: A plausible model. J Mol Biol 12:88–118, 1965

33. Koshland DE Jr., Némethy G, Filmer D: Comparison of experimental binding data and theoretical models in proteins containing subunits. Biochemistry 5:365–385, 1966

34. Fletcher JE, Spector AA: Alternative models for the analysis of drug-protein binding. Mol Pharmacol 13:387–399

35. Frieden C: Treatment of enzyme kinetic data. II. The multisite case: Comparison of allosteric models and a possible new mechanism. J Biol Chem 242:4045–4052, 1967

36. De Meyts P, Bianco AR, Roth J: Site-site interactions among insulin receptors: Characterization of the negative cooperativity. J Biol Chem 251:1877–1888, 1976

37. Paton WDM: A theory of drug action based on the rate of drug-receptor combination. Proc R Soc B 154:21–69, 1961

38. Levitzki A: Negative co-operativity in clustered receptors as a possible basis for membrane action. J Theor Biol 44:367–372, 1974

39. Rodbell M, Krans HMJ, Pohl SL, Birnbaumer L: The glucagon-sensitive adenyl cyclase system in plasma membranes of rat liver. IV. Effects of guanyl nucleotides on binding of ^{125}I-glucagon. J Biol Chem 246:1872–1876, 1971

40. Salomon Y, Lin MC, Londos C, Rendell M, Rodbell M: The hepatic adenylate cyclase system. I. Evidence for transition states and structural requirements for guanine nucleotide activation. J Biol Chem 250:4239–4245, 1975

41. Rodbell M, Birnbaumer L, Pohl SL: Hormones, receptors and adenyl cyclase activity in mammalian cells. Edited by TW Rall, M Rodbell, P Condliffe: The Role of Adenyl Cyclase and Cyclic 3',5'-AMP in Biological Systems. NIH Fogarty International Center Proceedings No. 4. Bethesda, Md, National Institutes of Health, 1969, pp 59–102

42. Tolbert MEM, Butcher FR, Fain JN: Lack of correlation between catecholamine effects on cyclic adenosine 3',5'-monophosphate and gluconeogenesis in isolated rat liver cells. J Biol Chem 248:5686–5692, 1973

43. Perkins JP: Adenyl cyclase. Adv Cyclic Nucleotide Res 3:1–64, 1973

44. Cuatrecasas P: Membrane receptors. Annu Rev Biochem 43:169–214, 1974

45. de Haën C: The non-stoichiometric floating receptor model for hormone sensitive adenylyl cyclase. J Theor Biol 58: 383–400, 1976

46. Schimke RT: Turnover of membrane proteins in animal cells. Edited by ED Korn: Methods in Membrane Biology. New York, Plenum, 1975, pp 201–236

47. Raff M: Self regulation of membrane receptors. Nature (London) 259:265–266, 1976

48. Posner BI: Regulation of lactogen specific binding sites in rat liver: Studies on the role of lactogens and estrogen. Endocrinology 99:1168–1177, 1976

49. Ginsberg BH: The insulin receptor: Properties and regulation. Edited by G Litwack: Biochemical Actions of Hormones. Vol. IV. Academic Press, New York, 1977, pp 313–349

50. Jacobs S, Schecter Y, Bissell K, Cuatrecasas P: Purification and properties of insulin receptors from rat liver membranes. Biochem Biophys Res Commun 77:981–988, 1977

51. Flier JS, Kahn CR, Roth J, Bar RS: Antibodies that impair insulin receptor binding in an unusual diabetic syndrome with se-

vere insulin resistance. Science 190:63–65, 1975

52. Kahn CR, Freychet P, Roth J, Neville DM Jr: Quantitative aspects of the insulin-receptor interaction in liver plasma membranes. J Biol Chem 249:2249–2257, 1974

53. Soll AH, Kahn CR, Neville DM Jr: Insulin binding to liver plasma membranes in the obese hyperglycemic (ob/ob) mouse: Demonstration of a decreased number of functionally normal receptors. J Biol Chem 250:4702–4707, 1975

54. Wisher MH, Dron DI, Sonksen PH, Thomas JH: The insulin-degrading activity of plasma-membrane fractions from rat liver. Biochem Soc Trans 5:313–316, 1977

55. Olefsky JM, Johnson J, Liu F, Edwards P, Bauer S: Comparison of ^{125}I-insulin binding and degradation to isolated rat hepatocytes and liver membranes. Diabetes 24:801–810, 1975

56. Terris S, Steiner DF: Binding and degradation of ^{125}I-insulin by rat hepatocytes. J Biol Chem 250:8389–8398, 1975

57. Terris S, Steiner DF: Retention and degradation of ^{125}I-insulin by perfused livers from diabetic rats. J Clin Invest 57:885–896, 1976

58. Dial LK, Miyamoto S, Arquilla ER: Modulation of ^{125}I-insulin degradation by receptors in liver plasma membranes. Biochim Biophys Res Commun 74:545–552, 1977

59. Freychet P, Roth J, Neville DM Jr; Insulin receptors in the liver: Specific binding of [^{125}I]insulin to the plasma membrane and its relation to insulin bioactivity. Proc Natl Acad Sci USA 68:1833–1837, 1971

60. Freychet P, Brandenburg D, Wollmer A: Receptor-binding assay of chemically modified insulins: Comparison with in vitro and in vivo bioassays. Diabetologia 10:1–5, 1974

61. Simon J, Freychet P, Rosselin G, De Meyts P: Enhanced binding affinity of chicken insulin in rat liver membranes and human lymphocytes: Relationship to the kinetic properties of the hormone receptor interaction. Endocrinology 100:115–121, 1977

62. Pullen RA, Lindsay DG, Wood SP, Tickle IJ, Blundell TL, Wollmer A, Drail G, Brandenburg D, Zahn H, Gliemann J, Gammeltoft S: Receptor-binding region of insulin. Nature (London) 259:369–373, 1976

63. Bergeron JJM, Levine G, Sikstrom R, O'Shaughnessy D, Kopriwa B, Nadler NJ, Posner NI: Polypeptide hormone binding sites in vivo: Initial localization of ^{125}I-labeled insulin to hepatocyte plasmalemma as visualized by electron microscope radioautography. Proc Natl Acad Sci USA 74:5051–5055, 1977

64. Orci L, Rufener C, Malaisse-Lagae F, Blondel B, Amherdt M, Bataille D, Freychet P, Perrelet A: A morphologic approach to surface receptors in islet and liver cells. Isr J Med Sci 11:639–655, 1975

65. Cuatrecasas P: Unmasking of insulin receptors in fat cells and fat cell membranes. Perturbation of membrane lipids. J Biol Chem 246:6532–6542, 1971

66. Gliemann S, Gammaltoft S, Vinten J: Time course of insulin-receptor binding and insulin-induced lipogenesis in isolated rat fat cells. J Biol Chem 250:3368–3374, 1975

67. Ginsberg BH, Cohen RM, Kahn CR: Insulin-induced dissociation of receptors into subunits: Possible molecular concommitant of negative cooperativity. Diabetes 25 (Suppl 1):322, 1976

68. Kahn CR, De Meyts P, Ginsberg BH, Roth J: Cooperative properties of hormone receptors. Edited by S Bonfils, P Fromageot, G Rosselin: Hormonal Receptors in Digestive Tract Physiology. Amsterdam, North-Holland, 1977, pp 103–111

69. Lee AG, Birdsall NJM, Metcalfe JC, Toon PA, Warren GB: Clusters in lipid bilayers and the interpretation of thermal effects in biological membranes. Biochemistry 13:3699–3705, 1974

70. Shimshick EJ, McConnell HM: Lateral phase separations in binary mixtures of cholesterol and phospholipids. Biochem Biophys Res Commun 53:446–451, 1973

71. Kahn CR, Neville DM, Roth J: Insulin-receptor interaction in the obese-hyperglycemic mouse. J Biol Chem 248:244–250, 1973

72. Karakash C, Assimacopoulos-Jeannet F, Jeanrenaud B: An anomaly of insulin removal in perfused livers of obese-hyperglycemic (ob/ob) mice. J Clin Invest 57:1117–1124, 1976

73. Baxter D, Lazarus NR: The control of insulin receptors in the New Zealand obese mouse. Diabetologia 11:261–267, 1975

74. Soll AH, Kahn CR, Neville DM Jr, Roth J: Insulin receptor deficiency in genetic and

acquired obesity. J Clin Invest 56:769–780, 1975

75. Garrison MM, Bates RW: Decreased binding of insulin to its receptors in rats with hormone induced insulin resistance. Biochem Biophys Res Commun 53:852–857, 1973

76. Olefsky JM, Johnson J, Liu F, Jen P, Reaven GM: The effect of acute and chronic dexamethasone administration on insulin binding to isolated rat hepatocytes and adipocytes. Metabolism 20:517–527, 1975

77. Soman V, Felig P: Glucagon and insulin binding to liver membranes in a partially nephrectomized uremic rat model. J Clin Invest 60:224–232, 1977

78. Simon J, Freychet P, Rosselin G: A study of insulin binding sites in the chicken tissues. Diabetologia 13:219–228, 1977

79. Hepp KD, Langley J, von Funcke HJ, Renner R, Kemmler W: Increased insulin binding capacity of liver membranes from diabetic Chinese hamsters. Nature (London) 258:154, 1975

80. Davidson MB, Kaplan SA: Increased insulin binding by hepatic plasma membranes from diabetic rats. Normalization by insulin therapy. J Clin Invest 59:22–30, 1977

81. Sun JV, Tepperman HM, Tepperman J: A comparison of insulin binding by liver plasma membranes of rats fed a high glucose diet or a high fat diet. J Lipid Res 18:533–539, 1977

82. Kahn CR, Flier JS, Jarrett D, Roth J: Use of antireceptor antibodies as probes of receptor structure and function. Edited by S Bonfils, P Fromageot, G Rosselin: Hormonal Receptors in Digestive Tract Physiology. Amsterdam, North-Holland, 1977, pp 69–78

83. van Wyk JJ, Underwood LE, Hintz RL, Clemmons DR, Voina SJ, Weaver RP: The somatomedins: A family of insulin-like hormones under growth hormone control. Recent Prog Horm Res 30:259–318, 1974

84. Megyesi K, Kahn CR, Roth J, Neville DM Jr, Nissley PS, Humbel RE, Froesch ER: The NSILA-s receptor in liver plasma membranes: Characterization and comparison with the insulin receptor. J Biol Chem 250:8990–8996, 1975

85. Kahn CR, Megyesi K, Roth J: Nonsuppressible insulin-like activity of human serum. A potent inhibitor of insulin degradation. J Clin Invest 57:526–529, 1976

86. Giorgio NA, Johnson CB, Blecher M: Hormone receptors. III. Properties of glucagon-binding proteins isolated from liver plasma membranes. J Biol Chem 249:428–437, 1974

87. Bregman MD, Levy D: Labeling of glucagon binding components in hepatocyte plasma membranes. Biochem Biophys Res Commun 78:584–590, 1977

88. Pohl SL, Krans HMJ, Kozyreff V, Birnbaumer L, Rodbell M: The glucagon-sensitive adenyl cyclase system in plasma membranes of rat liver. VI. Evidence for a role of membrane lipids. J Biol Chem 246:4447–4454, 1971

89. Rubalcava B, Rodbell M: The role of acidic phopholipids in glucagon action on rat liver adenylate cyclase. J Biol Chem 248:3831–3837, 1973

90. Pohl SL, Krans HMJ, Birnbaumer L, Rodbell M: Inactivation of glucagon by plasma membranes of rat liver. J Biol Chem 247:2295–2301, 1972

91. Desbuquois B, Cuatrecasas P: Independence of glucagon receptors and glucagon inactivation in liver cell membranes. Nature (New Biol) 237:202–204, 1972

92. Bataille DP, Freychet P, Kitabgi PE, Rosselin GE: Gut glucagon: A common receptor site with pancreatic glucagon in liver cell plasma membranes. FEBS Lett 30:215–218, 1973

93. Houslay MD, Metcalfe JC, Warren GB, Hesketh TR, Smith GA: The glucagon receptor of rat liver plasma membrane can couple to adenylate cyclase without activating it. Biochim Biophys Acta 436:489–494, 1976

94. Rodbell M, Birnbaumer L, Pohl SL, Sundby F: The reaction of glucagon with its receptor: Evidence for discrete regions of activity and binding in the glucagon molecule. Proc Natl Acad Sci 68:909–913, 1971

95. Lin MC, Wright DE, Hruby VJ, Rodbell M: Structure-function relationships in glucagon: Properties of highly purified des-his[1], monoiodo-, and [des-asn[28],thr[29]] (homoserine lactone[27])-glucagon. Biochemistry 14:1559–1563, 1975

96. Birnbaumer L, Pohl SL: Relation of glucagon-specific binding sites to glucagon-dependent stimulation of adenylyl cyclase activity in plasma membranes of rat liver. J Biol Chem 248:2056–2061, 1973

97. Rodbell M, Birnbaumer L, Pohl SL, Krans HMJ: The glucagon-sensitive adenyl cyclase system in plasma membranes of rat

liver. V. An obligatory role of guanyl nucleotides in glucagon action. J Biol Chem 246:1877–1882, 1971

98. Rodbell M, Lin MC, Salomon Y: Evidence for interdependent action of glucagon and nucleotides on the hepatic adenylate cyclase system. J Biol Chem 249:59–65, 1974

99. Lin MC, Nicosia S, Lad PM, Rodbell M: Effects of GTP on binding of [³H]glucagon to receptors in rat hepatic plasma membranes. J Biol Chem 252:2790–2792, 1977

100. Makman MH, Sutherland EW: The use of liver adenyl cyclase for assay of glucagon in human gastro-intestinal tract and pancreas. Endocrinology 75:127–134, 1964

101. Birnbaumer L, Pohl SL, Rodbell M: The glucagon-sensitive adenylate cyclase system in plasma membranes of rat liver. IV. Hormonal stimulation: Reversibility and dependence on concentration of free hormones. J Biol Chem 247:2038–2043, 1972

102. Bataille D, Freychet P, Rosselin G: Interactions of glucagon, gut glucagon, vasoactive intestinal polypeptide and secretin with liver and fat cell plasma membranes: Binding to specific cyclase. Endocrinology 95:713–721, 1974

103. Strikant CB, McCorkle K, Unger RH: Properties of immunoreactive glucagon fractions of canine stomach and pancreas. J Biol Chem 252:1847–1851, 1977

104. Pohl SL, Birnbaumer L, Rodbell M: The glucagon-sensitive adenyl cyclase system in plasma membranes of rat liver: Properties. J Biol Chem 246:1849–1856, 1971

105. Strikant CB, Freeman D, McCorkle K, Unger RH: Binding and biologic activity of glucagon in liver cell membranes of chronically hyperglucagonemic rats. J Biol Chem 252:7434–7436

106. Kreiner PW, Keirne JJ, Bitensky MW: A temperature-sensitive change in the energy of activation of hormone-stimulated hepatic adenyl cyclase. Proc Natl Acad Sci USA 70:1785–1789, 1973

107. Shlatz L, Marinetti GV: Hormone calcium interactions with the plasma membrane of rat liver cells. Science 176:175–177, 1972

108. Storm DR, Chase RA: Exploitation of hormone-induced conformational changes to label selectively a component of rat liver plasma membranes. J Biol Chem 250:2539–2545, 1975

109. Houslay MD, Hesketh TR, Smith GA, Warren GB, Metcalfe JC: The lipid environment of the glucagon receptor regulates adenylate cyclase activity. Biochim Biophys Acta 436:495–504, 1976

110. Blazquez E, Rubalcava B, Montesano R, Orci L, Unger RH: Development of insulin and glucagon binding and the adenylate cyclase response in liver membranes of the prenatal, postnatal and adult rat. Evidence of glucagon "resistance." Endocrinology 98:1014–1023, 1976

111. Leffert H, Alexander NM, Faloona G, Rubalcava B, Unger R: Specific endocrine and hormonal receptor changes associated with liver regeneration in adult rats. Proc Natl Acad Sci USA 72:4033–4036, 1975

112. De Rubertis RF, Craven P: Reduced sensitivity of the hepatic adenylate cyclase-cyclic AMP system to glucagon during sustained hormonal stimulation. J Clin Invest 57:435–443, 1976

113. Broer Y, Freychet P, Rosselin G: Insulin and glucagon-receptor interactions in the genetically obese Zucker rat: Studies of hormone binding and glucagon-stimulated cyclic AMP levels in isolated hepatocytes. Endocrinology 101:236–249, 1977

114. Soman V, Felig P: Glucagon binding and adenylate cyclase activity in liver membranes from untreated and insulin treated diabetic rats. J Clin Invest 61:552–560, 1978

115. Desbuquois B: The interaction of vasoactive intestinal polypeptide and secretin with liver cell membranes. Eur J Biochem 46:439–450, 1974

116. Moore WV, Leppert P: Binding of native and reduced and carbamidomethylated hGH to rabbit liver plasma membranes. J Clin Endocrinol Metab 45:569–575, 1977

117. Ranke MB, Stanley CA, Rodbard D, Baker L, Bongiovanni A, Parks JS: Sex differences in binding of human growth hormone to isolated rat hepatocytes. Proc Natl Acad Sci USA 73:847–851, 1976

118. Ranke MB, Stanley CA, Tenore A, Rodbard D, Bongiovanni AM, Parks JS: Characterization of somatogenic and lactogenic binding sites in isolated rat hepatocytes. Endocrinology 99:1033–1045, 1976

119. Herrington AC, Veith NM: The presence of lactogen but not growth hormone binding sites in isolated rat hepatocytes. J Endocrinol 74:323–334, 1977

120. Saitoh Y, Ui M: Stimulation of glycogenolysis and gluconeogenesis by epinephrine

independent of its beta-adrenergic function in perfused rat liver. Biochem Pharmacol 25:841–845, 1976

121. Hanoune J, Pecker F, Lacombe M-L, Rene E: The liver cyclic AMP system and its sensitivity to catecholamines. Edited by S Bonfils, P Fromageot, G Rosselin: Hormonal Receptors in Digestive Tract Physiology. Amsterdam, North-Holland, 1977, pp 141–154

122. Hutson MJ, Brumley FT, Assimacopoulos FD, Harper SC, Exton JH: Studies on the α-adrenergic activation of hepatic glucagon output. I. Studies on the α-adrenergic activation of phosphorylase and gluconeogenesis and inactivation of glycogen synthetase in isolated rat liver parenchymal cells. J Biol Chem 251:5200–5208, 1976

123. Wolfe BB, Harden TK, Molinoff PB: β adrenergic receptors in rat liver: Effects of adrenalectomy. Proc Natl Acad Sci USA 73:1343–1347, 1976

124. Rao GS, Eckel J, Rao ML, Brewer H: Uptake of thyroid hormones by isolated rat liver cells. Biochem Biophys Res Commun 73:98–104, 1976

125. Pliam NB, Goldfine ID: High affinity thyroid hormone binding sites on purified rat liver plasma membranes. Biochem Biophys Res Commun 79:166–172, 1977

126. Smigel M, Fleischer S: Characterization and localization of prostaglandin E_1 receptors in rat liver plasma membranes. Biochim Biophys Acta 332:358–372, 1974

127. Smigel M, Fleischer S: Characterization of Triton X-100-solubilized prostagladin E binding protein of rat liver plasma membranes. J Biol Chem 252:3689–3696, 1977

128. Tomasi V: Prostaglandin E_1 as an intercellular regulator of cyclic AMP levels. Exp Cell Biol 44:260–277, 1976

129. Okamura N, Terayama H: Prostaglandin receptor—adenylate cyclase system in plasma membranes of rat liver and ascites hepatomas, and the effect of GTP upon it. Biochim Biophys Acta 465:54–67, 1977

130. Baker PF: The sodium pump in animal tissues and its role in the control of cellular metabolism and function. Edited by LE Hokin: Metabolic Pathways (ed 3). Vol. 6. New York, Academic Press, 1972, pp 243–268

131. Hokin LE, Dahl JL: The sodium-potassium adenosinetriphosphatase. Edited by LE Hokin: Metabolic Pathways (ed 3). Vol. 6. New York, Academic Press, 1972, pp 269–315

132. Boyer JL, Reno D: Properties of $(Na^+ + K^+)$-activated ATPase in rat liver plasma membranes enriched with bile canaliculi. Biochim Biophys Acta 401:59–72, 1975

133. Layden TJ, Boyer JL: The effect of thyroid hormone on bile salt-independent bile flow and Na^+,K^+-ATPase activity in liver plasma membranes enriched in bile canaliculi. J Clin Invest 57:1009–1018, 1976

134. Reichen J, Paumgartner G: Relationship between bile flow and Na^+,K^+-adenosinetriphosphatase in liver plasma membrane enriched in bile canaliculi. J Clin Invest 60:429–434, 1977

135. Simon FR, Sutherland E, Accatino L: Stimulation of hepatic Na^+,K^+-ATPase activity by phenobarbital: Its possible role in regulation of bile flow. J Clin Invest 59:849–861, 1977

136. Samuels AM, Carey MC: Effects of chlorpromazine hydrochloride and its metabolites on Mg^{2+} and Na^+,K^+-ATPase activities of canalicular-enriched rat liver plasma membranes. Gastroenterology 74:1183–1190, 1978

137. Wannagat FJ, Adler RD, Ockner RK: Bile acid-induced increase in bile acid-independent flow and plasma membrane NaK-ATPase activity in rat liver. J Clin Invest 61:297–307, 1978

138. Blitzer BL, Boyer JL: Cytochemical localization of Na^+,K^+-ATPase in the rat hepatocytes. J Clin Invest 62:1104–1108, 1978

139. Graf J, Peterlik M: Ouabain-mediated sodium uptake and bile formation by the isolated perfused rat liver. Am J Physiol 230:876–885, 1976

140. Diamond JM, Bossert WH: Standing-gradient osmotic flow. A mechanism for coupling of water and solute transport in epithelia. J Gen Physiol 50:2061–2083, 1967

141. Schultz SG: The role of paracellular pathways in isotonic fluid transport. Yale J Biol Med 50:99–113, 1977

142. Williams TF, Exton JH, Park CR, Regen DM: Stereo-specific transport of glucose in the perfused rat liver. Am J Physiol 215:1200–1209, 1968

143. Goresky CA, Bach GG, Nadeau BE: On the uptake of materials by the intact liver. The transport and net removal of galactose. J Clin Invest 52:991–1009, 1973

144. Goresky CA, Nadeau BE: Uptake of materials by the intact liver. The exchange of glucose across the cell membranes. J Clin Invest 53:634–646, 1974

145. Hooper RH, Short AH: The hepatocellular uptake of glucose, galactose and fructose in conscious sheep. J Physiol (London) 264:523–539, 1977

146. Bachmann W, Challoner D: D-glucose uptake by a rat liver plasma membrane preparation. Biochim Biophys Acta 443:254–266, 1976

147. LeFevre PG: Transport of carbohydrates by animal cells. Edited by LE Hokin: Metabolic Pathways (ed 3). Vol. 6. New York, Academic Press, 1972, pp 385–454

148. Heinz E: Transport of amino acids by animal cells. Edited by LE Hokin: Metabolic Pathways (ed 3). Vol. 6. New York, Academic Press, 1972, pp 445–501

149. Christensen HN: Some special kinetic problems of transport. Adv Enzymol 32:1–20, 1969

150. LeCam A, Freychet P: Neutral amino acid transport. Characterization of the A and L systems in isolated rat hepatocytes. J Biol Chem 252:148–156, 1977

151. Ayala E, Canonico PG: Aminoisobutyric acid transport in primary cultures of normal adult rat hepatocytes. Proc Soc Exp Biol Med 149:1019–1022, 1975

152. Chen CP, Lee RH: Active transport of alpha-aminoisobutyric acid in freshly prepared rat hepatocytes. Life Sci 21:577–584, 1977

153. Edmondson JW, Lumeng L, Li TK: Direct measurement of active transport systems for alanine in freshly isolated liver cells. Biochem Biophys Res Commun 76:751–757, 1977

154. Kletzien RF, Pariza MW, Becker JE, Potter VR, Butcher FR: Induction of amino acid transport in primary cultures of adult rat liver parenchymal cells by insulin. J Biol Chem 251:3014–3020, 1976

155. McGivan JD, Bradford NM, Mendes-Mourao J: The transport of branched chain amino acids into isolated rat liver cells. FEBS Lett 80:380–384, 1977

156. Sperber I: Secretion of organic anions in the formation of urine and bile. Pharmacol Rev 11:109–134, 1959

157. Glasinovic JC, Dumont M, Duval M, Erlinger S: Hepatocellular uptake of bile acids in the dog: Evidence for a common carrier-mediated transport system. An indicator dilution study. Gastroenterology 69:973–981, 1975

158. Reichen J, Paumgartner G: Uptake of bile acids by perfused rat liver. Am J Physiol 231:734–742, 1976

159. Schwarz LR, Burr R, Schwenk M, Pfaff E, Greim H: Uptake of taurocholic acid into isolated rat liver cells. Eur J Biochem 55:617–623, 1975

160. Alpert S, Mosher M, Shanske A, Arias IM: Multiplicity of hepatic excretory mechanisms for organic anions. J Gen Physiol 53:238–247, 1969

161. Paumgartner G, Reichen J: Different pathways for hepatic uptake of taurocholate and indocyanine green. Experientia 31:306–308, 1975

162. Scharschmidt, BF, Waggoner JG, Berk PD: Hepatic organic anion uptake in the rat. J Clin Invest 56:1280–1292, 1975

163. Paumgartner G, Reichen J: Kinetics of hepatic uptake of unconjugated bilirubin. Clin Sci Mol Med 51:169–176, 1976

164. Schwenk M, Burr R, Schwarz L, Pfaff E: Uptake of bromosulphophthalein by isolated liver cells. Eur J Biochem 64:189–197, 1976

165. Accatino L, Simon FR: Identification and characterization of a bile acid receptor in isolated liver surface membranes. J Clin Invest 57:496–508, 1976

166. Goresky CA: The hepatic uptake and excretion of sulfobromophthalein and bilirubin. Can Med Assoc J 92:851–857, 1965

167. Paumgartner G, Probst P, Kraines R, Leevy CM: Kinetics of indocyanine green removal from the blood. Ann NY Acad Sci 170:134–147, 1970

168. Levi AJ, Gatmaitan Z, Arias IM: Two hepatic cytoplasmic protein fractions, Y and Z, and their possible role in the hepatic uptake of bilirubin, sulfobromophthalein and other anions. J Clin Invest 48:2156–2167, 1969

169. Meuwissen JATP, Ketterer B, Heirwegh KPM: Role of soluble binding proteins in

overall hepatic transport of bilirubin. Edited by PD Berk and NI Berlin: Chemistry and Physiology of Bile Pigments. U.S. DHEW Publication no. 77-1100. Washington, DC, Government Printing Office, 1977, pp 323–337

170. Reichen J, Blitzer BL, Berk PD: The binding of organic anionic dyes to hepatocellular plasma membranes. Clin Res 25:268A, 1977

171. Reichen J, Berk PD: Isolation of an organic anionic dye binding protein from rat liver plasma membrane. Gastroenterology 73:1242, 1977

172. Tiribelli C, Lunazzi G, Luciani M, Panfili E, Gassin B, Liut G, Sandri G, Sottocasa G: Isolation of a sulfobromophthalein-binding protein from hepatocyte plasma membrane. Biochim Biophys Acta 532:105–112, 1978

173. Meijer DKF: The mechanism for hepatic uptake and biliary excretion of organic cations. Excerpta Medica 391:196–207, 1976

174. Schanker LS: Transport of drugs. Edited by LE Hokin: Metabolic Pathways (ed 3). Vol. 6. New York, Academic Press, 1972, pp 543–571

175. Rao GS, Schulze-Hagen K, Rao ML, Brewer H: Kinetics of steroid transport through cell membranes: Comparison of the uptake of cortisol by isolated rat liver cells with binding of cortisol to rat liver cytosol. J Steroid Biochem 7:1123–1129, 1976

176. Rao ML, Rao GS, Eckel J, Brewer H: Factors involved in the uptake of corticosterone by rat liver cells. Biochim Biophys Acta 500:322–332, 1977

177. Riordan JR, Alon N: Binding of [³H]cytochalasin B and [³H]-colchicine to isolated liver plasma membranes. Biochim Biophys Acta 464:547–561

178. Jung CY, Rampal AL: Cytochalasin B binding sites and glucose transport carrier in human erythrocyte ghosts. J Biol Chem 252:5456–5463, 1977

179. Reichen J, Berman MD: The role of microfilaments and microtubules in bile salt uptake by isolated rat hepatocytes. Gastroenterology 74:1167, 1978

180. van Obberghen E, De Meyts P, Roth J: Cell surface receptors for insulin and growth hormone. Effect of microtubule and microfilament modifiers. J Biol Chem 251:6844–6851, 1976

181. Gregory DH, Vlahcevic ZR, Prugh MF, Swell L: Mechanism of secretion of biliary lipids: Role of microtubular system in hepatocellular transport of biliary lipids in the rat. Gastroenterology 74:93–100, 1978

182. Le Marchand Y, Patzelt C, Assimacopoulos-Jeannet F, Loten EG, Jeanrenaud B: Evidence for a role of the microtubular system in the secretion of newly synthesized albumin and other proteins by the liver. J Clin Invest 53:1512–1517, 1974

183. Goldman ID, Fyfe MJ, Bowen D, Loftfield S, Schafer JA: The effect of microtubular inhibitors on transport of α-aminoisobutyric acid. Inhibition of uphill transport without changes in transmembrane gradients of Na^+, K^+ or H^+. Biochim Biophys Acta 467:185–191, 1977

184. van Bockxmeer F, Hemmapbardh D, Morgan EH: Studies in the binding of transferrin to cell membrane receptors. Edited by RR Crichton: Proteins of Iron Storage and Transport in Biochemistry and Medicine. Amsterdam, North-Holland, 1975, pp 111–119

185. Grohlich D, Morley CGD, Miller JR, Bezkorovainy A: Iron incorporation into isolated rat hepatocytes. Biochem Biophys Res Commun 76:682–690, 1977

186. Grohlich D, Morley CGD, Miller RJ, Bezkorovainy A: The incorporation of iron into isolated rat hepatocytes. Edited by EB Brown, P Aisen, J Fieling, RR Crichton: Proteins of Iron Metabolism. New York, Grune & Stratton, 1977, pp 335–340

187. Beamish MR, Keay L, Okigaki T, Brown EB: Uptake of transferrin-bound iron by rat cells in tissue culture. Br J Haematol 31:479–491, 1975

188. Zimelman AP, Zimmerman HJ, McLean R, Weintraub LR: Effect of iron saturation of transferrin on hepatic iron uptake: An in vitro study. Gastroenterology 72:129–131, 1977

189. Fidler-Nagy C, Rowley GR, Coffey JW, Miller ON: Binding of vitamin B_{12}-rat transcobalamin II and free vitamin B_{12} to plasma membranes isolated from rat liver. Br J Haematol 31:311–321, 1975

190. Horne DW, Briggs W: Transport of methotrexate, folic acid and 5-methyltetrahydrofolic acid by freshly isolated hepatocytes. Fed Proc 35:581, 1976

191. Zamierowski MM, Wagner C: Identification of folate binding proteins in rat liver. J Biol Chem 252:933–938, 1977

192. van den Hamer, CJA, Morell AG, Scheinberg IH, Hickman J, Ashwell G: Physical and chemical studies on ceruloplasmin. IX. The role of galactosyl residues in the clearance of ceruloplasmin from the circulation. J Biol Chem 245:4397–4402, 1970

193. Morell AG, Gregoriadis G, Scheinberg IH, Hickman J, Ashwell G: The role of sialic acid in determining the survival of glycoproteins in the circulation. J Biol Chem 246:1461–1467, 1971

194. Pricer WE Jr, Ashwell G: The binding of desialylated glycoproteins by plasma membranes of rat liver. J Biol Chem 246:4825–4833, 1971

195. Hudgin RL, Pricer WE Jr, Ashwell G, Stockert RJ, Morell AG: The isolation and properties of a rabbit liver binding protein specific for asialoglycoproteins. J Biol Chem 249:5536–5543, 1974

196. Kawasaki T, Ashwell G: Chemical and physical properties of an hepatic membrane protein that specifically binds asialoglycoproteins. J Biol Chem 251:1296–1302, 1976

197. Jones EA, Vergalla J, Steer CJ, Bradley-Moore PR, Vierling JM: Metabolism of intact and desialylated α-1-antitrypsin. Clin Sci Mol Med, 55:139–148, 1978

198. Emerson WA, Vuch R: Isolation and characterization of human liver asialo-glycoprotein binding proteins. Clin Res 26:318A, 1978

199. Hutchinson DW, Kabayo JP: Current thoughs on neuraminidase. Trends Biochem Sci 2:1–3, 1977

200. La Badie JH, Chapman KP, Aronson NN Jr: Glycoprotein catabolism in rat liver. Lysosomal digestion of iodinated asialo-fetuin. Biochem J 152:271–279, 1975

201. Marshall JS, Green AM, Pensy J, Williams S, Zinn A, Carlson DM: Measurement of circulating desialylated glycoproteins and correlation with hepatocellular damage. J Clin Invest 54:555–562, 1974

202. Stockert RJ, Morell AG, Scheinberg IH: The existence of a second route for the transfer of certain glycoproteins from the circulation into the liver. Biochem Biophys Res Commun 68:988–993, 1976

203. Stahl P, Six H, Rodman JS, Schlesinger P, Tulsiani DRP, Touster O: Evidence for specific recognition sites mediating clearance of lysosomal enzymes in vivo. Proc Natl Acad Sci USA 73:4045–4049, 1976

204. Stahl P, Rodman JS, Schlesinger P: Clearance of lysosomal hydrolases following intravenous infusion. Arch Biochem Biophys 177:594–605, 1976

205. Schlesinger P, Rodman JS, Frey M, Lang S, Stahl P: Clearance of lysosomal hydrolases following intravenous infusion. Arch Biochem Biophys 177:606–614, 1976

206. Kawasaki T, Etoh R, Ramashina I: Isolation and characterization of a mannan-binding protein from rat liver. Biochem Biophys Res Commun 81:1018–1024, 1978

207. Furbish FS, Steer CJ, Barranger JA, Jones EA, Brady RO: The uptake of native and desialylated glucocerebrosidase by rat hepatocytes and Kupffer cells. Biochem Biophys Res Commun 81:1047–1053, 1978

208. Steer CJ, Furbish FS, Barranger JA, Brady RO, Jones EA: The uptake of agalacto-glucocerebrosidase by rat hepatocytes and Kupffer cells. FEBS Lett 91:202–205, 1978

209. Bachoric PS, Livingston JN, Cooke J, Kwiterovich PO: The binding of low density lipoprotein by liver membranes in the pig. Biochem Biophys Res Commun 69:927–935, 1976

210. Carella M, Cooper A: Demonstration of specific receptor for chylomicron remnants on rat liver plasma membranes. Gastroenterology 74:1018, 1978

211. Frank MM, Schreiber AD, Atkinson JP, Jaffee CJ: Pathophysiology of immune hemolytic anemia. Ann Intern Med 87:210–222, 1977

212. Schreiber AD, Frank MM: Role of antibody and complement in the immune clearance and destruction of erythrocytes. I. In vitro effects of IgG and IgM complement fixing sites. J Clin Invest 51:575–582, 1972

213. Schreiber AD, Frank MM: Role of antibody and complement in the immune clearance and destruction of erythrocytes. II. Molecular nature of IgG and IgM complement-fixing sites and effects of their interaction with serum. J Clin Invest 51:583–589, 1972

214. Atkinson JA, Frank MM: Studies on the in vivo effects of antibody: interaction of IgM antibody and complement in the immune clearance and destruction of erythrocytes in man. J Clin Invest 54:339–348, 1974

215. Jaffe CJ, Atkinson JP, Frank MM: The role of complement in the clearance of cold agglutinin sensitized erythrocytes in man. J Clin Invest 58:942–949, 1976

216. Brown DL, Lachmann PJ, Dacie JV: The in vivo behavior of complement-coated red cells: Studies in C6-deficient, C3-depleted and normal rabbits. Clin Exp Immunol 7:401–422, 1970

217. Reynolds HY, Atkinson JP, Newball HH, Frank MM: Receptors for immunoglobulin and complement on human alveolar macrophages. J Immunol 114:1813–1819, 1975

218. Jaffe CJ, Vierling JM, Jones EA, Lawley T, Frank MM: Receptor specific clearance by the reticuloendothelial system in chronic liver diseases: Demonstration of defective C3b specific clearance in primary biliary cirrhosis. J Clin Invest, 62:1069–1077, 1978

219. Vierling JM, Jaffe CJ, Lawley TJ, Frank MM, Jones EA: Compartmental analysis of hepatic reticuloendothelial clearance in chronic liver disease. Gastroenterology 72:1183, 1977

220. Jones EA, Frank MM, Jaffe CJ, Vierling JM: Primary biliary cirrhosis and the complement system. Ann Intern Med 90:72–84, 1979

221. Munthe-Kaas AC, Kerg T, Seglen PO, Seljelid R: Mass isolation and culture of rat Kupffer cells. J Exp Med 141:1–10, 1975

222. Munthe-Kaas AC: Phagocytosis in rat Kupffer cells in vitro. Exp Cell Res 99:319–327, 1976

223. Munthe-Kaas AC, Kaplan G, Seljelid R: On the mechanism of internalization of opsonized particles by rat Kupffer cells in vitro. Exp Cell Res 103:201–212, 1976

224. Stossel TP: Phagocytosis: Recognition and ingestion. Semin Hematol 12:83–116, 1975

225. Griffen FM Jr, Bianco C, Silverstein SC: Characterization of the macrophage receptor for complement and demonstration of its functional independence from the receptor for the Fc portion of immunoglobulin G. J Exp Med 141:1269–1277, 1975

226. Bianco C, Griffen FM, Silverstein SC: Studies of the macrophage complement receptor: Alteration of receptor function upon macrophage activation. J Exp Med 141:1278–1290, 1975

227. Ross GD, Polley MJ: Specificity of human lymphocyte complement receptors. J Exp Med 141:1163–1180, 1975

228. Hopf U, Meyer zum Buschenfelde K-H, Dierich MP: Demonstration of binding sites for IgG, Fc and the third complement component (C3) on isolated hepatocytes. J Immunol 117:639–645, 1976

229. Novogrodsky A, Ashwell G: Lymphocyte mitogenesis induced by a mammalian liver protein that specifically binds desialylated glycoproteins. Proc Natl Acad Sci USA 74:676–678, 1977

230. Vierling JM, Steer CJ, Hickman JW, James SJ, Jones EA: Cell-mediated cytotoxicity of desialylated human lymphocytes induced by a mitogenic mammalian liver protein. Gastroenterology, 75:456–461, 1978

231. Woodruff JJ, Gesner BM: The effect of neuraminidase on the fate of transfused lymphocytes. J Exp Med 129:551–567, 1969

232. Woodruff JJ, Woodruff JF: Influenza A virus interaction with murine lymphocytes. I. The influence of influenza virus A/Japan 305 (H2N2) on the pattern of migration of recirculating lymphocytes. J Immunol 117:852–858, 1976

233. Woodruff JJ, Woodruff JF: Influenza A virus interaction with murine lymphocytes. II. Changes in lymphocyte surface properties induced by influenza virus A/Japan 305 (H2N2). J Immunol 117:859–864, 1976

234. Winchester RJ, Fu SM, Winfield JB, Kunkel HG: Immunofluorescent studies on antibodies directed to a buried membrane structure present in lymphocytes and erythrocytes. J Immunol 114:410–414, 1975

235. Popper H: Summary. Edited by H Popper, L Bianchi, W Reutter: Membrane Alterations as Basis of Liver Injury. Lancaster, MTP Press, 1977, pp 371–377

Chapter 4

Electron Microscopy of Mitochondria and Peroxisomes of Human Hepatocytes

By IRMIN STERNLIEB, M.D.

ANY REVIEW of pathologic changes in organelles must necessarily be incomplete, overambitious, and in all likelihood, controversial. The absence of a single specialized medium for communication and the consequent scattering of reports about electron microscopy in a wide range of publications has done little to enhance interest in our understanding of human hepatic ultrastructure. Therefore, I welcomed the editors' invitation to present this review and have attempted to synthesize some of the information presently available in the hope of generating a more critical appraisal of the pathologic changes observed in mitochondria and peroxisomes of human hepatocytes. I have also tried to emphasize the diversity and the lack of specificity of these changes and the consequent difficulty in determining their functional significance in the absence of correlated biochemical and cytochemical studies. The task is complicated because the events that cause the configurational changes seen under the electron microscope are probably genetically controlled and influenced by multiple factors such as age, nutrition, and exposure to drugs or toxins. They are influenced more directly by intracellular changes in ionic content; by the ratios of phospholipids to proteins in the membranes; and by alterations in the availability of precursors or substrates from the cytosol to the endoplasmic reticulum. Although progress has been made in defining some characteristics of human mitochondria and peroxisomes and the ways in which they differ from those of rats, much remains to be learned on this subject.

MITOCHONDRIA

Normal Mitochondria

Mitochondria are easily recognizable in thin sections because of their characteristic structure. They appear as spheres or as ovoid or ellipsoid bodies,

Divisions of Genetic Medicine and Gastroenterology, and Liver Research Center, Department of Medicine, Albert Einstein College of Medicine, Bronx, New York.

Supported in parts by grants AM 1059 and AM 17702 from the National Institute of Arthritis, Metabolism, and Digestive Diseases, 5M01RR50 from the General Clinical Research Center, CA 06576 from the National Cancer Institute and from the Foundation for the Study of Wilson's Disease, Inc.

with diameters ranging from 0.5 to 1.0 μ. Those located in the periportal area are more oval or oblong, while the mitochondria in centrolobular cells are more frequently spherical.[1] These organelles are limited by a snugly fitting outer membrane that encloses a homogeneous, moderately electron-dense matrix compartment limited by the mitochondrion's inner membrane (Fig.1*). Irregularly distributed, narrow cristae, which may be slitlike, straight, or sinuous, are formed by infoldings of the inner membrane and dissect the matrix. These cristae communicate with the intermembranous space. A few discrete, electron-dense, calcium-containing granules are freely scattered throughout the matrix. There are about 2200 mitochondria in an average hepatocyte, occupying 17.6% of its volume.[2]

Abnormalities of Mitochondria

Changes in Number

A decrease in the number of mitochondria per hepatocyte seems to take place after 60 years of age. This is first compensated by an increase in the size of the cristae and later by an augmentation of the volume of the average mitochondrion.[3] A similar decrease in numbers of small mitochondria and a compensatory increase in the proportion of large mitochondria, resulting in a normal volume density of mitochondria, has been documented in patients with Gilbert's syndrome.[4] But conflicting data were reported for alcoholic liver disease in which the volume density was unaltered according to one study[5] and increased by as much as 23% in another.[6] An increased abundance of mitochondria was found in patients treated with clofibrate (CPIB).[7] Some hepatocellular carcinomas exhibit profound reductions[8] while others demonstrate increased numbers of mitochondria[9] (Fig. 7).

Changes in Shape

Some lack of uniformity of the outlines of mitochondria can be seen even in normal hepatocytes (Fig. 2), but striking pleomorphism, often associated with increased size, is more characteristic of pathologic hepatic changes (Figs. 3 to 5 and 15 to 18). There are ranges of pleomorphic changes, with extremes found among the tightly packed, interdigitating ameboid mitochondria in hepatocytes of patients with Reye's syndrome[11,12] (Fig. 6) and in some hepatocellular carcinomas. Peculiar buds or fingerlike projections have been reported in Hurler's syndrome,[13] Sanfilippo's syndrome,[14] and homocystinuria.[15]

---

*Figures 1 through 26 are electron micrographs of fine sections of liver biopsy specimens fixed in 1% osmium tetroxide in barbital buffer with 0.25 M sucrose, embedded in Epon, and stained with uranyl acetate and lead citrate. The normal biopsy specimens were obtained from apparently healthy adolescents or young adults suspected of, but subsequently shown not to have, Wilson's disease. The diagnoses indicated in the legends are for identification of the sources of the biopsy material and generally are not meant to imply specificity for the illustrated findings.

Abbreviations: D, desmosome; G, mitochondrial granule; H, hemosiderin; I, electron-dense inclusion; L, lipid droplet; M, mitochondrion; P, peroxisome; V, vacuole; c, crista; er, endoplasmic reticulum; g, glycogen; im, intermembranous space; pm, plasma membrane; ser, smooth endoplasmic reticulum.

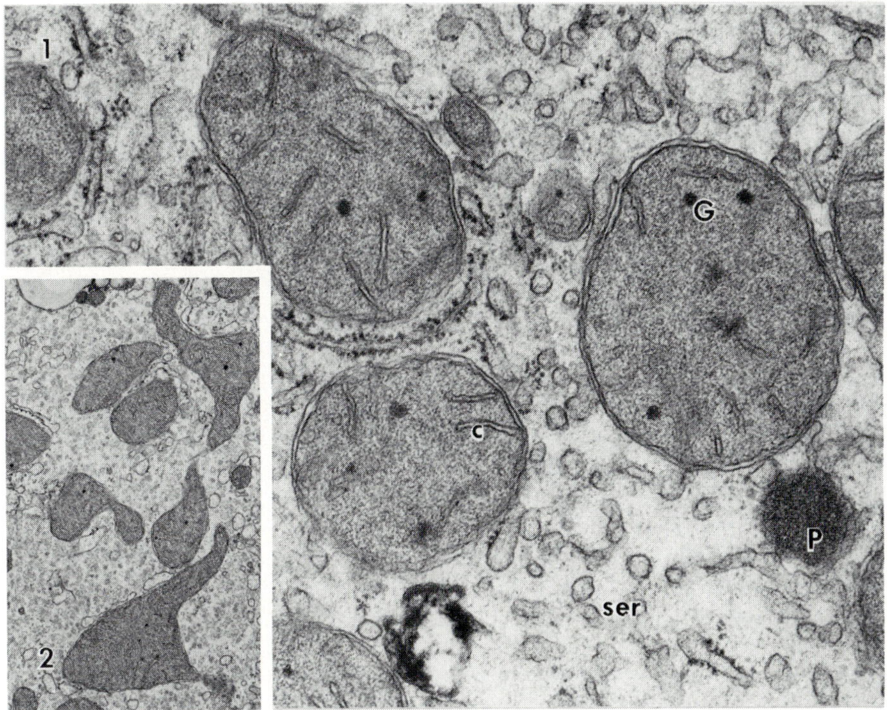

FIG. 1—Portion of hepatocyte from a 12-year-old boy that demonstrates the appearance of normal mitochondria. Note the regular outlines, the close apposition of the outer and inner membranes, the homogeneous appearance of the matrix, the size of normal dense granules (G), the scatter of the slitlike cristae (c), and the close association of the central mitochondria with a cisterna of rough endoplasmic reticulum (× 32,400).

FIG. 2—Some pleomorphism of mitochondria can be seen even in normal hepatocytes, as shown in the biopsy from a 27-year-old woman (× 7,250)

Changes in Size

A diminution of the average size of mitochondria has been reported only in neoplastic hepatocytes.[10] Whether or not similar diminution occurs in other conditions has not yet been documented by morphometric analysis. By contrast, enlarged mitochondria having globular, ellipsoid, greatly elongated, or other bizarre shapes are comparatively frequent in diseased hepatocytes.[16–21] One such abnormal pattern of enlargement usually predominates in any one specimen, but exceptions do occur. Except for the isolated augmentation of volume in the mitochondria of aged subjects[3] and patients with Gilbert's syndrome,[4] most giant or megamitochondria found in pathologic conditions display profound changes in the density of the matrix, in the arrangement of cristae, and in the size and appearance of the granules. This is seen particularly in alcoholic liver disease[16–20] (Fig. 5), in patients with halothane[22] or other forms of hepatitis,[23] systemic sclerosis,[24] Wilson's disease[25,26] (Fig. 18), or in the hepatocytes present in the vicinty of a hepatocellular carcinoma,[27] to name just a few. Although giant mitochondria are visible even by light microscopy,

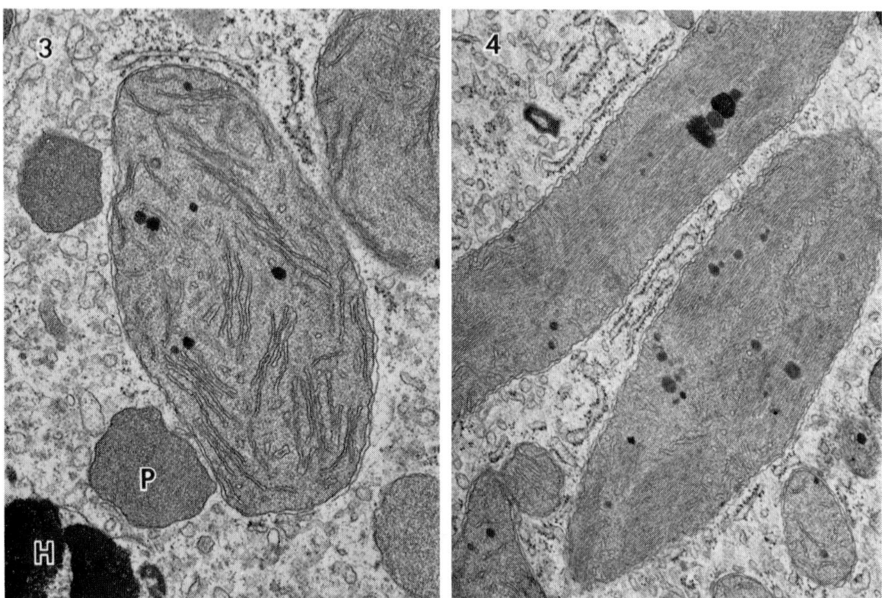

FIG. 3—Ellipsoid enlargement of a mitochondrion containing an increased number of elongated cristae in the hepatocyte of a 39-year-old man after 18 years of treatment with D-penicillamine for Wilson's disease. An incidental iron overload was present in the patient's hepatocytes (H) (× 22,000).

FIG. 4—Portion of a hepatocyte from a 64-year-old man with type V hyperlipoproteinemia. Only a portion of a greatly elongated mitochondrion (total length 8 μ) with electron-dense inclusions is shown next to an enlarged, ellipsoid mitochondrion. Both contain filamentous cristals aligned along the long axes of the organelles. Note the difference in size between the normal-sized organelles at the bottom of the picture and the two megamitochondria (× 18,000).

this finding is of little diagnostic value except for the globular megamitochondria with a reduced number of cristae (Fig. 5) that seem to be specific for alcoholic liver disease. The factors that control the organelle's growth have not been identified, but it can be assumed either that the translation or transcription of macromolecular synthesis of membrane components may be blocked, resulting in the generation of matrix-enriched organelles, or that fusion of small mitochondria takes place under abnormal circumstances.

Moderate to striking elongation of mitochondria, from 3 to 10 μ, occurs in numerous pathologic conditions, including alcoholic liver disease,[20] hyperlipoproteinemia[23,28] (Fig. 4), halothane hepatitis,[22] and systemic sclerosis,[24] among others. The filamentous crystals often present in the long axis of the mitochondrion[29] (Fig. 4) may be responsible for the shape and the elongation of the organelle, having an effect similar to that of sickle cell hemoglobin on the configuration of erythrocytes.

Outer Membranes

Generally the outer mitochondrial membrane is smooth and closely apposed to the inner membrane even when the shape and size of the matrix compart-

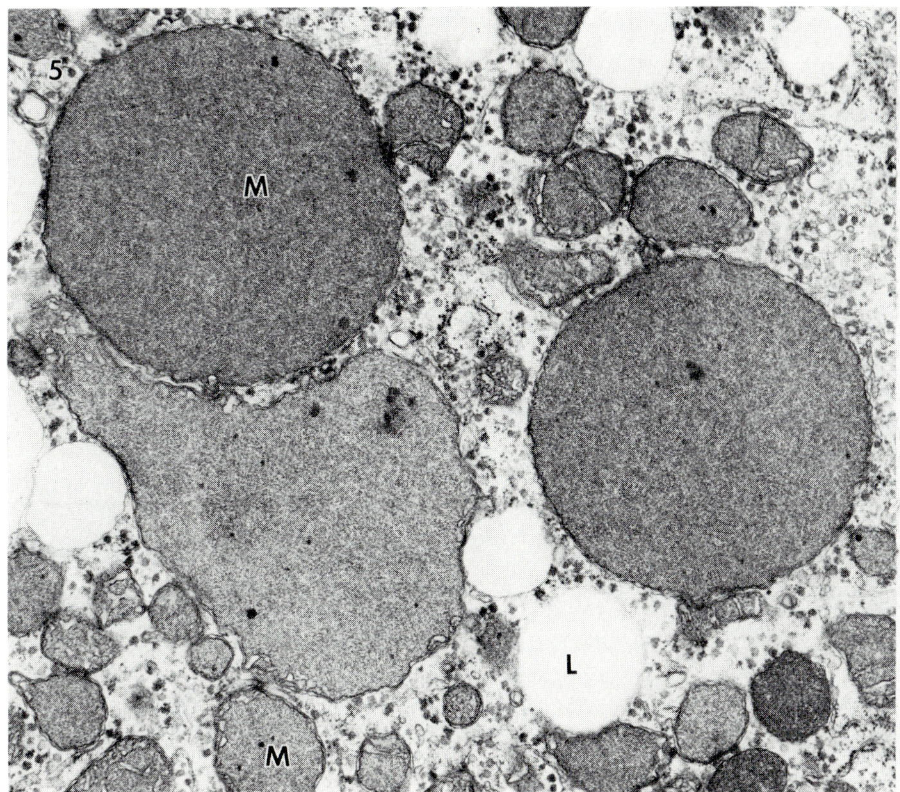

FIG. 5—Portion of a hepatocyte from a 38-year-old woman with florid alcoholic hepatitis containing one misshapen and two globular megamitochondria. There are striking differences in electron density of the matrices, as well as a striking paucity of cristae and granules ($\times$ 18,500).

ment has changed considerably (Figs. 1 and 2). The intactness of the outer membrane determines the accessibility of compounds to the inner compartment. When that membrane becomes ruffled, as seen in the mitochondria of young patients with Wilson's disease (Fig. 18), an abnormal, electron-lucent intermembranous space is created. The disappearance of portions of outer membranes, implying a specific mode of injury to the organelle, has been reported but is difficult to prove because membranes at a sufficient angle perpendicular to the plane of section are not apparent.

Inner Membranes and Cristae

The inner mitochondrial membrane contains the machinery responsible for most of the energy production in animal cells. This machinery consists of a multienzyme system that oxidizes pyruvate, amino acids, and fatty acids, generating movement of the electrons and protons that are the driving forces for the generation of ATP from ADP. Because of the critical role of the inner membrane in energy production, sufficient impairment of its function may affect the cell's viability. Configurational changes of the inner membranes are

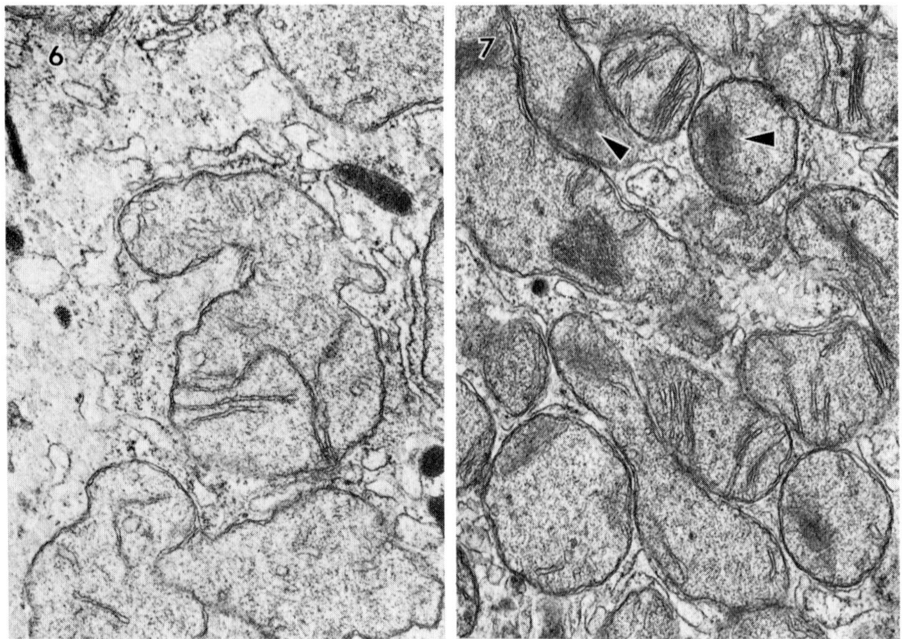

FIG. 6—Closely packed misshapen mitochondria with ameboid, interdigitating outlines; diminished electron density of the matrix; irregular cristae; and no demonstrable granules in the hepatocyte from a child with Reye's syndrome (× 25,800). (Courtesy J.C. Partin.)

FIG. 7—Tightly packed pleomorphic mitochondria exhibiting clustering of cristae and areas of condensation of the matrix (arrowhead) in the neoplastic hepatocyte of a 25-year-old man with hepatocellular carcinoma and HB_s Ag in the serum (× 20,000).

not recognizable, however, unless those displayed by the cristae are taken into consideration. Normally the cristae represent infoldings of the inner membranes that increase their surface and functional capacity.

A close look at different types of human hepatocellular mitochondria (Figs. 3 to 12) demonstrates that the cristal membrane has a considerable capacity to undergo configurational changes, giving rise to an almost limitless variety of alterations in the number, organization, shape, and size of cristae. There is also variability in the association of cristae with mitochondrial inclusions.

In some instances, a scatter of short cristae imparts a chaotic appearance to the organelle[24,30] (Fig. 3). This apparent lack of orderly arrangement contrasts with the remarkable organization of some cristae, which become stacked along the long mitochondrial axis[31] (Fig. 8), a phenomenon believed to be a sign of regeneration.[32] By contrast, in globular mitochondria the cristae occasionally arrange themselves concentrically at the periphery.[33] Some cristae form inclined rouleaux when they are associated with filamentous crystals[29,34] (Fig. 16) or become evenly spaced around the circumference of mitochondria, imparting the appearance of cartwheels to their cross sections[33,35] (Fig. 11). In an otherwise normal mitochondrion, an occasional widened cristal space may be insignificant, but widening of several cristae in nonperipheral hepatocytes is clearly abnormal (Figs. 18 and 25) provided the cells under study are at a distance from the edge of the tissue block, because in this location an artifactual swelling of mitochondria and widening of cristae may occur.[12,36]

Fragmentation of cristae occurs in patients with Reye's syndrome,[12] while an arrangement of cristae perpendicular to the long axis of the mitochondrion, traversing the width of the mitochondrial profile and apparently creating matrical compartments, occurs in hepatocytes affected by alcohol[19,20,33] (Fig. 10) and probably in other conditions as well. This arrangement contrasts with the peculiar curling of cristae that seems to be a characteristic of cholestasis.[36–38] The importance of this configurational change for cholestasis remains to be determined, since no detailed study of the frequency or regularity of this finding has been published. It is uncertain whether an alteration in the normal ratio of cholesterol to phospholipids in the cristal membranes, a likely cause of curling in cholestasis, is also responsible for this phenomenon in patients with gallstones[39] and in some patients with halothane hepatitis[40] or cryptogenic cirrhosis (Fig. 12). Conceivably, at some stage of cholestasis the cristae may be more affected than the biliary canaliculi.[38]

Quantitative data regarding the normal ratio of cristae to matrical volume in

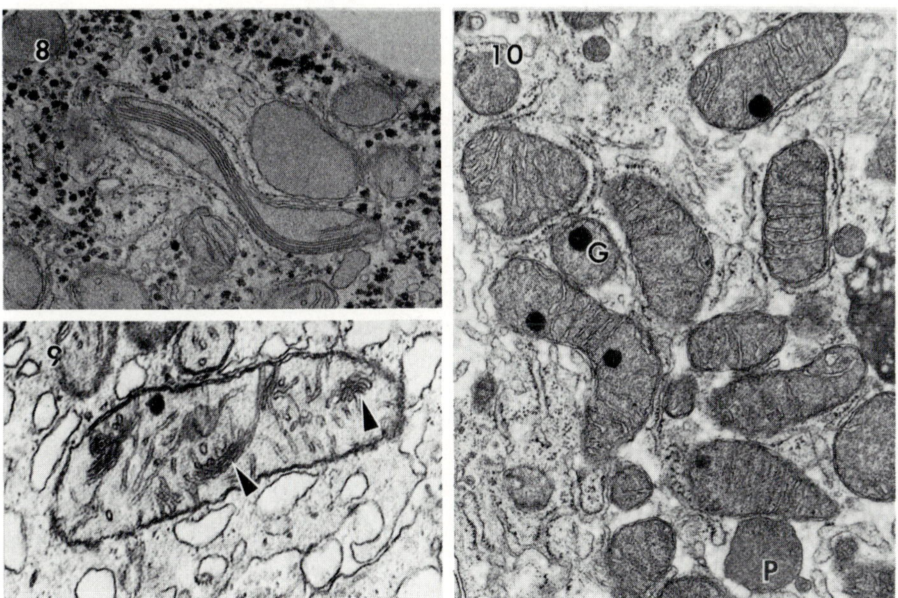

FIG. 8—Longitudinally stacked cristae in an elongated mitochondrion from the same patient as in Figure 4 (× 6,750).

FIG. 9—Helicoidally stacked cristae (arrowheads) in the mitochondrion of a patient with hyperlipoproteinemia after long-term treatment with clofibrate. This phenomenon was observed in 3 out of 19 treated subjects[7] (× 33,000). (Courtesy Dr. M. Hanefeld.)

FIG. 10—Portion of another hepatocyte from same biopsy shown in Figure 5. The mitochondria appear homogeneous, but their cristae are arranged perpendicularly to the outer membrane and seem to traverse the widths of the organelles. Note the presence of greatly enlarged granules (G) (× 12,300).

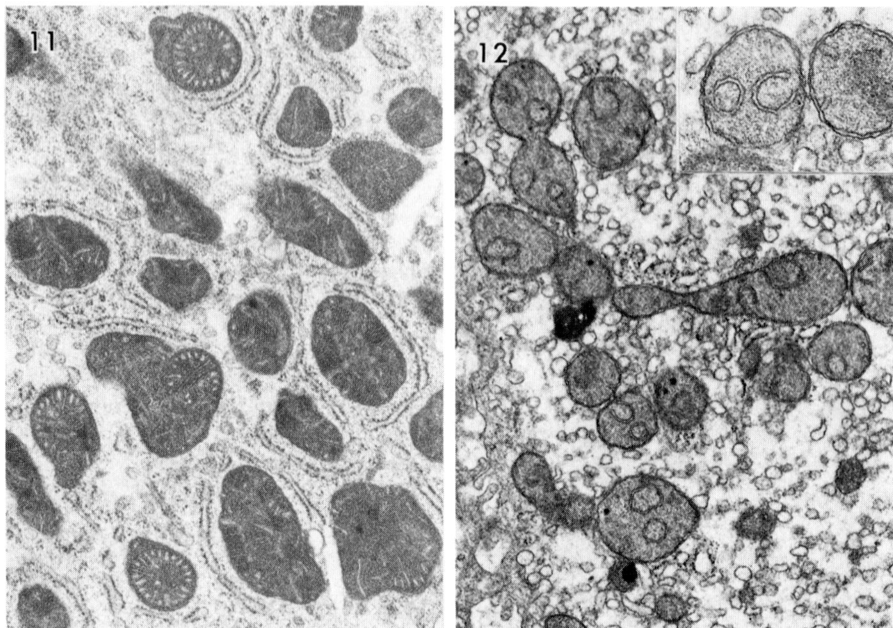

FIG. 11—Portion of hepatocyte from a 20-month-old child with Menkes' kinky or steely hair disease. Note the density of the matrix and the remarkable arrangement of the peripheral, regularly spaced cristae, which look like cartwheels, on transverse sections (× 18,300).

FIG. 12—Curled cristae characteristic of cholestasis in the mitochondria of a 52-year-old man with cryptogenic cirrhosis (× 7,400, inset × 23,400).

human hepatic mitochondria are scant. Stereologic analyses indicate that the surface density of the cristae is increased in the presence of cholestasis[41] or of cholesterol gallstones.[39] Age[3] and nutrition, e.g., vitamin B_{12} as well as extrahepatic hormonal factors also seem to determine the number of cristae. In hypothyroid rats, the surface of mitochondrial cristae per hepatocyte decreases to 38%, while in hyperthyroid rats it increases by 63% above the amount measured in specimens obtained from euthyroid littermates.[43] These results are consistent with the observations made on patients with different degrees of thyroid dysfunction in whom changes in the diameters of mitochondria were noted.[44] In some pathologic conditions, e.g., in alcoholic livers containing globular mitochondria (Fig. 5), mere inspection reveals a drastic reduction in the number of cristae.

Consistency of Matrix

Variations in the electron density of the matrix are common in pathologic specimens. As an isolated occurrence, a diminished density of the matrix may reflect aging, a physiologic degenerative process. Pronounced swelling of many mitochondria with apparent disintegration of the matrix is clearly pathologic, however. Examples of this kind of degeneration are seen in viral hepatitis,[45] in an occasional hepatocellular carcinoma,[46] and in chronic passive congestion of the liver.[47] The changes can be even more pronounced during certain stages of Reye's syndrome, when expansion and flocculation of the matrix supervene while the mitochondria take on irregular shapes and become disfigured and almost ameboid[11,12] (Fig. 6). Similar changes have been reported in patients suffering from acute fatty liver of pregnancy.[48]

Increases in electron density suggest condensation of matrical proteins. Such increases are difficult to interpret in micrographs because of variations in specimen fixation, staining, and contrast. Glutaraldehyde-fixed liver specimens stained with uranyl and lead salts always appear to be denser than those fixed in osmium tetroxide alone or those stained exclusively with lead. In mitochondria isolated from liver homogenates and in liver specimens obtained after death, general or patchy condensation of the matrix, with or without concomitant dilatation of the intercristal spaces, is readily seen.[49,50] In vitro, this appearance is reversible when the respiratory stage of the organelle is changed experimentally, but the relevance of the in vitro observations to the interpretation of similar images observed in sections is unclear. Nor is it evident whether the patchy condensation observed in postmortem specimens and that illustrated in Figs. 7 and 13, apparently consisting of tangled fibrils (Fig. 14), are identical. Condensation of the matrix has been observed in alcoholic liver disease,[33] viral hepatitis,[45] halothane hepatitis,[22] Wilson's disease[25,26] citrullinemia,[51] and other conditions.[52]

Mitochondrial Granules

Mitochondrial granules, which are spherical, electron-dense structures, contain calcium, magnesium, inorganic phosphate, carbonate, and a substantial amount of organic material. Since they are relatively few and are irregularly scattered in the matrix, they are difficult to quantitate. Nonetheless, their absence from the mitochondria of some hepatocellular carcinomas[46] and from those of patients with Reye's syndrome[11,12] (Fig. 6) is easy to determine, as is the reduction in the number of granules in the giant mitochondria shown in Figure 5 or the increased abundance of granules noted in hyperthyroid patients.[44] Striking enlargement of the mitochondrial granules and the occasional appearance of electron-lucent vacuoles in them[33,37] are seen in alcoholic liver disease (Figs. 10 and 19), in Wilson's disease[26] (Fig. 18), in systemic sclerosis,[24] and in hyperlipoproteinemia (Fig. 15).

Mitochondrial Myelinlike Figures and Whorls

There may be merely quantitative differences between several types of concentric arrays of membranes encountered in a unique patient with Dubin-Johnson syndrome[53] and those described in some mitochondria of hepatocytes of victims of heatstroke.[54] These arrays are remarkably similar to the myelinlike figures observed in the mitochondria of fasted rats treated with insulin or with both insulin and glucose.[55]

Inclusions

Intramitochondrial bodies may develop through condensation or reorganization of normal constituents of the mitochondrial matrix or through the uptake

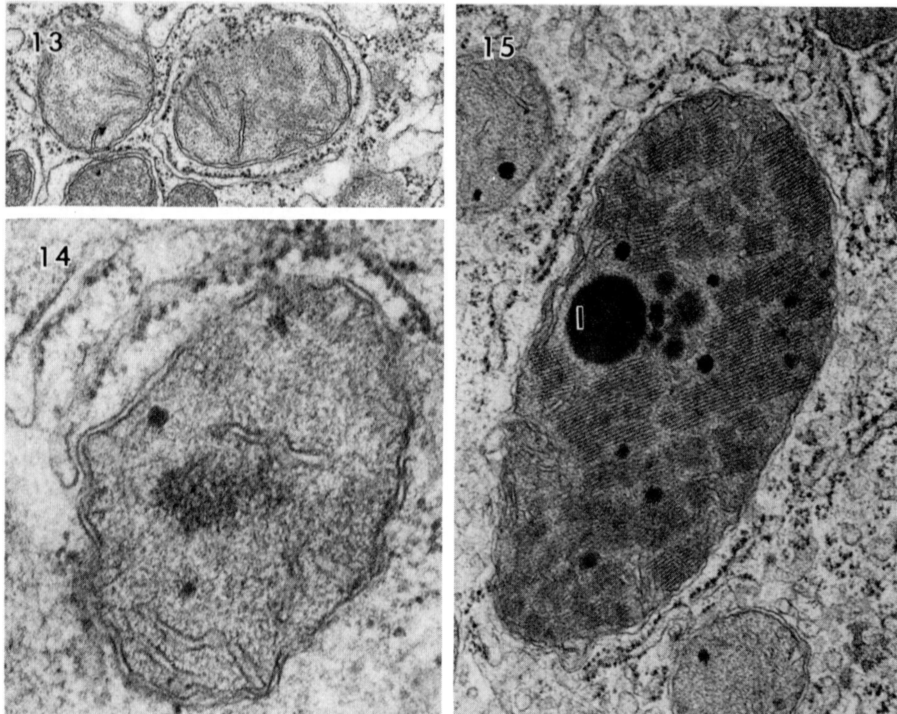

FIGS. 13 and 14—Amorphous condensation of the matrix, apparently containing tangled fibrils (Fig. 14) in the mitochondria of a 64-year-old man suffering from isoniazid-induced hepatitis (Fig. 13, × 17,800; Fig. 14, × 51,000).

FIG. 15—Giant mitochondrion with numerous filamentous crystals and large, round, electron-dense inclusions (I) in a hepatocyte from a patient with type V hyperlipoproteinemia (same as Figs. 4 and 8) (× 11,700).

of nonphysiologic compounds. Despite their frequency, no common denominator responsible for their development has been recognized. The inclusions appear as round or irregularly shaped electron-lucent vacuoles,[56] with or without loose granular contents (Fig. 18); spherical, homogeneous,[19,25,27,40] or laminated [33,57] electron-dense bodies (Figs. 4 and 15); flocculent densities;[49] tubular structures;[24] or orderly arrays of straight (Fig. 16) or helicoidal filaments (Fig. 17).

The most frequently seen inclusions are the filamentous crystals composed of regular arrays of short or long filamentous rods referred to as type A crystals in Table 1. They appear as regularly spaced groups of dots in cross section (Fig. 16). In ellipsoid or elongated mitochondria, the crystals are generally aligned parallel to the long axis (Fig. 4), while in spherical giant mitochondria, they are randomly oriented in the matrix. The numbers and dimensions of the filamentous crystals vary from single crystals, 2–7 μ long and about 0.5 μ wide, to as many as 65 smaller crystals within the section of a single profile.[106] Component filaments range in diameter from 3 to 12 nm, with center-to-center

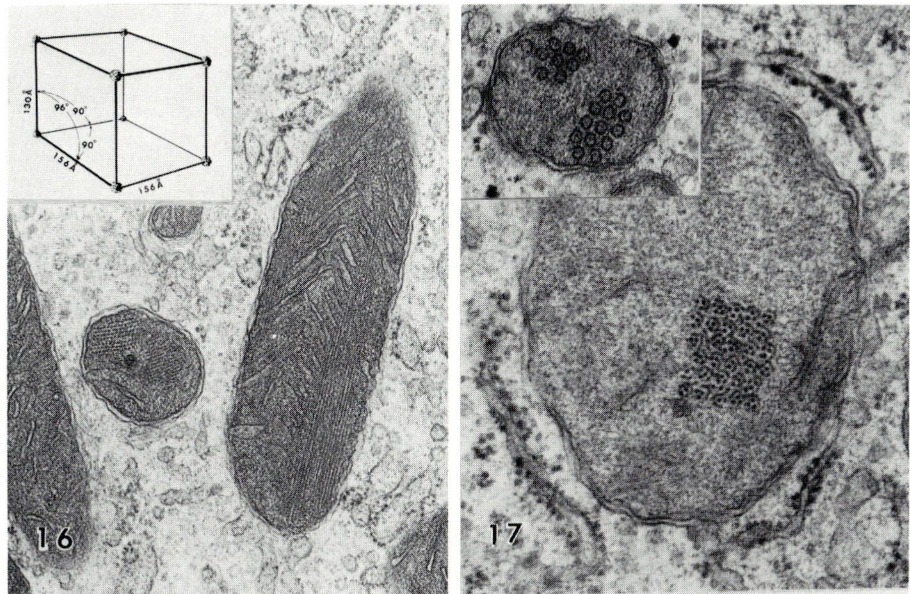

FIG. 16—Longitudinal and transverse section of filamentous (type A) crystals in two adjacent mitochondria from a 19-year-old woman with sickle cell hepatitis. Note the stacking and alignment of the cristae, which in this specimen formed angles of 126°–156° (mean ± SD, 134.6° ± 11.4) with the long axes of the crystals (× 36,000).

FIG. 17—Two sections of type B crystals with an annular appearance (inset) or an arrangement of dots and commas in the mitochondria of a 12-year-old girl suffering from Sydenham's chorea (× 41,500, inset, × 30,000), In longitudinal sections, these inclusions appear like loosely twisted bundles.[49,79]

separations of 5 to 20 nm. The unit cell, the smallest repeating unit of the crystal, is a monoclinic cell with dimensions of 130 × 156 × 156 Å and a face angle of 96° (Fig. 16). These dimensions, determined by optical diffraction analysis,[29,106] correspond to a minimum molecular weight for the crystalline material of about 200,000 daltons and a maximum value of about 1.5×10^6 daltons.[29] The constant 120°–140° angle of inclination formed by the spatial relationship of the stacked cristae to the filaments,[29,34] as well as observations made with the aid of a goniometric stage,[83] strongly suggests continuity between cristal membranes and filaments and the likelihood of a common origin.[35] There are no clues, however, to the nature of the factors or agencies by which the composition and configuration of the cristal membranes and the appearance of the crystals are effected.

Although type A crystals are common in the mitochrondria of pathologic specimens, they are not necessarily present in the most severely altered cells, as shown in a systematic stereologic study on patients with fatty livers following jejunoileal bypass.[35] Crystals and giant mitochondria tended to occur predominantly in juxtaportal hepatocytes, rather than in the centrally located cells containing excess fat. Despite this topographic dissociation and increased abundance of crystals in specimens with moderate rather than severe steatosis,

TABLE 1.—*Conditions Associated with Hepatic Mitochondrial Crystals**

	References	
	Type A Crystals	Type B Crystals
Physiologic Conditions		
Normal subjects	58	
Old age	3,59	
Pregnancy	60	
Hepatitis		
Viral hepatitis	23,34,49,64,65	
Chronic active hepatitis	93	
Disorders of bile secretion		
Biliary duct obstruction	64	
Cholesterol cholelithiasis	66	66
Intrahepatic cholestasis	32,34,67,104	
Primary biliary cirrhosis	68	
Toxic liver injury		
Alcohol	16,18–20,69–71	70
Amanita phalloides	72,73	
Lead	34	
Paraquat	74	
Vinyl chloride	75	
Metabolic diseases		
Amyloidosis	76	77
Diabetes mellitus	23,78	
Dubin-Johnson syndrome	80	79
Fucosidosis	81	
Gilbert's syndrome	82–85	85,86
Glycogenosis, type III	91	
Hyperlipoproteinemia, types I, IV, and V	23,28,71	
Hyperthyroidism	44,71	
Mucopolysaccharidosis (Sanfilippo type)	14	
Porphyria cutanea tarda	71,87,88	
Protein-calorie malnutrition	89	
Rotor's syndrome	82,90	
Steatosis associated with obesity	23	
Steatosis following jejunoileal bypass	35	
Wilson's disease	25,26,29,92	
Hematologic diseases		
Iron deficiency anemia	71	
Sickle cell disease	29	
Systemic infections		
Amebiasis	61	61
Leptospirosis	62,71	
Plasmodium vivax malaria	63	
Pneumococcal meningitis	34	
Collagen diseases		
Disseminated lupus erythematosus	34	
Systemic sclerosis	24	24
Neoplastic disorders		
Hepatic adenomas	52	
Hepatocellular carcinoma	10	
Metastatic liver disease	46,71,94	
Waldenström's disease	95	

TABLE 1.—*Conditions Associated with Hepatic Mitochondrial Crystals* (cont'd)*

	References	
	Type A Crystals	Type B Crystals
Drugs		
Acetylsalicylic acid	96	
Bishexestrol dihydrochloride	97	
Chlorpropamide	98	
Clofibrate	7	
Contraceptive pills	99,100	100
Diphenylhydantoin	101	
Halothane	22,40,102	
Lidoflazine	103	
Nicotinic acid	104	
Phenothiazine	34	
Miscellaneous conditions		
Cachexia	49	
Heatstroke	54	
Sydenham's chorea	Fig. 17	

**I apologize to all the authors whose reports on other conditions associated with mitochondrial crystals may have been overlooked.*

a clear temporal relation was present between steatosis and the occurrence of crystals. Moreover, with diminishing steatosis the latter tended to disappear, a phenomenon also observed in patients with Wilson's disease following treatment with D-penicillamine.[107]

Less frequent, although quite distinctive, are type B crystals, which are composed of bundles of tubules that have an annular appearance in some sections (Fig. 17) and in other sections appear either as several dots and a small arc of a fibril, resembling an asterisk (Fig. 17), or as undulating lines.[70,100] These crystals, occur in some of the same disorders, but usually not in the same specimen, as type A crystals (Table 1). These structures may be composed of helices, an interpretation supported by observations on similar structures composed of nine helical fibrils forming a tubular structure in the hepatic mitochondria of rhesus monkeys.[108]

To what extent do crystals signal the presence of a pathologic process? Because of their occurrence in so many disorders, while being an inconstant finding in any one of them, mitochondrial crystals have no diagnostic value. Nonetheless, they seem to be indicators of a disordered metabolic state, even though, on occasion, they are seen in livers that superficially fulfill the clinical and light-microscopic criteria of normality. Possibly, the liver of the alleged "normal" subject with mitochondrial crystals may have been affected by nutrition, drugs, or inapparent toxins, because in a systematic study in which mitochondrial crystals were looked for in liver biopsy specimens obtained at laparotomy from 77 adults, 32 of whom had gallbladder disease, crystals were found only in two specimens.[109] This observation is in stark contrast with results reported from an earlier study conducted in Spain in which a high

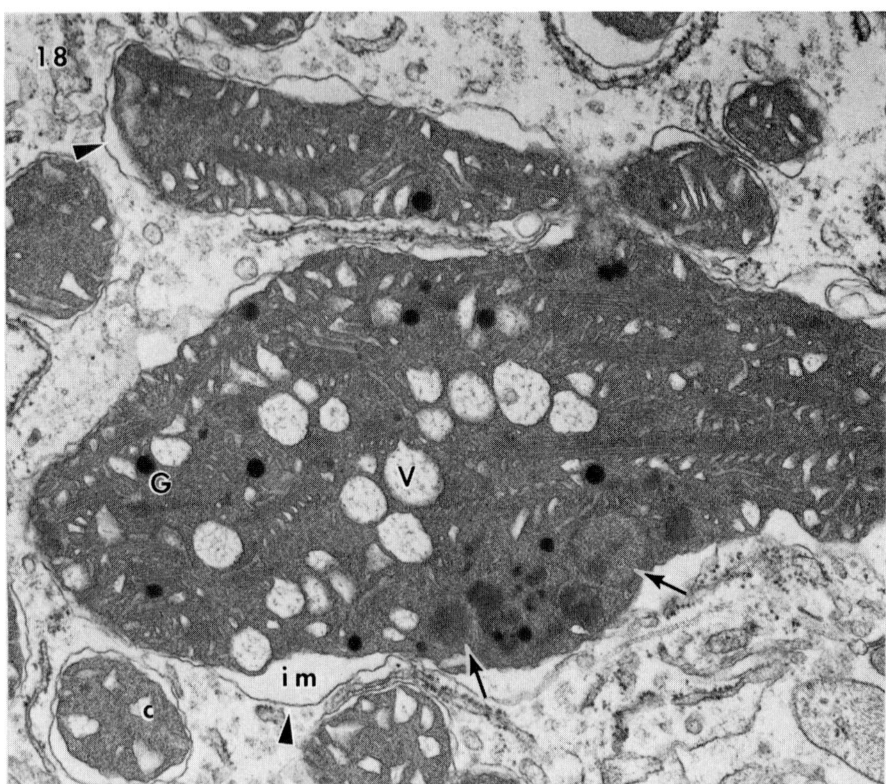

FIG. 18—Portion of hepatocyte from a 28-year-old woman with Wilson's disease, hepatic steatosis, and a copper content of 1039 μg/g dry liver. Note the separations of the redundant outer
membranes (arrowhead) creating dilated intermembranous spaces (im). Some cristal spaces (c) are
dilated both in the normal-sized and in the giant mitochondria. The latter also display filamentous
crystals, vacuoles with granular contents (V), round inclusions of varying electron density (arrows), and enlarged granules ($\times$ 17,000).

incidence of mitochondrial crystals was observed in liver biopsy specimens
from similar patients.[66] Obviously, factors other than gallstones must contribute to this high incidence of crystals in the Spanish patients. No comparable
data on the incidence of mitochondrial crystals in most of the conditions listed
in Table 1 are available, because the observation for several of these crystals
are based on single case reports.

Interactions with Other Cytoplasmic Organelles and Membranes

Mitochondria interact metabolically with most of the components of the
cell's cytoplasm. This is evident from the virtually constant topographical relationship of cisternae of rough endoplasmic reticulum that partially envelop
the mitochondria. This structural closeness seems to be required for cytochrome P-450 synthesis.[110] It is common for the same cisterna to be in close
relationship to a peroxisome as well, suggesting that the three organelles form
a functional unit.[111]

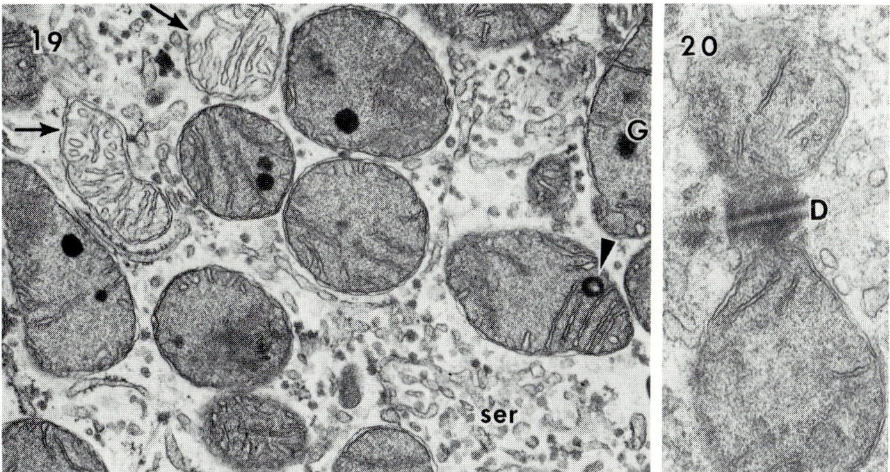

FIG. 19—Portion of hepatocyte from a patient with alcoholic hepatitis (same as in Figs. 5 and 10) with some mitochondria with parallel arrays of cristae. The granules contained in the other mitochondria are enlarged, and one of them is vacuolated (arrowhead). Note the presence of shrunken, degenerated mitochondria (arrows), having a ghostlike appearance without indication of autophagy (× 21,600).

FIG. 20—Mitochondrion-desmosome complex involving two hepatocytes from a normal subject (× 35,000).

An entirely different relationship is that of mitochondria with desmosomes. As shown in Figure 20, mitochondria may get trapped in the filaments on both sides of a desmosome, suggesting that the desmosomes may serve as routes of intercellular communication.[112] This phenomenon is seen in other tissues and other species as well.

PEROXISOMES

Normal Peroxisomes

Under the electron microscope, peroxisomes or microbodies are fairly easily recognizable in human hepatocytes as intracellular bodies with round, ellipsoid, slightly angular or occasionally elongated, irregular, and even misshapen outlines. They contain a homogeneous, amorphous, finely granular or flocculent, noncompartmentalized matrix, surrounded by a single tripartite membrane (Figs. 21 and 23). They are randomly distributed in the cytoplasm or arrange themselves in clusters. Their numbers vary from section to section and from cell to cell even in normal specimens. On average, there are about 1,000 peroxisomes,[2] with diameters ranging from 0.25 to 1.34 μ and a mean of 0.62 μ per hepatocyte.[111] In both normal and pathologic specimens, certain peroxisomes display peripheral electron-dense bands, approximately 27 nm wide and up to 0.4 μ long, which flatten the organelle's profile (Fig. 23). In other peroxisomes, the matrix contains an array of regularly spaced, electron-dense rods of uniform diameter, arranged in parallel and supported by fine

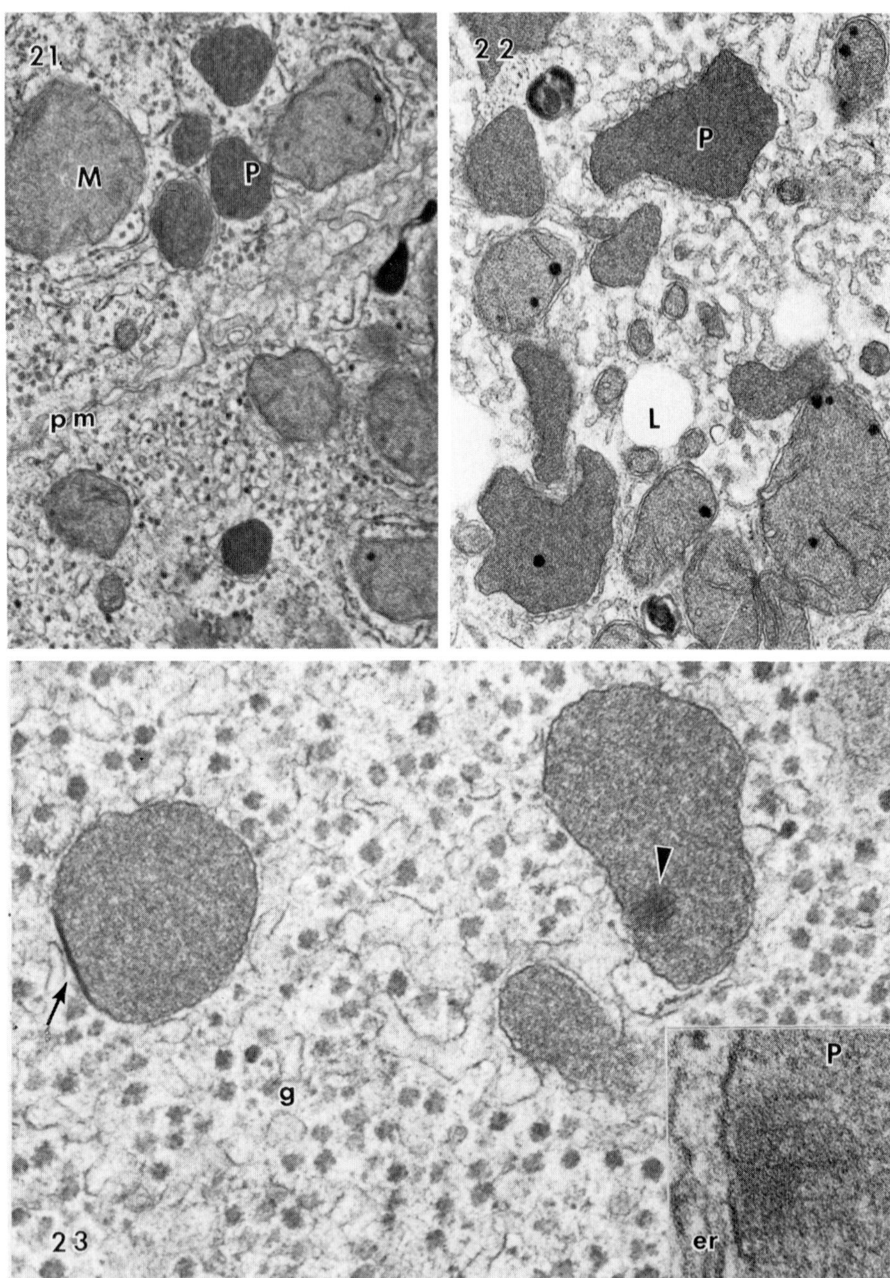

FIG. 21—Portions of two hepatocytes from a 15-year-old normal boy containing peroxisomes with diameters that are smaller than those of the neighboring mitochondria ($\times$ 13,200).

FIG. 22—Greatly enlarged misshapen peroxisomes in the hepatocyte of a patient with HB_s Ag-positive chronic active hepatitis ($\times$ 16,900).

FIG. 23—Portion of a hepatocyte of a normal subject (same as Fig. 21) demonstrates a marginal plate (arrow) and a peripheral crystalline inclusion (arrowhead) in different peroxisomes. ($\times$ 40,500) Another crystalline inclusion is also shown in detail ($\times$ 97,000).

transversely oriented filamentous bands (Fig. 23, insert). These crystalline inclusions, with their perpendicularly oriented longitudinal axis, seem either to be attached to or to arise from the periphery of the organelle and seem to favor the area of apposition of the endoplasmic reticulum.[111] So far, it has not been possible to resolve the discrete components of these inclusions.

The peroxisomes appear to be integrated with other cytoplasmic organelles, particularly with the endoplasmic reticulum, both through direct continuities and through intimate apposition of endoplasmic reticulum along a portion of the body's outline (Figs. 23 and 24). The cisternae that envelop part of a peroxisome are devoid of ribosomes at the level of apposition (Fig. 24). Occasionally, a single cisterna seems to form a bridge by wrapping itself around neighboring peroxisomes and mitochondria (Fig. 21). Apparent multiplication of peroxisomes, through budding, is observed infrequently[111] (Fig. 24).

Abnormalities of Peroxisomes

Changes in Number

An absence of hepatocellular peroxisomes is characteristic of Zellweger's cerebrohepatorenal syndrome.[113] In many other pathologic conditions the peroxisomes become more numerous, being distribued throughout the cytoplasm or aggregating in clusters. This phenomenon is seen in various forms of hep-

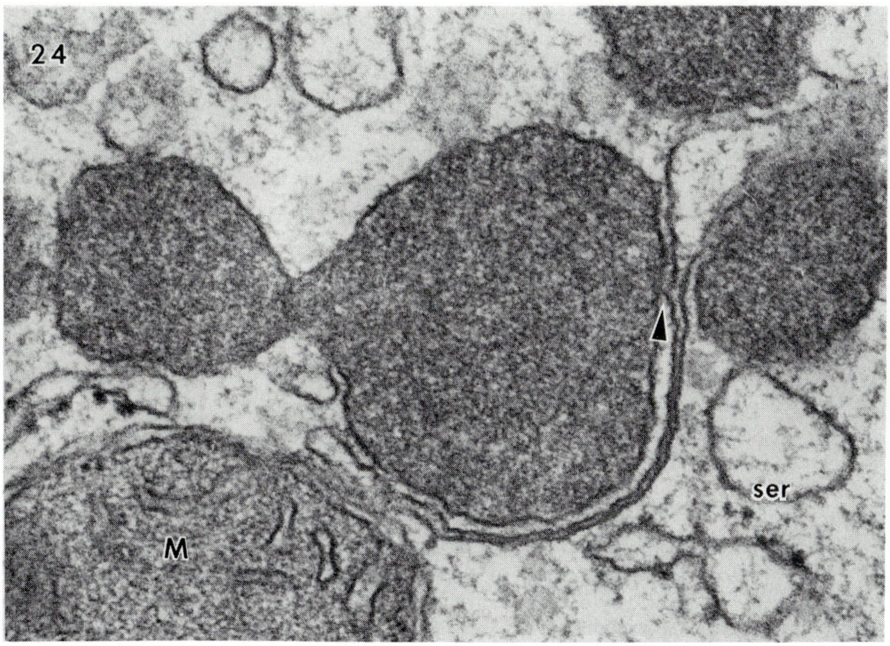

FIG. 24—High-power electron micrograph of portion of a hepatocyte from a 34-year-old man with chronic active hepatitis after treatment with prednisone. The central peroxisome seems to be in the process of dividing. Note the presence of threadlike junctions (arrowhead) between the peroxisome and the membrane of the cisterna of the endoplasmic reticulum ($\times$ 52,000).

atitis,[114,115] in Reye's syndrome,[12,116] in alcoholic liver disease, [117] in cholestatic jaundice of pregnancy[105] and following therapy with clofibrate[7] or 6-mercaptopurine.[118] By contrast with the rat, however, in which clofibrate induces a remarkable proliferation of hepatocellular peroxisomes, in human hepatocytes, the drug seems to predominantly affect the mitochondria.[7]

Changes in Size and Shape

Either a reduction or an increase in the average size of peroxisomes is likely to occur in pathologic conditions. In our study of a series of 16 pathologic specimens we found only 2 with normal-sized organelles. Moderate to striking increases were noted in chronic active hepatitis, familial cholestatic cirrhosis, isoniazid hepatitis, and untreated Wilson's disease.[111] Enlargement was also noted in a patient with cholestasis.[119] The shapes of the peroxisomes are also affected, resulting in irregular outlines (Fig. 22) or ballooning (Fig. 26) of the organelles. The frequency of marginal plates that partially flatten the outlines of the peroxisomes is increased in some pathologic specimens.

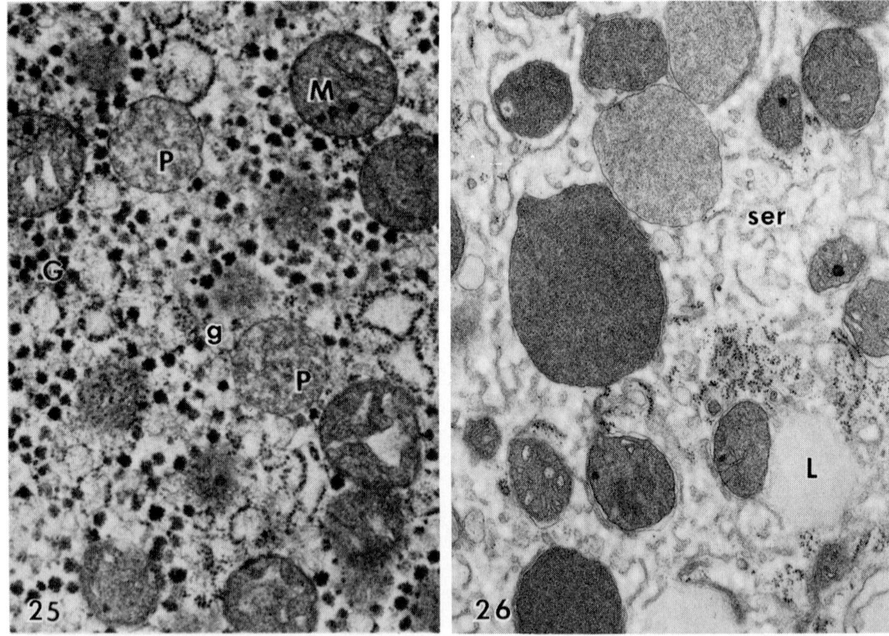

FIG. 25—Portion of hepatocyte from a 36-year-old woman with alcoholic liver disease. Some of the cristal spaces of mitochondria (M) are dilated, and the peroxisomal (P) matrix appears flocculent (× 20,500).

FIG. 26—Portion of hepatocyte from a 9-year-old boy with Wilson's disease containing pleomorphic, greatly enlarged peroxisomes with different matrical densities (cf. diameters with those of the mitochondria) (× 10,500).

Consistency of Matrix

A reduction or an increase in the electron density of the matrix, suggesting either swelling or condensation, can be seen in ballooned peroxisomes. The latter is more frequent in diseased hepatocytes, as noted in viral hepatitis, Wilson's disease, hepatocellular carcinoma, and other disorders.[111] Flocculation of the matrix is seen in alcoholic liver disease (Fig. 25), in familial cholestatic cirrhosis, and occasionally in Wilson's disease.[111]

Inclusions

Amorphous electron-dense inclusions are seen in the peroxisomes of normal hepatocytes[1,111] but are more common and more prominent in pathologic specimens.[26,41,111] Unique inclusions that resemble the uricase-containing core of rat peroxisomes were encountered in the peroxisomes of a patient with benign recurrent cholestatis.[120]

INTERPRETATION OF MITOCHONDRIAL AND PEROXISOMAL ABNORMALITIES

In a departure from traditions, this review has focused on the component elements of mitochondria and peroxisomes rather than on the disease processes that affect these organelles. What emerged is a kaleidoscopic series of images that indicate that an amazing range of reactions is elicited when the hepatocyte's homeostatic mechanisms are disrupted. Some reactions may represent attempts at adaptation[35,121] or, conversely, may signal a mobilization of the cell's defenses against injury.

Among the changes reviewed, the mitochondrial crystals illustrate how difficult it is to define the line that separates organelle health from organelle disease. Yet such a definition is crucial to the understanding of the significance of the observed changes. Although the descriptions provide little insight into the pathogenesis of hepatocellular lesions, they indicate that a multiplicity of molecular processes is involved in the observed configurational changes. Many of these changes cannot be reproduced in animals because of species-specificity. Therefore, human biopsy material is required for the identification of the biochemical events that underlie the ultrastructural changes. However, the average value obtained from enzymatic assays of homogenates of either surgical[122,123] or needle biopsy specimens[124] are incapable of identifying abnormalities of components of heterogeneous populations of organelles. New approaches, including a more intensive use of electron dispersion microanalysis and cytochemistry are required for the clarification of the puzzling events that are uncovered by the electron microscope when hepatocellular injury takes place.

ACKNOWLEDGMENTS

The superb technical assistance of Nelson Quintana and Phyllis Grushoff is gratefully acknowledged. Photographs were prepared by Marianne Van-Hooren.

REFERENCES

1. Ma MH, Biempica L: The normal human liver cell. Cytochemical and ultrastructural study. Am J Pathol 62:353–390, 1971
2. Rohr HP, Luthy J, Gudat F, Oberholzer M, Gysin C, Stalder G, Bianchi L: Stereology: A new supplement to the study of human liver biopsy specimens. Edited by H Popper and F Schaffner: Progress in Liver Diseases. Vol. V. New York, Grune & Stratton, 1976, pp 24–34
3. Sato T, Tauchi H: The formation of enlarged and giant mitochondria in the aging process of human hepatic cells. Acta Pathol Jap 25:403–412, 1975
4. Slabodsky-Brousse N, Feldmann G, Brousse J, Dreyfus P: Stereological study on the frequency of hepatic giant mitochondria in patients with Gilbert's disease as compared with a normal control group. Biol Gastroenterol (Paris) 7:179–186, 1974
5. Koch OR, Gamboni M: Alteraciones ultraestructurales de las mitochondrias del higado en alcoholistas sin enfermedad hepatica. Medicina (Buenos Aires) 37:351–357, 1977
6. Oudéa MC, Colette M, Dedieu P, Oudéa P: Morphometric study of the ultrastructure of human alcoholic fatty liver. Biomedicine 19:455–459, 1973
7. Hanefeld M, Kemmer C, Leonhardt W, Jaross W: Der Effekt der Regardin (CPIB)-therapie von Hyperlipoproteinämien (HLP) auf die Leber. Dtsch Gesundh-Wesen 32:2267–2270, 1977
8. Toker C, Trevino N: Ultrastructure of human primary hepatocellular carcinoma. Cancer 19:1594–1606, 1966
9. Ruebner BH, Gonzalez-Licea A, Slusser RJ: Electron microscopy of some human hepatomas. Gastroenterology 53:18–30, 1967
10. O'Conor GT, Tralka TS, Henson E, Vogel CL: Ultrastructural survey of primary liver cell carcinomas from Uganda. J Natl Cancer Inst 48:587–603, 1972
11. Partin JC, Schubert WK, Partin JS: Mitochondrial ultrastructure in Reye's syndrome (encephalopathy and fatty degeneration of viscera) N Engl J Med 285:1339–1343, 1971
12. Iancu TC, Mason WH, Neustein HB: Ultrastructural abnormalities of liver cells in Reye's syndrome. Hum Pathol 8:421–431, 1977
13. Haust MD: Mitochondrial budding and morphogenesis of cytoplasmic vacuoles in hepatocytes of children with the Hurler syndrome and Sanfilippo disease. Exp Mol Pathol 9:242–257, 1968
14. Haust MD: Crystalloid structures of hepatic mitochondria in children with heparitin sulphate mucopolysaccharidosis (Sanfilippo type) Exp Mol Pathol 8:123–134, 1968
15. Gaull GE, Schaffner F: Electron microscopic changes in hepatocytes of patients with homocystinuria. Pediatr Res 5:23–32, 1971
16. Porta EA, Bergman BJ, Stein AA: Acute alcoholic hepatitis. Am J Pathol 46:657–689, 1965
17. Iseri OA, Gottlieb LS: Alcoholic hyalin and megamitochondria as separate and distinct entities in liver disease associated with alcoholism. Gastroenterology 60:1027–1035, 1971
18. Albot G, Parturier-Albot M: Les mégamitochondries de l'hépatocyte. Ann Gastroenterol Hépatol 8:1–12, 1972
19. Oudéa P, Feldmann G, Domart-Oudéa MC: L'hépatite alcoholique. Etude au microscope électronique. Rev Int Hépatol (Paris) 18:155–170, 1968
20. Ma MH: Ultrastructural pathologic findings of the human hepatocyte. I. Alcoholic liver disease. Arch Pathol 94:554–571, 1972
21. Hug G, Schubert WK: Idiopathic cardiomyopathy. Mitochondrial and cytoplasmic alterations in heart and liver. Lab Invest 22:541–552, 1970
22. Uznalimoglu B, Yardley JH, Boitnott JK: The liver in mild halothane hepatitis. Am J Pathol 61:457–478, 1970
23. Bhagwat AG, Ross RC: Hepatic intramitochondrial crystalloids. Arch Pathol 91:70–77, 1971
24. Feldmann G, Maurice M, Husson JM, Fiessinger JN, Camilleri JP, Benhamou JP, Housset E: Hepatocyte giant mitochondria: An almost constant lesion in systemic scleroderma. Virchows Arch Pathol 374:215–227, 1977
25. Sternlieb I: Mitochondrial and fatty changes in hepatocytes of patients with Wilson's disease. Gastroenterology 55:354–367, 1968
26. Sternlieb, I: Evolution of the hepatic lesion in Wilson's disease (hepatolenticular degeneration). Edited by H Popper and F

Schaffner: Progress in Liver Diseases. Vol. IV. New York, Grune & Stratton 1972, pp 511–525

27. Ghadially FN, Parry EW: Ultrastructure of a human hepatocellular carcinoma and surrounding non-neoplastic liver. Cancer 19:1989–2004, 1966

28. Kovacs K, Lee R, Little JA: Ultrastructural changes of hepatocytes in hyperlipoproteinaemia. Lancet 1:752–753, 1972

29. Sternlieb I, Berger JE: Optical diffraction studies of crystalline structures in electron micrographs. II. Crystalline inclusions in mitochondria of human hepatocytes. J Cell Biol 43:448–455, 1969

30. Klion FM, Schaffner F: Ultrastructural studies in alcoholic liver disease. Digestion 1:2–14, 1968

31. Balazs M, Varkonyi S, Pinter A: Electron microscopic study of alcoholic liver disease with special attention to the changes of mesenchymal cells of the liver. Exp Pathol 14:340–350, 1977

32. Claude A: Mitochondrial cristae during liver regeneration. Protoplasma 63:275–282, 1967

33. Horvath E, Kovacs K, Ross RC: Alcoholic liver lesion. Frequency and diagnostic value of the fine structural alterations of hepatocytes. Beitr Pathol 148:67–85, 1972

34. Spycher MA, Rüttner JR: Kristalloide Einschlüsse in menschlichen Lebermitochondrien. Virchows Arch [Zellpathol] 1:211–221, 1968

35. Friedman HI, Chandler JG, Nemeth TJ: Hepatic intramitochondrial filaments in morbidly obese patients undergoing intestinal bypass. Gastroenterology 73:1353–1361, 1977

36. Jézéquel AM, Orlandi F: Fine morphology of the human liver as a tool in clinical pharmacology. Edited by F Orlandi and JM Jezequel: Liver and Drugs. New York, Academic Press, 1972, pp 145–192

37. Tanikawa K: Ultrastructural Aspects of the Liver and Its Disorders. New York, Springer, 1968

38. Popper H, Schaffner F: The pathophysiology of cholestasis. Hum Pathol 1:1–24, 1970

39. Koch MM, Jézéquel AM, Capurso L, Freddara U, Lorenzini I, Orlandi F: The ultrastructure of hepatocytes in cholestrol cholithiasis patients: A quantitative study before and during chenodeoxycholic (CDCA) therapy. Rendic Gastroenterol 9:243, 1977

40. Wills EJ, Walton B: A morphologic study of unexplained hepatitis following halothane anesthesia. Am J Pathol 91:11–32, 1978

41. Jézéquel AM, Capurso L, Freddara U, Orlandi F: Cholestasis in man. Reevaluation of ultrastructural data. Fegato 20:299–314, 1974

42. Frenkel EP, Mukherjee A, Hackenbrock CR, Srere PA: Biochemical and ultrastructural hepatic changes during vitamin B12 deficiency in animals and man. J Biol Chem 251:2147–2154, 1976

43. Jakovcic S, Swift HH, Gross NJ, Rabinowitz M: Biochemical and stereological analysis of rat liver mitochondria in different thyroid states. J Cell Biol 77:887–901, 1978

44. Klion FM, Segal R, Schaffner F: The effect of altered thyroid function on the ultrastructure of the human liver. Am J Med 50:317–324, 1971

45. Pavel I, Bonaparte H, Petrovici A: Involution of liver mitochondria in viral hepatitis. Arch Pathol 91:294–301, 1971

46. Ma MH, Blackburn CRB: Structure of primary liver tumors and tumor-bearing livers in man. Cancer Res 33:1766–1774, 1973

47. Safran AP, Schaffner F: Chronic passive congestion of the liver in man. Am J Pathol 50:447–463, 1967

48. Bertram PD, Anderson GD, Kelly S, Sabesin SM: Ultrastructural alterations in acute fatty liver of pregnancy: Similarity to Reye's syndrome. Gastroenterology 74:1008, 1978

49. Ruffolo R, Covington H: Matrix inclusion bodies in the mitochondria of the human liver. Am J Pathol 51:101–116, 1967

50. Trump BF, Kim KM, Jones RT, Valigorsky JM: Pathology of organelles. Edited by H Popper and F Schaffner: Progress in Liver Diseases. Vol. V. New York, Grune & Stratton, 1976, pp 51–68

51. Mihatsch MJ, Riede UN, Ohnacker H, Wick H, Bachmann C: Liver morphology in a case of citrullinemia (a light and electron microscopic study). Beitr Pathol 151:200–207, 1974

52. Horvath E, Kovacs K, Ross RC: Ultrastructural findings in a well-differentiated hepatoma. Digestion 7:74–82, 1972

53. Enat R, Barzilai D: Mitochondrial pathology in the liver in a patient with Dubin-Johnson syndrome. Isr J Med Sci 13:1197–1205, 1977

54. Kew MC, Minick OT, Bahu RM, Stein RJ, Kent G: Ultrastructural changes in the liver in heatstroke. Am J Pathol 90:609–618, 1978

55. LeBeux Y, Hetenyi G Jr, Phillips MJ: Mitochondrial myelinlike figures: A non-specific reactive process of mitochondrial phospholipid membranes to several stimuli. Z Zellforsch 99:491–506, 1969

56. Ancla A, Beaumont V: Etude du foie au microscope électronique dans deux variétés d'hyperlipidemies majeures. Pathol Biol (Paris) 14:23–24, 1966

57. Burns W, Vander Weide G, Chan C: Laminated mitochondrial inclusions in hepatocytes of liver biopsies. Arch Pathol 94:74–80, 1972

58. Wills EJ: Crystalline structures in the mitochondria of normal human liver parenchymal cells. J Cell Biol 24:511–514, 1965

59. Findor J, Perez V, Bruch Igartua E, Giovanetti M, Fioravantti N: Structure and ultrastructure of the liver in aged persons. Acta Hepato gastroenterol (Stuttg) 20:200–204, 1973

60. Gonzalez-Angulo A, Aznar-Ramos R, Marquez-Monter H, Bierzwinsky G, Martinez-Manautou J: The ultrastructure of liver cells in women under steroid therapy. Acta Endocrinol 65:193–206, 1970

61. Tandon BN, Tandon HD, Puri BK: An electron microscopic study of liver hepatomegaly presumably caused by amebiasis. Exp Mol Pathol 22:118–132, 1975

62. Sandborn EB, Cote C, Viallet A: Electron microscopy of a human liver in Weil's disease (leptospirosis icterohaemorrhagica). J Pathol Bacteriol 92:369–374, 1966

63. Brito T, Barone AA, Faria RM: Human liver biopsy in *P. falciparum* and *P. vivax* malaria. A light and electron microscopy study. Virchows Arch [Pathol Anat] 348:220–229, 1969

64. Jézéquel AM: Dégénérescence myélinique des mitochondries du foie humain dans un épithelioma du choledoque et un ictère viral. Etude au microscope électronique. J Ultrastruct Res 2:210–215, 1959

65. Wills EJ: Acute infective hepatitis. Fine structural and cytochemical alterations in human liver. Arch Pathol 86:184–207, 1968

66. Gomez Lazara C, Caro-Paton A, Coca MC: Intramitochondrial paracrystalline inclusions in hepatocytes of patients with biliary lithiasis. Lancet 2:1417–1418, 1972

67. Orlandi F: Electron microscope observation on human liver during cholestasis. Acta Hepatosplenol 9:155–164, 1962

68. Chedid A, Spellberg MA, DeBeer RA: Ultrastructural aspects of primary biliary cirrhosis and other types of cholestatic liver disease. Gastroenterology 67:858–869, 1974

69. Lane BP, Lieber CS: Ultrastructural alterations in human hepatocytes following ingestion of ethanol with adequate diets. Am J Pathol 49:593–603, 1966

70. Svoboda DJ, Manning RT: Chronic alcoholism with fatty metamorphosis of the liver. Am J Pathol 44:645–662, 1964

71. Mandel EM, Lewiniski V, Gafter U, Weiss S, Djaldetti M: The presence of hepatic intramitochondrial crystalline inclusions in routine liver biopsies. Am J Med Sci 274:61–67, 1977

72. Panner BJ, Hanss RJ: Hepatic injury in mushroom poisoning. Electron microscope observations of two nonfatal cases. Arch Pathol 87:35–45, 1969

73. Kisilevsky R: Hepatic nuclear and nucleolar changes in *Amanita* poisoning. Arch Pathol 97:253–258, 1974

74. Borchard F, Grabensee B, Jax W, Huth F: Morphologische Befunde bei Paraquatvergiftungen. Klin Wochenschr 52:657–671, 1974

75. Schattenberg P-J, Totovic V, Gedigk P, Marsteller HJ: Die Ultrastruktur der Leberschädigung bei der chronischen Vinylchlorid-Intoxikation. Virchows Arch [Pathol Anat] 373:233–247, 1977

76. Thiéry JP, Caroli J: Etude au microscope électronique de l'amylose hépatique primaire de l'homme. Semain Hôp (Paris) 37:29–40, 1961

77. Oudéa P, Domart-Oudéa M-C, Fauvert R: L'ultrastructure hépatique. II. Le foie pathologique. Rev Fr Etud Clin Biol 12:641–665, 1967

78. Laguens R, Bianchi N: Fine structure of the liver in human idiopathic diabetes mellitus. I. Parenchymal cell mitochondria. Exp Mol Pathol 2:203–214, 1963

79. Minio F, Magnenat P, Gardiol D, Gautier A: L'ultrastructure du foie humain lors d'ictères idiopathiques chroniques. I. Z Zellforsch 65:47–56, 1965

80. Minio F, Gautier A: L'ultrastructure du foie humain lors d'ictères idiopathiques chroniques. IV. Mitochondries de morphologie inhabituelle et "inclusions cyto-

plasmiques paracristallines'' hépatocytaires. Z Zellforsch 78:267–279, 1967

81. Freitag F, Kuchemann K, Blumcke S, Spranger J: Hepatic ultrastructure in fucosidosis. Virchows Arch [Pathol Anat] 7:99–113, 1971

82. Novikoff AB, Essner E: The liver cell, some new approaches to its study. Am J Med 29:102–131, 1960

83. Schaff Z, Lapis K, André J: Study of the tridimensional structure of intramitochondrial crystalline inclusions. J Microsc 20:259–264, 1974

84. Schaff Z, Lapis K, André J: Effect of proteolytic digestion on mitochondrial crystalline inclusions in Gilbert's syndrome. J Microsc 20:265–270, 1974

85. Feldmann G, Oudéa P, Domart-Oudéa MC, Molas G, Fauvert R: L'ultrastructure hépatique au cours de la maladie de Gilbert. Pathol Biol (Paris) 16:943–953, 1968

86. Barth RF, Grimley PM, Berk PD, Bloomer JR, Howe RB: Excess lipofuscin accumulation in constitutional hepatic dysfunction (Gilbert's syndrome). Arch Pathol 91:41–47, 1971

87. Waldo ED, Tobias H: Needle-like cytoplasmic inclusions in the liver in porphyria cutanea tarda. Arch Pathol 96:368–371, 1973

88. Moreno A, Navarro V, Oliva H: Lesiones granulomatosas con inclusiones cristalinas en la porfiria hepatocutanea. Rev Clin Esp 146:117–120, 1977

89. Tandon BN, Ramanujan RA, Tandon HD, Puri BK, Gandhi PC: Liver injury in protein-calorie malnutrition: an electron microscopic study. Am J Clin Nutr 27:550–558, 1974

90. Brito T, Borges A, daSilva LC: Electron microscopy of the liver in non hemolytic acholuric jaundice with kernicterus (Crigler-Najjar) and in idiopathic conjugated hyperbilirubinemia (Rotor). Gastroenterologia (Basel) 106:325–335, 1966

91. Leung TK, Feroldi J: Etude au microscope électronique du foie et du muscle de deux cas de glycogénose type III. Pathol Eur 7:112–125, 1972

92. Feldmann G, Groussard O, Fauvert R: L'ultrastructure hépatique au cours de la maladie de Wilson. Biol Gastroenterol 2:137–160, 1969

93. Gerlach U, Manitz G, Themann H: Feinstrukturelle Untersuchungen bei aktiver chronischer Hepatitis unter besonderer Berücksichtigung des Mesenchymes. Acta Hepatosplenol 16:90–105, 1969

94. Albukerk J, Duffy JL: Ultrastructural alterations in livers in metastasis. Arch Pathol Lab Med 100:168–171, 1976

95. Rouiller C, Jézéquel AM: Electron microscopy of the liver. Edited by C Rouiller: The Liver. Vol. 1. New York, Academic Press, 1963, pp 195–232

96. Iancu T, Elian E: Ultrastructural changes in aspirin hepatotoxicity. Am J Clin Pathol 66:570–575, 1976

97. De La Iglesia FA, Feuer G, Takada A, Matsuda Y: Morphologic studies on secondary phospholipidosis in human liver. Lab Invest 30:539–549, 1974

98. Reichel J, Goldberg SB, Ellenberg M, Schaffner F: Intrahepatic cholestasis following administration of chlorpropamide. Am J Med 28:654–660, 1960

99. Perez V, Gorodisch S, De Martina J, Nicholson R, Di Paola G: Oral contraceptives: Long-term use produces fine structural changes in mitochondria. Science 165:805–807, 1969

100. Martinez-Manautou J, Aznar-Ramos R, Bautista-O'Farrill J, Gonzalez-Angulo A: The ultrastructure of liver cells in women under steroid therapy. II Contraceptive therapy. Acta Endocrinol 65:207–221, 1970

101. Hoyumpa AM, Kim OJ, Scott WT, Schiff L: Electron microscopic changes in dilantin hepatitis. Gastroenterology 52:317, 1969

102. Klion FM, Schaffner F, Popper H: Hepatitis after exposure to halothane. Ann Intern Med 71:467–477, 1969

103. Verheyen A, Borgers M, Blaton H, Sowa H: The ultrastructure of human livers after prolonged lidoflazine therapy. Toxicol Appl Pharmacol 34:224–232, 1975

104. Baggentoss AH, Christensen NA, Berge KG, Baldus WP, Spiekerman RE, Ellefson RD: Fine structural changes in the liver in hypercholesteremic patients receiving long-term nicotinic acid therapy. Mayo Clin Proc 42:385–399, 1967

105. VanHaelst U, Bergstein N: Electron microscopic study of the liver in so-called idiopathic jaundice of late pregnancy. Pathol Eur 5:198–215, 1970

106. Themann H, von Bassewitz DB: Parakristalline Einschlusskorper der Mitochondrien des menschlichen Leberparenchysms. Elektonenmikroskopische und

histochemische Untersuchungen. Cytobiologie 1:135–151, 1969

107. Sternlieb I, Feldmann G: Effects of anticopper therapy on hepatocellular mitochondria in patients with Wilson's disease. Gastroenterology 71:457–461, 1976

108. Ruebner BH, Aguirre J, Brayton MA, Watanabe K: Inclusions with helical substructure in hepatocyte mitochondria of rhesus monkeys. J Ultrastr Res 35:499–507, 1971

109. Burnett W, Furnival C, Holland P, Molyneus G, Beer B, Green M: Intramitochondrial inclusion bodies in cholelithiasis. Lancet 2:148–149, 1977

110. Meier PJ, Spycher MA, Meyer JA: Isolation of a subfraction of rough endoplasmic reticulum closely associated with mitochondria. Exp Cell Res 111:479–483, 1978

111. Sternlieb I, Quintana N: The peroxisomes of human hepatocytes. Lab Invest 36:140–149, 1977

112. Sternlieb I: Mitochondrion-desmosome complexes in human hepatocytes. Z Zellforsch 93:249–253, 1969

113. Goldfischer S, Moore CL, Johnson AB, Spiro AJ, Valsamis MP, Wisniewski HK, Ritch R-H, Norton WT, Rapin I, Gartner LM: Peroxisomal and mitochondrial defects in the cerebro-hepatorenal syndrome. Science 182:62–64, 1973

114. Schaffner F: Intralobular changes in hepatocytes and the electron microscopic mesenchymal response in acute viral hepatitis. Medicine (Baltimore) 45:547–552, 1966

115. Brito T, Penna DO, Hoshino S, Pereira VG, Caldas ACPG, Rothstein W: Cholestasis in human leptospirosis: A clinical, histochemical, biochemical and electron microscope study based on liver biopsies. Beitr Pathol Anat 140:345, 1970

116. Schubert WK, Partin JC, Partin JS: Encephalopathy and fatty liver (Reye's syndrome). Edited by H Popper and F Schaffner: Progress in Liver Diseases. Vol. IV. New York, Grune & Stratton, 1972, pp 489–510

117. Rubin E, Lieber CS: Early fine structural changes in the human liver induced by alcohol. Gastroenterology 52:1–13, 1967

118. Orlandi F, Jézéquel AM: A comparative study of liver response to 6-Mercaptopurine in patients with normal liver or with chronic aggressive hepatitis. Digestion 4:169–170, 1971

119. Schubert WK, Partin JS, Partin JC: Congenital cholestasis: Clinical and ultrastructural study. Edited by S Berenberg: Liver Diseases in Infancy and Childhood. The Hague, Martinus Nijhoff, 1976, pp 148–162

120. Biempica L: Human hepatic microbodies with crystalloid cores. J Cell Biol 29:383–386, 1966

121. Petersen P: Abnormal mitochondria in hepatocytes in human fatty liver. Acta Pathol Microbiol Scand 85:413–420, 1977

122. Toader C, Acalovschi I, Toader I, Manta I, Hodarnau A, Benga G: Factors influencing the establishment of the normal values of the respiratory activities of human liver mitochondria. Enzyme 21:232–242, 1976

123. Sato N, Kamada T, Abe H, Suematsu T, Kawano S, Hayashi N, Matsumura T, Hagihara B: Stimultaneous measurement of mitochondrial and microsomal cytochrome levels in human liver biopsy. Clin Chim Acta 80:243–251, 1977

124. Peters TJ, Seymour CA: Analytical subcellular fractionation of needle-biopsy specimens from human liver. Biochem J 174:435–446, 1978

Chapter 5

Cytoskeleton of the Hepatocyte

By M.M. FISHER *and* M.J. PHILLIPS

THE TERM "CYTOSKELETON" is used to describe that dynamic and highly coordinated system of proteins which in their filamentous and nonfilamentous forms collaborate with other cell structures to help define the shape and motile functions of the cell. The system is labile and dependent upon complete cellular harmony. The structural role of other cell components, e.g., the plasma membrane, is obvious, and the occurrence of noncytoskeletal movement is certain.

The definition and regulation of cell structure and motility is one of the most active areas of cell biology, and our understanding of the morphology involved is much more advanced than our understanding of the chemistry. Few nonmuscle systems have been studied rigorously. The cytoskeleton of the liver cell has been investigated very little.

Therefore, this review involves dogma at its best. Not only has the field extrapolated from the muscle cell to the nonmuscle cell, but we have extrapolated from the nonhepatocyte to the hepatocyte. Such extrapolation, when qualified, is reasonable if not justified. Most of the major components of the muscle cytoskeleton, including actin, myosin, tropomyosin, and α-actinin, have been found in most eukaryotic cells. Although the same highly ordered cytoskeleton is generally not found in nonmuscle cells and although there are certain presumably important differences in the primary structure of the proteins involved in the muscle and nonmuscle cytoskeletons, the interaction of actin and myosin may provide the basis for the general mechanisms whereby cells convert chemical energy into force and movement. The use of the data generated on the cytoskeleton of the muscle cell as a framework for characterizing the analogous proteins in other cells is reasonable. The major components of the system are present and highly conserved over a broad evolutionary segment.

This chapter presents an overview of our understanding of the cytoskeleton of eukaryotic cells other than muscle cells and, where possible, focuses on the hepatocyte. The literature review, up to July 1978, is by no means exhaustive, and much relevant material, e.g., the role of the cytoskeleton in cell division and carcinogenesis and cells in tissue culture, has been omitted for the sake of brevity. It should be noted, however, that several important reviews on the cytoskeleton have recently been published.[1-14]

ACTIN AND THIN FILAMENTS

Actin has been found in all eukaryotic cells studied, and it provides the greatest continuity among the various cytoskeletal systems.[15] The recoveries

From the Departments of Pathology and Medicine, University of Toronto, Toronto, Ontario.

of purified actin are generally very poor,[16,17] but it probably comprises 1% to 2% of the protein of the mammalian liver.[17-20] This actin has not been fully characterized, but in view of the remarkable evolutionary conservation of the protein, it is probably structurally similar to other actins. Therefore, its monomeric form (globular or G-actin) has a molecular weight of approximately 42,000 daltons, and each mole contains 1 mole of bound adenine nucleotide and 1 mole of the unusual amino acid, 3-methylhistidine. Two isoactins, β and γ, are involved, and these are separable by isoelectric focusing.

G-actin has an unusually high proportion of acidic and basic amino acids, and through ionic interactions, it polymerizes in an appropriate environment to a filamentous form, F-actin.[1-3,6,13,17,21] These thin filaments, or microfilaments, are double-stranded helical structures with a width of 5–7 nm, a half-pitch of 35 nm, and an indeterminate length. One mole of bound ATP is converted to ADP for every monomeric actin subunit polymerized, and the process results in a product whose only known nonstructural function is the activation of the Mg^{2+}-ATPase activity of myosin (discussed later in the chapter). Although the distribution and positioning of these microfilaments within the cell are not understood much better than is their function,[22] they are usually associated with cell plasma membranes[8,23-25] and have been seen in this section in the hepatocyte.[24-27] Furthermore, most of the cellular functions that involve the microfilaments also involve the plasma membranes. The microfilaments are not associated only with the plasma membranes, however. For example, they extend throughout the entire cytoplasm of the hepatocyte in an organized manner, intersecting with each other and with other intracellular organelles,[24,28] and high-voltage electron microscopy has revealed microfilaments in contact with all cell organelles except the mitochondria.[29]

The binding of heavy meromyosin (HMM) by the microfilaments is not only specific but also demonstrates that the filaments possess an intrinsic polarity.[1,30] Along their entire length the arrowhead complexes resulting from the HMM binding all point to one end of the filament. In intestinal microvilli, e.g., the filaments are so oriented that the HMM arrowheads all point toward the center of the cell.[31] Only by physical anchoring can microfilaments perform useful work, and as in muscle, α-actinin is an important component of these attachment sites.[3,10,32-35]

The degree of the polymerization of actin in situ is difficult to quantitate. As mentioned above, its recovery from cells is generally poor,[16,17] and the extraction procedures possibly alter the physical state of the actin.[16] For example, the form of F-actin extracted from chicken gizzard muscle when calcium ions are present in the preparation medium is different from that extracted without calcium ions.[36] Not all cytoplasmic actin is filamentous, and all nonmuscle cells have specific mechanisms for maintaining actin in a nonpolymerized, nonfilamentous state.[32] Profilactin is the name given to the nonfilamentous, presumably storage form, of unpolymerized actin in cells.[30] Profilin, an actin-binding protein with a molecular weight of approximately 16,000, appears to be responsible for maintaining the profilactin.[30] The binding of profilin to actin prevents nucleotide from binding to the actin and at the same time stabilizes it in its unpolymerized form. This may be one of the mechanisms for maintaining an intracellular concentration of G-actin that is greater than the critical concentration above which it nucleates and elongates to form F-actin. None of the proteins that interact with actin has been isolated from the hepatocyte.

A high-molecular-weight actin-binding protein first purified from rabbit pulmonary macrophages[37] is associated with actin filaments in a wide range of cells.[13] This protein, an asymmetric dimer of two identical polypeptide subunits with an approximate molecular weight of 240,000–250,000 daltons, is apparently similar to, if not identical with, filamin, the actin-binding protein of smooth muscle.[38,39] Filamin interacts with and promotes the aggregation of F-actin, and it inhibits the ability of actin to activate myosin Mg^{2+}-ATPase.[40] Actin filaments associated with this protein may thereby be restricted to a purely structural role, but the exact function of this protein remains to be established.

The in vivo organization of the actin of nonmuscle cells differs from that of muscle cells in that the microfilaments of the former can aggregate with each other. These aggregates, called bundles, form through proteins associated with the microfilaments and possibly under the influence of ATP.[2,22] The bundles, 0.1–0.2 μ in diameter, tend to form near and perhaps in association with the plasma membrane. Although these bundles appear to be transient phenomena, they can form a gel through the influence of yet other actin-binding proteins,[6] and possibly this gel extends throughout the cytoplasm. Several of these gel-promoting actin-binding proteins have been isolated from nonmuscle cells.[17] The networks of microfilaments commonly seen in nonmuscle cells probably are artifactual. Actin filaments are fragmented during exposure to osmium tetroxide.[41]

Actin is ubiquitous and plays an important role in many cell processes.[2,3,6,13] Through its association with myosin, it provides the energy for cell movement, phagocytosis, secretion, cell division, and both intracellular and intercellular communication. To adapt to these various needs, it must be capable of continuous, rapid, and specific reorganization and this it achieves through its capacity to assume different physical states.[17] It appears, however, that it is the heterogeneous group of actin-binding proteins that controls the physical state and distribution of actin, the size and aggregation of actin filaments, the association of actin with other cellular organelles, and the ability of actin to activate myosin ATPase. Human smooth muscle antibodies of the IgG class directed against actin are common in chronic active liver diseases[27,42,43] but their determination is not of real clinical value. Actin may also have a role in the regenerative response of the hepatocyte, but studies are still at the documentary stage.[44,45] Microfilaments may be involved in biliary secretion[14,46] (See Chapter 25).

INTERMEDIATE FILAMENTS

The intermediate filaments are distinct and ubiquitous, but very little has been established about their role, composition, or organization.[47,48] They are approximately 10 nm in diameter and involve four subunits with molecular weights approximating 55,000 daltons and measuring 60 nm in length and 3.5

nm in diameter. Although the intermediate filaments are closely associated with actin and myosin, they seem not to be involved in the interaction of actin and myosin or in the regulation of this interaction by calcium. Furthermore, their distribution is not localized. They form a continuous network throughout certain cells and have an evenly distributed attachment to the plasma membrane.[47] Therefore, they perform a primarily structural role and are not an integral part of the contractile machinery of the cell. The compact network that they form around the cell nucleus of certain cells in situ or in response to microtubular inhibitors and their apparently tight association with the nucleus suggest that the intermediate filaments constrain the nucleus in its position in the cell.[48] The intermediate filament network can be rather labile,[48] however, and a complementary nonstructural role for these filaments is possible.

Skeletin and desmin are the names gives to the subunit polypeptides of these still poorly characterized filaments.[47,48] Like the filaments of Mallory bodies (see Chapter 31), the intermediate filaments have a branching architecture and do not bind HMM.[49,50]

MYOSIN AND THICK FILAMENTS

Myosin has been found in most eukaryotic cells, but in cells other than muscle it has been characterized even less well than actin[51] for the following reasons: (1) sufficient quantities of purified myosin are difficult to obtain, (2) myosin is not easily visualized electron-microscopically, and (3) the myosins of nonmuscle cells vary from cell to cell.[51-54] The pattern of distribution of myosin in human cells using immunofluorescent techniques is similar to that of actin.[55] The intimate association of myosin with cellular plasma membranes has been confirmed.[56,57]

Isolated, purified, and partially characterized myosin of the hepatocyte is similar to that obtained from other sources.[56,58] A noteworthy feature is its lack of methylated histidine.

The subunit of most myosins is an asymmetric protein with a molecular weight of approximately 500,000. It has ATPase activity that is stimulated when the myosin and actin interact under physiologic conditions involving low ionic strength and magnesium. The subunit has two heavy chains with molecular weights of approximately 215,000 daltons and two pairs of light chains with molecular weights approximating 17,000–20,000 daltons. Each heavy chain is a rod with a pear-shaped globular head approximately 19 nm long at one end. Each head region contains a site for actin binding, and it is also the head region of the heavy chains with which the light chains are associated. Although the globular head regions also contain the sites for ATPase activity, the exact location of these sites is controversial. Even though the two head regions of the myosin subunit interact, they seem to be functionally nonidentical, with only one containing ATPase activity.[59] The rod portions of the heavy chains are stranded together to form an α-helical unit approximately 150 nm long. A region of this helix is susceptible to mild proteolytic cleavage by trypsin or papain.[60] Two fragments are produced: HMM, which contains the two head regions,[61] and light meromyosin (LMM), which is insoluble at low ionic strength and considered responsible for the aggregation of myosin into a filamentous form.[62] Each light chain is bound noncovalently to the heavy chains and can be easily dissociated.[63] Skeletal myosin has two classes of light chains, the alkali light chains, which are dissociable from the myosin at alkaline pH, and the DTNB light chains, which are selectively removed by treatment of the myosin with 5,5'-dithio-bis-(2-nitrobenzoic acid) and EDTA. The alkali light chains are apparently necessary for the ATPase activity of myosin, while the DTNB light chains participate in the interaction of actin and myosin in the presence of ATP.[63]

Like actin, the myosin subunits of skeletal muscle form filaments at low ionic strength,[64] and in vitro nonmuscle myosin also forms "thick filaments." These latter filaments are also 16–17 nm in diameter but are usually shorter than those formed by striated muscle myosin, which are approximately 300–350 nm in length.[16,54,56] The thick filaments of smooth muscle myosin do not have the central "bare zone" that characterizes the thick filaments of skeletal muscle myosin,[51] and the structural organization of the thick filaments of nonmuscle myosin is probably not the same as that of skeletal muscle myosin. Unfortunately, these filaments are few in number and labile after tissue fixation. Therefore, they have been extremely difficult to find in situ in nonmuscle cells,[16,51] and we know little concerning their size and stability in such cells.

Because myosin filaments can form without accessory proteins, they could be the stable structural components of the cytoskeleton.[16] Myosin-linked regulation of motility has not been demonstrated in nonmuscle cell systems.[8]

INTERACTION OF ACTIN AND MYOSIN

Actin probably functions in force generation only in combination with myosin,[15] and the regulation of this interaction in nonmuscle cells has been the subject of much recent work[32,63,65,66] While contractile events similar to those of muscle probably occur in nonmuscle cells, evidence is accumulating that qualitatively different and other contractile mechanisms exist in these cells. An actomyosin system has not yet been reconstituted with characterized components from any nonmuscle cell.[8,65,66]

The regulation of motile events in nonmuscle cells is likely to involve a number of different mechanisms, and a cell may employ more than one mechanism. Skeletal and cardiac muscle cell motility is regulated by the calcium-binding tropomyosin-troponin system.[67] Troponin via tropomyosin regulates the ability of actin to interact with myosin. Similar proteins have been isolated from nonmuscle vertebrate cells, but there is no convincing evidence that nonmuscle cells contain a troponin complex like that found in muscle. Furthermore, in certain nonmuscle cells studied, the tropomyosin has not been distributed uniformly with the actin. The tropomyosin in nonmuscle cells may therefore be associated primarily with structural actin.

Different requirements dictate the development of different systems, however, and posttranslational events probably influence the interaction of actin and myosin in nonmuscle cells. For example, platelet myosin, phosphorylated by a specific kinase, has higher activation by actin than does unphosphorylated myosin.[68] Other actin-associated proteins have similar effects in other systems and as in the tropomyosin-troponin system, the concentration of intracellular calcium appears to play a key regulatory role. Other variables are involved, but they, too, may exert their influence through changes in calcium concentration. For example, both actin and myosin are present as long filaments in solutions with a low ionic strength and low concentration of ATP. The addition of ATP induces the formation of a network of actin and myosin filaments as a consequence of cross-linkages between these filaments.[64]

Therefore, myosin and other contractile proteins probably exist in some form wherever actin is found, and the basic control of the physical, chemical, and functional state of the system is dependent upon associated proteins that respond to changes in the intracellular concentration of calcium, other ions, and ATP.

TUBULIN AND MICROTUBULES

Tubulin is a protein that, in its native state, is a heterodimer.[69] This unit, known as 6S tubulin, has a molecular weight of approximately 115,000 daltons. Each dimer binds 2 moles of guanine nucleotide; one is rapidly exchangeable with the guanine nucleotide in the surrounding medium, while the other is not so exchangeable. The GTP at the exchangeable site appears to be essential for the efficient polymerization of tubulin (discussed later).[70,71] The two subunits that comprise the 6S tubulin of nonnervous tissue cells have molecular weights of approximately 55,000 daltons and have been designated α and β tubulin.[7,72]

The tubulin from various nonnervous tissue cells is similar and differs from nervous tissue tubulin. It has a lower molecular weight, it is not associated with accessory proteins (microtubule-associated protein), and it has a different nucleation pathway.[73] Differences in experimental methodology produce conflicting data in this and other areas of the cytoskeletal field.[74] High-affinity colchicine binding sites resembling tubulin represent approximately 1% of the soluble protein of isolated rat hepatocytes.[75] In these studies, most of the nonparticulate tubulin, approximately 85%, was present in the cell in its dimeric, nonpolymerized form. Estimates of 70% in rat liver and 60% in mouse liver have been obtained.[76,77] Major problems remain in measuring the native state of tubulin.[78] Furthermore, the physical state of tubulin in the hepatocyte changes with physiologic factors such as nutritional status.[79]

Under the influence of certain other proteins, tubulin polymerizes into microtubules—straight, hollow, cylindrical structures with walls 5 nm thick, an outer diameter of 25 nm, and an indefinite length.[72,80-82] The walls of the microtubules are made up of 13 helical protofilaments lying parallel to each other and to the long axis of the cylinder. The microtubules traverse the cytoplasm for long distances and in general are especially prominent between the perinuclear area and the plasma membrane.[83]

Microtubules are the best-studied components of the cytoskeleton[84,85] and have been tentatively assigned a role in many cell processes.[80] Because of their functional versatility the microtubules must be subject to highly specific and precisely controlled assembly and disassembly, both in space and time. Therefore, a great deal of work has focused on the regulation of polymerization and depolymerization of tubulin as one of the mechanisms by which microtubules might exert their various functions. A dynamic equilibrium is thought to exist between free tubulin and its polymerized forms.[77] Tubulin polymers other than microtubules may also exist.

Microtubules have an intrinsic polarity,[86] and this could either explain or be explained by a microtubule assembly–disassembly equilibrium that involves a steady state of two different reactions occurring at opposite ends of the microtubule. In vitro, the assembly reaction is strongly favored at one end of the microtubule and disassembly at the other end.[87]

Various cofactors, including nucleotides, protein, and glutathione, are involved in the maintenance of this equilibrium. Much attention has been paid to posttranslational modifications of tubulin as the initial event in its polymerization, because microtubules form and disappear rapidly at times when the total cell content of tubulin appears constant.[88] Therefore, transcriptional or translational events are unlikely to exert the obviously necessary fine control of the monomer-polymer equilibrium.[69,89]

One of these modifications involves the binding of nucleotides to tubulin, and it has been suggested that cyclic AMP inhibits polymerization of tubulin and cyclic GMP promotes the process.[70,72] Experiments have failed to support the concept that the phosphorylation of tubulin inhibits its assembly into microtubules.[90]

Another possible regulator in the polymerization process is the reversible addition of tyrosine to the carboxyl terminus of the alpha chain of tubulin under the influence of the enzyme tyrosine-tubulin ligase.[88,89,91,92] It has been suggested that the loss of tyrosine is linked to microtubule assembly.[92] However, both tyrosylated and detyrosylated tubulin can polymerize in vitro, the true substrate of the enzyme is unknown, and it is not known whether tubulin is tyrosylated in vivo.[88] Although the biologic significance of the reaction is unknown, such a modification of the primary structure of tubulin would produce two different populations of tubulin in the cell, and the balance between them could control the assembly maintenance and function of the microtubules. This enzyme is widely distributed in eukaryotic cells, including the hepatocyte.[93]

Several microtubule-associated proteins, i.e., proteins that copolymerize with tubulin during successive cycles of assembly and disassembly, induce and are required for microtubule formation in vitro.[94] Tau protein, with an approximate molecular weight of 60,000–70,000 daltons, has been found in several nonnervous tissue cells. Tau protein is both necessary and sufficient for the nucleation and elongation of microtubules in their tau protein-tubulin reconstituted system.[82,95] The microtubule-associated proteins that control the in vitro assembly of microtubules of neuronal origin are proteins with molecular weights ranging from 271,000 to 345,000 daltons.[96,97] Other proteins may induce microtubule assembly, but none of these has been purified.[80] Tubulin assembly protein (TAP) binds stoichiometrically to tubulin.[80] It activates tubulin for polymerization, appears to have a role in the initiation of microtubule assembly, and is structurally incorporated along the entire length of the growing microtubule. TAP and tau protein are probably identical. Considerable controversy continues concerning the nature, distribution, and relative importance of the various microtubule-associated proteins.[98-100]

Intact sulfydryl groups also appear to be essential for the monomer-polymer equilibrium, and microtubule function is impaired by oxidized glutathione, the concentration of which can be influenced by the redox state of the cell.[101,102] Temperature, calcium, and other influences on the monomer-polymer equilibrium and tubulin-binding agents like colchicine have been studied.[70,103-105]

Although cytoplasmic microtubules are found in hepatocytes, the role they play in liver cell structure and function is not clear.[7,106] Furthermore, liver tubulin has not been polymerized in vitro.[77]

NUCLEAR CYTOSKELETON

Although actin has been found in association with eukaryotic nuclei, the association is not tight, and it does not seem to have a role in nuclear function.[107,108] Actin does not bind to DNA,[109] and there appears to be no need to involve the actin-myosin system in the mitotic process. Actin may be present in nuclei only because of free movement of actin between the cytoplasm and the nucleus. However, differences in their solubilities suggest that there may be structural differences between cytoplasmic and nuclear actin.[110]

Myosin binds to DNA with high affinity,[109] but its role in nuclear structure and function has not been defined. Instead, other acidic proteins appear to determine the internal organization and overall form of cell nuclei.[111] A residual fibrillar matrix or nucleoskeleton isolated from rat liver nuclei[112-115] contains 98.2% protein and accounts for 12% of the total nuclear protein. It maintains the essential spherical form of the nucleus and is composed of three major acidic, nonhistone polypeptides with approximate molecular weights of 60,000–70,000 daltons.[112] This nucleoskeleton extends from the nuclear envelope and forms a distinctive internal matrix that connects to the nucleolus. The DNA associated with the nucleoskeleton is rapidly labeled during the DNA synthesis that accompanies hepatic regeneration, and it has been postulated that the structure plays an important role in DNA metabolism.[113] Although this nuclear matrix does express reversible contractility in vitro, whether it represents a contractile system independent of actomyosin is not clear.

Although the molecular mechanism of mitosis in higher eukaryotic cells is largely unknown,[87,116] microtubules are involved. In fact, the formation of the spindle of the mitotic apparatus, whereby the chromosomes are separated in the anaphase of mitosis, is perhaps the best-defined function of the microtubules. The relative roles of the microtubules and the microtubule-associated protein remain to be defined. Tubulin itself does not appear to interact with DNA, whereas microtubule associated proteins do.[117] Therefore, the nuclei of certain cells have a cytoskeleton,[118] but some of it may just be imported from the cytoplasm in time of need and some of it appears to be functionally independent of the actomyosin system. The special role of microtubules in mitosis is beyond the scope of this review.

THE ORGANIZATION AND OPERATION
OF THE CYTOSKELETON

Comments on the organization and operation of the cytoskeleton should be cautious. An organization must exist, and it must be controlled by mechanisms that are very finely tuned and rigorously maintained. Various components of the cytoskeleton probably interact in one form or another with each other as well as with all other cell organelles. The following discussion merely reflects the most attractive possibilities, because so little is known about the cytoskeleton of the nonmuscle cell.

Actin, myosin, and related proteins of the eukaryotic cell interact with cell membranes, microtubules, and other organelles to create many diverse activities. The interaction between these various agents is precisely regulated, and although the mechanism for this regulation is unknown, probably calcium, other ions, and guanine nucleotides are important.

The role of the nonfilamentous forms of the cytoskeletal proteins in maintaining cell shape and organizing cell function has not been established. Virtually all attention has been directed toward the study of the linear elements and especially of the microfilaments and microtubules.

In order for actin, myosin, and their related proteins to convert chemical energy to motile force, the contractile elements must be anchored, and as in muscle, α-actinin has been assigned the role of the anchoring protein for the microtubules.[34,35] Studies by electron microscopy and those on isolated cell fractions suggest that the most important anchoring sites may be the plasma membranes of the cell and the microtubules.

The association of actin filaments with plasma membranes is a well-recognized and apparently universal phenomenon in animal cells.[23] Dialysis of plasma membranes against ATP at low ionic strengths removes only part of this actin. Extraction of the remaining actin with Triton X-100 suggests that this residual actin is either directly inserted into the membrane or is attached to other molecules that are so inserted, but actin is not the only component involved in the interaction between the cytoskeleton and the plasma membrane.

The cytoskeleton appears to control the movements of cell surface receptors.[4,5] Much of the evidence for this comes from experiments with drugs that alter the activity of cytoskeletal components.[119-121]

Cell surface receptors control several fundamental cell functions,[122] and this depends on their lateral mobility in the membrane. Inhibition of this lateral mobility by lectins led to the concept of anchorage modulation.[120,123,124] Basic to this concept is a surface modulating assembly involving the microfilaments and microtubules. The surface receptor molecules apparently penetrate the lipid bilayer of the membrane and interact with the microtubules by the microfilaments and their associated proteins. Evidence for such an assembly comes from several areas. The region of a lymphocyte lying beneath an antigen cap contains an accumulation of actin, myosin, and tubulin, and aggregation of the plasma membrane surface proteins may create a new link with the actin.[125] Concanavalin A (ConA) receptors may be structurally related to actin, since α-actinin appears to occur in closely related sites in a variety of cells and since ConA binding to surface receptors actually changes the physical state of the associated F-actin.[126]

Plasma membrane particles (PMP) visualized by electron microscopy and freeze-fracture techniques are important structures in biologic membranes and are associated with hydrophobic regions of intrinsic proteins of certain membranes, e.g., the erythrocyte and retinal rod.[127] The interaction of plasma membranes and the cytoskeleton appears to influence PMP topography.[127] The role of the intercellular junction, specifically of the desmosomes, in connecting the cytoskeletons of adjacent cells has been reviewed.[128]

The potential for surface receptor-cytoskeleton interaction was seen when a transformation-sensitive membrane glycoprotein was copurified with a protein identified as an intermediate filament-forming protein of hamster embryo fibroblasts.[129] These two proteins coprecipitated when the intermediate filament-forming protein was polymerized to form intermediate filaments.

Actin and tubulin, which probably have different functions, move concurrently along the cell membrane with a single class of surface receptors.[119] Evidence has been provided for attachment of surface immunoglobulins (Ig) to cellular actin.[130] Surface receptors for ConA were linearly redistributed on normal rat kidney (NRK) cell surfaces by the addition of fluorescent conjugated ConA.[131] These linear arrays were superimposed on actomyosinlike filaments as revealed by antimyosin antibody. Microtubules were apparently not involved in this phenomenon. Finally, in at least one system, the major histocompatibility antigen H2 forms a stable transmembrane association with actin.[132] This association occurs in situ and does not depend on the presence of the plasma membrane.

Therefore, a surface modulating assembly that physically links the cytoskeleton and the plasma membrane and that regulates the movement arrangement and function of cell surface proteins[119] is an attractive concept. The precise physical and chemical nature of the interactions between the various components of the surface modulating assembly remains to be defined.[133]

Perhaps not sufficiently stressed is the interaction between the microtubules and the rest of the cytoskeleton.[105] In general, the microtubules radiate from the center of the cell toward the plasma membrane,[134,135] while the microfilaments are mostly distributed peripherally in association with the plasma membrane.[134] Although the proof of a skeletal role for microtubules is only available for systems with large bundles of parallel and interconnecting microtubules,[86] the microtubules are probably the structural elements on which the other components of the cytoskeleton are anchored.[50] The microtubules may well exist in a gel of actin, however, and to assign a particular role to any of the components of the cytoskeleton of any nonmuscle eukaryotic cell is probably not wise.

This note of caution is particularly applicable to the function of the cytoskeleton, which has been tentatively assigned a role in the secretion of bile[136,137] and of biliary lipids,[138] in the movement of secretory vesicles to the liver cell plasma membranes,[139,140] and in the secretion of albumin, lipoproteins, and other proteins across the liver cell plasma membranes.[139,141-149] These studies on function have all involved cytoskeletal inhibitors like colchicine, cytochalasin B, and phalloidin. Colchicine binds to soluble 6S tubulin and prevents its polymerization.[150-153] Cytochalasin B, a metabolite of the fungus, *Helminthosporium dematioideum*, weakens the structure of actin filaments.[16] Phalloidin, a cyclic peptide from the poisonous mushroom *Amanita phalloides*, stabilizes actin filaments against polymerization by KCl.

Unfortunately, these agents influence other organelles and especially the plasma membrane on whose receptors they can have various and even contradictory effects.[86] For example, the binding of colchicine to tubulin is not specific.[90] Colchicine binds to plasma membranes, and it exerts effects on cell processes that are not dependent upon microtubule integrity. At least two specific binding sites exist for cytochalasin B on the liver cell plasma membrane.[150] Furthermore, cytochalasin B alters the function of the plasma membrane at doses lower than those required to affect the microfilaments.[127] Therefore, caution must be exercised in interpreting studies of cell function that involve cytoskeleton-inhibiting agents. A colchicine binding protein system was postulated to be crucial in the transmission of information from cell membrane to nucleus.[154] Such transmission may involve only certain types of information, however.[155]

Microtubules are probably necessary for the optimal function of the vacuolar system and endogenous lysosomal proteolysis[156] and for the movement of secretory products to the plasma membrane[90] but are not necessary for the movement and cellular discharge of lysosomal granules.[90] The secretion of microsomal β-glucuronidase by the hepatocyte does not depend on microtubular function.[157] There may be a fundamental difference between the secretion of proteins like β-glucuronidase, which are largely stored by the hepatocyte, and that of proteins like albumin and fibrinogen, which are normally secreted soon after their synthesis.[157] Antimicrotubular agents actually increase hormonally stimulated steroid secretion by adrenal tumor cells in culture,[158] and participation of microtubules in hepatic VLDL secretion has been questioned.[159] Therefore, the precise role of the cytoskeleton in the secretory process has not been defined, and although the microtubules may exert primarily a structural role and the microfilaments primarily a contractile role, the precise role of any component of the cytoskeleton of any nonmuscle cell has not been defined.

OUTLOOK

This incomplete review of a very active field gave little attention to some of the more clinical and functional problems that may involve the cytoskeleton. The review emphasizes that our understanding of the cytoskeleton is fragmentary at best. There is a cytoskeleton in all cells, and its organization is dynamic, constantly changing according to the immediate needs of the cell.[16] However, no nonmuscle cell has had its cytoskeleton thoroughly characterized from either the structural or the functional point of view. The descriptive phase is largely over, although further revelations can be anticipated on the basis of more advanced technology. What remains is the need for the systematic identification and purification of each component of the cytoskeleton and the reconstruction of these components into fundamental assemblies.

REFERENCES

1. Pollard TD, Weihing RR: Actin and myosin and cell movement. CRC Crit Rev Biochem 2:1–65, 1974

2. Pollard TD: Functional implications of the biochemical and structural properties of cytoplasmic contractile proteins. Edited by S Inoue and RE Stephens: Molecules and Cell Movement. New York, Raven Press, 1975, pp 259–286

3. Tilney LG: The role of actin in nonmuscle cell motility. Edited by S Inoue and RE Stephens: Molecules and Cell Movement. New York, Raven Press, 1975, pp 339–388

4. Nicolson, GL: Transmembrane control of the receptors on normal and tumor cells. I. Cytoplasmic influence over cell surface components. Biochim Biophys Acta 457:57–108, 1976

5. Nicholson GL: Trans-membrane control of the receptors on normal and tumor cells. II. Surface changes associated with transformation and malignancy. Biochim phys Acta 458:1–72, 1976

6. Poilard TD: Cytoskeletal functions of cytoplasmic contractile proteins. J Supramol Struct 5:317–334, 1976

7. Stephens RE, Edds KT: Microtubules: structure, chemistry and function. Physiol Rev 56:709–777, 1976

8. Hitchcock SE: Regulation of motility in nonmuscle cells. J Cell Biol 74:1–15, 1977

9. Kamiya N: Introductory remarks. Edited by BR Brinkley and KR Porter: International Cell Biology. New York, Rockefeller University Press, 1977, pp 361–366

10. Pollard TD: Cytoplasmic contractile proteins. Edited by BR Brinkley and KR Porter: International Cell Biology. New York, Rockefeller University Press, 1977, pp 378–387

11. Taylor DS: Dynamics of cytoplasmic structure and contractility. Edited by BR Brinkley and KR Porter: International Cell Biology. New York, Rockefeller University Press, 1977, pp 367–377

12. Tilney LG: Actin: Its association with membranes and the regulation of its polymerization. Edited by BR Brinkley and KR Porter: International Cell Biology. New York, Rockefeller University Press, 1977, pp 388–406

13. Stossel TP: Contractile proteins in cell structure and function. Annu Rev Med 29:427–457, 1978

14. Phillips MJ, Oda M, Funatsu K: Reactions of the liver to injury: Cholestasis, ultrastructural aspects. Edited by E Farber and MM Fisher: Toxic Injury of the Liver. New York, Marcel Dekker (in press)

15. Lu RC, Elzinga M: Partial amino acid sequence of brain actin and its homology with muscle actin. Biochemistry 16:5801–5806, 1977

16. Clarke M, Spudich JA: Nonmuscle contractile proteins: The role of actin and myosin in cell motility and shape determination. Annu Rev Biochem 46:797–822, 1977

17. Gordon DJ, Boyer JL, Korn ED: Comparative biochemistry of non-muscle actins. J Biol Chem 252:8300–8309, 1977

18. Weihing RR: Occurrence of microfilaments in non-muscle cells and tissues. Edited by PC Altman and DD Katz: Cell Biology. Bethesda, Md, FASEB, 1976, pp 341–356

19. Weihing RR, Korn ED: Acanthamoeba actin. Isolation and properties. Biochemistry 10:590–600, 1971

20. Gordon DJ, Eisenberg E, Korn ED: Characterization of cytoplasmic actin isolated from Acanthamoeba castellanii by a new method. J Biol Chem 251:4778–4786, 1976

21. Dos Remedios CG, Barden JA: Effects of Gd(III) on G-actin: Inhibition of polymerization of G-actin and activation of myosin ATPase activity by Gd-G-actin. Biochem Biophys Res Commun 77:1339–1346, 1977

22. Edds KT: Microfilament bundles. I. Formation with uniform polarity. Exp Cell Res 108:452–456, 1977

23. Tannenbaum J, Tannenbaum SW, Godman GC: The binding sites of cytochalasin D. J Cell Physiol 91:225–238, 1977

24. French SW, Davies PL: Ultrastructural localization of actin-like filaments in rat hepatocytes. Gastroenterology 68:765–774, 1975

25. Neifakh SA, Vasilets IM: Actomyosin-like protein in outer membrane of liver cells. Fed Proc 24:T561-T562, 1965

26. Trump EF, Dees JH, Shelburne JD: The ultrastructure of the human liver cell and its common pattern of reaction to injury. Edited by EA Gall and FK Mostofi: The Liver. Baltimore, Williams & Wilkins, 1973, pp 80–120

27. Gabbiani F, Ryan GB, Lamelin JP, Vassalli P, Majno G, Bouview CA, Cruchaud A,

Lüscher EF: Human smooth muscle autoantibody: Its identification as antiactin antibody and a study of its binding to "nonmuscular" cells. Am J Pathol 72: 473–484, 1973

28. Miettinen A, Virtanen I, Linder E: Cellular actin and junction formation during reaggregation of adult rat hepatocytes into epithelial cell sheets. J Cell Sci 31:341–353, 1978

29. Wolosewick JJ, Porter KR: Stereo high-voltage electron microscopy of whole cells of the human diploid line, W1–38, Am J Anat 147:303–324, 1976

30. Carlsson L, Myström LE, Sundkvist I, Markey F, Lindberg U: Actin polymerizability is influenced by profilin, a low molecular weight protein in non-muscle cells. J Mol Biol 115:465–483, 1977

31. Mooseker M, Tilney LG: Organization of an actin filament-membrane complex. J Cell Biol 67:725–743, 1975

32. Korn ED: Biochemistry of actomyosin-dependent cell motility (a review). Proc Natl Acad Sci USA 75:588–599, 1978

33. Jockusch BM, Burger MM, DaPrada M, Richards JG, Chaponnier C, Gabbiani G: α-Actinin attached to membranes of secretory vesicles. Nature 270:628–629, 1977

34. Puszkin S, Puszkin E, Maimon J, Rouault C, Schook W, Ores C, Kochwa S, Rosenfield R: α-Actinin and tropomyosin interactions with a hybrid complex of erythrocyte·actin and muscle·myosin. J Biol Chem 252:5529–5537, 1977

35. Lazarides E, Burridge K: α-Actinin: Immunofluorescent localization of a muscle structural protein in nonmuscle cells. Cell 6:289–298, 1975

36. Suzuki K, Yamaguchi M, Sekine T: Two forms of chicken gizzard F-actin depending on preparation with or without added calcium. J Biochem 83:869–878, 1978

37. Hartwig JH, Stossel TP: Isolation and properties of actin, myosin and a new actin-binding protein in rabbit alveolar macrophages. J Biol Chem 250:5696–5705, 1975

38. Wang K: Filamin, a new high-molecular-weight protein found in smooth muscle and nonmuscle cells. Purification and properties of chicken gizzard filamin. Biochemistry 16:1857–1865, 1977

39. Davies PJA, Wallach D, Willingham MC, Pastan I, Yamaguchi M, Robson RM: Filamin-actin interaction. Dissociation of binding from gelatin by Ca^{2+}-activated proteolysis. J Biol Chem 253:4036–4042, 1978

40. Davies P, Bechtel P, Pastan I: Filamin inhibits actin activation of heavy meromyosin ATPase. FEBS Lett 77:228–232, 1977

41. Maupin-Szamier P, Pollard TD: Actin filament destruction by osmium tetroxide. J Cell Biol 77:837–852, 1978

42. Kurki P, Linder E, Miettinen A, Alfthan O: Smooth muscle antibodies of actin and "nonactin" specificity. Clin Immunol Immunopathol 9:443–453, 1978

43. Trenchev P, Sneyd P, Holborow EJ: Immunofluorescent tracing of smooth muscle contractile protein antigens in tissues other than smooth muscle. Clin Exp Immunol 16:125–136, 1974

44. Toh BH, Cauchi MN, Muller HK: Actin-like contractile protein in carbon tetrachloride-induced cirrhosis in the rat. Pathology 9:187–194, 1977

45. Lampert IA, Trenchev P, Holborow EJ: Contractile protein changes in the regenerating rat liver. Virchows Arch [Zellpathol] 15:351–355, 1974

46. French SW: Is cholestasis due to microfilament failure? Hum Pathol 7:243–244, 1976

47. Small JV, Sobieszek A: Studies on the function and composition of the 10-NM (100-Å) filaments of vertebrate smooth muscle. J Cell Sci 23:243–268, 1977

48. Small JV, Celis JE: Direct visualization of the 10-nm (100-Å)-filament network in whole and enucleated cultured cells. J Cell Sci 31:393–409, 1978

49. Sim JS, Franks KE, French SW, Caldwell MG: Mallory bodies compared with microfilament hyperplasia. Arch Pathol Lab Med 101:401–404, 1977

50. Petersen P: Alcoholic hyalin, microfilaments and microtubules in alcoholic hepatitis. Acta Pathol Microbiol Scand [A] 85:384–394, 1977

51. Small JV: Studies on isolated smooth muscle cells: The contractile apparatus. J Cell Sci 24:327–349, 1977

52. Takahashi K: Topography of the myosin molecule as visualized by an improved negative staining method. J Biochem 83: 905–908, 1978

53. Cooke P: A filamentous cytoskeleton in vertebrate smooth muscle fibers. J Cell Biol 68:539–556, 1976

54. Burridge K, Bray D: Purification and structural analysis of myosins from brain and other non-muscle tissues. J Mol Biol 99:1–14, 1975

55. Fujiwara K, Pollard TD: Fluorescent anti-

body localization of myosin in the cytoplasm, cleavage furrow, and mitotic spindle of human cells. J Cell Biol 71:848–875, 1976

56. Brandon DL: The identification of myosin in rabbit hepatocytes. Eur J Biochem 65:139–146, 1976

57. Rikihisa Y, Mizuno D: Demonstration of myosin on the cytoplasmic side of plasma membranes of guinea pig polymorphonuclear leukocytes with immunoferritin. Exp Cell Res 110:87–92, 1977

58. Brandon DL: Myosin-like polypeptides in plasma membrane preparations. FEBS Lett 58:349–352, 1975

59. Yoshida M, Morita F: Isolation of intramolecularly uncleaved myosin subfragment-1 and its heterogeneous properties on substrate binding. J Biochem 82:1135–1144, 1977

60. Lowey S, Slayter HS, Weeds AG, Baker H: Substructure of the myosin molecule. I. Subfragments of myosin by enzymic degradation. J Mol Biol 42:1–29, 1969

61. Offer G, Elliott A: Can a myosin molecule bind to two actin filaments? Nature 271:325–329, 1978

62. Chowrashi PK, Pepe FA: Light meromyosin paracrystal formation. J Cell Biol 74:136–152, 1977

63. Hozumi R, Hotta K: Effect of myosin DTNB light chain on the actin-myosin interaction in the presence of ATP. J Biochem 83:671–676, 1978

64. Hozumi T, Hotta K: Presence of a unit for actin-myosin interaction during the superprecipitation of actomyosin. J Biochem 81:1141–1146, 1977

65. Adelstein RS: Myosin phosphorylation, cell motility and smooth muscle contraction. Trends Biochem Sci 3:27–30, 1978

66. Pollard TD: Introductory remarks: Myosin and control mechanisms. Edited by R Goldman, T Pollard, and J Rosenbaum: Cell Motility. Vol 3. Cold Spring Harbor Conference on Cell Proliferation, 1976, pp 685–687

67. Gergely J: Troponon-tropomyosin-dependent regulation of muscle contraction by calcium. Edited by R Goldman, T Pollard, and J Rosenbaum: Cell Motility. Vol. 3. Cold Spring Harbor Conference Cell Proliferation, 1976, pp 137–149

68. Adelstein RS, Conti MA: Phosphorylation of platelet myosin increases actin-activated myosin ATPase activity. Nature (Lond) 256:597–598, 1975

69. Luduena RF, Shooter EM, Wilson L: Structure of the tubulin dimer. J Biol Chem 252:7006–7014, 1977

70. Arai T, Kaziro Y: Role of GTP in the assembly of microtubules. J Biochem 82:1063–1071, 1977

71. Maccioni R, Seeds NW: Stoichiometry of GTP hydrolysis and tubulin polymerization. Proc Natl Acad Sci USA 74:462–466, 1977

72. Snyder JA, McIntosh JR: Biochemistry and physiology of microtubules. Annu Rev Biochem 45:699–720, 1976

73. Nagle BW, Doenges KH, Bryan J: Assembly of tubulin from cultured cells and comparison with the neurotubulin model. Cell 12:573–586, 1977

74. Hains FO, Dickerson RM, Wilson L, Owellen RJ: Differences in the binding properties of vinca alkaloids and colchicine to tubulin by varying protein sources and methodology. Biochem Pharmacol 27:71–76, 1978

75. Reaven EP, Cheng Y, Miller MD: Quantitative analysis of tubulin and microtubule compartments in isolated rat hepatocytes. J Cell Biol 75:731–742, 1977

76. Pipeleers DG, Pipeleers-Marichal MA, Kipnis DM: A sensitive method for measuring polymerized and depolymerized forms of tubulin in tissues. J Cell Biol 74:341–350, 1977

77. Patzelt C, Singh A, LeMarchand Y, Orci L, Jeanrenaud B: Colchicine-binding protein of the liver. Its characterization and relation to microtubules. J Cell Biol 66:609–620, 1975

78. Barton JS: Polymerization and colchicine binding. Two independent properties of tubulin. Biochim Biophys Acta 532:155–160, 1978

79. Pipeleers DG, Pipeleers-Marichal MA, Kipnis DM: Physiological regulation of total tubulin and polymerized tubulin in tissues. J Cell Biol 74:351–357, 1977

80. Lockwood AH: Tubulin assembly protein: Immunochemical and immunofluorescent studies on its function and distribution in microtubules and cultured cells. Cell 13:613–627, 1978

81. DeBrabander M, DeMey J, Joniau M, Geuens S: Immunocytochemical visualization of microtubules and tubulin at the light- and electron-microscopic level. J Cell Sci 28:283–301, 1977

82. Fellous A, Francon J, Lennon AM, Nunez

J: Microtubule assembly in vitro. Purification of assembly-promoting factors. Eur J Biochem 78:167–174, 1977

83. Osborn M, Webster RE, Weber K: Individual microtubules viewed by immunofluorescence and electron microscopy in the same PtK2 cell. J Cell Biol 77:R27–R34, 1978

84. Soifer D (editor): The biology of cytoplasmic microtubules. Ann NY Acad Sci 253:1–848, 1975

85. DeMey J, Hoebeke J, DeBrabander M, Geuens G, Joniau M: Immunoperoxidase visualisation of microtubules and microtubular proteins. Nature 264:273–275, 1976

86. DeBrabander M, DeMey J, Van de Veire R, Aerts F, Geuens G: Microtubules in mammalian cell shape and surface modulation: An alternative hypothesis. Cell Biol Int Rep 1:453–461, 1977

87. Margolis RL, Wilson L, Kiefer BI: Mitotic mechanism based on intrinsic microtubule behaviour. Nature 272:450–452, 1978

88. Raybin D, Flavin M: An enzyme tyrosylating α-tubulin and its role in microtubule assembly. Biochem Biophys Res Commun 65:1088–1095, 1975

89. Raybin D, Flavin M: Modification of tubulin by tyrosylation in cells and extracts and its effect on assembly in vitro. J Cell Biol 73:492–504, 1977

90. Deporter DA: Microtubules, cyclic AMP and lysosomal enzyme release. A review. Biomedicine 28:5–8, 1978

91. Deanin GG, Thompson WC, Gordon MW: Tyrosyltubulin ligase activity in brain, skeletal muscle, and liver of the developing chick. Dev Biol 57:230–233, 1977

92. Thompson WC: Post-translational addition of tyrosin to alpha tubulin in vivo in intact brain and in myogenic cells in culture. FEBS Lett 80:9–13, 1977

93. Deanin GG, Gordon MW: The distribution of tyrosyltubulin ligase in brain and other tissues. Biochem Biophys Res Commun 71:676–683, 1976

94. Cleveland DW, Hwo SY, Kirschner MW: Physical and chemical properties of purified tau factor and the role of tau in microtubule assembly. J Mol Biol 116:227–247, 1977

95. Cleveland DW, Hwo SY, Kirschner MW: Purification of tau, a microtubule-associated protein that induces assembly of microtubules from purified tubulin. J Mol Biol 116:207–225, 1977

96. Vallee RB, Borisy GG: The non-tubulin component of microtubule protein oligomers. J Biol Chem 253:2834–2845, 1978

97. Scheele RB, Borisy GG: Electron microscopy of metal-shadowed and negatively stained microtubule protein. J Biol Chem 253:2846–2851, 1978

98. Weatherbee JA, Luftig RB, Weihing RR: In vitro polymerization of microtubules from HeLa cells. J Cell Biol 78:47–57, 1978

99. Himes RH, Burton PR, Gaito JM: Dimethyl sulfoxide-induced self-assembly of tubulin lacking associated proteins. J Biol Chem 252:6222–6228, 1977

100. Murphy DB, Vallee RB, Borisy GG: Identity and polymerization-stimulatory activity of the nontubulin proteins associated with microtubules. Biochemistry 16:2598–2605, 1977

101. Editorial: Malfunctioning microtubules. Lancet 1:697–698, 1978

102. Oliver JM, Albertini DF, Berlin RD: Effects of glutathione-oxidizing agents on microtubule assembly and microtubule-dependent surface properties of human neutrophils. J Cell Biol 71:921–932, 1976

103. Kuriyama R: In vitro polymerization of marine egg tubulin into microtubules. J Biochem 81:115–1125, 1977

104. Nishida E, Sakai H: Calcium-sensitivity of the microtubule reassembly system. J Biochem 82:303–306, 1977

105. Fuller GM, Brinkley BR: Structure and control of assembly of cytoplasmic microtubules in normal and transformed cells. J Supramol Struct 5:497–514, 1976

106. Olmsted JB, Borisy GG: Microtubules. Annu Rev Biochem 42:507–540, 1973

107. Goldstein L, Rubin R, Ko C: The presence of actin in nuclei: A critical appraisal. Cell 12:601–608, 1977

108. Goldstein L, Ko C, Errick J: Nuclear actin: An apparent association with condensed chromatin. Cell Biol Int Rep 1:511–515, 1977

109. Corces VG, Avila J: Interaction of contractile proteins with DNA. Eur J Biochem 83:529–535, 1978

110. Rubin RW, Goldstein L, Ko C: Differences between nucleus and cytoplasm in the degree of actin polymerization. J Cell Biol 77:698–701, 1978

111. Wunderlich F, Herlan G: A reversibly contractile nuclear matrix. J Cell Biol 73:271–278, 1977

112. Berezney R, Coffey DS: Identification of

a nuclear protein matrix. Biochem Biophys Res Comm 60:1410–1417, 1974

113. Berezney R, Coffey DS: Nuclear protein matrix: Association with newly synthesized DNA. Science 189:291–293, 1975

114. Berezney R, Coffey DS: Nuclear matrix: Isolation and characterization of a framework structure from rat liver nuclei. J Cell Biol 73:616–637, 1977

115. Berezney R, Coffey DS: The nuclear protein matrix: Isolation, structure and functions. Adv Enzyme Regul 14:63–100, 1976

116. Wilson L, Anderson K, Chin D: Nonstoichiometric poisoning of microtubule polymerization: A model for the mechanism of action of the vinca alkaloids, podophyllotoxin and colchicine. Edited by R Goldman, T Pollard, and J Rosenbaum: Cell Motility. Vol. 3. Cold Spring Harbor Conference Cell Proliferation, 1976, pp 1051–1064

117. Corces VG, Salas J, Salas ML, Avila J: Binding of microtubule proteins to DNA: Specificity of the interaction. Eur J Biochem 86:473–479, 1978

118. Lestourgeon WM, Totten R, Forer A: The nuclear acidic proteins in cell proliferation and differentiation. Edited by IL Cameron and JR Jeter, Jr: Acidic Proteins of the Nucleus. New York, Academic Press, 1974, pp 159–190

119. Gabbiani G, Chaponnier C, Zumbe A, Vassalli P: Actin and tubulin co-cap with surface immunoglobulins in mouse B lymphocytes. Nature 269:697–698, 1977

120. Edelman GM: Surface modulation in cell recognition and cell growth. Science 192:218–226, 1976

121. Berlin RD, Oliver JM, Ukena TE, Yin HH: Control of cell surface topography. Nature 247:45–46, 1974

122. Schlessinger J, Elson EL, Webb WW, Yahara I, Rutishauser U, Edelman GM: Receptor diffusion on cell surfaces modulated by locally bound concanavalin A. Proc Natl Acad Sci USA 74:1110–1114, 1977

123. Yahara I, Edelman GM: Electron microscopic analysis of the modulation of lymphocyte receptor mobility. Exp Cell Res 91:125–142, 1975

124. Virtanen I, Miettinen A, Wartiovaara J: Lectin-binding sites are found in rat liver cell plasma membrane only on its extracellular surface. J Cell Sci 29:287–296, 1978

125. Bray D: Membrane movements and microfilaments. Nature 273:265–266, 1978

126. Toh BH, Hard GC: Actin co-caps with concanavalin A receptors. Nature 269:695–696, 1977

127. Scott RE, Maercklein PB, Furcht LT: Plasma membrane intramembranous particle topography in 3T3 and SV3T3 cells: The effect of cytochalasin B. J Cell Sci 23:173–192, 1977

128. Staehelin LA, Hull BE: Junctions between living cells. Scientific American 238:140–152, 1978

129. Carter WG, Hakomori S: A protease-resistant, transformation-sensitive membrane glycoprotein and an intermediate filament-forming protein of hamster embryo fibroblasts. J Biol Chem 253:2867–2874, 1978

130. Flanagan J, Koch GLE: Cross-linked surface Ig attaches to actin. Nature 723:278–281, 1978

131. Ash JF, Singer SJ: Concanavalin-A-induced transmembrane linkage of concanavalin A surface receptors to intracellular myosin-containing filaments. Proc Natl Acad Sci USA 73:4575–4579, 1976

132. Koch GLE, Smith MJ: An association between actin and the major histocompatibility antigen H2. Nature 273:274–278, 1978

133. Loor F: Cell surface design. Nature 264:272–273, 1976

134. Cheung HT, Cantarow WD, Sundharadas G: Colchicine and cytochalasin B (CB) effects on random movement, spreading and adhesion of mouse macrophages. Exp Cell Res 111:95–103, 1978

135. Bhisey AN, Freed JJ: Ameboid movement induced in cultured macrophages by colchicine or vinblastine. Exp Cell Res 64:419–429, 1971.

136. Phillips MJ, Oda M, Yousef I, Fisher MM, Jeejeebhoy KN, Funatsu K: Microfilaments and cholestasis: Selected electron microscopic and cytochemical observations. Edited by H Popper, L Bianchi, and W Reutter: Membrane Alterations as Basis of Liver Injury. Lancaster, England, MTP Press, 1977, pp 343–352

137. Phillips MJ, Oda M, Mak E, Fisher MM, Jeejeebhoy KN: Microfilament dysfunction as a possible cause of intrahepatic cholestasis. Gastroenterology 69:48–58, 1975

138. Gregory DH, Vlahcevic ZR, Prugh MF,

Swell L: Mechanism of secretion of biliary lipids: Role of a microtubular system in hepatocellular transport of biliary lipids in the rat. Gastroenterology 74:93–100, 1978

139. Redman CM, Manerjee D, Howell K, Palade GE: Colchicine inhibition of plasma protein release from rat hepatocytes. J Cell Biol 66:42–59, 1975

140. Redman CM, Manerjee D, Howell K, Palade GE: The step at which colchicine blocks the secretion of plasma protein by rat liver. Ann NY Acad Sci 253:780–788, 1975

141. Orci L, LeMarchand Y, Singh A, Assimacopoulos-Jeannet F, Rouiller C, Jeanrenaud B: Role of microtubules in lipoprotein secretion by the liver. Nature 244:30–32, 1973

142. Stein O, Sanger L, Stein Y: Colchicine-induced inhibition of lipoprotein and protein secretion into the serum and lack of interference with secretion of biliary phospholipids and cholesterol by rat liver in vivo. J Cell Biol 62:90–103, 1974

143. LeMarchand Y, Jeanrenaud B: Role of microtubules in hepatic secretory processes, and metabolic consequences of colchicine administration in vivo. Edited by J Dumont and J Nunez: Hormones and Cell Regulation. Vol 1. Amsterdam, Elsevier, 1977, pp 77–90

144. Baraona E, Leo MA, Borowsky SA, Lieber CS: Pathogenesis of alcohol-induced accumulation of protein in the liver. J Clin Invest 60:546–554, 1977

145. LeMarchand Y, Singh A, Assimacopoulos-Jeannet F, Orci L, Rouiller C, Jeanrenaud B: A role for the microtubular system in the release of very low density lipoproteins by perfused mouse livers. J Biol Chem 248:6862–6870, 1973

146. LeMarchand Y, Patzelt C, Assimacopoulos-Jeannet F, Loten EG, Jeanrenaud B: Evidence for a role of the microtubular system in the secretion of newly synthesized albumin and other proteins by the liver. J Clin Invest 53:1512–1517, 1974

147. Feldman G, Maurice M, Sapin C, Benhamou JP: Inhibition by colchicine of fibrinogen translocation in hepatocytes. J Cell Biol 67:237–243, 1975

148. Chajek T, Friedman G, Stein O, Stein Y: Effect of colchicine, cycloheximide and chloroquine on the hepatic triacylglycerol hydrolase in the intact rat and perfused liver. Biochim Biophys Acta 488:270–279, 1977

149. Jeanrenaud B, LeMarchand Y, Patzelt C: Role of microtubules in hepatic secretory processes. Edited by H Popper, L Bianchi, and W Reutter: Membrane Alterations as Basis of Liver Injury. Lancaster, England, MTP Press, 1977, pp 247–255

150. Riordan JR, Alon N: Binding of [^{3}H]cytochalasin B and [^{3}H]colchicine to isolated liver plasma membranes. Biochim Biophys Acta 464:547–561, 1977

151. Margolis RL, Wilson L: Addition of colchicine-tubulin complex to microtubule ends: The mechanism of substoichiometric colchicine poisoning. Proc Natl Acad Sci USA 74:3466–3470, 1977

152. Wilson L, Bamburg JR, Mizel SB, Grisham LM, Creswell KM: Interaction of drugs with microtubule proteins. Fed Proc 33:158–166, 1974

153. Borisy GG, Taylor EW: The mechanism of action of colchicine. Binding of colchicine-^{3}H to cellular protein. J Cell Biol 34:525–533, 1967

154. Edelman GM, Yahara I, Wang JL: Receptor mobility and receptor-cytoplasmic interactions in lymphocytes. Proc Natl Acad Sci USA 70:1442–1446, 1973

155. Rasmussen SA, Davis RP: Effect of microtubular antagonists on lymphocyte mitogenesis. Nature 269:249–251, 1977

156. Amenta JS, Sargus MJ, Baccino FM: Effect of microtubular or translational inhibitors on general cell protein degradation. Biochem J 168:223–227, 1977

157. Mandell BF, Stahl PD: Demonstration of microtubule independent protein secretion from rat liver. Experientia 33:1464–1465, 1977

158. Temple R, Wolff J: Stimulation of steroid secretion by antimicrotubular agents. J Biol Chem 248:2691–2698, 1973

159. Reaven EP, Reaven GML: Dissociation between rate of hepatic lipoprotein secretion and hepatocyte microtubule content. J Cell Biol 77:735–742, 1978

Chapter 6

Regulation of Growth of Hepatocytes by Sodium Ions

By H. L. LEFFERT *and* K. S. KOCH

ENVIRONMENTAL CONTROL of hepatocyte proliferation depends on complex steady-state interactions among many factors. These consist of defined peptides, their cellular receptors, and other low-molecular-weight substances, including amino acids.[1-5] This view is somewhat compelling because it is supported by observations from many different approaches (Table 1). These have led to findings that at least six classes of substances directly regulate the frequencies with which hepatocytes synthesize DNA and/or divide (Table 2). Detailed discussions have been presented on how these factors interact; how their in vivo blood and intrahepatic levels change during proliferative transitions; how they may exert their effects; and how hepatocellular specificity, if it exists, may be controlled.[3-5,10,19,24,27,32]

THE "COUPLING" PROBLEM

One aspect of hepatocyte growth regulation is the phenomenon of "retrodifferentiation."[33] This process occurs during well-regulated proliferative transitions[34] and involves the transient regression of the adult cell toward a more primitive state. When growth regulation fails, e.g., during chemical hepatocarcinogenesis, retrodifferentiation tends to be irreversible, although to differing degrees.[35]

The molecular mechanisms that "couple" retrodifferentiation to normal proliferation are unknown. Recently, we simulated retrodifferentiation patterns observed during liver regeneration[34,36,37] using a novel adult rat hepatocyte culture system.[8,9] The preliminary results, described here, suggest that altered monovalent cation ion fluxes bear upon the "coupling" problem.

PROLIFERATIVE PROPERTIES OF NORMAL ADULT RAT HEPATOCYTES IN PRIMARY MONOLAYER CULTURE

Adult hepatocytes (Fig. 1) from "quiescent" tissue proliferate in vitro.[3,8-10] DNA synthesis rates increase strikingly within 48 hr after plating,[8] and cell

From the Cell Biology and Molecular Biology Laboratories, the Salk Institute for Biological Studies, San Diego, California.

Supported by National Cancer Institute Grant CA 21230 and National Institute on Alcohol Abuse and Alcoholism Grant P50AA03504.

123

TABLE 1.—*Systems Used to Study Growth Regulation of Hepatocytes*

System	Comments	References
Hepatocyte tissue culture	Primary euploid monolayers	3, 6–11
	Fetal or adult	
	Proliferation-competent	
	Prominent differentiated function	
Chronic infusion	Intact animal	12, 13
	Hormones and nutrients	
	Evisceration; 70% hepatectomy	14, 15
	Repletion with specific hormones	
	70% hepatectomy	16
	Anti-insulin serum	
Split portacaval transposition	Long-term	17
	Specific hormone addition	
Nutritional	Intact animal	13, 18
	Amino acid deficiency	
	Intact animal or 70% hepatectomy	5, 10
	choline/methionine deficiency (lipotrope)	
Nutritional/cell culture	Lipotrope deficiency	3
	Primary adult hepatocyte monolayers	
Animal mutants	"Fatty" Zucker rats	19
	Hypertriglyceridemia	

division begins after a 2- to 3-day lag (Fig. 2A). Population growth proceeds slowly, with a doubling time of 60 to 70 hr. Proliferation occurs in arginine-free medium, but only if ornithine is present; a functioning urea cycle[8-10] probably enables this growth under these conditions.[7] Proliferation is further limited by deficient levels of insulin, glucocorticoid, and other serum factors.[3,8-10] During the growth cycle, DNA synthesis is not further stimulated by the addition of glucagon or epidermal growth factor.[8]

Nine to eleven days after plating, a stationary phase is reached (Fig. 2A). This probably results from the depletion of growth factors from the medium, increased cell density, and the increased buildup of nonspecific (e.g., lactic acid and ammonium ion) and specific (e.g., very low density lipoprotein [VLDL][19]) growth inhibitors. Studies with fetal hepatocyte cultures and with different in vivo animal models predict that cultured adult hepatocytes should produce less VLDL during the growth cycle and more during "resting" states.[5,10,19,27] Preliminary observations of triglyceride synthesis, a putative marker for VLDL production, are consistent with this prediction (Fig. 2E). Similar conclusions have been reached from direct studies of VLDL synthesis and secretion using a porcine hepatocyte system (J. C. Williams and D. B. Weinstein, personal communication).

Stationary phase conditions are partly reversible because fluid changes to fresh growth media promote DNA synthesis initiation after a 12-hr delay (Fig. 3). Using this assay, under chemically defined conditions, synergistic stimulation of DNA synthesis by nanogram levels of insulin, glucagon, and epidermal growth factor is now observed (H. Leffert and T. Moran, unpublished observations).

TABLE 2.—*Factors Regulating Hepatocyte Proliferation*

Class	Substance	Action*	References†
Peptide	Somatomedin C	+	1
	Epidermal growth factor	+	16,20
Peptide hormone	Insulin	+	1–3,8,15,17,20–24
	Glucagon	− and +	1,10,12,13,15,20–23
	Parathyroid hormone‡	? +	25
	Hydrocortisone	+/−	1,3,8–10,24,26
	Triiodothyronine; thyroxine	+/−	1,10,12,13,24
Nutrient	Amino acids	+	2,3,12,13,18,21
Lipid	"Conditioning factor"	+	2
	Prostaglandin E_1	+/−	27
	Fatty acid(s)	+/−	K.S.Koch, unpublished
Serum macromolecule	Fetal bovine "SFI"	+	28
	Fetal bovine "SFII"	−	28
	Rat "SFI"	+	19
	Rat "SFII"	+	19
	Rat very low density lipoprotein	−	5,10,19,27
Purine	Cyclic GMP	+	1,23,29
	Cyclic AMP	+/−	1,23,29
	Hypoxanthine (? highly phosphorylated nucleotide)	+	4,27,30,31

*The symbols +, − indicate direct in vitro stimulatory or inhibitory effects, respectively; the symbol − and + indicates results with fetal and adult system, respectively; and +/− indicates mixed actions at low to high molar concentrations.

†References refer to in vitro and in vivo studies.

‡In vivo hepatic proliferation absolutely requires parathyroid hormone, but direct in vitro effects have yet to be demonstrated.

Carcinogen metabolism, reflected by cytochrome P-450 activation of *N*-acetylaminofluorene (AAF) and binding of its metabolites to cellular macromolecules,[3] shows a dose-related growth-cycle pattern (Fig. 2F). How this metabolism is related to malignant transformation, if at all, is poorly understood.

RETRODIFFERENTIATION IN VITRO

Five additional properties have been measured during the growth cycle. These include the expression of the "adult" and "fetal" isozymic forms of pyruvate kinase (Fig. 2B); albumin (Fig. 2C) and α_1-fetoprotein secretion (Fig. 2D); and the levels of glutathione S-transferase B ("ligandin," Fig. 2G), an anion-binding cytosol protein involved with nonoxidative detoxification reactions[38] (see Chapter 11).

The data show that the "adult" phenotype, defined by high cellular levels of pyruvate kinase L-type activity and ligandin, is transiently "lost" during logarithmic growth but reappears as the system enters a stationary phase. The "fetal" phenotype, defined by high cellular levels of pyruvate kinase K-type activity and α_1-fetoprotein secretion, appears only after proliferation begins. Details of these findings have been published.[9]

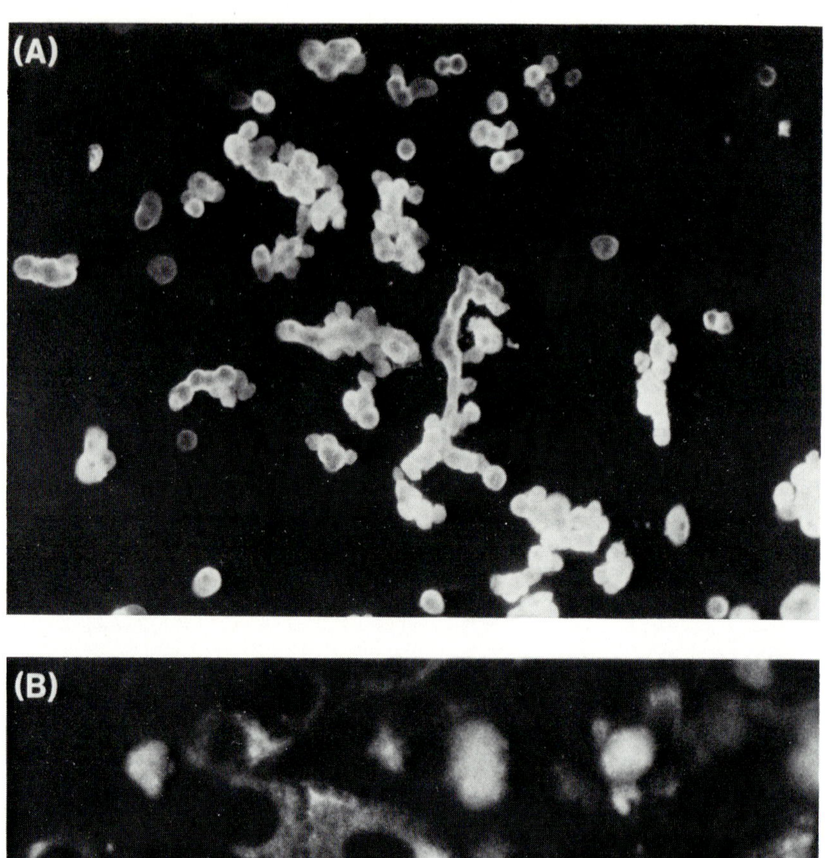

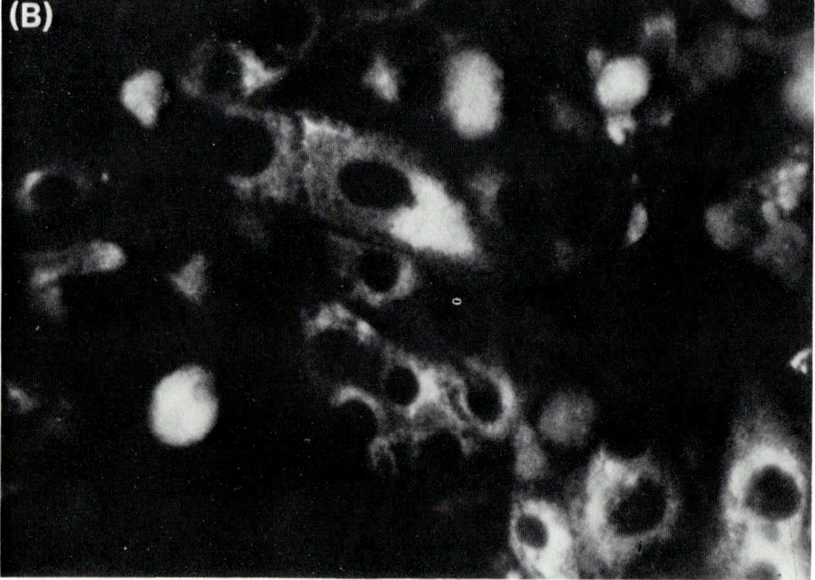

FIG. 1—Immunofluorescent visualization of albumin-containing adult rat hepatocytes in primary monolayer culture. These photomicrographs were made by D. Bostwick in this laboratory, in collaboration with S. Sell. The cells were fixed, after extensive washing, in 100% ethanol. Staining methodology has been discussed elsewhere.[10] Culture ages were 1 to 2 hr (panel A, × 100); 4 to 5 days (panel B, × 400); and 11 to 12 days (panel C, × 100) postplating.

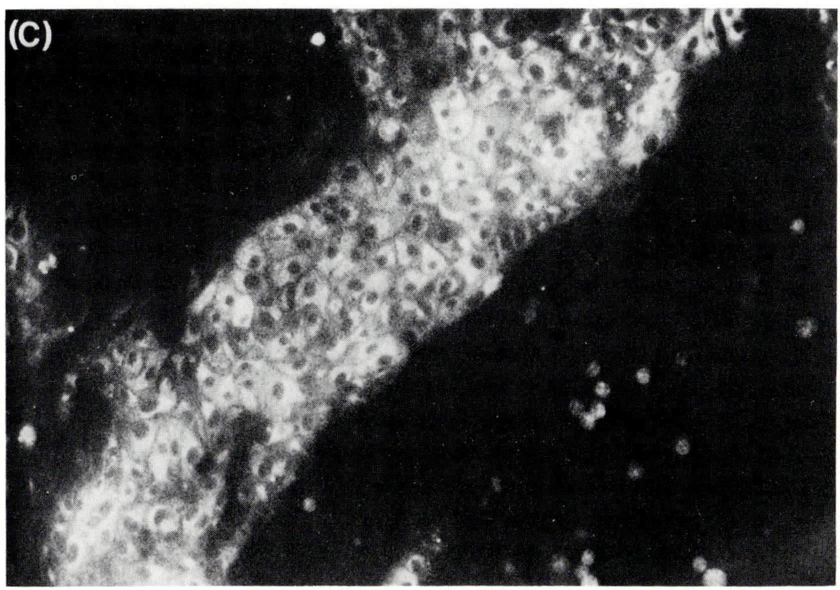

MONOVALENT CATION FLUXES REGULATE
HEPATOCYTE PROLIFERATION

Potassium and sodium ion influxes are inhibited by ouabain, a specific inhibitor of (Na^+, K^+) ATPase,[39] and by amiloride, a potassium-sparing diuretic thought to interact specifically with cell-surface sodium ion binding sites.[40] Both drugs inhibit hepatic DNA synthesis initiation after 70% hepatectomy; amiloride is four times more effective than ouabain under these conditions (Table 3).

This inhibition could result from indirect effects. Similar results, however, are obtained with cultured adult hepatocytes (Table 3; Fig. 3). The data do not show that unstimulated basal rates (e.g., laparotomy or no medium change) are significantly less inhibited (about 30%), whereas stimulated DNA synthesis rates can be inhibited more than 99%. Tetrodotoxin, a sodium ion influx inhibitor specific for excitable cells, fails to detectably inhibit hepatocyte DNA synthesis.

Amiloride and ouabain are ineffective when administered 22 hr after initial stimulation (Table 3). In culture, amiloride washout is not followed immediately by increased DNA synthetic rates but rather by a constant delay of 12 hr before these rates change (Fig. 3). These results imply that altered monovalent cation fluxes are very early and continuously required prereplicative changes necessary to initiate hepatocyte DNA synthesis. Full details will be reported (H. Leffert and K. S. Koch, in preparation).

Number of Cells per Culture
10⁶
A
PYRUVATE KINASE (L-Isozyme)
I.U. per Culture
B
0.14
0.12
0.10
0.08
0.06
0.04
0.02
0
0.7
0.6
0.5
0.4
0.3
0.2
0.1
0
I.U. per Culture
PYRUVATE KINASE (K-Isozyme)
PYRUVATE KINASE (L-Isozyme)
I.U. per mg protein
0.5
0.4
0.3
0.2
0.1
0
L-TYPE (I)
K-TYPE (II)
3
2
1
0
I.U. per mg protein
PYRUVATE KINASE (K-Isozyme)
DAYS AFTER PLATING
ALBUMIN
(ng Secreted per Culture / 24 hrs.)
C
2000
1500
1000
500
0
Cycloheximide
0   2   4   6   8   10   12
DAYS AFTER PLATING
D
[³H]-Leucine
Incorporation
Cycloheximide
5
4
3
2
1
[³H]-Leucine Uptake into α₁-Fetoprotein
(cpm Secreted per
Culture / 24 hrs. X 10⁻³)
0   2   4   6   8   10   12
DAYS AFTER PLATING

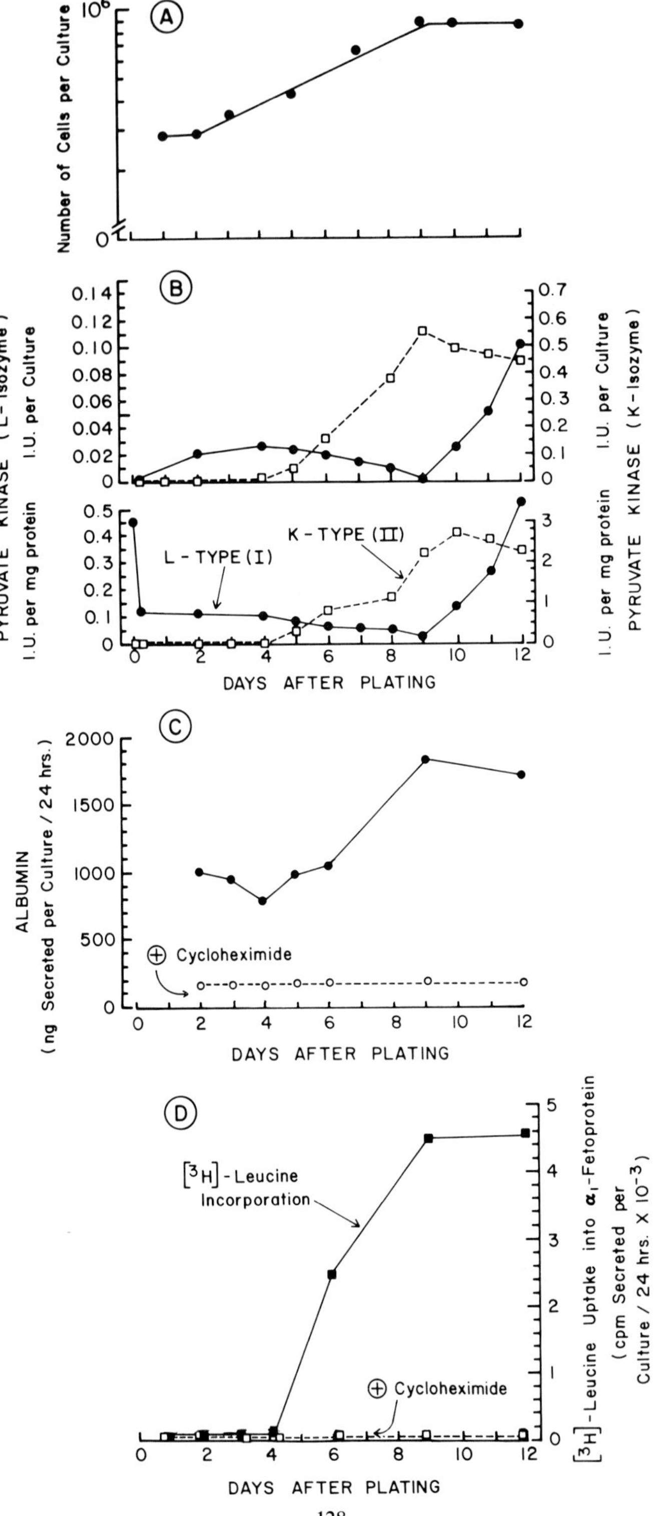

128

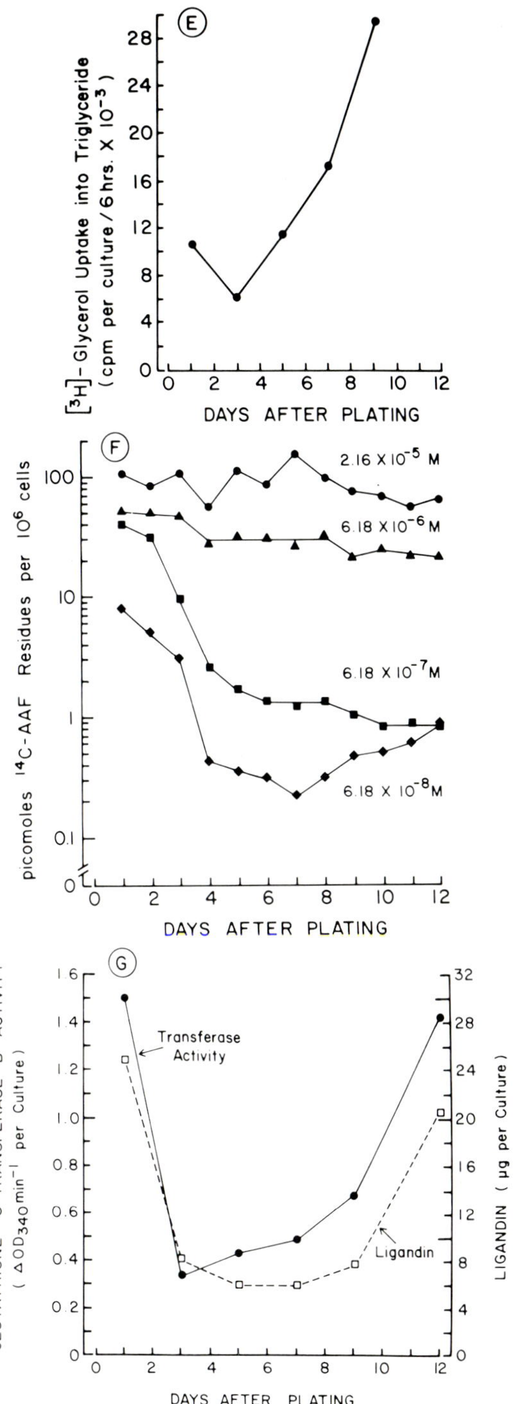

FIG. 2—Phenotypic patterns during the growth cycle of adult rat hepatocytes in primary monolayer culture. Experimental details are given in references 3 and 9. Molar values shown in panel F are initial AAF concentrations; labeling was for 24 hr.[3]

129

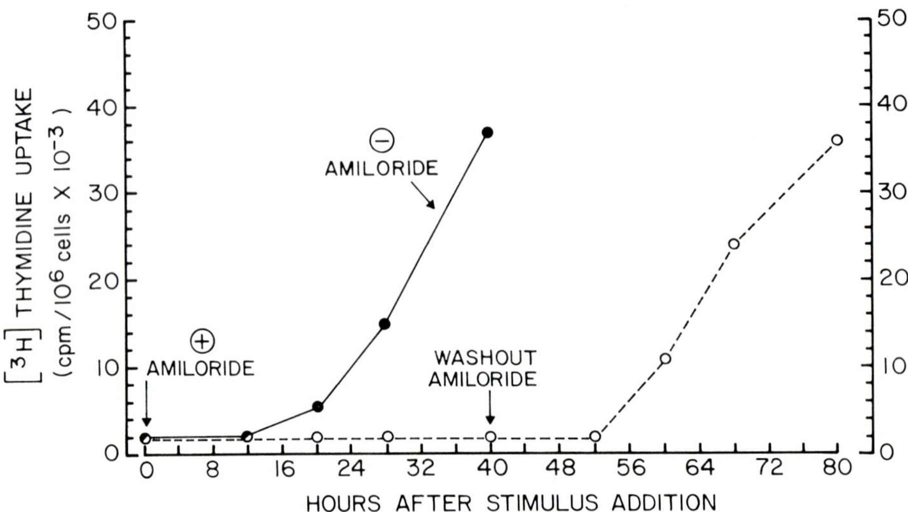

FIG. 3—Amiloride effects upon DNA synthesis initiation in primary monolayer cultures of adult rat hepatocytes. Twelve-day-old cultures (Fig. 2A) were stimualted by a change to fresh arginine-minus ornithine-supplemented medium containing insulin, hydrocortisone, and 15% v/v dialyzed fetal bovine serum.[8] DNA synthesis was measured with [³H]thymidine.[1] The label was present continuously in unchanged cultures 12 hr prior to "zero-time" ("zero hour" point) or added again at the time of the medium change. Amiloride (3×10^{-4} M) was present as indicated; "washout" consisted of a change to fresh medium plus label. Similar results were obtained if fresh arginine-minus ornithine-supplemented medium contained *only* insulin, glucagon, and epidermal growth factor (each present at 50 nanograms ml⁻¹) instead of insulin, hydrocortisone, and 15y serum, as stated above.

TABLE 3.—*Effects of Amiloride and Ouabain on Adult Hepatocyte DNA Synthesis Initiation**

Addition	Dose†	Hours after Stimulus†	% Inhibition‡
Amiloride	1.0, in vivo	0	36
	50.0, in vivo	0	>99
	50.0, in vivo	22	0
	0.3 mM, in vitro	0	>99
	0.3 mM, in vitro	22	0
Ouabain	50.0, in vivo	0	23
	50.0, in vivo	22	0
	0.15 mM, in vitro	0	>99
	0.15 mM, in vitro	22	0

*Hepatocyte DNA synthesis was initiated in vivo by 70% hepatectomy and in vitro using adult cells as described in the legend to Figure 3.

†Drugs were administered intramuscularly as saline suspensions in vivo (mg/250 g body weight) and as aqueous solutions in vitro (final molariconcentrations in medium) at the indicated times. Time-zero is defined as the time of applying the stimulus.

‡In vivo DNA synthesis was measured between 22 and 24 hr after the operation[19] and is expressed as [³H]thymidine counts per minute incorporated per milligram of DNA per 2 hr (laparotomy = 500-1000 cpm, 70% hepatectomy = 140,000 cpm; input [³H] = 40 μCi/250 g, 40 Ci/mM). In vitro DNA synthesis, expressed as [³H]thymidine cpm incorporated/10⁶ cells/24 hr, was measured as described in the legend to Figure 3 (no change = 2500 cpm; change to fresh medium = 28,000 cpm). Control values (0% inhibition) are the numerical differences between stimulated and unstimulated values. Errors of measurement were ± 10%.

TABLE 4.—*Effects of Amiloride and Ouabain on Cultured Adult Rat Hepatocyte Protein Synthesis**

| | % Inhibition | | | | | | | | |
| | Secreted | | | Intracellular | | | Total[†] | | |
Addition[‡]	Total	Albumin	α_1F	Total	Albumin	α_1F	Total	Albumin	α_1F
Amiloride	49	31	75	69	66	76	64	40	76
Ouabain	9	13	41	23	22	33	20	15	40

*Hepatocyte cultures were those described in the legend to Figure 3. Total protein synthesis and specific protein synthesis represent [³H]leucine uptake into hot acid-insoluble protein or into a specific immunoprecipitate, respectively (for details, see reference 9).
†These numbers are based on the (raw data) sum of "intracellular" plus "secreted" values.
‡Additions were made at "zero-time"; control = saline vehicle; amiloride and ouabain at final concentrations of 3.0 and 1.5×10^{-4} M, respectively. Control values (0% inhibition) were, from left to right (nine columns): 4.5, 0.9, 0.146; 14.2, 0.330, 0.072; 18.7, 1.23, and 0.218 ([³H]leucine cpm/culture/24 hr $\times 10^{-6}$). Errors of measurement ranged ± 10% ($N=3$); cell numbers per culture were invariant.

MONOVALENT CATION FLUXES REGULATE HEPATOCYTE-DIFFERENTIATED FUNCTION

Alpha$_1$-fetoprotein (α_1F) synthesis in vitro is selectively inhibited, compared to albumin, by amiloride and ouabain (Table 4). This is seen with respect to total protein synthesis or to synthesized material secreted by the cells. In both cases, α_1F synthesis is two- to threefold more sensitive than albumin to inhibitory effects. Neither drug appears to inhibit secretion per se because a coordinated inhibition of secreted total protein and secreted albumin or α_1F is not observed. Inhibition of overall total protein synthesis also does not account for these findings because ouabain is 69% less effective than amiloride. Anomalous values for inhibition of "intracellular" albumin production (66% and 22%, for amiloride and ouabain, respectively) as compared to values observed for "secretion" (31% and 13%, respectively) may result partly from albumin compartmentalization.[41] Precise interpretations must await detailed molecular studies.

POSSIBLE SIGNIFICANCE OF THESE FINDINGS TO HEPATOCYTE GROWTH REGULATION

An association between cellular proliferation and increased nutrient utilization has been known for many years. One prevailing idea is that growth factors regulate proliferation partly by stimulating cellular uptake of growth-limiting nutrients (for review, see reference 24).

In this regard, blood and intrahepatic hormone level alterations following 70% hepatectomy seem consistent with increased solute transport being one of the early changes required for liver regeneration.[3,27] Solute transport is energized by sodium ion gradients.[42] Furthermore, sodium ions selectively increase rates of initiation of protein synthesis.[43]

These considerations and the findings described above suggest to us that one mechanism for proliferation-retrodifferentiation coupling may occur at the level of cell membrane systems regulating sodium flux. This hypothesis can be tested in several ways, including measurements of intracellular sodium levels and of membrane potential, especially after treatments with DNA-initiating hormones.

We cannot help but wonder if high intracellular sodium levels represent a chemical symbol of primitive evolutionary existence. It may not be fortuitous that sodium ions also regulate the initiation of DNA replication in the fertilized egg[44] and the initiation of amphibian limb regeneration.[45]

ACKNOWLEDGMENTS

Invaluable technical assistance from T. Moran and H. Skelly is gratefully appreciated. Amiloride® was a generous gift from Dr. C. Stone of Merck, Sharpe and Dohme; EGF was provided by Dr. S. Potter (the Salk Institute).

REFERENCES

1. Leffert HL: Growth control of differentiated fetal rat hepatocytes in primary monolayer culture. VII. Hormonal control of DNA synthesis and its possible significance to the problem of liver regeneration. J Cell Biol 62:792–801, 1974

2. Koch KS, Leffert HL: Growth control of differentiated fetal rat hepatocytes in primary monolayer culture. VI. Studies with conditioned medium and its functional interactions with serum factors. J Cell Biol 62:780–791, 1974

3. Leffert HL, Koch KS: Proliferation of hepatocytes. Ciba Foundation Symposium 55 (new series): Hepatotrophic Factors. Amsterdam, Elsevier/Excerpta Medica/North-Holland, 1978, pp 61-94

4. Koch KS, Leffert HL: Control of hepatic proliferation: A working hypothesis involving hormones, lipoproteins, and novel nucleotides. Metabolism 25:1419-1422, 1976

5. Leffert HL: Glucagon, insulin and their hepatic receptors: An endocrine pattern characterizing hepatoproliferative transitions in the rat. Edited by PP Foá, JS Bajaj, and NL Foá: Glucagon, Its Role in Physiology and Clinical Medicine. New York, Springer-Verlag, 1978, pp 305-319

6. Leffert HL, Paul D: Studies on primary cultures of differentiated fetal liver cells. J Cell Biol 52:559-568, 1972

7. Leffert HL, Paul D: Serum dependent growth of primary cultured differentiated fetal rat hepatocytes in arginine-deficient medium. J Cell Physiol 81:113-124, 1973

8. Leffert HL, Moran T, Boorstein R, Koch KS: Procarcinogen activation and hormonal control of cell proliferation in differentiated primary adult rat liver cell cultures. Nature 267:58–61, 1977

9. Leffert H, Moran T, Sell S, Skelly H, Ibsen K, Mueller M, Arias I: Growth state-dependent phenotypes of adult hepatocytes in primary monolayer culture. Proc Natl Acad Sci USA 75:1834–1838, 1978

10. Leffert HL, Koch KS, Rubalcava B, Sell S, Moran T, Boorstein, R: Hepatocyte growth control: In vitro approach to problems of liver regeneration and function. J Natl Cancer Inst 48:87–101, 1978

11. Leffert HL, Koch KS, Moran T, Williams M: [47] Liver cells. Edited by WB Jakoby and IH Pastan: Methods in Enzymology: Tissue Culture. Vol. 58. New York, Academic Press, 1979, pp 536–544

12. Short J, Brown RF, Husakova A, Gilbertson JR, Zemel R, Lieberman I: Induction of DNA synthesis in the liver of the intact animal. J Biol Chem 247:1757–1766, 1972

13. Short J, Armstrong NB, Kolitsky MA, Mitchell RA, Zemel R, Lieberman I: Amino acids and the control of nuclear DNA replication in liver. Edited by B Clarkson and R Baserga: Control of Proliferation in Animal Cells. Vol. I. Cold Spring Harbor Laboratory, NY, Cold Spring Harbor, 1974, pp 37–48

14. Whittemore AD, Kasuya M, Voorhees AB Jr, Price JB Jr: Hepatic regeneration in the absence of portal viscera. Surgery 77:419–426, 1975

15. Bucher NLR, Swaffield MN: Regulation of hepatic regeneration by synergistic action of insulin and glucagon. Proc Natl Acad Sci USA 72:1156–1160, 1975

16. Bucher NLR, Patel U, Cohen S: Hormonal factors concerned with liver regeneration. Ciba Foundation Symposium 55 (new series): Hepatotrophic Factors. Amsterdam, Elsevier/Excerpta Medica/North-Holland, 1978, pp 95–100

17. Starzl TE, Porter KA, Kashiwagi N, Putnam CW: Portal hepatotrophic factors, diabetes mellitus and acute liver atrophy, hypertrophy and regeneration. Surg Gynecol Obstet 141:843–858, 1975

18. Short J, Armstrong NB, Zemel R, Lieberman I: A role for amino acids in the induction of deoxyribonucleic acid synthesis in liver. Biochem Biophys Res Commun 50:430–437, 1973

19. Leffert HL, Weinstein DB: Growth control of differentiated fetal rat hepatocytes in primary monolayer culture. IX. Specific inhibition of DNA synthesis initiation by very low density lipoprotein and possible significance to the problem of liver regeneration. J Cell Biol 71:20–32, 1976

20. Richman RA, Claus TH, Pilkis SJ, Friedman DL: Hormonal stimulation of DNA synthesis in primary cultures of adult rat hepatocytes. Proc Natl Acad Sci USA 73:3589–3593, 1976

21. Paul D, Walter S: Growth control in primary fetal rat liver cells in culture. J Cell Physiol 85:113–123, 1975

22. Price JB Jr: Insulin and glucagon as modifiers of DNA synthesis in the regenerating rat liver. Metabolism 25:1427-1428, 1976

23. Armato U, Draghi E, Andreis PG: Effects of purine nucleotides on the growth of neonatal rat hepatocytes in primary tissue culture. Exp Cell Res 105:337–347, 1977

24. Leffert HL, Koch KS: Control of animal cell proliferation. Edited by G Rothblat and V Cristofalo: Growth, Nutrition and Metabolism of Cells in Culture. Vol. III. New York, Academic Press, 1977, pp 225–294

25. Rixon RH, Whitfield JF: The control of liver regeneration by parathyroid hormone and calcium. J Cell Physiol 87:147–157, 1976

26. Henderson C, Fischel RE, Loeb JN: Suppression of liver DNA synthesis by cortisone. Endocrinology 88:1471–1476, 1971

27. Leffert HL, Koch KS, Rubalcava B: Present paradoxes in the environmental control of hepatic proliferation. Cancer Res 36:4250–4255, 1976

28. Leffert HL: Growth control of differentiated fetal rat hepatocytes in primary monolayer culture. V. Occurrence in dialyzed fetal bovine serum of macromolecules having both positive and negative growth regulatory functions. J Cell Biol 62:767–779, 1974

29. Short J, Tsukada K, Rudert WA, Lieberman I: Cyclic adenosine 3':5'-monophosphate and the induction of deoxyribonucleic acid synthesis in liver. J Biol Chem 250:3602–3606, 1975

30. Koch KS, Leffert HL, Moran T: Hepatic proliferation control by purines, hormones, and nutrients. Edited by W Fishman and S Sell: Onco-Developmental Gene Expression. New York, Academic Press, 1976, pp 21-33

31. Rapaport E, Bucher NLR: Two new adenine nucleotides in normal and regenerating liver. Edited by W Fishman and S Sell: Onco-Developmental Gene Expression. New York, Academic Press, 1976, pp 13–20

32. Ciba Foundation Symposium 55 (new series): Hepatotrophic Factors. Amsterdam, Elsevier/Excerpta Medica/North-Holland, 1978, pp 1–405

33. Uriel J: Cancer, retrodifferentiation and the myth of Faust. Cancer Res 36:4269–4275, 1976

34. Sell S, Nichols M, Becker FF, Leffert HL: Hepatocyte proliferation and alpha₁-fetoprotein in pregnant, neonatal, and partially hepatectomized rats. Cancer Res 34:865–871, 1974

35. Advances in Experimental Medicine and Biology. Vol. 92. Edited by HP Morris and WE Criss: Morris Hepatomas. New York, Plenum Press, 1978, pp 1–775

36. Bonney RJ, Walker PR, Potter VR: Isozyme patterns in parenchymal and nonparenchymal cells isolated from regenerating and regenerated rat liver. Biochem J 136:947–954, 1973

37. Arias I, Fleischner G, Kirsch R, Mishkin S, Gatmaitan Z: On the structure, regulation and function of ligandin. Edited by IM Arias and WG Jakoby: Glutathione: Metabolism and Function. New York, Raven, 1976, pp 175–188

38. Habig W, Pabst M, Fleischner G, Gatmaitan Z, Arias IM, Jakoby W: The identity of glutathione transferase B with ligandin, a major binding protein of liver. Proc Natl Acad Sci USA 71:3879–3882, 1974

39. Perrone JR, Blostein R: Asymmetric interaction of inside-out and right-side out erythrocyte membrane vesicles with ouabain. Biochim Biophys Acta 291:680–689, 1973

40. Benos DJ, Mandel LJ: Irreversible inhibition of sodium entry sites in frog skin by a photosensitive amiloride analog. Science 199:1205-1206, 1978

41. Judah JD, Quinn PS: Calcium ion-dependent vesicle fusion in the conversion of proalbumin to albumin. Nature 271:384-385, 1978

42. Schultz SG, Curran PF: Coupled transport of sodium and organic solutes. Physiol Rev 50:637–718, 1970

43. Christman JK: Effect of elevated potassium level and amino acid deprivation on polysome distribution and rate of protein synthesis in L cells. Biochim Biophys Acta 294:138–152, 1973

44. Johnson JD, Epel D, Paul M: Intracellular pH and activation of sea urchin eggs after fertilization. Nature 262:661–664, 1976

45. Borgens RB, Vanable JW Jr, Jaffe LF: Bioelectricity and regeneration. I. Initiation of frog limb regeneration by minute currents. J Exp Zool 200:403–416, 1977

Chapter 7

Hepatotrophic Substances

By THOMAS E. STARZL, M.D., Ph.D.
and
JOHN TERBLANCHE, Ch.M., F.R.C.S. (Eng), F.C.S. (S.A.)

BLOOD returning from the nonhepatic splanchnic organs via the portal venous system can specifically influence the morphologic features, regenerative capacity, and function of the liver. The portal blood constituents responsible for these effects have collectively been termed portal hepatotrophic factors. Much of the in vivo evidence about portal hepatotrophic factors has been obtained by seeing what happens to the liver when it is deprived of all or part of the portal venous return, by surgically removing nonhepatic splanchnic viscera, or by infusing hormones or other substances systemically or directly into the liver circulation.

In this review, the effects of hepatotrophic substances upon hepatocytic structure and function are treated separately from their influence upon the regeneration that follows partial hepatectomy. The failure to make this distinction has probably been responsible for many of the controversies about new developments in portal hepatotrophic physiology. This was clear in the discussions of a symposium on this subject held in May 1977.[1]

HEPATOTROPHIC EFFECTS EXCLUDING REGENERATION

The most easily achieved portaprival state occurs when all the splanchnic venous return is diverted around the liver via an anastomosis to the vena cava, leaving the liver with only an arterial supply. This procedure of portacaval shunt is also called Eck's fistula, after the Russian military surgeon who described it in dogs more than 100 years ago.[2] Based on the short-term survival of one of his eight dogs, Eck thought that a completely diverting portacaval shunt in dogs was compatible with prolonged good health. In 1893, however, Hahn, Massen, Nencki, and Pavlov[3] showed that dogs with Eck's fistula developed anorexia, weight loss, hepatic atrophy, and encephalopathy.

The atrophy of hepatocytes caused by Eck's fistula, as well as other

From the Departments of Surgery, Denver Veterans Administration Hospital and University of Colorado Medical Center, Denver, Colorado; University of Cape Town, South Africa.

The work was supported by research grants MRIS 8118-01 and 7227-01 from the Veterans Administration; by grant numbers AM-17260 and AM-07772 from the National Institutes of Health; and by grant numbers RR-00051 and RR-00069 from the General Clinical Research Centers Program of the Division of Research Resources, National Institutes of Health; and the Medical Research Council, South Africa.

structural changes, occurs with great rapidity, being 90% complete within 4 days.[4-6] Ultrastructurally, the most striking and specific changes are depletion and disruption of the rough endoplasmic reticulum and reduction in the membrane-bound ribosomes. The same general light- and electron-microscopic changes occur after portal diversion in the livers of rats, dogs, swine, baboons, and man, with some variations in degree.[7] Thus the hepatic injury of Eck's fistula is common to all species studied.

What is the explanation of the changes caused by portacaval shunt? When Bollman[8] summarized the situation of Eck's fistula in 1961, the flow hypothesis was widely accepted. It stated that Eck's fistula syndrome was caused by a suboptimal volume as opposed to quality of hepatic blood flow. This conclusion was apparently incontrovertibly supported by experiments in which the portal flow lost after portacaval shunt was replaced with vena caval and arterial blood, respectively.[9,10] With this portal blood replacement, most of the adverse effects of Eck's fistula in dogs were avoided. Thus, portal blood seemed to possess no physiologically important special qualities.

The fallacy of the flow hypothesis became evident during efforts to define the necessary conditions for successful auxiliary liver transplantation.[11] With two livers present, the organ given blood returning from the nonhepatic splanchnic organs remained healthy, whereas the liver deprived of such nourishment atrophied in spite of adequate portal flow from nonsplanchnic sources.[12] Apparently, the liver with first access to the splanchnic venous blood was extracting something efficiently enough so that the second organ suffered from its absence.

The transplant preparations that had made the foregoing physiologic effect apparent had a flaw that prevented complete acceptance of what had become known as the hepatotrophic concept. There was a potential inequality of the two organs in that the homograft was under immunologic attack despite host immunosuppression, whereas the animal's own liver was not. Consequently, other experiments were designed.

At first, a split or partial transposition was developed that, in effect, divided the dog's own liver into two fragments.[13,14] With this operation, splanchnic venous blood was provided for one portal branch of the liver, whereas the other portal branch was detached and supplied with blood from the inferior vena cava. The quantity of flow was measured in many of these experiments[13,14] and found to be generally greater on the side perfused by vena caval blood. The lobes supplied with systemic venous blood atrophied grossly and histopathologically, whereas the lobes given normal portal blood hypertrophied.

The two sides had other easily quantifiable differences. The splanchnic-fed lobes had more glycogen and glucokinase activity and lower concentrations of cyclic AMP and active phosphorylase. The biochemical dissociation was shown in many other ways[15] that are beyond the scope of this review, but the reasonable inference was that these two liver sides were living in different metabolic worlds in which hormone control played a dominant role. The nature of the biochemical differences suggested that endogenous insulin, which was being efficiently extracted by the first liver tissue to which it was exposed, played an important role. The significance of endogenous insulin was further highlighted when the advantages enjoyed by the lobes perfused by splanchnic venous blood were greatly reduced, although not eliminated, by either total pancreatectomy or alloxan diabetes.[16,17] While emphasizing the role of insulin, these investigations showed equally clearly that nonpancreatic hormones or other substances also contributed to the total hepatotrophic effect of splanchnic venous blood. Although the influence of these extrapancreatic factors remains unchallenged, they have not been identified.

Eventually, another kind of double liver fragment model provided much more decisive information.[15,17,18] In these experiments, one portion of the liver was fed by the effluent of hormone-rich blood returning from the pancreas, duodenum, stomach, and spleen, while the opposite lobes were perfused via a venous graft with nutrition-rich blood returning from the intestine (Fig. 1A).

The histopathologic results in 60-day experiments or even as early as 4 days were dramatic. The lobules in liver lobes receiving pancreaticoduodenal venous effluent became bigger and crammed with glycogen in contrast to the shrunken deglycogenated lobules in lobes receiving intestinal venous return.

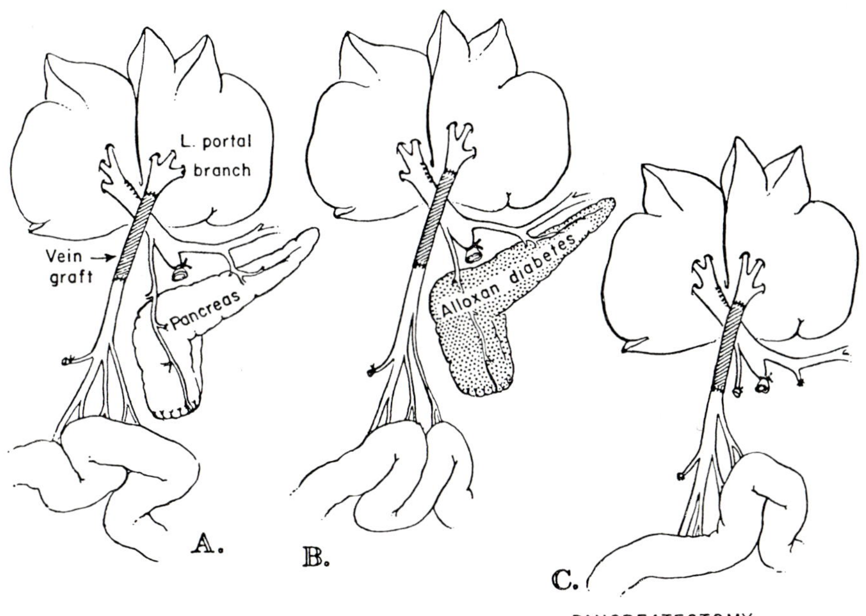

Splanchnic division

FIG. 1—Splanchnic division experiments. In these dogs, the right liver lobes received venous return from the pancreaticogastroduodenosplenic region, and the left liver lobes received venous blood from the intestines. In other experiments, the intestinal blood was directed into the right lobes with pancreatic flow to the left side. (A) Nondiabetic dogs. (B) Alloxan-induced diabetic dogs. (C) Dogs with total pancreatectomy. (By permission of Surgery, Gynecology, and Obstetrics 140:549–562, 1975.)

An accurate way to quantitate hepatocytic size was developed for such experiments.[15] With light-microscopic tracing, hepatocytes were drawn on a standard thickness paper and weighed. The weights were called size units. In Figure 2, the right lobar hepatocytes, which had pancreatic input, had an obvious advantage as compared to those on the left, which were fed with intestinal venous return. The cell size data could then be summarized in graphs or tables.

In splanchnic division experiments (Fig. 1), the previously mentioned possibility that insulin was the major cause for the kind of cell size difference seen in Figure 2 was strengthened by additional 60-day experiments in which alloxan diabetes (Fig. 1B) and pancreatectomy (Fig. 1C) were superimposed.[16,17] The animals were treated daily with subcutaneous insulin, which presumably was delivered to both sides of the liver without preference. The size advantages for the right-sided hepatocytes were cancelled about equally in the animals subjected to alloxan diabetes or pancreatectomy. In all such experiments, the nearly equal effects of alloxan poisoning and pancreatectomy have tended to minimize any major role of glucagon as a hepatotrophic factor, at least as far as cell size was concerned.

At the same time, these experiments emphasized that insulin was not the only factor. When endogenous insulin was removed from the splanchnic division experiments in which subcutaneous exogenous insulin was given, the dominant hepatic tissue became that supplied by intestinal venous return. Translating these findings into more practical terms, the most favorable condition for portal perfusion was with splanchnic venous blood that contained normal amounts of endogenous insulin. The least favorable condition was perfusion with systemic venous blood. Intermediate in quality was splanchnic

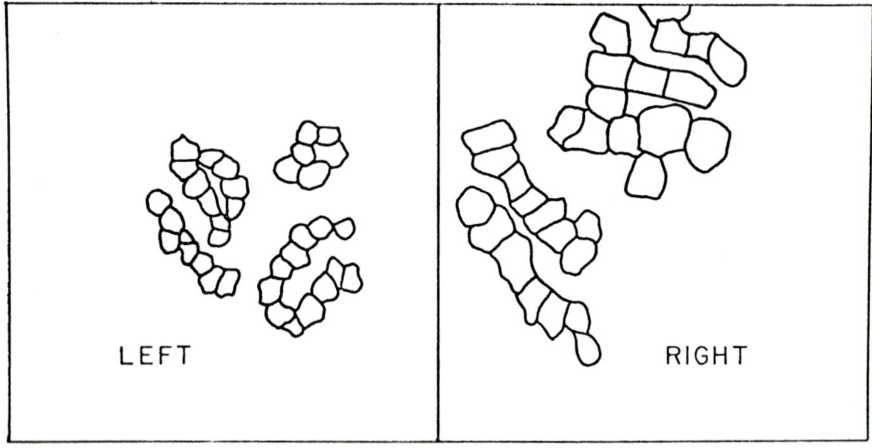

FIG. 2—Hepatocyte shadows traced during histopathologic examination. These were later cut out on standard paper and weighed as an index of hepatocyte size. The right lobes with the large hepatic cells received venous blood from the pancreas, stomach, duodenum, and spleen. The relatively shrunken left lobes with the small hepatocytes received intestinal blood. (By permission of Surgery, Gynecology, and Obstetrics 137:179–199, 1973.)

TABLE 1.—*Number of Labeled Hepatocytes per 1,000 Hepatocytes in Livers of Normal Dogs and Dogs with Splanchnic Division*

Type Dog	Number of Experiments	Right Lobes Mean SD	Left Lobes Mean SD
Normal	11	1.6 ± 0.5	1.5 ± 0.4
Splanchnic division (nondiabetic)	6	17.3 ± 3.8	4.0 ± 1.0
Splanchnic division (alloxan)	4	4.9 ± 0.4	17.8 ± 3.6
Splanchnic division (pancreatectomy)	5	5.1 ± 1.0	17.5 ± 3.9

venous blood that was deficient in endogenous insulin but rich in other as yet unknown elements.

An insulin effect on cell proliferation was also convincingly unmasked by the divided liver experiments[16,17] (Table 1). The liver lobes receiving pancreatic blood (the right lobes in the experiments shown, Table 1) of nondiabetic dogs submitted to splanchnic division had autoradiographic evidence of hepatocyte hyperplasia relative to the lobes receiving intestinal blood, although both sides had greater cell renewal than normal after 60 days. This right lobar dominance was eliminated, being transferred to the left side by either alloxan or pancreatectomy diabetes in those animals being treated with subcutaneous regular insulin. The emergence of dominant left lobes (Table 1) after the elimination of endogenous insulin indicated, as previously emphasized from other lines of evidence, the presence of potent but unknown additional intestinal portal factors.

The full implications of portal blood deprivation on liver function are not known, since whatever changes occur in the portaprival state are undoubtedly subtle. Liver function after Eck's fistula, or after the better tolerated portacaval transposition of Child, was long thought to be essentially normal, the main deficiency being inefficient clearance of ammonia.[19,20] With the striking organelle changes described earlier after portal blood deprivation, however, the effects are apt to be wide ranging. An example is the striking antilipidemic effect of portacaval shunt in dogs,[16,21–24] rats,[25,26] baboons,[7,15] pigs,[27,28] and man.[29,30] The consequent falls in cholesterol phospholipids and possibly triglycerides may be due in part to reduced hepatic lipid synthesis.[16,25,27,28,31,32]

The effect of portal factors upon hepatic lipid synthesis has been demonstrated in the same splanchnic division models shown in Figure 1, after 60 days.[16] Lipid synthesis in normal unaltered dogs measured either with in vitro or in vivo techniques was the same on both sides of the liver (Fig. 3). After splanchnic division in nondiabetic animals, the liver perfused with blood from the pancreas and upper splanchnic organs synthesized more cholesterol than the other liver portion perfused with venous return from the intestine. This advantage in cholesterol synthesis was reversed with alloxan diabetes and total pancreatectomy. As before, these results (Fig. 3) indicated the dependence of normal cholesterol synthesis upon the pancreas, but the reversal effect demonstrated a major contribution by nonpancreatic venous blood as well. The same conclusions were reached in other experiments in which hepatic choles-

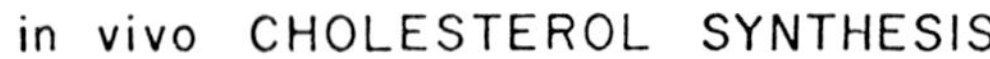

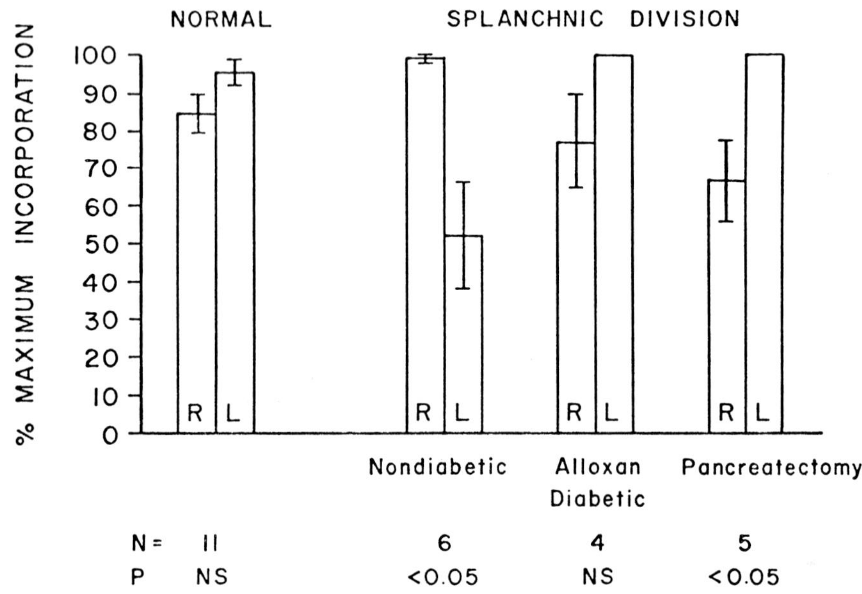

FIG. 3—In vivo cholesterol synthesis in the right and left liver lobes in normal dogs and in dogs submitted to splanchnic division. In all the splanchnic division experiments, the right lobes received pancreaticogastroduodenosplenic blood, while the left lobes were nourished with intestinal venous blood. The animals with splanchnic division were nondiabetic, alloxan-diabetic, or diabetic as the result of total pancreatectomy. The *p* values compare the synthesis rates for the two sides, the greater rate of synthesis being assigned a value of 100%. For the other side, a proportionately lower percentage was calculated. (By permission of Surgery, Gynecololgy, and Obstetrics 140:381–396, 1975.)

terol synthesis was measured after stepwise portacaval shunt in which intestinal flow was diverted at a first stage followed by secondary diversion of the pancreaticogastroduodenosplenic blood.[16]

We now return from the double liver fragment models full cycle to Eck's fistula. If insulin was a vital portal hepatotrophic factor, the reason for its unmasking by the double liver fragment experiments became understandable. The well-known efficiency of insulin's removal during a first pass through hepatic tissue[33] made the insulin relatively unavailable for a second liver or liver fragment. At the same time the protection afforded after portal diversion by flow augmentation procedures such as Child's portacaval transposition[9] or Fisher's portal arterialization[10] was explained. If insulin and other hepatotrophic substances were bypassed around a single liver, they would be returned to it in diluted form in direct relation to the total hepatic blood flow that these procedures increased.

If the secrets of Eck's fistula were explained mainly by depriving the liver of direct access to endogenous insulin, the experiment shown in Figure 4 should be a direct test of that hypothesis. Nonhypoglycemic infusions of insulin

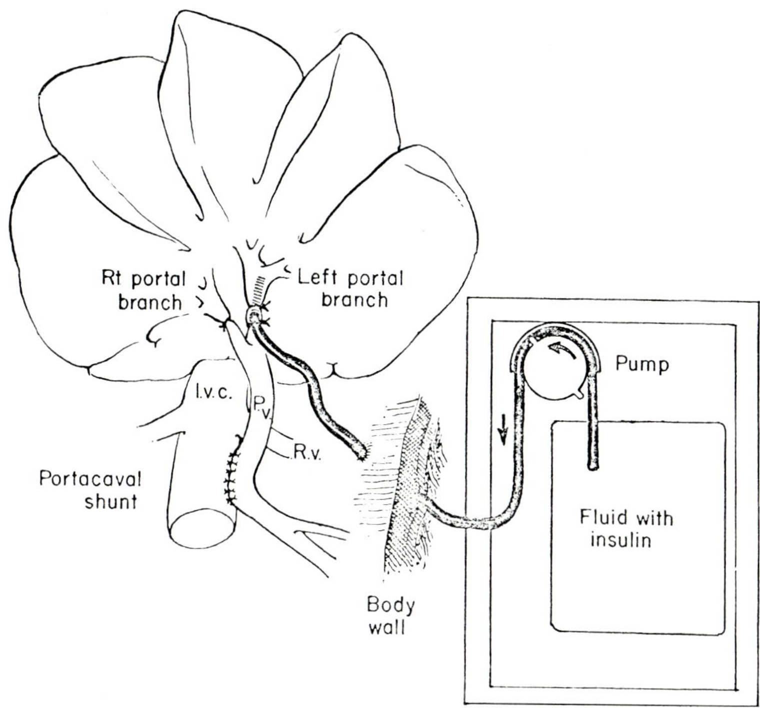

FIG. 4—Experiments in which Eck's fistula is performed and postoperative infusions are made into the left portal vein. (By permission of the Lancet 1:821–825, 1976.)

and other substances were made for 4 days into the ligated left portal vein after Eck's fistula.[5,6] The experiment was designed to evaluate any direct protective effect on the left lobar hepatic tissue, as well as to assess a spillover effect on the right lobes after recirculation. The results were unequivocal. Insulin greatly reduced the acute atrophy that otherwise halved the size of the cells, and it preserved hepatocytic ultrastructure. In small doses, glucagon did not potentiate the action of insulin, and in large doses, it may have reduced the insulin benefit. Glucagon alone in either small or large doses had no effect.[5,6]

The effect of insulin on hepatocytic proliferation was also striking. After Eck's fistula, the mitotic rate was already increased to about three times normal (from 1.6 to 4.8 per 1000 cells). Insulin more than tripled this cell renewal, with no spillover to the contralateral lobes. Glucagon alone had no effect, nor did it potentiate the action of insulin.[5,6]

Thus, relative "hepatic insulinopenia" was established as the most important element in the liver injury of Eck's fistula. It would be regrettable if the very clarity with which insulin has emerged as a principal portal hepatotrophic substance were to obscure the search for contributory factors. The observation that the insulin protection in our infusion experiments was not complete was interpreted as a reflection of missing ancillary substances. The same multifactorial theme has been consistent in all work from our laboratory on the hepatotrophic subject. However, the fact that the multifactorial control of hepatocytic integrity has not deemphasized the central role of insulin in maintaining liver cells was recently redemonstrated after removal of all the nonhepatic splanchnic viscera including the pancreas.[34] The intraportal infusion of insulin alone prevented most of the atrophy and other structural deterioration of hepatocytes, and it preserved the rate of spontaneous liver cell renewal which was otherwise depressed. The hepatic protection in eviscerated animals was almost identical to that observed with intraportal insulin therapy after portacaval shunt described above and was indistinguishable from the hepatotrophic effect of insulin in diabetic rats.[35] In hepatocyte tissue culture systems, many investigators have described analogous insulin effects.[36-39] The role of insulin in maintaining hepatocytic mitochondrial metabolism has also been emphasized.[40,41] No potentiating effect of glucagon has been demonstrated in any of these nonregeneration models.

PORTAL BLOOD FACTORS AND REGENERATION

From the information in the foregoing section, portal blood factors are indisputably important in maintaining healthy liver cells. The assumption was a natural one that portal blood might have a specific effect on the hepatic regeneration that follows partial hepatectomy. This possibility was purely speculative, however, since hepatectomies were not performed in any of our early studies. However, a portal blood effect on regeneration after liver resection in rats was soon demonstrated.[42-44]

The nature of the regeneration-promoting substances and their origin remain in dispute. An additional question is whether they initiate regeneration or merely permit the process to proceed and, in either case, by what means. The conflicting conclusions reached in various laboratories on these issues result in part from the use of different experimental models and in part from the way in which data have been interpreted or the time after hepatectomy when the data have been acquired.

Much information about the origin of regeneration-promoting (or permitting) factors has come from evisceration procedures introduced in dogs[45] in conjunction with partial hepatectomy and adapted for rats.[46] An artifact existed in this early work in that exogenous insulin was incidentally administered as part of the postoperative parenteral fluid therapy. Later studies showed a striking depression and delay of regeneration after complete evisceration that could be restored toward or even to normal by treatment with a combination of insulin and glucagon in high doses.[47-49]

The crucial splanchnic factors did not seem to be from the intestine. Although an obtunded regeneration response was found after intestinal resection,[50] this could not be confirmed.[51,52] By contrast, an almost complete absence of liver regeneration after total pancreatectomy in rats and dogs was reported,[51,53,54] and this could be restored to normal by treatment with insulin and glucagon.[54] The crucial splanchnic organ for hepatic regeneration was concluded to be the pancreas, and insulin and glucagon were the most critical elements in a pancreatic role, while the other nonhepatic splanchnic organs were of minor importance.[54]

Evidence that this was an excessively simplified view was available from older work,[55] recently confirmed,[56] that liver resection in diabetic rats is followed by vigorous regeneration. Our own investigations with split liver preparations (Fig. 1) plus hepatectomy in diabetic and nondiabetic dogs emphasized the importance of pancreatic blood in supporting regeneration, but they also showed important similar qualities in nonpancreatic splanchnic blood.[4] Although their data were not so interpreted by them, Broelsch et al. demonstrated with clever isotransplantation experiments that venous effluent from the jejunum, ileum, and duodenum supported hepatic regeneration, albeit less well than blood from the pancreas.[57]

The results of a recent study have again demonstrated the complexity of control of regeneration by portal hepatotrophic factors and have strengthened our original multifactorial hypothesis by clearly differentiating pancreatic influences from those originating in the rest of the intra-abdominal gastrointestinal tract.[58] In these investigations, the removal of all the nonhepatic splanchnic viscera resulted in severe inhibition of DNA synthesis and essentially complete elimination of the histopathologic expression of liver regeneration. Leaving the distal colon in place did not significantly improve the eviscerated animals' response to hepatic resection, as measured with autoradiography, despite the fact that plasma pancreaticlike glucagon was thereby kept at a nearly normal concentration. Nor did the infusion of exogenous glucagon, insulin, or glucagon and insulin in combination into the portal vein have a striking restorative effect upon regeneration.

Concomitant or prior removal of the pancreas alone reduced but did not abolish the response to 44% hepatectomy. The response to 72% hepatic resection was likewise dampened by pancreatectomy. Most importantly, extirpation of the rest of the nonhepatic splanchnic viscera, while preserving the pancreas, reduced the response to hepatic resection even more than did pancreatectomy alone. Thus, removal of the pancreas and other viscera had a subtractive effect on regeneration.

Bucher and Malt[59] and more recently Leffert and Koch[60] have similarly proposed regeneration as a complex series of events under multifactorial control. If hormones play an important regulatory role, precise delineation of their contributions may be difficult with any of the presently available experimental models, since a hormone-free environment is hard to achieve in intact animals, particularly dogs.[56] Small amounts of hormones could have major physiologic effects, since the regenerating hepatocytes may have changing sensitivity to insulin and/or glucagon.[61-63] The same probably applies to other hormones.

Do Portal Factors Initiate Regeneration?

Hormone interactions conceivably could be responsible for growth initiation as well as control.[64] After partial hepatectomy in rats or dogs, well-ordered biphasic changes occur in liver cyclic AMP and adenyl cyclase prior to and during regeneration.[63,65–67] The various nonhepatic splanchnic eviscerations (pancreatectomy, extirpation of all organs except the pancreas, total eviscer- ation) which resulted in retarded regeneration caused severe pertubations in these hormonally controlled "messenger" components.[63] Whether these de- viations have a cause-and-effect relation to the defective regeneration that was observed or are merely coincidental remains speculative.

The potential link between multiple hormone changes and regeneration is strengthened by the intriguing studies of MacManus et al.,[65] who had previ- ously shown with cultured thymus cells that increases in cyclic AMP levels induced with epinephrine, parathormone, prostaglandins, and calcium imme- diately preceded the initiation of DNA synthesis and active cell proliferation. The same early biphasic rises in cyclic AMP occur in rat livers 2½ and 12 hr after partial hepatectomy with a return toward normal as DNA synthesis be- gan.[65] These findings have been confirmed in rats,[66,67] and similar but less well defined changes have been noted in regenerating dog livers.[63] In addition, in- creased cyclic-AMP-dependent protein kinases correlated perfectly in regen- erating rat livers with the induction of ornithine decarboxylase.[67]

Ornithine decarboxylase has been implicated[68–70] as the rate-limiting enzyme in the polyamine biosynthetic pathways active in regeneration. Intravenous solutions containing triiodothyronine, amino acids, glucagon, and heparin in- duced nuclear DNA formation and mitosis in the whole livers of unoperated nondiabetic rats,[71] and enhanced ornithine decarboxylase activity followed treatment with this solution.[72] Glucagon in this stimulatory solution could be completely replaced with a butyryl derivative of cyclic AMP, leading to the conclusion that cyclic nucleotide plays a critical role in the induction of hepatic DNA synthesis and cell mitosis.[73]

Do Nonportal Factors Initiate Regeneration?

While portal blood factors clearly influence regeneration, they may not ini- tiate this process but merely play a permissive role. The actual genesis of regeneration may have a quite different explanation and could even start in the liver itself. This possibility has not been fully explored, even though the lit- erature is replete with reports compatible with such a hypothesis.

Publications between 1931 and 1953 suggested that liver mitosis could be stimulated in intact experimental animals by homologous liver mash injected intraperitoneally[74–76] or by intravenous injections of liver fractions.[77] McJunkin and Breuhaus were the first to demonstrate increased mitosis in a model using the already regenerating partially hepatectomized liver of the rat.[74] However, the first truly convincing evidence of a liver-specific mitotic stimulator was that a single administration of liver mash prepared from weanling rat livers and given intraperitoneally to adult rats caused hepatocyte proliferation that was maximum at 48 hr.[78,79] Although adult liver mash was not stimulatory, striking stimulatory activity was found when the regenerating remnant of an adult rat liver, 48 hr after partial hepatectomy, was used to prepare the liver mash.[79] Even after a year of twice-weekly injections, regenerating adult liver mash still had a hepatic mitotic stimulatory effect. Furthermore, in these chronically treated rats, intra-abdominal tumors developed at a 67% rate, presumably because of the specific stimulus to proliferation. Only one of these tumors was a liver tumor, however, while the majority were intraperitoneal reticular sarcomas. Rats chronically treated with nonregenerating adult liver mash did not develop intra-abdominal tumors.[79]

The concept of a stimulatory substance originating in the regenerating liver itself lay dormant until 1971.[80,81] Then in 1975, a regenerative stimulator substance was demonstrated in the supernatant after high-speed centrifugation of an extract of rat liver mash. This regenerative stimulator substance was present in very young rat livers but only appeared after partial hepatectomy in adult livers. The extract from intact adult rat livers actually inhibited regeneration in the assay system used (34% hepatectomized rats).[82]

Meanwhile, evidence was accumulating that there was a circulating plasma or serum stimulatory factor in animals with regenerating livers. The relevant experiments were diverse and ingenious. Regenerative activity was increased in the intact liver of the unresected partner of a pair of parabiotic rats after partial hepatectomy in the parabiotic twin.[83] Although confirmed by some,[84,85] the concept remained in dispute until clarified by the more efficient cross-circulation experiments.[86–88] As total hepatectomy in one rat stimulated significant DNA synthesis in the cross-circulated partner with an intact liver, the source of the humoral factor was postulated not to be in the resected liver remnant,[88] but the rationale of this contention has subsequently been challenged.[80]

Although suggested earlier,[89] the stimulatory effect of serum from animals with a regenerating liver was first convincingly demonstrated in a cell culture system in 1952.[90] This finding has been confirmed and extended.[91–93] Serum or plasma also increased mitotic activity in vivo,[94–98] while hepatocytes proliferated in normal rats subjected to multiple exchange transfusions with blood from partially hepatectomized rats.[99] Finally, mitotic activity was increased in small liver autografts in partially hepatectomized animals.[100–103] The stimulating substance in the serum of rats with regenerating livers was characterized as a heat-stable protein of low molecular weight (approximating 26,000).[104]

The first convincing suggestion that such humoral factors came from the liver itself was made by Blomqvist.[79] Fisher, however, based on the experiments already discussed, did not favor this concept.[88] Then Levi and Zeppa[80,81] appeared to establish the link between the serum-stimulating factors and the liver by direct investigation with an isolated perfused rat liver system. They demonstrated increased DNA synthesis in normal livers perfused for 1 hr (after a 20-min stabilization period), using the effluent of a regenerating rat liver that had been subjected to a 70% partial hepatectomy 18 or 24 hr previously and testing this by either direct cross-circulation or perfusion of the normal liver with reconstituted effluent. Nonregenerating intact rat livers caused no increase in DNA synthesis in this system.[80] They subsequently showed that the cells synthesizing new DNA were mostly hepatic parenchymal cells situated predominantly in the peripheral region.[81] Unfortunately, this work could not be confirmed in carefully conducted studies.[105,106] The major objection was the short time (1 hr) of exposure of the normal liver to the partially hepatectomized liver effluent. Attention has once again been directed to a liver source for the humoral factors, however,[82] and, if confirmed, would strongly support a liver-plasma physiologic axis that is important in liver regeneration.

By contrast, an inhibitor of liver regeneration remains an intriguing and controversial question despite investigation over the past half century. The controversy is highlighted in a number of excellent reviews.[107–110] Both serum and liver extract from intact adult rats have been shown to inhibit regeneration in the already regenerating liver,[82,98,110] while this inhibitor disappears within 2 hr of partial hepatectomy and is, in fact, replaced by a stimulatory substance.[82]

At this time, the true role of portal blood or liver factors in initiating or potentiating or in stimulating or inhibiting liver regeneration remains to be fully elucidated.

CLINICAL IMPLICATIONS

Decisions in patients for or against portacaval shunt, as well as the type of shunt, should take into consideration the hepatotrophic concept. If hepatopetal flow is still present in the portal vein, the Warren-Zeppa shunt[111] preserves this flow while at the same time decompressing esophageal varices. The long-term results of controlled trials of this ingenious procedure are awaited with interest. If portacaval shunting does not prove to be of benefit in cirrhotic patients with bleeding esophageal varices,[112] the evaluation of nonshunt procedures will assume increasing importance.[113]

We believe that preservation of portal flow is a vital concern in patients with liver disease. However, the fact that man is resistant to the more serious metabolic consequences of Eck's fistula[7] has made it feasible to perform the procedure with benefit in patients suffering from glycogen storage disease. These patients have had correction of a number of preexisting metabolic abnormalities, as well as amazing growth spurts.[29,114,115] Continuous feeding may be an even better way of treating these children or at least is an ancillary measure that can be used with shunting.[116]

Lately, our greatest interest in portal diversion has been in homozygous type II hyperlipidemia,[29,30] a disorder that leads to lethal cardiovascular complications by adolescence. More than 20 patients throughout the world (3 in our personal experience) have had their serum lipids lowered by portacaval shunt. Only two outright failures of response have been recorded, and in both (one from Europe and one from South Africa) the shunts had clotted. The serum cholesterol concentration in our original case fell from 800 mg/dl to nearly normal, probably as a result, at least in part, of reduced hepatic cholesterol synthesis, as mentioned earlier. The falls in serum cholesterol in our patients 2 and 3 were also dramatic, the range of reduction being 40% to 60%. The unsightly xanthomas in the skin and tendons melted away with time. Relief of angina in some of these patients and diminution of aortic stenosis in others have suggested that resorption of the same material is occurring from the damaged vascular system.

The hepatotrophic concept has suggested new lines of inquiry in a more general way about the pathogenesis and/or treatment of several human disease processes, including a variety of liver disorders and even diabetes mellitus, for which subcutaneous insulin therapy may be the right drug by an inappropriate route.[1]

Saunders and co-workers,[117] in Volume IV of this series, pointed out that the ability of the liver to regenerate in the setting of fulminant hepatic failure had been overemphasized in the past. In their view the available methods of treatment would not influence mortality unless sufficient regeneration occurred spontaneously or could be stimulated therapeutically. As no major breakthrough has been made in the management of fulminant hepatic failure, the hope remains that with a better understanding of the controlling mechanisms of regeneration (initiators and potentiators), methods of stimulating regeneration in these patients will become available. Possible therapeutic modalities include hormone therapy, as suggested in the past.[17] Whether the answer will be in complicated mixtures[71,73] or in pharmacologic doses of insulin and glucagon, as suggested by the study in mice with murine hepatitis,[118] still remains to be proven. Alternatively, future therapy may well be with as yet unidentified initiators of regeneration, which might even originate from the damaged or regenerating liver itself.

REFERENCES

1. Porter R, Whelan J (Editors): Hepatotrophic Factors (Ciba Foundation Symposium 55). Amsterdam, Elsevier Excerpta Medica, 1978, pp 1–405
2. Eck NVK: Concerning ligation of the vena porta. Voen Med Zh 130:1. (English translation: Child CG: Eck's fistula. Surg Gynecol Obstet 96:375–376, 1953)
3. Hahn M, Massen O, Nencki M, Pavlov J: Die Eck'sche Fistel zwischen der unteren Hohlvene und der Pfortader und ihre Folgen für den Organismus. Arch Exp Pathol Pharmakol 32:161–210, 1893
4. Starzl TE, Porter KA, Kashiwagi N, Putnam CW: Portal hepatotrophic factors, diabetes mellitus, and acute liver atrophy, hypertrophy, and regeneration. Surg Gynecol Obstet 141:843–858, 1975
5. Starzl TE, Porter KA, Putnam CW: Intraportal insulin protects from the liver injury of portacaval shunt in dogs. Lancet 2:1241–1242, 1975
6. Starzl TE, Porter KA, Watanabe K, Putnam CW: The effects of insulin, glucagon and insulin/glucagon infusions upon liver morphology and cell division after complete portacaval shunt in dogs. Lancet 1:821–825, 1976
7. Putnam CW, Porter KA, Starzl, TE: Hepatic encephalopathy and light and electron micrographic changes of the baboon liver after portal diversion. Ann Surg 184:155–161, 1976
8. Bollman JL: The animal with an Eck fistula. Physiol Rev 41:607–621, 1961
9. Child CG, Barr D, Holswade GR, Harrison CS: Liver regeneration following portacaval transposition in dogs. Ann Surg 138:600–608, 1953
10. Fisher B, Russ C, Updegraff H, Fisher ER: Effect of increased hepatic blood flow upon liver regeneration. Arch Surg 69:263–272, 1954
11. Starzl TE, Marchioro TL, Rowlands DT Jr, Kirkpatrick CH, Wilson WEC, Rifkind D, Waddell WR: Immunosuppression after experimental and clinical homotransplantation of the liver. Ann Surg 160:411–439, 1964
12. Marchioro TL, Porter KA, Dickinson TC, Faris TD, Starzl TE: Physiologic requirements for auxiliary liver homotransplantation. Surg Gynecol Obstet 121:16–31, 1965
13. Marchioro TL, Porter KA, Brown BI, Faris TD, Herrmann TJ, Sudweeks A, Starzl TE: The specific influence of non-hepatic

splanchnic venous blood flow on the liver. Surg Forum 16:280–282, 1965

14. Marchioro TL, Porter KA, Brown BI, Otte J-B, Starzl TE: The effect of partial portacaval transposition on the canine liver. Surgery 61:723–732, 1967

15. Starzl TE, Francavilla A, Halgrimson CG, Francavilla FR, Porter KA, Brown TH, Putnam CW: The origin, hormonal nature, and action of hepatotrophic substances in portal venous blood. Surg Gynecol Obstet 137:179–199, 1973

16. Starzl TE, Lee IY, Porter KA, Putnam CW: The influence of portal blood upon lipid metabolism in normal and diabetic dogs and baboons. Surg Gynecol Obstet 140:381–396, 1975

17. Starzl TE, Porter KA, Kashiwagi N, Lee IY, Russell WJI, Putnam CW: The effect of diabetes mellitus on portal blood hepatotrophic factors in dogs. Surg Gynecol Obstet 140:549–562, 1975

18. Pouyet M, Berard Ph, Ruckebusch Y, Grivel ML, Bousquet G, Vauzelle JL: Derivations portohepatiques selectives origine pancreatique du facteur hepatotrophique portal. Ann Chir 23:393–402, 1969

19. Silen W, Mawdsley DL, Weirich WL, Harper HA: Studies of hepatic function in dogs with Eck fistula or portacaval transposition. AMA Arch Surg 74:964–973, 1957

20. Owsley JQ, Goin JM, Clarke JC, Harper HA, McCorkle HJ: A comparison of galactose clearance by the liver following portacaval transposition or Eck fistula. Surg Forum 9:515–518, 1958

21. Winter IC, van Dolah HE, Crandell LA: Lowered serum lipid levels in the Eck fistula dog. Am J Physiol 133:566–571, 1941

22. Coyle JJ, Schwartz MZ, Marubbio AT, Varco RL, Buchwald H: The effect of portacaval shunt on plasma lipids and tissue cholesterol synthesis in the dog. Surgery 80:54–60, 1976

23. Horak W, Gangl A, Funovics J, Grabner G: Effect of portacaval shunt and arterialization of the liver on bile acid metabolism. Gastroenterology 69:338–341, 1975

24. Guzman IJ, Coyle JJ, Schneider PD, Varco RL, Buchwald H: The effect of selective visceral caval shunt on plasma lipids and cholesterol dynamics. Surgery 82:42–50, 1977

25. Edwards KDG, Herz R, Sealey JE, Bradley SE: Lowering of blood pressure, plasma renin substrate, cholesterol and triglyceride by portacaval anastomosis in rats fed on a 60% sucrose/5% lard diet. Clin Sci Mol Med (Suppl) 51:145–146, 1976

26. Magide AA, Press CM, Myant NB, Mitropoulos KA, Balasubramaniam S: The effect of portacaval anastomosis on plasma lipoprotein metabolism in rats. Biochim Biophys Acta 411:302–307, 1976

27. Chase HP, Morris T: Cholesterol metabolism following portacaval shunt in the pig. Atherosclerosis 24:141–148, 1976

28. Carew TE, Saik RP, Johansen KH, Dennis CA, Steinberg D: Low density and high density lipoprotein turnover following portacaval shunt in swine. J Lipid Res 17:441–450, 1976

29. Starzl TE, Chase HP, Putnam CW, Porter KA: Portacaval shunt in hyperlipoproteinaemia. Lancet 2:940–944, 1973

30. Starzl TE, Putnam CW, Koep LJ: Portacaval shunt and hyperlipidemia. Arch Surg 113:71–74, 1978

31. James J, Soeters PB, Fischer JE: In vivo demonstration of impaired cholesterol and fatty acid synthesis following portacaval shunt (PCS) (abstracted). Gastroenterology 72:1075, 1977

32. Bilheimer DW, Goldstein JL, Grundy SM, Brown MS: Reduction in cholesterol and low density lipoprotein synthesis after portacaval shunt surgery in a patient with homozygous familial hypercholesterolemia. J Clin Invest 56:1420–1430, 1975

33. Field JB: Extraction of insulin by liver. Annu Rev Med 24:309–314, 1973

34. Starzl TE, Francavilla A, Porter KA, Benichou J: The effect upon the liver of evisceration with or without hormone replacement. Surg Gynecol Obstet 146:524–531, 1978

35. Reaven EP, Peterson DT, Reaven GM: The effect of experimental diabetes mellitus and insulin replacement on hepatic ultrastructure and protein synthesis. J Clin Invest 52:248–262, 1973

36. Gerschenson LE, Okigaki T, Andersson M, Molson J, Davidson MB: Fine structural and growth characteristics of cultured rat liver cells: Insulin effects. Exp Cell Res 71:49–58, 1972

37. Wagle SR, Ingebretsen WR, Jr, Sampson L: Studies on the effects of insulin on glycogen synthesis and ultrastructure in isolated rat liver hepatocytes. Biochem Biophys Res Commun 53:937–943, 1973

38. Junge U, Nagamori S: Effect of insulin and

glucagon on the DNA synthesis of hepatocyte cultures. Verh Dtsch Ges Inn Med 82(1):385–386, 1976

39. Bernaert D, Wanson J-C, Drochmans P, Popowski A: Effect of insulin on ultrastructure and glycogenesis in primary cultures of adult rat hepatocytes. J Cell Biol 74:878–900, 1977

40. Ozawa K, Yamada T, Honjo I: Role of insulin as a portal factor in maintaining the viability of liver. Ann Surg 180:716–719, 1974

41. Ozawa K, Yamaoka Y, Nanbu H, Honjo I: Insulin as the primary factor governing changes in mitochondrial metabolism leading to liver regeneration and atrophy. Am J Surg 127:669–675, 1974

42. Lee S, Keiter JE, Rosen H, Williams R, Chandler JG, Orloff M: Influence of blood supply on regeneration of liver transplants. Surg Forum 20:369–371, 1969

43. Fisher B, Szuch P, Fisher ER: Evaluation of a humoral factor in liver regeneration utilizing liver transplants. Cancer Res 31:322–331, 1971

44. Chandler JG, Lee S, Krubel R, Rosen H, Nakaji NT, Orloff MJ: The interliver competition and portal blood in regeneration of auxiliary liver transplants. Surg Forum 22:341–343, 1971

45. Price JB, Jr, Takeshige K, Max MH, Voorhees AB, Jr: Glucagon as the portal factor modifying hepatic regeneration. Surgery 72:74–82, 1972

46. Bucher NLR, Swaffield MN: Regeneration of liver in rats in the absence of portal splanchnic organs and a portal blood supply. Cancer Res 33:3189–3194, 1973

47. Bucher NLR, Swaffield MN: Regulation of hepatic regeneration in rats by synergistic action of insulin and glucagon. Proc Natl Acad Sci USA 72:1157–1160, 1975.

48. Price JB, Jr: Insulin and glucagon as modifiers of DNA synthesis in the regenerating rat liver. Metabolism 25(11, Suppl 1): 1427–1428, 1976

49. Whittemore AD, Voorhees AB, Jr, Price JB, Jr: Hepatic blood flow and pancreatic hormones as modifiers of hepatic regeneration. Surg Forum 27:363–365, 1976

50. Fisher B, Szuch P, Levine M, Saffer E, Fisher ER: The intestine as a source of a portal blood factor responsible for liver regeneration. Surg Gynecol Obstet 137: 210–214, 1973

51. Sgro J-C, Charters AC, Chandler JG, Grambort DE, Orloff MJ: Site of origin of the hepatotrophic portal blood factor involved in liver regeneration. Surg Forum 24:377–379, 1973

52. Poirier RA, Cahow CE: Role of the small intestine in liver regeneration. Am Surg 40:555–557, 1974

53. Duguay LR, Orloff MJ: Regulation of liver regeneration by the pancreas in dogs. Surg Forum 27:355–357, 1976

54. Duguay LR, Orloff MJ: Role of the pancreas in regulation of liver regeneration in dogs. Surg Forum 28:387–390, 1977

55. Younger LR, King J, Steiner DF: Hepatic proliferative response to insulin in severe alloxan diabetes. Cancer Res 26:1408–1413, 1966

56. Barra R, Hall JC: Liver regeneration in normal and alloxan-induced diabetic rats. J Exp Zool 201(1):93–99, 1977

57. Broelsch CE, Lee S, Charters AC, III, Chandler JG, Grambort DE, Orloff MJ: Regeneration of liver isografts transplanted in continuity with splanchnic organs. Surg Forum 25:394–397, 1974

58. Starzl TE, Francavilla A, Porter KA, Benichou J, Jones AF: The effect of splanchnic viscera removal upon canine liver regeneration. Surg Gynecol Obstet 147:193–207, 1978

59. Bucher NLR, Malt RA: The nature of the problem. Edited by NLR Bucher and RA Malt: Regeneration of Liver and Kidney. Boston, Little, Brown, 1971, pp 17–21

60. Leffert H, Koch K: Control of animal cell proliferation. Edited by GH Rothblat and VJ Cristofalo: Growth, Nutrition and Metabolism of Cells in Culture. Vol. 3. New York, Academic Press, 1977, pp 226–294

61. Bucher NLR: Insulin, glucagon, and the liver. Adv Enzyme Regul 15:221–230, 1976

62. Leffert H, Alexander NM, Faloona G, Rubalcava B, Unger R: Specific endocrine and hormonal receptor changes associated with liver regeneration in adult rats. Proc Natl Acad Sci USA 72:4033–4036, 1975

63. Francavilla A, Porter KA, Benichou J, Jones AF, Starzl TE: Liver regeneration in dogs: Morphologic and chemical changes. J Surg Res (in press)

64. Holley RW: Control of growth of mammalian cells in cell culture. Nature 258:487–490, 1975

65. MacManus, JP, Franks DJ, Youdale T, Braceland BM: Increases in rat liver cyclic AMP concentrations prior to the initiation

of DNA synthesis following partial hepatectomy or hormone infusion. Biochem Biophys Res Commun 49(5):1201–1207, 1972

66. Thrower S, Ord MG: Hormonal control of liver regeneration. Biochem J 144:361–369, 1974

67. Byus CV, Hedge GA, Russell DH: The involvement of cyclic AMP-dependent protein kinase(s) in the induction of ornithine decarboxylase in the regenerating rat liver and in the adrenal gland after unilateral adrenalectomy. Biochim Biophys Acta 498(1):39–45, 1977

68. Cohen SS: Introduction to the Polyamines. Englewood Cliffs, NJ, Prentice-Hall, 1971, pp 1–179

69. Jänne J, Raina A: Stimulation of spermidine synthesis in the regenerating rat liver: Relation to increased ornithine decarboxylase activity. Acta Chem Scand 22:1349–1351, 1968

70. Russell D, Snyder SH: Amine synthesis in rapidly growing tissues: Ornithine decarboxylase activity in regenerating rat liver, chick embryo and various tumors. Proc Natl Acad Sci USA 60:1420–1427, 1968

71. Short J, Brown RF, Husakova A, Gilbertson JR, Zemel R, Lieberman I: Induction of deoxyribonucleic acid synthesis in the liver of the intact animal. J Biol Chem 247:1757–1766, 1972

72. Gaza DJ, Short J, Lieberman I: On the possibility that the prereplicative increases in ornithine decarboxylase are related to DNA synthesis in liver. FEBS Lett 32:251–253, 1973

73. Short J, Tsukada K, Rudert WA, Lieberman I: Cyclic adenosine 3':5'-monophosphate and the induction of deoxyribonucleic acid synthesis in liver. J Biol Chem 250:3602–3606, 1975

74. McJunkin FA, Breuhaus HC: Homologous liver as a stimulus to hepatic regeneration. Arch Pathol 12:900–908, 1931

75. Wilson JW, Leduc EH: Mitotic rate in mouse liver following intraperitoneal injection of liver, kidney and egg yolk. Anat Rec 97:471–493, 1947

76. Kelly LS, Jones HB: Influence of homologous tissue factors on DNA turnover and radiation protection. Am J Physiol 172:575–578, 1953

77. Marshak A, Walker AC: Effect of liver fractions on mitosis in regenerating liver. Am J Physiol 143:226–234, 1945

78. Teir H, Ravanti K: Mitotic activity and growth factors in the liver of the whole rat. Exp Cell Res 5:500–507, 1953

79. Blomqvist K: Growth stimulation in the liver and tumor development following intraperitoneal injections of liver homogenates in the rat. Acta Pathol Microbiol Scand [Suppl] 121, 1957

80. Levi JU, Zeppa R: Source of the humoral factor that initiates hepatic regeneration. Ann Surg 174:364–370, 1971

81. Levi JU, Zeppa R: The response of normal rat hepatocytes when exposed to humoral (regenerating) factor. J Surg Res 12:114–119, 1972

82. LaBrecque DR, Pesch LA: Preparation and partial characterization of hepatic regenerative stimulator substance (SS) from rat liver. J Physiol 248:273–284, 1975

83. Christensen BG, Jacobsen E: Studies on liver regeneration. Acta Med Scand [Suppl] 234:103–108, 1949

84. Wenneker AS, Sussman N: Regeneration of liver tissue following partial hepatectomy in parabiotic rats. Proc Soc Exp Biol Med 76:683–686, 1951

85. Bucher NL, Scott JF, Aub JC: Regeneration of liver in parabiotic rats. Cancer Res 11:457–465, 1951

86. Moolten FL, Bucher NLR: Regeneration of rat liver. Transfer of humoral agent by cross-circulation. Science 158:272–274, 1967

87. Sakai A: Humoral factor triggering DNA synthesis after partial hepatectomy in the rat. Nature 228:1186–1187, 1970

88. Fisher B, Szuch P, Levine M, Fisher ER: A portal blood factor as the humoral agent in liver regeneration. Science 171:575–577, 1971

89. Akamatsu N: Über Gewebskulturen von Lebergewebe. Virchows Arch [Pathol Anat] 240:308–311, 1923

90. Glinos AD, Gey GO: Hormone factors involved in the induction of liver regeneration in the rat. Proc Soc Exp Biol Med 80:421–425, 1952

91. Wrba H, Rabes H, Ripoll-Gómez M, Ranz H: Die stoffwechselsteigernde Wirkung von Serum teilhepatektomierter Tiere auf Leberkulturen. Exp Cell Res 26:70–77, 1962

92. Grisham JW, Kaufman DG, Alexander RW: ^{3}H-thymidine-labeling of rat liver cells cultured in plasma from sham-or partially-hepatectomized rats (abstracted). Fed Proc 26:624, 1967

93. Hays DM, Tedo I, Matsushima Y: Stimulation of in vitro growth of rat liver cells

with calf serum drawn following partial hepatectomy. J Surg Res 9:133–137, 1969

94. Friedrich-Freksa H, Zaki FG: Spezifische Mitose-auslosung in normaler Rattenleber durch Serum von partiell hepatektomierten Ratten. Z Naturforsch 9b:394–397, 1954

95. Smythe RL, Moore RO: A study of possible humoral factors in liver regeneration in the rat. Surgery 44:561–569, 1958

96. Adibi S, Paschkis KE, Cantarow A: Stimulation of liver mitosis by blood serum from hepatectomized rats. Exp Cell Res 18:396–398, 1959

97. Zimmerman M, Celozzi E: Stimulation of cell division in normal rat liver by a factor in serum from hepatectomized rats (abstracted). Fed Proc 19:139, 1960

98. Stich HF, Florian ML: The presence of a mitosis inhibitor in the serum and liver of adult rats. Can J Biochem Physiol 36:855–859, 1958

99. Grisham JW: Hepatocytic proliferation in normal rats after multiple exchange transfusions with blood from partially hepatectomized rats. Cell Tissue Kinet 2:277–282, 1969

100. Sigel B, Acevedo FJ, Dunn MR: The effect of partial hepatectomy on autotransplanted liver tissue. Surg Gynecol Obstet 117:29–36, 1963

101. Sigel B, Baldia LB, Dunn MR, Menduke H: Humoral control of liver regeneration. Surg Gynecol Obstet 124:1023–1031, 1967

102. Leong GF, Grisham JW, Hole BV, Albright ML: Effect of partial hepatectomy on DNA synthesis and mitosis in heterotopic partial autografts of rat liver. Cancer Res 4:1496–1501, 1964

103. Virolainen M: Mitotic response in liver autograft after partial hepatectomy in rat. Exp Cell Res 33:588–591, 1964

104. Morley CGD, Kingdon HS: The regulation of cell growth. 1. Identification and partial characterization of a DNA synthesis stimulating factor from the serum of partially hepatectomized rats. Biochim Biophys Acta 308:260–275, 1973

105. Compagno J, Grisham JW: Do regenerating liver cells release a substance that shortens G1? (abstracted) Fed Proc 32:837, 1973

106. Lloyd EA, Crozier N, Pamphlet G, Wells M, Saunders SJ: Some observations on liver cell proliferation in the isolated perfused rat liver. Br J Exp Pathol 55:251–259, 1974

107. Brues AM, Subbarow Y, Jackson EB, Aub J: Growth inhibition by substances in the liver. J Exp Med 71:423–438, 1940

108. Weinbren K: Regeneration of the liver. Gastroenterology 37:657–668, 1959

109. Bucher NLR: Experimental aspects of hepatic regeneration. N Engl J Med 277:686–696, 738–746, 1967

110. Bradbrook RA, Newcombe RG, Thatcher J, Blumgart LH: The inhibition of the uptake of ^{3}H-thymidine into liver DNA by the intraportal infusion of fresh serum after partial hepatectomy in the rat. Eur Surg Res 6:364–374, 1974

111. Warren WD, Zeppa R, Fomon JJ: Selective trans-splenic decompression of gastroesophageal varices by distal splenorenal shunt. Ann Surg 166:437–455, 1967

112. Conn HO: Therapeutic portacaval anastomosis: To shunt or not to shunt. Gastroenterology 67:1065–1073, 1974

113. Terblanche J, Northover JMA, Bornman P, Kahn D, Silber W, Barbezat GO, Sellars S, Campbell JAC, Saunders SJ: A prospective controlled trial of injection sclerotherapy in the long-term management of patients after esophageal variceal bleeding: A preliminary report. Surg Gynecol Obstet (in press)

114. Starzl TE, Marchioro TL, Sexton A, Illingworth B, Waddell WR, Faris T, Herrmann TJ: The effect of portacaval transpgsition upon carbohydrate metabolism: Experimental and clinical observations. Surgery 57:687–697, 1965

115. Starzl TE, Putnam CW, Porter KA, Halgrimson CG, Corman J, Brown BI, Gotlin RW, Rodgerson DO, Greene HL: Portal diversion for the treatment of glycogen storage disease in humans. Ann Surg 178:525–539, 1973

116. Crigler JF, Folkman J: Glycogen storage disease: New approaches to therapy. Edited by R Porter and J Whelan: Hepatotrophic Factors (Ciba Foundation Symposium 55). Amsterdam, Elsevier Excerpta Medica, 1978, pp 331–356

117. Saunders SJ, Hickman R, MacDonald R, Terblanche J: The treatment of acute liver failure. Edited by H Popper and F Schaffner: Progress in Liver Disease. Vol. IV. New York, Grune & Stratton, 1972, pp 333–344

118. Farivar M, Wands JR, Isselbacher KJ, Bucher NLR: Effect of insulin and glucagon on fulminant murine hepatitis. N Engl J Med 295:1517–1519, 1976

The Investigation of Sinusoidal Cells: A New Approach to the Study of Liver Function

By E. WISSE *and* D. L. KNOOK

OUR KNOWLEDGE of specific functions of sinusoidal cells of the liver is limited in relation to what is known about parenchymal cells (hepatocytes). One reason for this is that sinusoidal cells are smaller than hepatocytes, so they are easily overlooked in the microscope or neglected in biochemical experiments. The methods for collecting evidence on sinusoidal cells are more or less complementary and can be summarized as follows: (1) microscopic methods, studying morphologic features such as reactions of the cells to experimental conditions, specific staining reactions, enzyme cytochemistry, or intravital light microscopy; (2) biochemical methods, especially with isolation, purification, and culture of different cell types for further biochemical investigations.

Indirect data have been collected by studying reticuloendothelial system (RES) clearance, for instance, under normal and many experimental conditions. These more physiologic data are of importance in increasing knowledge about sinusoidal cells, although they also concern reactions of many cells, including the RES cells in other organs such as the spleen and the bone marrow.

The morphologic peculiarities of sinusoidal cells were elegantly demonstrated in a morphometric study of sinusoidal and parenchymal cells in per-

TABLE 1—*Morphometric Data on Cell Organelles in Sinusoidal Cells and Parenchymal Cells**

	Endothelial Cell	Kupffer Cell	Fat-storing Cell	Parenchymal Cells
Total cytoplasm	3.0	2.3	1.5	93.2
Mitochondria	0.5	0.4	0.3	98.8
Peroxisomes	—	—	—	100
Lipid droplets	—	—	54.7	45.3
Plasma membrane†	15.2	4.2	7.1	73.5
Pinocytotic vesicles	45.2	12.0	0.7	42.1
Lysosomes	14.5	22.1	1.0	62.4

*Data from Blouin et al.,[8] expressed as % of aggregate organelle volume.
†Expressed as % of aggregate membrane surface area.

From the Laboratory for Electron Microscopy, University of Leiden, Rijnsburgerweg, Leiden and the Institute for Experimental Gerontology TNO, Lange Kleiweg, Rijswijk (Z.H.), The Netherlands.

fusion-fixed rat livers[8] (see Table 1). Sinusoidal cells comprise only 6% of the volume of the liver lobule, but contribute 26.5% to the total surface of plasma membranes; they contain 37.6% of the total volume of lysosomes, 54.7% of all lipid droplets, and 57.9% of all pinocytotic vesicles. Since the volume of a certain structure can be related to its functional capacity, it is interesting to compare the volume percentages of the above-mentioned organelles with the volume percentage of, for instance, biliary canaliculi (as a well-known functional entity within the liver lobule), which contributes only 0.43% to the volume of the liver lobule.

FIXATION

For morphologic and cytochemical studies on sinusoidal cells, successful chemical fixation is of great importance. Four different methods for fixing liver tissue are available:

1. Immersion fixation of small (1 mm³) pieces of liver tissue, either in aldehyde or osmic acid solution. This type of fixation may give good results for parenchymal cells, but it is disastrous for sinusoidal cells because they lose characteristic fine structural details and their histologic arrangement is disturbed.
2. Perfusion fixation with glutaraldehyde[27,114] through the portal vein. This is a prerequisite for good preservation of sinusoidal cells.
3. Semiperfusion or transparenchymal perfusion of excised liver tissue (surgical biopsies) by the injection of the tissue with glutaraldehyde with a hypodermic needle. This method can give excellent results in those parts of the tissue not mechanically disturbed by the introduction of the needle.[121]
4. Puncture-perfusion of human needle biopsies of about 2.0 mm diameter can be obtained by wrapping the tissue in plastic film and perfusing it with saline, followed by glutaraldehyde through a very thin needle.[70,71]

MORPHOLOGY

The four different types of sinusoidal cells (Fig. 1) can be characterized by morphologic, cytochemical, and functional criteria which result in the distinction of endothelial, Kupffer, fat-storing, and pit cells.

Endothelial Cells

Endothelial cells form an integral but fenestrated lining of the sinusoids. The fenestrae, with a pore size of 0.1 μ, are arranged in so-called sieve plates also found (Figs. 2 and 4) in the human liver.[71] A basement membrane is lacking. Specific fine structural details of these cells include a spheridium (nuclear body) and a specialized endoplasmic reticulum. The rough endoplasmic reticulum (RER) sometimes parallels the plasma membrane and connects with a network of tubular smooth endoplasmic reticulum. Numerous vesicles can be found within the cytoplasm; most of them belong to the vacuolar apparatus of the

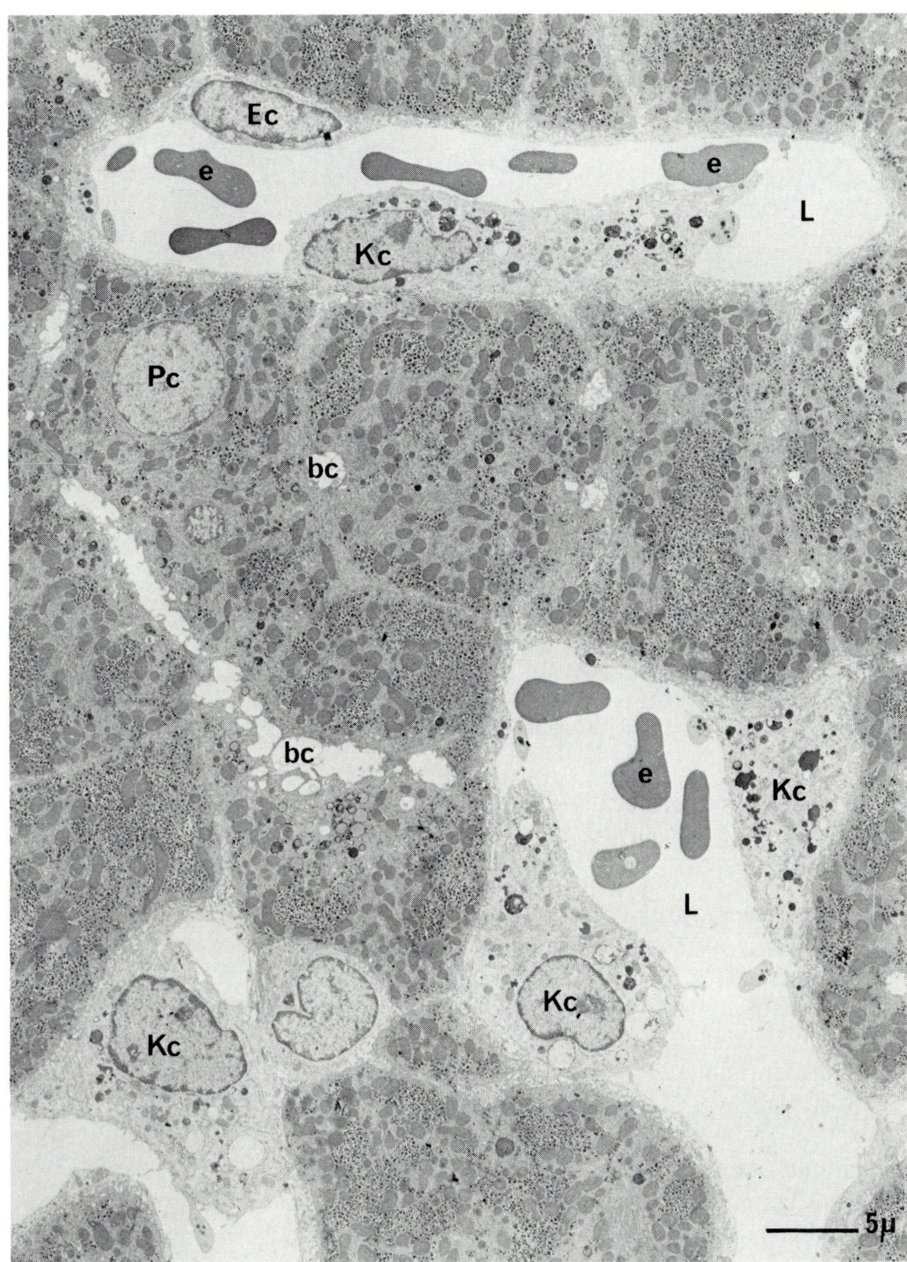

FIG. 1—Transmission electron micrograph of peripheral part of rat liver lobule. Several Kupffer cells (Kc) are seen. These cells show characteristics of macrophages, such as an irregular surface and many dense bodies (lysosomes). Endothelial cells (Ec) form the sinusoidal wall. Erythrocytes cells (e) are not completely washed away, in spite of the perfusion fixation. Pc, hepatocyte; bc, bile canaliculus; L, sinusoidal lumen.

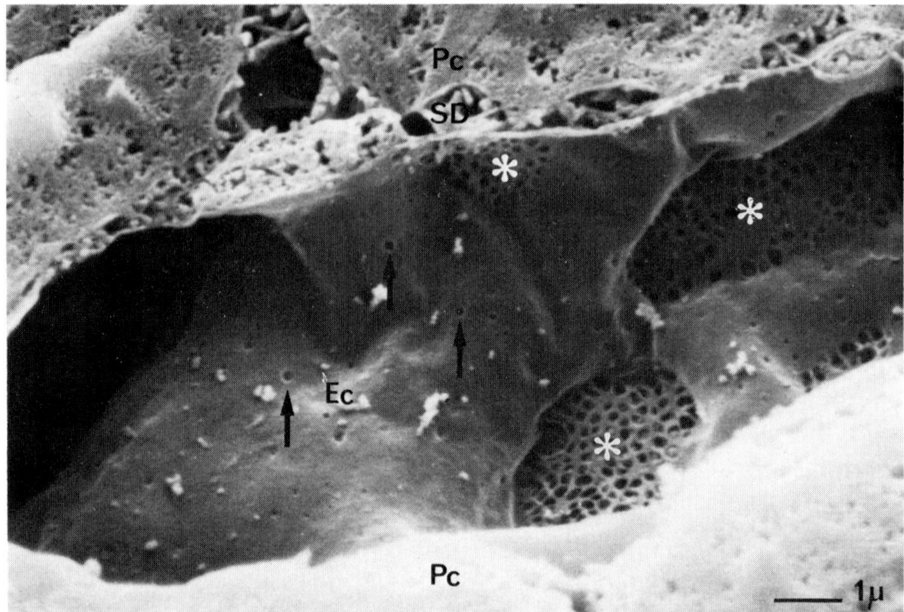

FIG. 2—Scanning electron micrograph of an endothelial cell (Ec) in rat liver. The cell body, containing the nucleus, shows small indentations (arrows), corresponding to bristle-coated micropinocytotic vesicles. Cytoplasmic processes surround sieve plates, composed of many endothelial fenestrations (asterisks). Pc, hepatocyte; SD, space of Disse.

cell, which can be specifically stained with phosphotungstic acid.[16] The vesicles can be classified as follows:

1. Bristle-coated micropinocytotic vesicles (0.1 μ), which pinch off from the plasma membrane. Presumably, these vesicles lose their coat rather soon after their formation so that they become smooth vesicles of about the same diameter.
2. Macropinocytotic vesicles (0.7 μ), known for their endocytotic capacity.[115]
3. Small bristle-coated vesicles pinching off from the Golgi apparatus.
4. Transfer tubules, probably Golgi-derived or arising from the fusion of other vesicles.[16]

Endothelial cells have well-developed lysosomes, which show reaction product after staining for acid phosphatase. No transitional stages between endothelial cells and Kupffer cells are seen either normally or under experimentally altered conditions.

Kupffer Cells

Macrophages located on or embedded in the endothelial lining (Fig. 3) tend to occur around the branches of the portal vein. Although Kupffer cells are basically stellate, they have an irregular shape, suggesting a capacity for movement. Much of the fuzzy-coated surface is exposed to the bloodstream. Foreign particles attach to this surface and are engulfed by hyaloplasmic pseudopodia

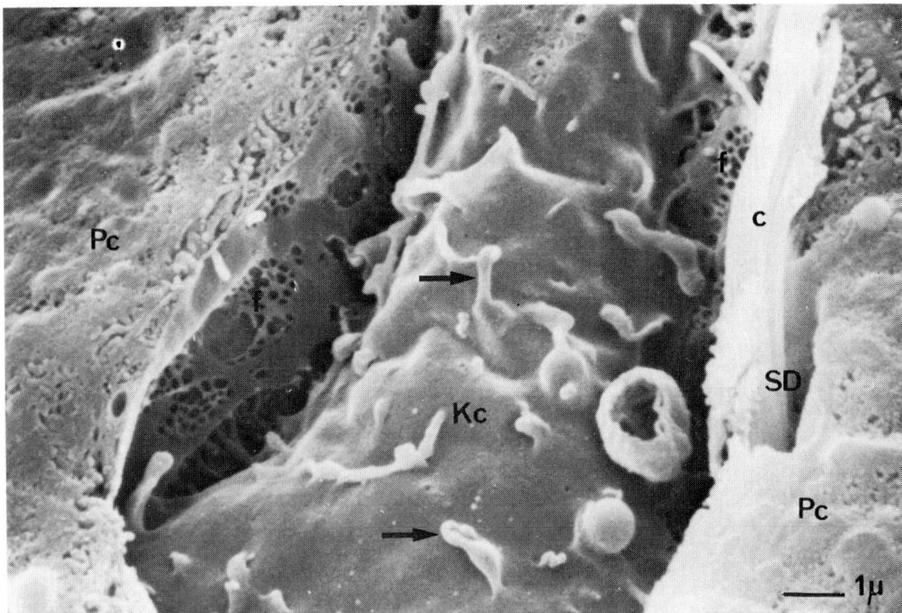

FIG. 3—Scanning electron micrograph of a Kupffer cell (Kc) from rat liver showing microvilli (arrows). Pc, hepatocyte; f, fenestrae; SD, space of Disse; C, collagen bundle.

(phagocytosis). Cytochemically, Kupffer cells can be stained specifically with a peroxidase medium[28,110,115,116,122] and can be recognized by either light or electron microscopy. Peculiar fine structural details can be found in Kupffer cells. Wormlike structures are invaginations of the cell surface and contain a dense midline, probably formed during invagination by the doubling of the 70-nm-thick fuzzy coat. These structures may be involved in endocytosis. They might, however, also be regarded as plasma membrane reservoirs, the membrane becoming available by simple reevagination.[94,117] Sometimes annulate lamellae, connected with RER, can be found in the cytoplasm, together with an abundance of dense bodies (lysosomes) that vary in density, shape, and diameter. Electron-lucent vacuoles, sometimes with a preserved 70-nm fuzzy coat on the inner side, may also be seen in the cytoplasm. We have not found transitional stages between Kupffer cells and other cell types, such as other sinusoidal cells, monocytes, or lymphocytes.[45,94,110,116-118]

Fat-storing Cells

Fat-storing cells lie within the space of Disse.[45,107] Characteristic fat droplets occur in the cytoplasm, which morphologically resemble fibroblasts because of the widened RER. These cells store vitamin A.[107] Fat-storing cell processes underlie the endothelial lining and therefore can be regarded as a special type of pericyte. Fat-storing cells may play a role in the attachment of endothelial cells.[114] Probably, fat-storing cells are involved in collagen synthesis, since they show transitions into fibroblasts and therefore may participate in hepatic fibrogenesis (see chapter 9).[48]

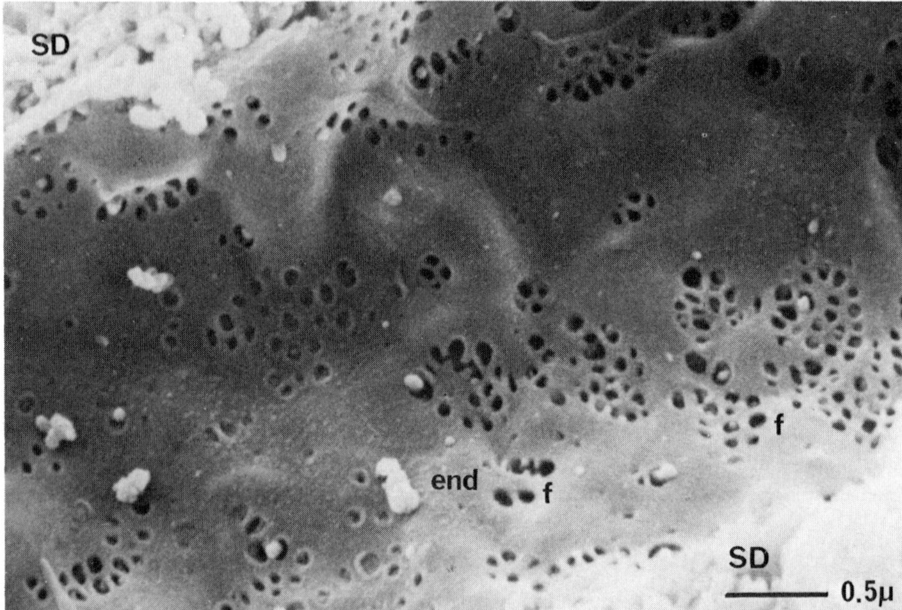

FIG. 4—Surface view of the endothelial lining (end) of a rat liver sinusoid, as seen by the scanning electron microscope. Fenestrae (f) are grouped into sieve plates. SD, space of Disse.

Pit Cells

The pit cell has only recently been described.[123] These cells are located or embedded in the endothelial lining in much the same way as are Kupffer cells. They contain highly characteristic granules resembling those found in cells known to have an endocrine function. The cell is often seen in sinusoidal cell isolates and can also be found in buffy coat preparations of peripheral blood. Pit cells are nonphagocytic and show a high degree of polarity; i.e., all organelles are mostly grouped at one side of the nucleus. The function of pit cells is unclear. Their presence in human liver has not been confirmed.[123]

Characteristics of Sinusoidal Cells

The characteristics of the different liver cells are listed in Table 2. Most of the criteria for the distinction of cell types require the use of an electron microscope. A few characteristics, however, can be used for the light-microscopic recognition of rat liver Kupffer cells, i.e., the phagocytosis of large (0.8 μ) latex particles and specific peroxidase staining.[110] Recently, peroxidase has also been found in endothelial cells of mouse liver.[92]

The question can be asked whether the different sinusoidal cell types represent specific, autochthonous cells not found in other organs. Kupffer cells have been reported to migrate to the lungs;[86] cells comparable to pit cells have been described in the epididymis;[42] and fat-storing cells and transitional stages to fibroblasts can also be found in the kidney, adrenals, lung, and small intestine.[48] The endothelial cells seem to be unique, however, because of their fenestrations, the lack of a basement membrane, the presence of the two types of pinocytotic vesicles (bristle-coated micropinocytosis, macropinocytosis),

TABLE 2.—*Characteristics of Different Cell Types in the Hepatic Parenchyma*

	Endothelial Cell	Kupffer Cell	Fat-storing Cell	Pit Cell	Parenchymal Cell
Fenestrated processes	+	−	−	−	−
Macropinocytotic vesicles (0.7 μ)	+	−	−	−	−
Spheridium	+	−	−	−	−
Annulate lamellae	−	+	−	−	−
Fuzzy coat	−	+	−	−	−
Pinocytosis (fuzzy coat vacuole)	−	+	−	−	−
Wormlike structures	−	+	−	−	−
Phagocytosis by pseudopodia	−	+	−	−	−
Phagocytosis of 0.8 μ latex	−	+	−	−	−
Peroxidase in RER	−	+	−	−	−
Situated in the space of Disse	−	−	+	−	−
Fat droplets in cytoplasm	−	−	+	−	+
Endocrine type of granules	−	−	−	+	−
Peroxisomes with catalase	−	−	−	−	+
Glycogen particles	−	−	−	−	+
Bristle-coated micropinocytosis	+	+	+	−	+
Fixed shape of the cell	+	−	+	−	+
Flat surface	+	−	+	−	−
Smooth ER	+	−	−	−	+
Dense bodies (lysosomes)	+	+	+	−	+
Multivesicular bodies	−	−	+	+	+

and the absence of some characteristics found in other types of endothelial cells.[115] Also, the simultaneous occurrence of the four cell types and their histologic arrangement is not found in any other organ. The occurrence of nerve cell processes within the liver lobule was demonstrated by the use of different staining techniques.[89] Specific staining on the electron-microscopic level would be needed to distinguish these processes from fat-storing cell processes within the space of Disse. This would also allow the study of possible cell contacts between nerve cells and parenchymal cells or sinusoidal cells.

The further study of sinusoidal cells by intravital microscopy[7,56,57] might contribute considerably to the knowledge of reactions of living sinusoidal cells. A decrease in the diameter of sinusoids in response to lower blood pressures and to adrenergic agents was observed.[56,57] The occurrence of sphincters[71] controlling the flow of blood through the lobular parenchyma needs further study and correlation with scanning electron-microscopic observations.[9,65]

SOME FUNCTIONS OF SINUSOIDAL CELLS

One of the functions suggested by the morphologic appearance of endothelial cells concerns a possible filtration effect on particles through endothelial fenestrae.[114] One of the particles to be filtered by these pores is the chylomicron. Many authors have demonstrated that remnant chylomicrons, which are smaller than normal, are hepatotropic and are more easily taken up by hepatocytes than are native chylomicrons,[13,30,33,74,87] although hepatocytes have the capacity to take up native chylomicrons in cell cultures.[29] The filtering capacity of endothelial cells was demonstrated by injecting radio-labeled chylomicrons of varying diameters;[30] the smaller ones were more easily taken up. Chylomicrons in the serum of neonatal rats were larger than those present in the space of Disse.[73]

Single particles smaller than 0.1 μ may pass the fenestrae without hindrance; very low density lipoproteins (VLDLs) secreted by the hepatocytes or viral particles in certain diseases may belong in this category.

The question of larger gaps in the endothelial lining is subject to debate. Definite proof of their genuine or artifactual nature is lacking, but we think that they are artifacts. The fenestrae have been observed in ultrathin sections and freeze-etch preparations without chemical fixation[114] and in scanning EM preparations.[9,65,71] The size of fenestrations can apparently be influenced. Fenestrae enlarge as a result of irradiation, endotoxin exposure, and hypoxia.[75] Larger gaps may be formed by the fusion of smaller ones.[64] Endothelial fenestrations decrease after injection of some hormones.[102]

Another specialized function of both endothelial and Kupffer cells is endocytosis. This function is emphasized by morphometric data (Table 1), and more qualitative data such as the occurrence of five morphologically distinct endocytotic structures[118] are designated as follows (see Table 2):

1. Bristle-coated micropinocytotic vesicles
2. Macropinocytotic vesicles
3. Wormlike structures
4. Pinocytosis (fuzzy coat vacuole)
5. Phagocytosis by hyaloplasmic pseudopodia

Depending on the nature of the molecules or particles to be taken up, one or more of the above mechanisms may operate as an endocytotic carrier, either as a continuous process (pinocytosis) or initiated or accelerated by the interaction of a particle with the cell surface (phagocytosis). Mechanisms 1 through 4 can be found in normal liver without any particle or substance being injected. Sinusoidal cells, therefore, may be involved in a continuous process of endocytosis of molecular components. Further studies are needed to reveal the exact details of the events taking place during phagocytosis, such as the interaction of particles with opsonins[84] or specific antibodies such as IgG or IgM,[69] the subsequent attachment to the fuzzy-coated cell surface,[21,24,25,116,118] and the following hyaloplasmic transition of the peripheral cytoplasm in the process of pseudopodia formation[117,118] and the factors influencing lysosome-phagosome fusion.

Besides a well-developed endocytotic capacity, sinusoidal cells also possess a lysosomal apparatus enabling the cells to digest ingested materials.[118] The digestion process is rapid;[35] injected isolated mitochondria show structural breakdown at 20 min after endocytosis. The breakdown of ^{14}C leucine-labeled mitochondrial protein molecules had a half-life (T½) of 1½ hr.[35] A portion of the lysosomal hydrolases escape from the endocytosing cells during phagocytosis. Since lysosomal hydrolases were found in the blood during experimental blocking of the RES,[60] this enzyme loss is possibly parallel with or identical to the secretion of endogenous pyrogen by Kupffer cells after the endocytosis of bacteria or endotoxin.[38] Endocytosis and digestion can be further studied by isolation, purification, and culture of sinusoidal cells.

ISOLATION, PURIFICATION, AND CULTURE

Several procedures have been described for the isolation of sinusoidal cells from rat liver. Less than 40% of the cells can be characterized as Kupffer cells, whereas the majority of them are endothelial. The number of endothelial cells and Kupffer cells has been estimated to be, respectively, 4.2×10^7 and 1.2×10^7 per gram of liver tissue.[50] The identification of Kupffer cells can be based on peroxidase staining and the uptake of 0.8μ latex particles.[110] Endothelial cells can be identified only by ultrastructural morphologic features. No marker enzyme for this cell is known. The number of isolated endothelial cells can be estimated indirectly by subtracting the peroxidase positive cells from the total esterase positive cells.[23]

Several methods for the isolation and further purification of sinusoidal cells have been published (Table 3):

1. Cell suspensions of liver tissue may be obtained by collagenase and hyaluronidase perfusion. Kupffer cells can be loaded with iron particles and washed out of the liver; they are separated from cell suspensions by use of a magnet.[82] Drawbacks of this method include the low viability of the cells,[113] the contamination with other cells,[3] and the irreversibility of the iron loading.
2. Selective destruction of parenchymal cells is achieved by incubation with pronase.[62,81] Further purification of Kupffer cells is obtained by using their characteristic of attaching to glass during culture.[23,67] During attachment, however, the cells engulf a considerable amount of cellular debris,[5] which might influence further studies on endocytosis[10] and result in an increase in lysosomal enzyme activity.[5]
3. Metrizamide density-gradient centrifugation is applied to suspensions of sinusoidal cells loaded in vivo with substances such as triton WR-1339 or Jectofer density of Kupffer cells.[50] By selecting those endothelial cells in

TABLE 3.—*Yield of Kupffer and Endothelial Cells from Rat Liver Prepared by Various Methods*

Endothelial Cells per Gram of Liver	Kupffer Cells per Gram of Liver	Purification Method
—	9.0×10^6	Magnetic separation[113]
—	13.7×10^6	Magnetic separation[3]
—	6×10^6	Attachment in culture[67]
4×10^6	$6–7 \times 10^6$	Density gradient centrifugation[50,53]
$16–28 \times 10^6$	$4–8 \times 10^6$	Centrifugal elutriation[50,53]

the gradient that band at a density of 1.064 g/cm[3] or less, a highly purified endothelial cell suspension can be obtained.[50]

4. Centrifugal elutriation obtains 90% to 95% pure populations of Kupffer or endothelial cells, starting with pronase- or collagenase-prepared sinusoidal cell suspensions from untreated animals.[50,52,53]

Data concerning the diameter, volume, and DNA and protein content of sinusoidal and parenchymal cells prepared by different methods are summarized in Table 4. Endothelial cells are smaller than Kupffer cells, and the protein content of both cells is less than 10% of the protein content of hepatocytes.

Microscopic studies of isolated sinusoidal cells revealed lamellipodia on Kupffer cells[19] (Fig. 5), Fc and C3 receptors on cultured Kupffer cells,[69] and fenestrae on the surface of endothelial cells.[19] Ultrathin sections[10,19,23,50,62,92] showed similar fine structural detail in isolated and in situ Kupffer cells.[116] The absence of a 70-nm-thick fuzzy coat on isolated and cultured Kupffer cells, however, was striking.[23] Attachment of gold colloid to the fuzzy coat could be seen in intact livers[118] but not on cultured Kupffer cells.[66]

The activities of lysosomal hydrolases of isolated cells concern the primary function of two types of sinusoidal cells, i.e., endocytosis and digestion (see Table 5). All lysosomal enzyme activities per milligram of protein appear to be higher in endothelial and Kupffer cells than in hepatocytes. Some have a higher activity in endothelial cells (arylsulfatase) or in Kupffer cells (cathepsin D). Furthermore, hepatocytes contain multiple forms of acid phosphatase that are not found in Kupffer cells.[90] Preparation artifacts inducing enhanced cathepsin D activity in Kupffer cells by the uptake of proteases from the applied pronase mixture could be excluded.[50] During culture, the lysosomal enzyme activities might be subject to alteration, possibly from endocytosis of cell debris.[5]

Peroxidase activity was demonstrated in Kupffer cells cytochemically[28,110,122] and biochemically.[96,97] This peroxidase may be involved in a bactericidal mechanism.[79] Probably a substantial amount of H_2O_2 is formed from O_2 by super-

TABLE 4.—*Some Properties of Endothelial, Kupffer, and Nonparenchymal Cells and Parenchymal Cells from Rat Liver*

	Endothelial Cells	Kupffer Cells	Nonparenchymal Cells*	Parenchymal Cells†
Diameter (μ)	7.0[55]	8.7–9.1[91]	7.2[123]	19.0–28.5[20,43]
Volume (μ^3/cell)	179[55]	345–394[91]	904[68]	2500–11000[11]
				2710–6970[54,61,109]
				6186,[20] 9198[68]
μg DNA/10[6] cells	—	—	8,[123] 10[68]	15,[123] 18[68]
				18–31[43]
μg Protein/10[6] cells	47[50]	78–116,[91] 138[3] 154[67]	63,[52] 65[58] 109,[67] 141[68]	1600–2125[3,43,58,67,68,80,101]

*Values are highly variable as a result of the presence of various cell types in nonparenchymal cell suspension.

†Values are highly variable as a result of the presence of hepatocytes of various ploidy classes and of different size; furthermore, the degree of ploidy is strain- and age-dependent.

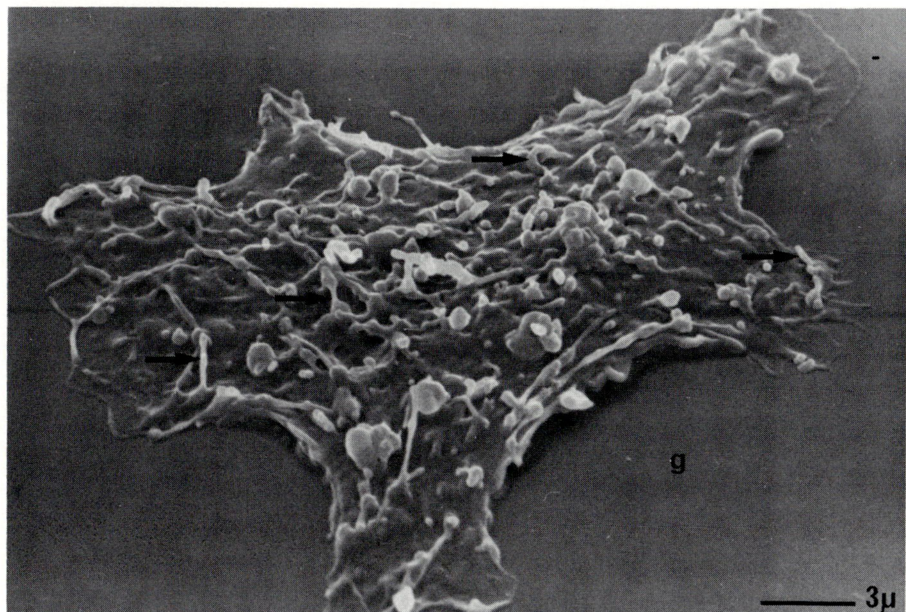

FIG. 5—Kupffer cell from rat liver, isolated by the pronase method, purified by centrifugal elutriation, and cultured for 20 hr on a glass surface (g). The surface features of the cell are comparable to Kupffer cells in situ (see Fig. 3); microvilli (arrows) are present.

oxide dismutase activity,[79,100] and the enzyme was demonstrated in a sinusoidal cell preparation[100] along with NADPH oxidase, another enzyme involved in H_2O_2 synthesis.[98] These results led to the postulate of a hypothetical series of events involved in H_2O_2 formation and catabolism of endocytotic material in sinusoidal cells.[98] However, the cytochemically demonstrable peroxidase of Kupffer cells localized in the RER nuclear envelope and annulate lamellae

TABLE 5.—*Some Lysosomal EnzymeActivities in Endothelial, Kupffer, and Nonparenchymal Cells and Parenchymal Cells from Rat Liver*[*]

Enzyme	Endothelial Cells	Kupffer Cells	Nonparenchymal Cells	Parenchymal Cells
Acid phosphatase	98[50]	87–108[50,91]	40–66[1,51,54,68,99]	20–38[1,51,54,68,99]
Arylsulfatase B	108[50]	34[50]	21–28[51,54,99]	7–12[51,54,99]
Cathepsin D 1[†]	6[49,50]	15–18[49,50,91]	8[49]	1[49]
II	—	—	42[99]	7[99]
III	—	273[‡][5]	63[68]	12[68]
Arginine naphthylamidase	9[49]	12–15[49,91]	11[49]	8[49]
Acid lipase	—	—	30[99]	5[99]
Acid DNAse	—	8–25[3,67]	28–35[54,67,68]	3–11[3,54,68]
β-Glucuronidase	—	11–41[3,53,67,91]	12–18[67,68]	4–9[3,67,68]
β-Acetylglucosaminidase	—	180[91]	88[68]	21[68]

[*]Activities expressed as nmoles/min/mg protein: the highest and lowest values of a range are given.
[†]I-III: different enzyme determinations.
[‡]Kupffer cells in culture.

does not fuse with phagosomes containing bacteria.[22] In polymorphonuclear leukocytes, however, the peroxidase-positive lysosomes fuse with phagosomes,[122] after which bacteria are killed by the halide-H_2O_2-peroxidase bactericidal system.[79]

MISCELLANEOUS FUNCTIONS

Another indication of the physiologic function of lysosomal hydrolases of sinusoidal cells was obtained by comparing the activity of three lysosomal hydrolases in parenchymal and sinusoidal cells isolated from germfree, monocontaminated, and conventional rats.[4] In the last, the activity was doubled, apparently because of the bacterial status of the animal. Since lysosomal hydrolase activity depends on endocytotic activity, in normal rat livers the sinusoidal cells presumably clear and break down bacteria and bacterial products such as endotoxin. The phagocytosis of bacteria by Kupffer cells[32,40,63,122] and their bactericidal activity[32,83] have been demonstrated. These observations apply to clinical situations; e.g., systemic endotoxemia of intestinal origin relates to Kupffer cell failure in different liver diseases[59] (see Chapter 10). Accurate and reproducible routine methods are needed for measuring hepatic RES activity in patients. In laboratory animals, endotoxin inhibits RES function simultaneously with stimulated ^{3}H-thymidine incorporation by sinusoidal cells.[36] ^{51}Cr-labeled endotoxin is cleared mainly by the liver.[76,124] The cellular and subcellular distribution remains unclear, however, because 45% of the labeled endotoxin was unexpectedly associated with nuclei and 75% was localized in hepatocytes.[124]

Kupffer cells are involved in several endocytotic events that may be of clinical relevance. The intravenous administration of artificial lipid emulsions for alimentation stimulates large-scale phagocytosis of fat droplets by Kupffer cells.[39,47,104] This property of Kupffer cells can also be used to measure RES function.[18,95]

In experimentally evoked disseminated intravascular coagulations, Kupffer cells attach fibrin but do not phagocytize it.[23] Fibrinolytic enzymes are apparently responsible for the disappearance of attached fibrin. Subsequent uptake of degradation products might occur, however.[26,88]

The injection of aluminium hydroxide particles has been reported to influence favorably the course of viral hepatitisA and B.[2] After injection into rats, we found the particles exclusively in Kupffer cells.

A direct interaction of Kupffer cells and tumor cells followed by phagocytosis and destruction of the latter cells was observed with significant differences among different tumor cell lines or even sublines.[80]

The interference of sinusoidal cells with viruses is an almost unexploited field of investigation. Very low doses of frog virus FV3 produce severe toxic reactions of sinusoidal cells shortly after injection.[34] Other highly toxic substances were described such as ricin (1.0 ng/100 g body weight)[17] and gadolinium chloride (0.5 mg/100 g body weight).[44]

The interaction of sinusoidal cells with hepatitis virus and the reactions of these cells during parenchymal cell necrosis remain to be investigated. The importance of the hepatic RES in the response to some hepatotropic viruses is assumed, and the capacity of viruses to replicate within Kupffer cells is considered to influence some forms of hepatitis.[85]

SINUSOIDAL CELLS IN PATHOLOGIC PROCESSES

The role of sinusoidal cells in many disease processes is still unclear[93] (Table 4). The light microscope barely distinguishes the different sinusoidal types, particularly in diseased tissue. Immersion fixation complicates the EM study of sinusoidal cells. Much can be expected from careful studies of the role of sinusoidal cells in diseases by using semiperfusion-fixed surgical biopsies[121] or puncture-perfused needle biopsies.[70,71]

The importance of a sharp distinction between endothelial and Kupffer cells, e.g., in lysosomal storage disease, is exemplified by the observation that in Morquio's disease, only the endothelial cells are modified into foamy cells, whereas earlier pathologic examinations had incriminated the Kupffer cells.[121]

The involvement of Kupffer and endothelial cells in iron storage has been demonstrated.[41] After infusion of saccharated iron oxide, Kupffer cells metabolized the ferritin-iron, whereas the endothelial cells still showed lysosomal iron storage long after application of the iron compound.

KINETICS OF SINUSOIDAL CELLS

We showed in early experiments that Kupffer cells undergo mitoses upon certain stimuli. Dividing Kupffer cells are found in normal liver,[111,118] after partial hepatectomy,[111,117] after RES stimulation with zymosan,[117] during RES blockade,[117] in fetal liver,[72] and in cell culture.[12,82] Endothelial cells proliferate after partial hepatectomy[111] or diethylstilbestrol treatment.[112] Partial hepatectomy as a model for rapid organ growth can be used to demonstrate the capacity for proliferation of all four types of sinusoidal cells.[118] Morphologic, cytochemical, and functional criteria on the EM level should, however, carefully characterize the cells. These results on the self-replicating capacity of sinusoidal cells conflict with the proposed concept of the mononuclear phagocyte system,[103] which postulates that blood monocytes, originating in the bone marrow, are precursor cells of all tissue macrophages, including Kupffer cells. Monocytes are present in normal rat liver sinusoids,[116,120] and they can locally develop into macrophages. There is no definite proof that Kupffer cells derive from monocytes; tagged cells are found in the liver after injection of ^{3}H-thymidine. Here, too, detailed cell recognition methods (fine structure, cytochemistry, latex phagocytosis) are needed to characterize the radio-labeled cells. Monocytes or monocyte-derived macrophages appear to be a different category of cells from Kupffer cells or tissue (resident) macrophages.[14,15,77,117,118] They seem to differ in fine structure and localization of the enzyme peroxidase,[14,15,116] as well as in their capacity to take up particles.[118] Moreover, cell labeling and kinetic studies do not support the idea of a transition of monocytes

TABLE 6.—*Functions of Sinusoidal Cells in the Liver*

Filtration of chylomicrons (endothelial cells)[30,73]
Particle phagocytosis (Kupffer cells)
Endocytosis of bacteria and endotoxin[32,40,63,122]
Erythrophagocytosis and iron metabolism[6,41]
Phagocytosis of circulating tumor cells[80]
Clearance of cellular debris after trauma[84] (surgery, burning, shock, hemorrhagia)
Storage of vitamin A[48,107]
Synthesis of collagen (fat-storing cells)[48]
Reactions in many diseases: kala-azar, malaria, amyloidosis, viral hepatitis, lysosomal storage
    diseases, iron storage diseases, thorotrast storage, infectious mononucleosis, Banti's
    syndrome, cholestasis, cholesterol ester storage, reticuloendotheliosis[93]
Clearance of antigens (spillover) and immune complexes
Turnover of (plasma) proteins
Secretion of:
  Endogenous pyrogen[38]
  Lysosomal hydrolases[60]
  Colony-stimulating factor[46]
  Erythropoietine[37,78]
  Collagenase
  Complement

into tissue macrophages.[105] Thus, we can conclude that tissue macrophages and monocyte-derived macrophages may very well coexist and have complementary or overlapping functions. Their reactions to experimental conditions and disease differ, and they have different origins and functions.

FUTURE STUDIES

Since the original publication of Carl von Kupffer in 1899,[106] light microscopy and systemic RES studies have contributed to the knowledge of sinusoidal cells. Powerful research tools such as electron microscopy, cytochemistry, and biochemistry have provided new results and permitted identification of four separate sinusoidal cell types: endothelial cells, Kupffer cells, fat-storing cells, and pit cells[118] (Table 2). Sinusoidal cells have been isolated and endothelial and Kupffer cell populations purified.[52,67] Kupffer cells have been cultured and biochemically investigated (Tables 4 and 5). Future studies should enable investigators to isolate, purify, and culture all four types of sinusoidal cells or even coculture them,[108] and modern cell biological methods should be used to study specific cell function in vivo,[7] in situ, and in vitro in order to extend the list of known sinusoidal cell functions (Table 6).

REFERENCES

1. Arborgh B, Berg T, Ericsson JLE: Quantitation of acid phosphatase and aryl sulphatase in rat hepatic parenchymal and Kupffer cells. FEBS Lett 35:51–54, 1973

2. Aron E: Traitement des hépatites virales par un adjuvant de l'immunité. Méd Chir Dig 5:231–234, 1976

3. Berg T, Boman D: Distribution of lysosomal enzymes between parenchymal and Kupffer cells of rat liver. Biochim Biophys Acta 321:585–596, 1973

4. Berg T, Midtvedt T: The influence of infection on the content of lysosomal enzymes in rat Kupffer cells and hepatocytes. Acta

Pathol Microbiol Scand[A] 84:415–420, 1976

5. Berg T, Munthe-KaasAC: Lysosomal enzymes in cultured rat Kupffer cells. Exp Cell Res 109:119–125, 1977

6. Bissell DM, Hammaker L, Schmid R: Liver phagocytes: Identification of a subpopulation for erythrocyte catabolism. J Cell Biol 54:107–119, 1972

7. Bloch EH, McCuskey RS: Biodynamics of phagocytosis: An analysis of the dynamics of phagocytosis in the liver by in vivo microscopy. Edited by E Wisse and DL Knook: Kupffer Cells and Other Liver Sinusoidal Cells. Amsterdam, Elsevier, 1977, pp 21–32

8. Blouin A, Bolender RP, Weibel ER: Distribution of organelles and membranes between hepatocytes and nonhepatocytes in the rat liver parenchyma. J Cell Biol 72:441–455, 1977

9. Brooks SEH, Haggis GH: Scanning electron microscopy of rat's liver. Application of freeze-fracture and freeze-drying techniques. Lab Invest 29:60–64, 1973

10. Brouwer A, Knook DL: Quantitative determination of endocytosis and intracellular digestion by rat liver Kupffer cells in vitro. Edited by E Wisse and DL Knook: Kupffer Cells and Other Liver Sinusoidal Cells. Amsterdam, Elsevier, 1977, pp 343–352

11. Castagna M, Chauveau J: Séparation des hépatocytes isolés de rat en fractions cellulaires métaboliquement distinctes. Exp Cell Res 57:211–222, 1969

12. Clark JM, Pateman JA: Long-term culture of chinese hamster Kupffer cell lines isolated by a primary cloning step. Exp Cell Res 112:207–217, 1978

13. Cooper AD: The metabolism of chylomicron remnants by isolated perfused rat liver. Biochim Biophy Acta 488:464–474, 1977

14. Daems WTh, Koerten HK, Soranzo MR: Differences between monocyte-derived and tissue macrophages. Advances in Experimental Medicine and Biology. Vol. 73A. Edited by SM Reichard, MR Escobar, and H Friedman: The RES in Health and Disease: Functions and Characteristics. New York, Plenum Press, 1976 pp 27–40

15. Daems WTh, Wisse E, Brederoo P, Emeis JJ: Peroxidatic activity in monocytes and macrophages. Edited by R van Furth: Mononuclear Phagocytes in Immunity, Infection and Pathology. Oxford, Blackwell, 1975, pp 57–77

16. De Bruijn PPH, Michelson S, Becker RP: PTH as a marker for the endocytic-lysosomal system (vacuolar apparatus) including transfer tubules of the living cells of the sinusoids in the bone marrow and liver. J Ultrastruct Res 58:87–95, 1977

17. Derenzini M, Bonetti E, Marinozzi V, Stirpe F: Toxic effects of ricin, studies on the pathogenesis of liver lesions. Virchows Arch [Zell pathol] 20:15–28, 1976

18. DiLuzio NR, Salky NK, Riggi SJ, Ladman AJ: Experimental and clinical evaluation of reticuloendothelial function by means of a specific lipid emulsion. Proceedings of IV International Symposium on RES, The Reticuloendothelial System, 1964, pp 389–404

19. Drochmans P, Sleyster ECh, Penasse W, Wanson JC, Knook DL: Morphology of isolated and cultured sinus-lining cells of rat liver. Edited by E Wisse and DL Knook: Kupffer Cells and Other Liver Sinusoidal Cells. Amsterdam, Elsevier, 1977, pp 131–139

20. Drochmans P, Wanson JC, Mosselmans R: Isolation and subfractionation on Ficoll gradients of adult rat hepatocytes. J Cell Biol 66:1–22, 1975

21. Emeis JJ: Morphological and cytochemical heterogeneity of the cell coat of rat liver Kupffer cells. J Reticuloendothel Soc 20:31–50, 1976

22. Emeis JJ, Lindeman J: Rat liver macrophages will not phagocytose fibrin during disseminated intravascular coagulation. Haemostasis 5:193–210, 1976

23. Emeis JJ, Planqué B: Heterogeneity of cells isolated from rat liver by pronase digestion: Ultrastructure, cytochemistry and cell culture. J Reticuloendothel Soc 20:11–29, 1976

24. Emeis JJ, Wisse E: Electron microscopic cytochemistry of the cell coat of Kupffer cells in rat liver. Advances in Experimental Medicine and Biology. Vol. 15. Edited by NR DiLuzio and K Flemming: The RES and Immune Phenomena. New York, Plenum Press, 1971, pp 1–12

25. Emeis JJ, Wisse E: On the cell coat of rat liver Kupffer cells. Edited by R van Furth: Mononuclear Phagocytes in Immunity, Infection and Pathology. Oxford, Blackwell, 1975, pp 315–325

26. Fabre J, Delsol G, Familiades J, Tapie C, Boneu B, Bierme R: Apport de la morphologie dans la mise en évidence des dérivés de fibrinogène. Pathol Biol 22 (Suppl): 53–59, 1974

27. Fahimi HD: Perfusion and immersion fix-

ation of rat liver with glutaraldehyde. Lab Invest 16:736, 1967

28. Fahimi DH: The fine structural localization of endogenous and exogenous peroxidase activity in Kupffer cells of rat liver. J Cell Biol 47:247–262, 1970

29. Florén CH, Nilsson Å: Degradation of chylomicron remnants cholesteryl ester by rat hepatocyte monolayers. Inhibition by chloroquine and colchicine. Biochem Biophys Res Commun 74:520–528, 1977

30. Fraser R, Bosanquet AG, Day WA: Filtration of chylomicrons by the liver may influence cholesterol metabolism and atherosclerosis. Atherosclerosis 29:113–123, 1978

31. Frenzel H, Kremer B, Mücker H: The liver sinusoids under various pathological conditions. A TEM and SEM study of rat liver after respiratory hypoxia, telecobalt-irradiation and endotoxin application. Edited by E Wisse and DL Knook: Kupffer Cells and Other Liver Sinusoidal Cells. Amsterdam, Elsevier, 1977, pp 213–222

32. Friedman RL, Moon RJ: Hepatic clearance of *Salmonella typhimurium* in silica-treated mice. Infect Immun 16:1005–1012, 1977

33. Gardner RS, Mayes PA: Comparison of the metabolism of chylomicrons and chylomicron remnants by the perfused liver. Biochem J 170:47–55, 1978

34. Gendrault JL, Steffan AM, Bingen A, Kirn A: Interaction of frog virus (FV3) with sinusoidal cells. Edited by E Wisse and DL Knook: Kupffer Cells and Other Liver Sinusoidal Cells. Amsterdam, Elsevier, 1977, pp 223–232

35. Glaumann H: Heterophagocytosis and lysosomal degradation of subcellular organelles. Edited by F Biering: Proceedings of the Ninth Congress of the Nordic Society for Cell Biology. Odense, Odense University Press, 1976, pp 101–112

36. Gospos Ch, Freudenberg N, Bank A, Freudenberg MA: Effect of endotoxin-induced shock on the reticuloendothelial system. Phagocytic activity and DNA-synthesis of reticuloendothelial cells following endotoxin treatment. Beitr Pathol 161:100–106, 1977

37. Gruber DF, Zucali JR, Mirand EA: Identification of erythropoietin producing cells in fetal mouse liver cultures. Exp Hematol 5:392–398, 1977

38. Haeseler F, Bodel P, Atkins E: Characteristics of pyrogen production by isolated rabbit Kupffer cells in vitro. J Reticuloendothel Soc 22:569–581, 1977

39. Hatae T: Electron microscopic observations on the mouse liver after intravenous administration of fat emulsion. Arch Histol Jpn 37:149–163, 1974

40. Hauser R, Matter BE: Localization of *E. coli* K-12 in livers of mice used for an intrasanguineous host-mediated assay. Mutat Res 46:45–48, 1977

41. Hausmann K, Wulfhekel U, Düllmann J, Kuse R: Iron storage in macrophages and endothelial cells. Blut 32:289–295, 1976

42. Hoffer AP, Hamilton DW, Fawcett DW: The ultrastructure of the principal cells and intraepithelial leucocytes in the initial segment of the rat epididymis. Anat Rec 175:169–202, 1973

43. Horsfall AC, Ketterer B: The fractionation of isolated liver cells from normal and carcinogen treated rats. Br J Cancer 33:96–104, 1976

44. Husztik E, Lazar G, Szilagyi S: Study on the mechanism of Kupffer cell phagocytosis blockade induced by gadolinium chloride. Edited by E Wisse and DL Knook: Kupffer Cells and Other Liver Sinusoidal Cells. Amsterdam, Elsevier, 1977, pp 387–395

45. Ito T: Recent advances in the study of the fine structure of the hepatic sinusoidal wall: A review. Gunma Rep Med Sci 6:119, 1973

46. Joyce RA, Chervenick PA: Stimulation of granulopoiesis by liver macrophages. J Lab Clin Med 86:112–117, 1975

47. Kajihara H, Totović V, Gedigk P: Zur Ultrastruktur und Morphogenese des Ceroidpigmentes. I. Fettphagocytose und Bildung von lipidhaltigen Lysosomen in den Kupfferschen Sternzellen der Rattenleber nach intravenöser Injektion hochungesättigter Lipide. VirchowsArch [Zell pathol] 19:221–237, 1975

48. Kent G, Gay S, Inouye T, Bahu R, Minick OT, Popper H: Vitamin A-containing lipocytes and formation of type III collagen in liver injury. Proc Natl Acad Sci USA 73:3719–3722, 1976

49. Knook DL: The role of lysosomal enzymes in protein degradation in different types of rat liver cells. Acta Biol Med Ger 36:1747–1752, 1978

50. Knook DL, Blansjaar N, Sleyster ECh: Isolation and characterization of Kupffer and endothelial cells from the rat liver. Exp Cell Res 109:317–329, 1977

51. Knook DL, Sleyster ECh: Lysosomal enzyme activities in parenchymal and nonparenchymal liver cells isolated from young, adult and old rats. Mech Ageing Dev 3:107–119, 1974

52. Knook DL, Sleyster ECh: Separation of Kupffer and endothelial cells of the rat liver by centrifugal elutriation. Exp Cell Res 99:444–448, 1976

53. Knook DL, Sleyster ECh: Preparation and characterization of Kupffer cells from rat and mouse liver. Edited by E Wisse and DL Knook: Kupffer Cells and Other Liver Sinusoidal Cells. Amsterdam, Elsevier, 1977, pp 273–288

54. Knook DL, Sleyster ECh, Van Noord M: Changes in lysosomes during ageing of parenchymal and non-parenchymal liver cells. Edited by VJ Cristofalo and E Holĕcková: Cell Impairment in Ageing and Development. New York, Plenum Press, 1975, pp 155–169

55. Knook DL, Van Doorn E: unpublished observations

56. Koo A, Liang IYS: Blood flow in hepatic sinusoids in experimental hemorrhagic shock in the rat. Microvasc Res 13:315–325, 1977

57. Koo A, Liang IYS, Cheng KK: Adrenergic mechanisms in the hepatic microcirculation in the rat. Q J Exp Physiol 62:199–208, 1977

58. Lentz PE, DiLuzio NR: Biochemical characterization of Kupffer and parenchymal cells isolated from rat liver. Exp Cell Res 67:17–26, 1971

59. Liehr H, Grün M: Clinical aspects of Kupffer cell failure in liver diseases. Edited by E Wisse and DL Knook: Kupffer Cells and Other Liver Sinusoidal Cells. Amsterdam, Elsevier, 1977, pp 427–436

60. Loegering DJ, Kaplan JE, Saba TM: Correlation of plasma lysosomal enzyme levels with hepatic RE function after trauma. Proc Soc Exp Biol Med 152: 42–46, 1976

61. Loud AV: A quantitative stereological description of the ultrastructure of normal rat liver parenchymal cells. J Cell Biol 37:27–46, 1968

62. Mills DM, Zucker-Franklin D: Electron microscopic study of isolated Kupffer cells. Am J Pathol 54:147–166, 1969

63. Mohelska H, Moluša R, Kubin M, Smetana K: Endocellular parasitism of *Mycobacterium avium* in rabbit liver. Exp Pathol 10:122–131, 1975

64. Montesano R, Nicolescu P: Fenestrations in endothelium of rat liver sinusoids revisited by freeze-fracture. Anat Rec 190: 861–870, 1978

65. Motta P: A scanning electron microscopic study of the rat liver sinusoid endothelial and Kupffer cells. Cell Tissue Res 164:371–385, 1975

66. Munthe-KaasAC: Uptake of macromolecules by rat Kupffer cells in vitro. Exp Cell Res 107:55–62, 1977

67. Munthe-Kaas AC, Berg T, Seglen PO, Seljelid R: Mass isolation and culture of rat Kupffer cells. J Exp Med 141:1–10, 1975

68. Munthe-Kaas AC, Berg T, Seljelid R: Distribution of lysosomal enzymes in different types of rat liver cells. Exp Cell Res 99:146–154, 1976.

69. Munthe-Kaas AC, Kaplan G, Seljelid R: On the mechanism of internalization of opsonized particles by rat Kupffer cells in vitro. Exp Cell Res 103:201–212, 1976

70. Murakami T: Puncture perfusion of small tissue pieces for scanning electron microscopy. Arch Histol Jpn 39:99–103, 1976

71. Muto M, Nishi M, Fujita T: Scanning electron microscopy of human liver sinusoids. Arch Histol Jpn 40:137–151, 1977

72. Naito M, Wisse E: Observation on the fine structure and cytochemistry of sinusoidal cells in fetal and neonatal rat liver. Edited by E Wisse and DL Knook: Kupffer Cells and Other Liver Sinusoidal Cells. Amsterdam, Elsevier, 1977, pp 497–505

73. Naito M, Wisse E: Filtration effect of endothelial fenestrations on chylomicron transport in neonatal rat liver sinusoids. Cell Tissue Res 190:371–382, 1978

74. Nilsson Å, Zilversmit DB: Distribution of chylomicron cholesteryl ester between parenchymal and Kupffer cells of rat liver. Biochim Biophys Acta 248:137–142, 1971

75. Nopanitaya W, Lamb JC, Grisham JW, Carsson JL: Effect of hepatic venous outflow obstruction on pores and fenestrations in sinusoidal endothelium. Br J Exp Pathol 57:604–609, 1976

76. Noyes HE, McInturf CR, Blahuta GJ: Studies on the distribution of E. coli endotoxin in mice. Proc Soc Exp Biol Med 100:65–68, 1959

77. Ogawa T, Koerten HK, Daems WTh: Peroxidatic activity in monocytes and tissue macrophages in mice. Cell Tissue Res 188:361–373, 1978

78. Peschle C, Marone G, Genovese A, Magli C, Condorelli M: Hepatic erythropoietin: Enhanced production in anephric rats with hyperplasia of Kupffer cells. Br J Haematol 32:105–111, 1976

79. Roos D: Oxidative killing of microorganisms by phagocytic cells. Trends Biochem Sci 2:61–64, 1977

80. Roos E, Dingemans KP: Phagocytosis of tumor cells by Kupffer cells in vivo and in the perfused mouse liver. Edited by E

Wisse and DL Knook: Kupffer Cells and Other Liver Sinusoidal Cells. Amsterdam, Elsevier, 1977, pp 183–190

81. Roser B: The distribution of intravenously injected Kupffer cells in the mouse. J Reticuloendothel Soc 5:455–471, 1968

82. Rous P, Beard JW: Selection with the magnet and cultivation of reticuloendothelial cells (Kupffer cells). J Exp Med 59:577–591, 1934

83. Ruggiero G, Utili R, Andreana A: Clearance of viable *Salmonella* strains by the isolated, perfused rat liver: A study of serum and cellular factors involved and of the effect of treatments with carbon tetrachloride or *Salmonella enteritidis* lipopolysaccharide. J Reticuloendothel Soc 21:79–88, 1977

84. Saba TM: Humoral control of Kupffer cell function after injury. Bull Kupffer Cell Found 1:12–22, 1978

85. Sabesin SM, Koff RS: Pathogenesis of experimental viral hepatitis. N Engl J Med 290:944–950, 1974

86. Schneeberger-Keeley EE, Burger EJ: Intravascular macrophages in cat lungs after open chest ventilation. Lab Invest 22:361, 1970

87. Sherill BC, Dietschy JM: Characterization of the sinusoidal transport process responsible for uptake of chylomicrons by the liver. J Biol Chem 253:1859–1867, 1978

88. Sherman LA, Lee J, Jacobson A: Quantitation of the reticuloendothelial system clearance of soluble fibrin. Br J Haematol 37:231–238, 1977

89. Skaaring P, Bierring F: On the intrinsic innervation of normal rat liver. Cell Tissue Res 171:141–155, 1976

90. Sleyster ECh, Knook DL: Multiple forms of acid phosphatase in rat liver parenchymal, endothelial and Kupffer cells. Arch Biochem Biophys (in press)

91. Sleyster ECh, Westerhuis FG, Knook DL: The purification of non-parenchymal liver cell classes by centrifugal elutriation. Edited by E Wisse and DL Knook: Kupffer cells and other liver sinusoidal cells. Amsterdam, Elsevier, 1977, pp 289–298

92. Stöhr G, Deimann W, Fahimi HD: Peroxidase-positive endothelial cells in sinusoids of the mouse liver. J Histochem Cytochem 26:409–411, 1978

93. Tanikawa K, Ikejiri N: Fine structural alterations of the sinusoidal lining cells in various liver diseases. Edited by E Wisse and DL Knook: Kupffer Cells and Other Liver Sinusoidal Cells. Amsterdam, Elsevier, 1977, pp 153–162

94. Tanuma J: Fine structure of the Kupffer cell in the bat, with special reference to the worm-like bodies. Arch Histol Jpn 41:113–127, 1978

95. Tonaki H, Saba TM, Mayron LW, Kaplan E: Phagocytosis of gelatinized ''R.E. Test Lipid Emulsion'' by Kupffer cells: EM observations. Exp Mol Pathol 25:189–201, 1976

96. Van Berkel ThJC: Difference spectra, catalase- and peroxidase activities of isolated parenchymal and non-parenchymal cells from rat liver. Biochem Biophys Res Commun 61:204–205, 1974

97. Van Berkel ThJC, Kruyt JK: Identity of peroxidatic activities in nonparenchymal rat liver cells in relation to parenchymal liver cells. Edited by E Wisse and DL Knook: Kupffer Cells and Other Liver Sinusoidal Cells. Amsterdam, Elsevier, 1977, pp 307–314

98. Van Berkel ThJC, Kruyt JK: Distribution and some properties of NADPH and NADH oxidase in parenchymal and non-parenchymal liver cells. Arch Biochem Biophys 179:8–14, 1977

99. Van Berkel ThJC, Kruyt JK, Koster JF: Identity and activities of lysosomal enzymes in parenchymal and non-parenchymal cells from rat liver. Eur J Biochem 58:145–152, 1975

100. Van Berkel ThJC, Kruyt JK, Stee RG, Koster JF: Identity and activities of superoxide dismutase in parenchymal and nonparenchymal cells from rat liver. Arch Biochem Biophys 179:1–7, 1977

101. Van Bezooijen CFA, Grell T, Knook DL: Albumin synthesis by liver parenchymal cells isolated from young, adult and old rats. Biochem Biophys Res Comm 71:513–519, 1976

102. Van Dierendonck JH, Wisse E: unpublished observations, 1978

103. Van Furth R: Origin and kinetics of mononuclear phagocytes. Am NY Acad Sci 278:161–175, 1976

104. Van Haelst UJGM: Effects of parenteral nutrition with lipids on the human liver. VirchowsArch [Zell pathol] 22:323–332, 1976

105. Volkman A: Disparity in origin of mononuclear phagocyte populations. J Reticuloendothel Soc 19:249–268, 1976

106. Von Kupffer C: Uber die sogenannten Sternzellen der Säugethierleber. Arch Mikrosk Anat 54:254, 1899

107. Wake K: "Sternzellen" in the liver: Perisinusoidal cells with specific reference to storage of vitamin A. Am J Anat 132:429, 1971

108. Wanson JC, Drochmans P, Mosselmans R, Knook DL: Symbiotic culture of adult hepatocytes and sinus-lining cells. Edited by E Wisse and DL Knook: Kupffer Cells and Other Liver Sinusoidal Cells. Amsterdam, Elsevier, 1977, pp 141–150

109. Weibel ER, Stäubli W, Griägi HR, Hess FA: Correlated morphometric and biochemical studies on the liver cell: I. Morphometric model, stereological methods and normal morphometric data for rat liver. J Cell Biol 42:68–91, 1969

110. Widmann JJ, Cotran RS, Fahimi HD: Mononuclear phagocytes (Kupffer cells) and endothelial cells. Identification of two functional cell types in rat liver sinusoids by endogenous peroxidase activity. J Cell Biol 52:159–170, 1972

111. Widmann JJ, Fahimi HD: Proliferation of mononuclear phagocytes (Kupffer cells) and endothelial cells in regenerating rat liver. Am J Pathol 80:349–360, 1975

112. Widmann JJ, Fahimi HD: Proliferation of endothelial cells in estrogen-stimulated rat liver. Lab Invest 34:141–149, 1976

113. Wincek TJ, Hupka AL, Sweat FW: Stimulation of adenylate cyclase from isolated hepatocytes and Kupffer cells. J Biol Chem 250:8863–8873, 1975

114. Wisse E: An electron microscopic study of the fenestrated endothelial lining of rat liver sinusoids. J Ultrastruct Res 31: 125–150, 1970

115. Wisse E: An ultrastructural characterization of the endothelial cell in the rat liver sinusoid under normal and various experimental conditions, as a contribution to the distinction between endothelial and Kupffer cells. J Ultrastruct Res 38:528–562, 1972

116. Wisse E: Observations on the fine structure and peroxidase cytochemistry of normal rat liver Kupffer cells. J Ultrastruct Res 46:393–426, 1974

117. Wisse E: Kupffer cell reactions in rat liver under various conditions as observed in the electron microscope. J Ultrastruct Res 46:499–520, 1974

118. Wisse E: Ultrastructure and function of Kupffer cells and other sinusoidal cells in the liver. Edited by E Wisse and DL Knook: Kupffer Cells and Other Liver Sinusoidal Cells. Amsterdam, Elsevier, 1977, pp 33–60

119. Wisse E: Ultrastructure and function of Kupffer cells and other sinusoidal cells in the liver. Méd Chir Dig 6:409–418, 1977

120. Wisse E, Daems WTh: Fine structural study on the sinusoidal lining cells of rat liver. Edited by R van Furth: Mononuclear Phagocytes, Oxford, Blackwell, 1970, pp 200–210

121. Wisse E, Emeis JJ, Daems WTh: Some fine structural considerations on the possible involvement of the liver RES in lysosomal storage diseases, with observations in a case of Morquio's disease. Edited by JM Tager et al: Enzyme Therapy in Lysosomal Storage Diseases. Amsterdam, North-Holland, 1974, pp 95–110

122. Wisse E, Giphart M, van der Meulen J, Roels F, Emeis JJ, Daems WTh: Peroxidatic activity in bacteria-phagocytizing Kupffer cells, demonstrated by a new method: Perfusion incubation. Proceedings of the Fifth Regional Conference on Electron Microscopy, Manchester, 1972, p 272

123. Wisse E, Van 't Noordende JM, van der Meulen J, Daems WTh: The pit cell: Description of a new type of cell occurring in rat liver sinusoids and peripheral blood. Cell Tissue Res 173:423–435, 1976

124. Zlydaszyk JC, Moon RJ: Fate of ^{51}Cr-labeled lipopolysaccharide in tissue culture cells and liver of normal mice. Infect Immun 14:100–105, 1976

Chapter 9

Experimental Aspects of Hepatic Fibrosis

By ROBERT STERN, M.D.

COLLAGEN COMPRISES 30% of the total protein of the mammalian body. Very small amounts, approximately 4%,[1] are present in the normal liver. In chronic liver disease and in cirrhosis, however, pathologic quantities of hepatic collagen are found. Although the mechanism of fibrosis in the liver is probably no different from collagen deposition elsewhere in the body, the fibrotic process is responsible for the serious sequelae of chronic disease more directly in the liver than in any other organ.

Some of the molecular mechanisms that underlie abnormal collagen deposition are beginning to be resolved. At least nine posttranslational enzymatic reactions have been identified that endow the collagen chain with secondary modifications, each of which is a potentially rate-limiting or regulatory step. Regulatory steps at the translational and transcriptional level must also exist, however. A single cell is able to synthesize at least two types of collagen simultaneously.[2] Changes in the ratio of collagen types, as well as levels of collagen synthesis have been observed, indicating modulation of synthesis.[3] Cyclic nucleotide effects have been shown,[4,5] as well as both an increase and a decrease following viral infection of cells.[6,7]

Collagen biochemistry has been well reviewed,[8–12] and the current status of the field has been described.[13,14] A survey of recent progress is presented in this chapter in areas relevant to hepatic fibrosis, with particular attention to in vitro experimental models. The understanding of the various steps in collagen deposition, isolated and assayed in tissue culture, may ultimately reveal a mechanism for controlling the fibrosis of chronic liver disease.

The purpose of this chapter is to develop new conceptual frameworks and potential model systems in order to stimulate research in hepatic fibrosis, rather than to supplement the excellent review of Rojkind in Volume V of this series. The current progress in culture techniques for liver cells, the advances in our ability to handle the collagen molecule, and the recently acquired ability to recognize various intermediates in the maturation of the molecule by chromatographic and other separatory techniques make it reasonable to address the question of hepatic fibrosis in several in vitro systems.

COLLAGEN STRUCTURE

Collagen is the product of multiple genes. The characteristic three α chains in a triple-stranded helix is common to all collagens. The strands contain the

From the Department of Pathology, University of California, San Francisco.

173

repeating triplet *gly-x-y*, in which *x* and *y* may be any amino acid but are proline or hydroxyproline 50% of the time. This answer to a structural problem has been utilized by nature a number of times. Examples are a fragment of the acetylcholinesterase molecule[15] and a component of complement Clq,[16] both of which contain triple helical collagenous segments. Only the supramolecular fibrous proteins of the extracellular matrix are the true "collagens," however.

The collagen monomers are aligned so that three glycines are at the cross point of the three strands, the only amino acid residue small enough to permit approximation of the chains to each other. This explains why such a sequence has been so highly conserved through evolution. No exception to the *gly-x-y* triplet has been found in the triple helical domain of collagens, ranging in nature from mammals down to the sponges.

Collagen is synthesized as a high-molecular-weight soluble precursor.[14] The three pro α chains, termed procollagen, contain nonhelical propeptide extensions at both their N- and C-termini. These peptides are removed through several scissions with specific proteases before deposition into the supramolecular insoluble matrix fiber can occur. The specific proteases have been partially purified.[17,18] Radioimmunoassays to detect such enzymes in the circulation, as well as their peptide cleavage products, may provide clinical tests for monitoring fibrosis in chronic liver disease. These may more accurately reflect the fibrotic process than liver biopsies with their attendant sampling errors and diversions of the needle by tenacious fibrous connective tissue.

Collagen is recognized as a family of closely related proteins, each a different gene product. Superimposed on this protein heterogeneity is a myriad of secondary modifications. On the basis of cyanogen bromide peptide map studies, separate collagens can be resolved and are now classified according to the following simplified scheme:

Type I—skin, bone, tendon
Type II—cartilage
Type III—smooth muscle, fetal, vascular
Type IV—basement membrane
Type V—smooth muscle

Further resolution of collagen types has been made possible, and heterogeneity of collagen is far greater than previously realized. Basement membrane collagens can be further resolved into several tissue specific types.[19] Many minor collagen species have also been detected[20,21] and are components of normal as well as pathologic tissues. The complexity of collagen types may soon surpass that of the hemoglobins. An evolution of collagen types in an organism, from the fetal to the adult state, is recognized, which also parallels the hemoglobin situation. Recapitulation of fetal collagens in malignant sarcomas and compensatory deposition of fetal collagens to supplant genetically defective adult collagens are areas of active research. Whether such collagens are relevant to the fibrosis of chronic liver disease must await future investigation.

The most useful distinguishing characteristics in separating the collagen types are the peptide patterns following cyanogen bromide cleavage. Cyanogen bromide cleaves specifically at methionine residues, and collagens, conveniently, contain seven to eight well-spaced methionines per α chain of 1,000 residues. A manageable array of convenient peptides is thus generated.

Progress in tissue culture techniques and use of protease inhibitors during isolation procedures have made it possible to detect various intermediates in the processing of the procollagen molecule. Such intermediates accumulate in the media of cultured cells. These precursor forms of the various type-specific collagens have greater differences between them than do the fully processed mature collagen chains. Such procollagens are also more amenable to ordinary biochemical investigations. Although these procollagens have only a transient existence in vivo, they tend to accumulate in the artificial in vitro tissue culture, since the normal cleavage reactions that occur in the processing of the molecule are much reduced. Instead, the procollagens are elaborated into the tissue culture medium and away from the cell surface, where most such cleavage reactions occur.

An area of potential investigation is the isolation of various cleavage products from the maturation process to determine if they play a regulatory feedback role in the biosynthesis of the molecule.

HUMAN HEPATIC FIBROSIS

Humans have a much more vigorous fibrotic response to injury than any other animal, both in the rapidity and the ease with which a fibrotic response can be induced. Even though excellent experimental animal models for liver injury are available, having the advantages of well-worked-out protein schemes and defined genetic systems, no animal other than man mounts the profound fibrous reaction in the liver, not even the lesser primates. In the study of human fibrosis the only relevant model appears to be man himself. For this reason, tissue culture systems for growing human liver cells take on increased importance in attempting to recreate the fibrous response in vitro.

One example is the mouse model of vinyl chloride exposure. In man the angiosarcoma that develops is accompanied by a vigorous fibrosis. In the mouse, only the angiosarcoma is found, with no fibrosis.[22]

COLLAGEN AND RETICULIN

In simple wound healing, type III collagen is deposited early in the process. This forms a temporary matrix for the future deposition of the firm, coarse, often doubly refractile type I collagen. The partial resorption of type III collagen and its replacement by type I collagen causes contraction of the wound and is the basis of the "proud flesh" phenomenon, the protrusion of scar tissue above the skin surface late in wound healing. It is also responsible for the contractures that occur in the surgical repair of severed tendons. The predominance of type III collagen in fetal skin and its gradual replacement with type I collagen with maturation is also consistent with a temporary nature for type III collagen.[23] From these observations in the biochemistry of skin collagen, it would be simple to make an extrapolation to fibrotic scarring in the liver and to suggest that the transition from reversible to irreversible scarring in chronic liver disease might correlate with the transition from type III to type I collagen. This is particularly tempting in light of the contracture of the liver in end-stage chronic disease. Indeed, data are available that type III collagen is present in higher concentrations in the early stages of hepatic fibrosis,[24,25] but a simple correlation between collagen types and chronicity is an oversimplification and probably incorrect.

Identity of type III collagen with the reticulin observed in the silver impregnation method of the histopathologist has been suggested. Increased levels of reticulin in the early phases of wound healing and in early hepatic fibrosis are consistent with such a suggestion. Some type III collagen may well be reticulin. Evidence that all reticulin is type III collagen remains tenuous, however, and again no simple relationship may exist. The carbohydrate moieties that are added to collagen in the course of the many secondary modifications of the molecule may reflect more accurately what the pathologist observes.

IMMUNOFLUORESCENT STUDIES

Major discrepancies are observed between immunofluorescent studies of collagen and biochemical analyses of the same tissue. In human skin, using human collagen type-specific antibodies, type III collagen appears concentrated in the papillary dermis, and the broad collagen bands of the deeper reticular dermis stain with monospecific type I immunofluorescent antiserum.[26] By biochemical analysis, however, type I and type III collagens are present at a constant ratio throughout all levels of the skin.[27] In cartilage, type II cartilage-specific collagen is undetectable in cartilagenous tissue unless proteoglycan is removed by prior digestion with hyaluronidase.[28] This digestion seems to expose antigenic combining sites that are otherwise unavailable.

Two apparent populations of hepatic collagen have been reported, one stainable by fluorescein-labeled antitype III collagen antibody and another not stainable by either antitype I or III collagen.[29,30] A theory has been proposed that liver contains a new undefined collagen type or that liver contains type I collagen that differs from the type I collagen of skin in its immunologic properties. However, biochemical investigations indicate that type I collagen is a major constituent of liver and that it is indistinguishable from type I collagen in other tissues [25,31] Even the carbohydrates or normal and cirrhotic liver collagens are indistinguishable from other organs. There is no explanation for such discrepancies.

Experiments performed perhaps with more defined antisera reveal that type III collagen is present as a fine meshwork in the hepatic parenchyma which parallels the distribution of reticulum fibers identified by the silver impregnation technique. Type I collagen fibers are present in the portal zone and in the central canal. In cirrhosis, type III collagen is present in the septa early. It is then replaced by type I in the nodular parenchyma and portal tracts. An increased deposition of type III collagens is found in experimental liver injury, such as in ethionine administration and following bile duct ligation around proliferated bile ductules and is followed subsequently by type I collagen. Increased amounts of basement membrane collagen stainability is noted around sinusoids in all cases of chronic liver injury.[29,32,33] These observations indicate the necessity of using antisera that has been vigorously characterized, and even then, it is not a quantitative procedure.

Extractable levels of actin, another structural protein (see Chapter 4), can be constant from several different tissue preparations by SDS-polyacrylamide gel electrophoresis criterion. The stainability of these same tissues by antiactin immune sera is highly variable, occasionally being absent altogether, and appears to reflect changes in the organization of cellular actin rather than differences in actin levels.[34]

Thus, data from immunofluorescent and possibly immunoperoxidase techniques on the histologic distribution of insoluble structural proteins and particularly matrix proteins such as collagen are difficult to interpret. Such studies can at best only confirm data already documented biochemically. When positive reactivity is achieved, subtle features of structural organization can be observed, and this is perhaps the chief function of such immunofluorescent studies.

CELL SURFACE PROTEINS

The major cell surface glycoprotein found in cultured fibroblasts has been the subject of intensive investigation.[35] Several other proteins that have been studied independently are identical or similar proteins, and all are related to cold insoluble globulin (CIg) of serum. Fibronectin, CAP (cell-attachment protein), CAF (cell adhesion factor), LETS (large external transformation sensitive) protein, and CSP (cell surface protein) are among the synonyms for this protein. The term "fibronectin" is used here, and CIg is used for the circulating form. No functional role is known for this protein, but because of its intriguing properties speculations abound.

Cells have a striking diminution of this surface protein following chemical or viral transformation. When transformed cells are given an exogenous source of this protein, they regain normal phenotypic appearance. Synthesis of this protein in cultured cells is dependent on the presence of epidermal growth factor, usually present in the serum.[36] This polypeptide, found in the murine salivary glands, has a site of origin in the human gastrointestinal tract that is yet to be detected.

Cells in vivo interact with each other, with neighboring cells, with the host immune system, and with circulating elements of the blood. Much of this interaction is at the cell surface. The cell surface is a complex assembly that can be viewed as having three components: (1) submembranous arrays of microfilaments and microtubules; (2) cell surface membrane proteins and receptors; and (3) the cytoexoskeleton. These form a modulating assembly that functions as a regulator of cell activity. Fibronectin and collagen comprise the cytoexoskeleton, the outermost part of this assembly constituting a microstroma about the cell. This microstroma is involved in the social behavior of cells,[37] i.e., cell-cell and cell-surface interactions. Both the internal and external cytoskeletons disappear during mitosis and are rapidly resynthesized in the daughter cells as soon as mitosis is completed. This may explain why cells in mitosis are much less adherent to their substrate.

Fibronectin is an integral part of connective tissue matrix and appears associated with connective tissues as well as with basal laminae throughout the body.[38,39] Fibronectin is also covalently bound to fibrin through blood coagulation factor XIII, the Hagemann factor which catalyzes a transglutaminase reaction.[40] Collagen, fibrinogen, and fibronectin all constitute this meshwork around the cell in this miniature stroma.

Stabilization also occurs by extensive disulfide bond formation between fibronectin monomers, probably type III collagen (R. Stern, unpublished observations), and other cell surface proteins.[41]

Fibronectin binds simultaneously to the cell surface and to the extracellular matrix collagen. Fibronectin binds to collagen at a very specific site. The binding site is close to or identical to the single collagenase cleavage site[42] three-quarters of the way from the amino terminal end of the molecule, in α I-CNBr 7, the region that also supports myoblast differentiation. In the other collagen chain types, the collagenase cleavage site and fibronectin binding occur on the homologous region of the chain. This region of the collagen molecule is obviously of critical importance to the cell.

One possible model of pathologic as well as normal collagen deposition involves the interaction of collagen with either collagenase or fibronectin. In a competition between fibronectin and collagenase for the same site, prior binding of fibronectin may prevent collagen degradation and permit its accumulation, while binding of collagenase causes collagen removal. Data to support this intriguing model of fibrosis have not been obtained.

The concept of stroma must be redefined, i.e., the immediate stroma of the cell, which alters with the cell cycle growth rate, with transformation, and perhaps in pathologic processes. In addition, there is the major stroma or fibrous connective tissue stroma that can be observed grossly. An interaction between these two stromas may exist, and determining whether coordination in their biosynthesis exists should become a major concern in the study of the fibrosis of chronic liver diseases. Disruptions of matrix organization through changes in collagen and fibronectin deposition on the liver cell surface may occur in various pathologic states. This is another area for future investigation.

For normal vascular endothelium, the vascular side of the cell is nonthrombogenic, but the undersurface that abuts on basement membrane is highly thrombogenic. The adhesion proteins, such as fibronectin, which binds the cell to its basement membrane, are critically important for the normal function of vascular endothelium. Fibronectin is a major component of the proteins synthesized by endothelial cells. Whether the endothelial cells of the liver sinusoids also synthesize fibronectin is not established, but possibly much of circulating CIg is the product of both liver sinusoidal endothelial cells and the vascular endothelium.

Fibronectin and collagen biosynthesis are not restricted to mesenchymal cells, but they are also elaborated by cells of epithelial origin, including the hepatocyte.[43,44] When rat hepatocytes are continuously passaged in culture, fibronectin undergoes a progressive decrease until it completely disappears.[42] It is intriguing to postulate that if hepatocytes were to be cultured in the continued presence of stromal cells, biosynthesis of hepatocyte fibronectin might be maintained, together with a basement membrane. Such examples of mesenchymal-epithelial interdependency are considered later.

The function of an adhesion protein on the surface of epithelial cells endowed with gap junctions, tight junctions, desmosomes, tonofibrils, and hemidesmosomes is not clear. Additional undefined functions may well exist. Fibronectin may be involved in the attachment of epithelial cells to their basement membrane, particularly the collagenous portion of the membrane. Suggestive evidence has been obtained from endothelial cells in culture and in teratocarcinoma cells as they differentiate into embryoid bodies.[45]

In invertebrates, such as the lobster, CIg and fibrinogen are related molecules.[46] Perhaps in vertebrates also a relationship exists between the cell surface fibronectin and the coagulation protein, fibrinogen. Peptide mapping and immunologic probes will provide evidence for such a model. Possibly the peptides in these two proteins, which are substrates for factor XIII, are homologous.

A model for the fibrotic response to liver cell injury can be developed from the preceding considerations. Proteases are known to participate in many areas of biologic control.[47] The transformed cell in culture and continuous lines of malignant cells have elevated levels of proteases at the cell surface. These proteolytic activities can be detected in the culture medium. When placed in culture the injured liver cell may also have elevated proteases associated with surface membranes. Such activities may cause perturbation of normal cell surfaces, of the collagen-fibronectin exoskeleton of stromal cells, or of hepatocytes. Partial cleavage of this meshwork about the cell may be a signal to initiate collagen synthesis or resynthesis of the exoskeleton matrix. The normal cell in mitosis has elevated proteases associated with the cell surface, and here also, matrix resynthesis is stimulated. Specific collagenases must be invoked for the disruption of the exoskeletal matrix. Whether such activities are present during mitosis in the normal cell has also not been tested. To test the cell layer and overlying media in the injured hepatocytic system would be of interest to see whether collagenase activity is paradoxically associated with increased levels of collagen synthesis. In testing such a scheme, it would be necessary to examine the culture media not only for intact strands of collagen or procollagen but also for partially cleaved digestion products.

EPITHELIAL-MESENCHYMAL INTERACTIONS

Epithelial-mesenchymal interactions in embryonic tissues and their interdependence in morphogenetic processes have been well described, including the major role that the collagenous stroma plays in that interaction.[48-50] The extrapolation can be made from embryonic tissues to a similar interplay between mesenchyme and epithelium in the fibrotic response to injury in the liver. Separation of the epithelial hepatocyte and the various stromal cells of mesenchymal origin, including the multiple cell types of the liver sinusoid, must be achieved so that they can be admixed, in a controlled manner, in cocultivation experiments.

Cooperation and even dependency have long been recognized in growth of cells in tissue culture. For the growth of human skin epithelial cells, irradiated 3T3 cells are required; the 3T3 cells may provide a specific connective tissue growth factor.[51] However, a trivial explanation may be that the irradiated 3T3 cells are providing a collagenous stroma for epithelial cell attachment.

Lens epithelial cells in culture are able to synthesize a basement membrane only when grown on frozen-killed lens stromal cells. This indicates that the connective tissue matrix, in this case of lens basal lamina, is elaborated by the epithelial cell but is dependent on the presence of a mesenchymal substratum.

A low level of stromal cell contamination in cultures of hepatocytes may be required for their attachment and survival. As liver culture systems become more refined, it will be necessary to quantitate levels of contamination in an attempt to resolve such phenomena. The degree of cooperation in stromal deposition following injury and the effect of mesenchyme on epithelial cells and epithelial cells on mesenchyme must be assessed, both in the normal state and following injury. Such interactions can perhaps be duplicated by conditioned media from the appropriate cell culture on the opposite cell type. The periductular fibrosis associated with bile duct obstruction may be the best example of an epithelial-mesenchymal interaction involved in a fibrous response. Focal accumulations of fibrous tissue such as around tumors, abscesses, or granulomas, may each have a different mechanism of fiber deposition.

THE DESMOPLASTIC RESPONSE TO METASTATIC TUMORS

An additional exploitable model of hepatic fibrosis is the scirrhous response to metastatic tumor, typified by lesions from the stomach, pancreas, prostate, and breast. The malignant epithelial cells in the liver induce a dense fibrous response. This is a variation of the theme on the interaction between epithelium and mesenchyme. Whether the collagen is elaborated by the tumors themselves or is a reaction of the host tissue has not been established. Convincing evidence has been provided to support each point of view.[52,53] An alternative explanation is that the response is dependent on an interaction between the two cell types. The question remains whether it is the liver epithelial or stromal cells that participate in the response to the malignant cells. The answer to that question may provide insight into the fibrosis of chronic liver disease. The dense stroma of scirrhous lesions represents a major commitment of a particular cell to connective tissue synthesis. The reaction may be transplanted to a tissue culture model in which liver slices or isolated cells can be cocultivated with malignant epithelial cells or cultivated in the presence of conditioned media from such cells. Examination of collagens and collagenase activities elaborated in the course of such incubations may uncover potential synthetic activities in the various populations of cells within the liver. Isolation of factors from such conditioned media may reveal the molecular mediators of hepatic fibrosis. From experiments using conditioned media, other tissues have generated a family of peptide factors. These include plasminogen activator,[54] plasminogen-independent fibrinolysins,[55] migration inhibitory factor,[56] migration-stimulating activity,[57] multiplication-stimulating activity-[58] and tumor angiogenesis factor.[59] It is appropriate to invoke such a factor from the conditioned media of malignant cells as the basis of this fibrotic response in the liver and to attempt to isolate this factor.

Alternatively, factors comparable to the mitogenic activities extracted from platelets[60] or macrophages[61] may be more accurate analogs of the putative fibroplasia-inducing factor that acts on the liver. Such a peptide from the injured liver, if isolated, would make it possible to develop an immune serum and eventually a radioimmunoassay, a clinical test to follow hepatic fibrosis. The literature is replete with suggestions of factors of this type in the injured and regenerating liver,[62,63] but most of these have remained hard to define because of the great difficulty in establishing bioassays to measure activity. The appropriate culture system may facilitate such an assay.

COLLAGENASES

Fibrosis may occur not only as a result of increased synthesis of collagen but also by its diminished removal. Collagenase research is an extraordinary difficult area. The assay is tedious and time-consuming, and the resulting data are not amenable to kinetic analysis.

The granulocyte has a type I-specific collagenase.[64] The classical animal collagenase of fibroblast origin can use as substrates types I, II, and III collagens.[65,66] A basement-membrane-specific collagenase has been observed that does not cleave other collagens (Liotta and Martin, personal communication). A collagenase specific for type III collagen, or one that degrades type III preferentially, has not been observed. Neutral proteases have been described that can cleave collagens at a tryptic sensitive site close to but not indentical to the collagenase cleavage site. Collagenase specificity has not been examined in relation to liver disease. The occurrence of a type III-specific collagenase should be present in hepatic fibrosis in the transition from early to late stages as type III collagen is replaced by type I. Such an activity has not been detected, but most investigators do not have the array of appropriate type-specific collagen to test their activities.

Collagenases from animal cells all have a similar mode of action, to cleave native triple helical collagen at a single site. Two fragments are produced which are three-quarters and one-quarter the length of the original molecule. The fragments are then easily attacked by nonspecific proteases to which the native collagen is impervious prior to that initial cut.

Collagenase may exist in a precursor form as a prozymogen that requires extracellular conversion to the active form of the enzyme.[67–70] Release of a specific protease may be required for this conversion. Again, from the studies of the biochemistry of skin collagen, information is available from which it is possible to extrapolate to the problem of hepatic fibrosis and to establish a testable model. In basal cell carcinomas of the skin, collagenase is found only in the stroma immediately surrounding islands of tumor cells.[71] This suggests that the tumor cells secrete a protease or a factor required for the activation of the latent collagenase. Such a model can be applied to the culture system of injured liver cells. Are the collagenases that are synthesized and secreted by macrophages and fibroblasts dependent on a product of the epithelial cell in cocultivation experiments, and is the hepatocyte that is derived from the injured liver a more effective source of such an activity?

IMMUNOLOGIC FACTORS IN HEPATIC FIBROSIS

Immunologic factors have been recognized as a component of chronic liver disease and are usually treated separately from the fibrotic reaction. These two reactions may be related to one another, however, and are not entirely separate phenomena.

Lymphokines from normal human peripheral blood monocytes stimulated with phytohemagglutinins increase collagen synthesis in cultured fibroblasts.[72] Lymphokines also stimulate collagenase production by macrophages.[73] Portal fibrosis is particularly striking around iron-laden macrophages in the case of iron overload from various causes. Additional evidence comes from schistosomiasis in which the collagen- and elastin-containing granuloma is thought to be a response to soluble antigens from the egg. Granuloma formation is diminished in immunosuppressed animals.

Chronic inflammation from any cause frequently leads to fibrosis. Perhaps all fibrosis is a response to inflammation, particularly since inflammatory cell infiltrates are often found in association with the fibrotic response. In the desmoplastic reaction to pancreatic tumors, however, inflammatory cells are completely absent, except in the presence of tissue necrosis or partial duct obstruction.

The human serum opsonic α_2 surface binding (α_2SB) glycoprotein is related to or perhaps identical to fibronectin. This serum protein has been considered a major mechanism by which reticuloendothelial cells phagocytize foreign and abnormal substances, and serum levels are a reflection of RES function. This defense process is depressed in patients following trauma, surgery, burn injury, advanced neoplastic disease, and rickettsial infection.

Opsonic α_2SB glycoprotein is a major product of endothelial cells.[74] One class of sinusoidal cell of the liver, the endothelial cell, synthesizes a product that enables another sinusoidal cell, the Kupffer cell, to accomplish its phagocytic function. The α_2SB is thus also a link between the immune system (the integrity of macrophage function) and the fibrotic response (fibronectin and collagen interaction).

UNANSWERED QUESTIONS

Several questions emerge from this review. What is the chief cell responsible for the deposition of pathologic quantities of collagen in the liver? We can now rephrase that question: What are the cellular interactions involved in collagen deposition? Is CIg or fibronectin involved in hepatic fibrosis? What other circulating factors are also involved in that process? And what is the role of collagenase in the overall process? Answers to some of these questions may somehow uncover an exploitable mechanism for the control of hepatic fibrosis.

REFERENCES

1. Grant ME, Prockop DJ: The biochemical synthesis of collagen. N Engl J Med 286:194–199, 242–249, 291–300, 1972
2. Gay S, Martin GR, Müller PK, Timpl R, Kühn K: Simultaneous synthesis of types I and III collagen by fibroblasts in culture. Proc Natl Acad Sci USA 73:4037–4040, 1976.
3. Rabson AS, Stern R, Tralka TS, Costa J, Wilczek J: Hexamethylene bisacetamide induces morphologic changes and increased synthesis of procollagen in cell line from glioblastoma multiforme. Proc Natl Acad Sci USA 74:5060–5064, 1977
4. Peterkofsky B, Prather WB: Increased collagen synthesis in Kirsten sarcoma virus-transformed BALB 3T3 cells grown in the presence of dibutyryl cyclic AMP. Cell 3:291–299, 1974
5. Baum BJ, Moss J, Breul SD, Crystal RG: Association in normal human fibroblasts of elevated levels of adenosine 3'5'-monophosphate with selective decrease in collagen production. J Biol Chem 253:3391–3394, 1978
6. Levinson W, Liu TZ, Bhatnagar RS: Loss of ability to synthesize collagen in fibroblasts transformed by Rous sarcoma virus. J Natl Cancer Inst 55:207, 1975
7. Banes AT, Smith RE, Mechanic GL: Increased collagen synthesis in myeloblastosis-associated virus-infected chicken embryo fibroblasts. Biochem Biophys Res Commun 82:723–726, 1978
8. Bornstein P: The biosynthesis of collagen. Ann Rev Biochem 43:567–603, 1974
9. Martin GR, Byer PH, Piez KA: Procollagen. Adv Enzymol 42:167–191, 1975
10. Gallop PM, Paz MA: Posttranslational protein modifications with special attention to collagen and elastin. Physiol Rev 55:418–487, 1975
11. Kivirikko KI, Risteli L: Biosynthesis of collagen and its alterations in pathological states. Med Biol 54:159–186, 1976
12. Hance AJ, Crystal RG: The connective tissue of lung. Am Rev Resp Dis 112:657–711, 1975
13. Popper H, Piez KA: Collagen metabolism in the liver. Am J Dig Dis 23:614–659, 1978
14. Fessler J, Fessler LL: Biosynthesis of procollagen. Annu Rev Biochem 47:129–162, 1978
15. Lwebuga-Mukusa JS, Lappi S, Tayler P: Molecular forms of acetylcholinesterase from *Torpedo californica*: Their relationship to synaptic membranes. Biochemistry 15:1425–1434, 1976
16. Reid KBM, Porter RR: Subunit composition and structure of component Clq of the first component of complement. Biochem J 155:19–23, 1976
17. Tuderman L, Kivirikko KI, Prockop J: Partial purification and characterization of a neutral protease which cleaves the N-terminal propeptides from procollagen. Biochemistry 17:2948–2954, 1978
18. Kessler E, Goldberg B: A method for assaying the activity of the endopeptidase which excises the non helical carboxyterminal extension from type I procollagen. Anal Biochem 86:463–469, 1978
19. Chung E, Rhodes RK, Miller EJ: Isolation of three collagenous components of probable basement membrane origin from several tissues. Biochem Biophys Res Commun 71:1167–1174, 1976
20. Jiminez SA, Yankowski R, Bashey RI: Identification of two new collagen α-chains in extracts of lathyritic chick embryo ten-

dons. Biochem Biophys Res Commun 81:1298–1306, 1978

21. Brown RA, Shuttleworth CA, Weiss JB: Three new α-chains of collagen from a non-basement membrane source. Biochem Biophys Res Commun 80:866–872, 1978

22. Thomas LB, Popper H, Berk PD, Selikoff I, Falk H: Vinyl chloride-induced liver disease N Engl J Med 292:17–22, 1975

23. Epstein EH Jr: αl (III) ₃ human skin collagen. J Biol Chem 249:3225–3231, 1974

24. Kent G, Gay S, Inouye T, Bahu R, Minick OT, Popper H: Vitamin A-containing lipocytes and formation of type III collagen in liver injury. Proc Natl Acad Sci USA 73:3719–3722, 1976

25. Rojkind M, Martinez-Palomo A: Increase in type I and type III collagens in human alcoholic liver cirrhosis. Proc Natl Acad Sci USA 73:539–543, 1976

26. Becker V, Nowack H, Gay S, Timpl R: Production and specificity of antibodies against the aminoterminal region in type III collagen. Immunology 31:57–65, 1976

27. Epstein EH Jr, Munderloh NH: Human skin collagen: Presence of type I and type III at levels of the dermis. J. Biol Chem 253:1336, 1978

28. Von der Mark K, Von der Mark H, Gay S: Study of differential collagen synthesis during development of the chick embryo by immunofluorescence. Dev Biol 53:153, 1976

29. Gay S, Fietzek PP, Remberger K, Eder M, Kuhn K: Liver cirrhosis: immunofluorescence and biochemical studies demonstrate two types of collagen. Klin Wochenschr 53:205–208, 1975

30. Remberger K, Gay S, Fietzek PP: Immunochistochemische untersuchungen zur kollagen characteristierung in lebereirrhosen. Virchows Arch [Pathol Anat] 367:231–240, 1975

31. Seyer JM, Hutcheson ET, Kang AH: Collagen polymorphism in normal and cirrhotic human liver. J Clin Invest 59:241–248, 1977

32. Kent G, Gay S, Inouye T: Type I and type III collagen in experimental liver injury. Gastroenterology 71:A-22/915, 1976

33. Gay S, Inouye T, Minick OT: Basement membrane formation in experimental hepatic injury. Gastroenterology 71:A-14/907, 1976

34. Norberg R, Biberfeld G, Fagracus A, Lidman K, Thortensson R, Utter G: Immunofluorescent studies on actin. Clin Exp Immunol 28:512–518, 1977

35. Vaheri A, Ruoslahti E, Mosher DF (eds): Fibroblast Surface Protein. Vol. 312. New York, Annals of the New York Academy of Science, 1978

36. Chen LB, Gudor RC, Sun T-T, Chen AB, Mosesson MW: Control of a cell surface major glycoprotein by epidermal growth factor. Science 197:776–778, 1977

37. Bornstein P, Ash JF: Cell surface-associated structural proteins in connective tissue cells. Proc Natl Acad Sci USA 74:2480–2484, 1977

38. Linder E, Vaheri A, Ruoslahti E, Wartioraara J: Distribution of fibroblast surface antigen in the developing chick embryo. J Exp Med 142:41–49, 1975

39. Wartiovaara J, Stenman S, Vaheri A: Changes in expression of fibroblast surface antigen (FFA) during cytodifferentiation and heterokaryon formation. Differentiation 5:85–89, 1976

40. Keski-Oja J, Mosher DF, Vaheri A: Cross-linking of a major fibroblast surface-associated glycoprotein (fibronectin) catalyzed by blood coagulation factor XIII. Cell 9:29–35, 1976

41. Hynes RO, Destree A: Extensive disulfide bonding at the mammalian cell surface. Proc Natl Acad Sci USA 74:2855–2859, 1977

42. Kleinman HK, McGoodwin EB, Martin GR, Klebe RJ, Fietzek PP, Wooley DE: Localization of the binding site for cell attachment in the αl(I) chain of collagen. J Biol Chem 253:5642–5646, 1978

43. Sakakibara K, Takaoka T, Katsuta H, Umeda M, Tsukada Y: Collagen fiber formation as a common property of epithelial liver cell lines in culture. Exp Cell Res 111:63–71, 1978

44. Marceau N, Robert A, Mailhot D: The major surface protein of epithelial cells from newborn and adult rat livers in primary culture. Biochem Biophys Res Commun 76:1092–1097, 1977

45. Wartiovaara J, Leivo I, Virtanen I, Vaheri A, Graham CF: Appearance of fibronectin during differentiation of mouse teratocarcinoma in vitro. Nature 272:355–356, 1978

46. Mosher DF: Cross-linking of cold-insoluble globulin by fibrin-stabilizing factor. J Biol Chem 250:6614–6621, 1977

47. Reich E, Rifkin DB, Shaw E (eds): Pro-

teases and Biological Control. New York, Cold Spring Harbor Laboratory, 1975

48. Grobstein C: Tissue interaction in the morphogenesis of mouse embryonic rudiments *in vitro*. In: Aspects of Synthesis and Order in Growth. Ed: D Rudnick, Princeton University Press, Princeton, 1955

49. Cohen AM, Hay ED: Secretion of collagen by embryonic neuroepithelium at the time of spinal cord-somite interaction. Dev Biol 26:578–605, 1971

50. Trelstad RL: The developmental biology of vertebrate collagens. J Histochem Cytochem 21:521–528, 1973

51. Rheinwald JG, Green H: Serial cultivation of strains of human epidermal keratinocytes: the formation of keratinizing colonies from single cells. Cell 6:331–344, 1975

52. Willis RA: In The Spread of Tumors in the Human Body. Butterworth, London, 1952, p 115

53. Al-Adnani MS, Kirrane JA, McGee JO: Inappropriate production of collagen and prolyl hydroxylase by human breast cancer cells in- vivo. Br J Cancer 31:653–660, 1975

54. Unkless JC, Tobia A, Ossowski L, Quigley JP, Rifkin DB, Reach E: An enzymatic function associated with transformation of fibroblasts by oncogenic viruses. J Exp Med 137:85–112, 1973

55. Chen LB, Buchanan JM: Plasminogen-independent fibrinolysis by proteases produced by transformed chick embryo fibroblasts. Proc Natl Acad Sci USA 72: 1132–1136, 1975

56. Hammond ME, Roblin RO, Dvorak AM, Selvaggio SS, Black PH, Dvorak HF: MIF-like activity in simian virus 40-transformed 3T3 fibroblast cultures. Science 185:955–957, 1974

57. Burk RR: A factor from a transformed cell line that affects cell migration: Proc Natl Acad Sci USA 70:369–372, 1973

58. Klagsbrun M, Knighton D, Folkman J: Tumor angiogenesis activity in cells grown in tissue culture. Cancer Res 36:110–113, 1976

59. Dulak NC, Temin HM: A partially purified polypeptide fraction from rat liver cell conditioned medium with multiplication-stimulating activity for embryo fibroblasts. J Cell Physiol 81:153–160, 1973

60. Rutherford RB, Ross R: Platelet factors stimulate fibroblasts and smooth muscle cells quiescent in plasma serum to proliferate. J Cell Biol 69:196–203, 1976

61. Leibovitch SJ, Ross R: A macrophage-dependent factor that stimulates the proliferation of fibroblasts in vitro. Am J Pathol 84:501–513, 1976

62. McGee JO, O'Hare RP, Patrick RS: Stimulation of the collagen biosynthesis pathway by factors isolated from experimentally-injured liver Nature [New Biol] 243:121–123, 1973

63. Pickart L, Thaler MM: Tripeptide in human serum which prolongs survival of normal liver cells and stimulates growth in neoplastic liver. Nature [New Biol] 243:85–87, 1973

64. Horwitz AL, Hance AJ, Crystal RG: Granulocyte collagenase: Selective digestion of type I relative to type III collagen. Proc Natl Acad Sci USA 74:897–901, 1977

65. Perez-Tamayo R: Pathology of Collagen Degradation. Am J Pathol 92:507–566, 1978

66. Harris ED Jr, Krane SM: Collagenases. N Engl J Med 291:557–563, 605–609, 652–659, 1974

67. Harper E, Bloch KJ, Gross J: The zymogen of tadpole collagenase. Biochemistry 10: 3035–3041, 1971

68. Vaes G: The release of collagenase as as inactive proenzyme by bone explants in culture. Biochem J 126:275–289, 1972

69. Bauer EA, Stricklin GP, Jeffrey JJ, Eisen AZ: Collagenase production by human skin fibroblasts. Biochem Biophys Res Commun 64:232–240, 1975

70. Bauer EA, Gedde-Dahl T Jr, Eisen AZ: The role of human skin collagenase in epidermolysis bullosa. J Invest Dermatol 68:119–124, 1977

71. Bauer EA, Gordon JU, Reddick ME, Eisen AZ: Quantitation and immunocytochemical localization of human skin collagenase in basal cell carcinoma. J Invest Dermatol 69:363–367, 1977

72. Johnson RL, Ziff M: Lymphokine stimulation of collagen synthesis. J Clin Invest 58:240–252, 1976

73. Wahl LM, Wahl SM, Mergenhagen SE, Martin GR: Collagenase production by lymphokine-activated macrophages. Science 187:261–263, 1975

74. Blumenstock F, Weber P, Sabe TM: Isolation and biochemical characterization of α-2-opsonic glycoprotein from rat serum. J Biol Chem 252:7156–7162, 1977.

Chapter 10

Current Concepts of Bilirubin Metabolism and Hereditary Hyperbilirubinemia

By BRUCE F. SCHARSCHMIDT, M.D.
and
JOHN L. GOLLAN, M.D., Ph.D.

THE COMPLEXITIES of bilirubin metabolism have piqued the curiosity of many generations of scientists, largely because accumulation of this orange-colored compound in tissues is such an obvious and frequent sign of liver dysfunction. This review is focused primarily on those aspects of bilirubin chemistry, formation, and disposition about which new information has become available to modify conventional thinking and, in many instances, to stimulate controversy. Many of these aspects of bilirubin metabolism also have broader implications regarding the handling by the liver of a variety of other organic anions including drugs, dyes, and hormones. The term "organic anion," as used here, includes many substances excreted in bile such as dyes (e.g., bilirubin, indocyanine green [ICG], rose bengal, and sulfobromophthalein [BSP]), as well as some anionic drugs, hormones, and their metabolites. Although bile acids are also organic anions, their hepatic metabolism differs from that of these other substances in many respects, and bile acids are therefore not included in the category of "organic anions" in this review.

The hereditary disorders of bilirubin metabolism have been outlined in Table 1 and are referred to in the text only with respect to the underlying metabolic defect(s). For a detailed clinical discussion of these inherited disorders, the reader is referred to several excellent reviews.[1-4]

BIOLOGIC IMPLICATIONS OF BILIRUBIN CHEMISTRY

Bilirubin IXα results from selective cleavage of ferroprotoporphyrin IX (heme) at the α-methene bridge and is the predominant bile pigment in mammals. Although the chemical structure (Fig. 1, top panel) of bilirubin IXα has been established beyond reasonable doubt for more than 35 years,[5] a reawakening of interest in this molecule with investigation of its stereochemistry and conformation has helped to explain many of its unusual physical properties, the biologic implications of which are only just being fully appreciated.[6] X-ray diffraction studies revealed that the rigid methene bridge double bonds adjacent

From the Department of Medicine and the Liver Center, University of California, San Francisco, California.

Supported in part by NIH grants P50 AM 18520 and Research Career Development Award 1 KO4 AM 00323 (Dr. Scharschmidt).

TABLE 1.—*The Hereditary Hyperbilirubinemias*

| | Unconjugated Hyperbilirubinemia | | | Conjugated Hyperbilirubinemia | |
| | | Crigler-Najjar Syndrome (Congenital Nonhemolytic Jaundice) | | | |
	Gilbert's Syndrome	Type I	Type II	Dubin-Johnson Syndrome	Rotor's Syndrome
Identified defects in bilirubin metabolism	(a) Decreased hepatic uptake,[121,125,126] (b) Decreased glucuronyl transferase activity[144,145]	Absent glucuronyl transferase activity[150,151]	Markedly decreased or absent glucuronyl transferase activity[147-150]	Impaired biliary excretion[213-216]	Impaired biliary excretion[122,212]
Plasma bilirubin concentration (mg/dl)	Total: ≤ 3 in absence of hemolysis or fasting Conjugated: ≤ 0.4[2,121,146,217,218]	Total: 17-50 (usually > 20) Conjugated: 0[4,150,224]	Total: 6-45 (usually < 20) Conjugated: 0[2,148,150]	Total: 1-25 (usually < 7) Conjugated: averages 60% of total[214-216]	Total: 1-20 (usually < 7) Conjugated: averages 60% of total[212,219]
Bile pigment	Diglucuronide decreased and monoglucuronide increased compared with normal[164,165]	Small amount of unconjugated bilirubin;[150] trace monoconjugates[164]	Predominantly monoglucuronide[148,149,169]	Not studied	Not studied
Incidence	$\leq 7\%$ of population[2,220,221]	Rare	Uncommon	Rare, up to 1:1300 in Iranian Jews[215]	Rare
Inheritance	? Autosomal dominant[218,222]	Autosomal recessive[150,223,224]	? Autosomal dominant with variable penetrance[150,225,226]	Autosomal recessive[209,215,227]	Autosomal recessive[212]
Age when hyperbilirubinemia recognized	Variable, usually by early adulthood (often during fasting)[2,217]	1-3 days after birth[150,224]	Usually during the first year of life, occasionally later[148,150]	Variable (birth to age 70), usually by early adulthood[213-215]	Variable, usually in childhood[219]

Associated hemolysis	Mild hemolysis is detectable in about half of patients[121,127,228,229]	No	No	No	No
Symptoms	Nonspecific or absent[2,218]	Those of kernicterus[150,224]	Usually none[148,150]	Nonspecific or absent[211,213]	Nonspecific or absent[212,219]
Physical Findings	Occasional scleral icterus	Jaundice, findings of kernicterus in infants;[150,224] seizures, myoclonus athetosis, incoordination, retardation in young adults[151]	Jaundice, findings of kernicterus only rarely present[148,150]	Jaundice, occasional hepatomegaly[214-216]	Jaundice[219]
Routine liver tests	Normal	Normal	Normal	Usually normal, minor abnormalities reported[214-216]	Usually normal[230]
Plasma BSP disappearance rate	Decreased in some patients (45 min retention ≤15%)[125,126]	Normal	Normal	Slow initial disappearance (45 min retention ≤20%); frequent secondary rise at 90–120 min[213-215]	Markedly slow initial disappearance (45 min retention 30%-50%); no secondary rise[212,231]
Oral cholecystography	Normal[121]	Normal [151]	Normal[149,225]	Faint or nonvisualization[213-215,227,232]	Usually normal[211,230]

Continued on next page

TABLE 1.—*The Hereditary Hyperbilirubinemias (continued)*

| | Unconjugated Hyperbilirubinemia | | | Conjugated Hyperbilirubinemia | |
	Gilbert's Syndrome	Crigler-Najjar Syndrome (Congenital Nonhemolytic Jaundice) Type I	Type II	Dubin-Johnson Syndrome	Rotor's Syndrome
Liver Macroscopic	Normal	Normal	Normal	Black[213,214,232]	Normal
Microscopic	Normal, lipofuscin may be increased[233]	Normal	Normal	Coarse dark pigment in centrolobular cells[213,214,232]	Normal[212,219,230]
Reduction in plasma bilirubin concentration by phenobarbital	Yes[153,154]	None[150,151]	Yes[148-150]	Variable and minimal[216]	Not studied
Diagnosis	Clinical and laboratory findings; response to fasting[217,234,235] or nicotinic acid[236] may be helpful; liver biopsy not routinely necessary[2]	Clinical and laboratory findings; no response to phenobarbital[150]	Clinical and laboratory findings; response to phenobarbital[150]	Clinical and laboratory findings including BSP disappearance and urinary coproporphyrins (see "Biliary Excretion"); liver biopsy	Clinical and laboratory findings including BSP disappearance and urinary coproporphyrins (see "Biliary Excretion); liver biopsy
Treatment	Phenobarbital rarely indicated	No generally effective, practical, and safe treatment available	Phenobarbital if indicated	No specific treatment available; avoid estrogens	No specific treatment available
Prognosis	Normal	Usually death in infancy; rarely, later onset of neurologic damage[150,151,224,237]	Usually normal; kernicterus occurs only rarely[148-150]	Probably good	Probably good

190

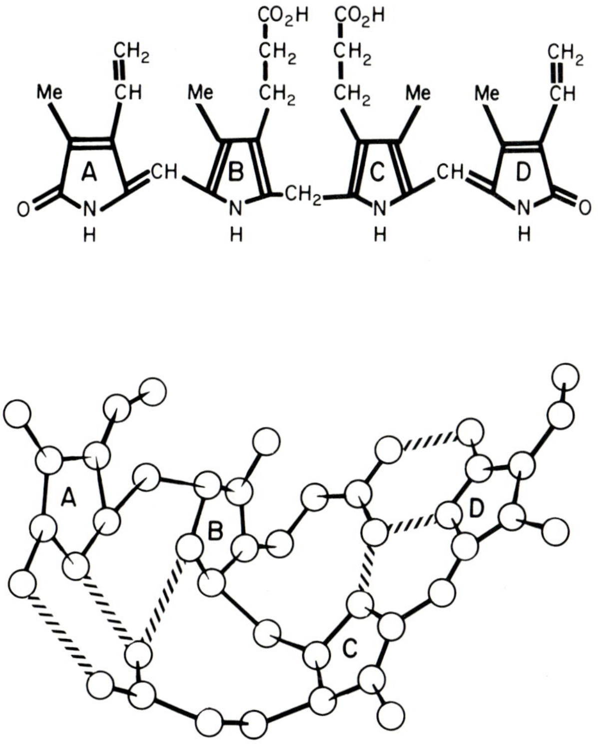

FIG. 1—Structure of bilirubin IXα. The conventionally written structure is shown in the top panel with the methene bridge double bonds adjacent to the outer pyrrole rings (A and D) in the Z-Z position. The other geometric isomers of bilirubin IXα (E-Z, Z-E, and E-E) can be written by "inverting" the methene bridge double bonds adjacent to the A, D, or A and D rings, respectively. The other structural isomers of bilirubin IX (IXβ, IXγ, and IXδ) are formed by rupture of the heme ring at the β, γ, or δ (rather than the α) methene bridge, respectively, and have the methyl, vinyl, and propionic acid side chains arranged differently on the pyrrole rings. The bottom panel shows the involuted internally hydrogen bonded structure of bilirubin IXα (Z-Z), in which the propionic acid groups of pyrrole rings B and C are linked by hydrogen bonds (broken lines) to the oxygen and nitrogens of the opposite pyrrole rings. (Reproduced by permission from Schmid R: Bilirubin metabolism: State of the art. Gastroenterology 74:1307–1312, 1978. Copyright 1978, American Gastroenterological Association.)

to the outer pyrrole rings have the configuration shown in Figure 1 (top panel).[7] Because the cis/trans terminology is not readily applicable to these asymmetric double bonds, this configuration is designated Z (as opposed to E).[7] The naturally occurring geometric isomer is thus bilirubin IXα (Z-Z). X-ray diffraction studies also indicate that bilirubin IXα (Z-Z) is not a "linear" tetrapyrrole as typically illustrated in Figure 1 (top panel). Rather, it has an involuted structure both in the solid state[7] and in solution, at least in nonpolar solvents[8] in which the propionic acid groups are linked by intramolecular hydrogen bonds to the nitrogens and oxygen of the opposite pyrrole rings (Fig. 1, bottom panel). Since this hydrogen bonding shields the polar sites that could otherwise interact with polar solvents, bilirubin IXα (Z-Z) is virtually water insoluble (approximately 0.1 μmole/liter at pH 7.4[9]). Disruption of these hydrogen bonds by alkaline solution exposes hydrophilic sites that greatly increase the solubility of bilirubin IXα in polar solvents. Esterification of the propionic acid groups with glucuronic acid apparently also prevents hydrogen bond formation. This raises the possibility that the absence of intramolecular hydrogen bonding, rather than glucuronide conjugation per se, facilitates the reaction of bilirubin with diazo reagent; i.e., accounts for the direct van den Bergh reaction.[6] This is supported by the observation that reaction of bilirubin with diazo reagent is also facilitated by methanol, ethanol, or 5 M urea, agents that are known to disrupt hydrogen and/or hydrophobic bonds.

Intramolecular hydrogen bonding occurs most readily when the two propionic acid groups are located on the central pyrrole rings, as in bilirubin IXα. Mammalian bile also contains trace amounts of the β, γ, and δ structural isomers.[10,11] These are formed by heme cleavage at the β, γ, or δ carbon bridges, respectively, and the sequence of propionic acid and other side groups on the pyrrole rings is different from that of bilirubin IXα. Since intramolecular hydrogen bonding is presumably altered or absent in these non-α isomers, they are more water soluble than bilirubin IXα and are excreted into rat bile largely in unconjugated form.[10] Bilirubin IXα (Z-Z) may, in part, undergo photoisomerization to its E-Z, Z-E, and/or E-E geometric isomers during phototherapy.[12-14] Formation of these geometric isomers, which are probably unable to form intramolecular hydrogen bonds, may account for the increased biliary excretion of unconjugated bilirubin IXα in Gunn rats[13,15] and jaundiced neonates[16] during phototherapy. These observations have important implications regarding the hepatic excretory mechanisms for organic anions, as discussed later under "Biliary Excretion."

SOURCES AND FORMATION OF BILIRUBIN

In adults the daily production of bilirubin as measured by turnover studies with radiolabeled bilirubin[17] or by endogenous carbon monoxide (CO) production[18] averages 250–350 mg or 3.8 ± 0.6 (± SE) mg/kg. Whereas CO production reflects total body heme degradation, plasma turnover studies measure only the bilirubin fraction that enters plasma prior to excretion and thus yield values for bilirubin production that are slightly lower than those calculated from CO production.[19,20]

The heme moiety of hemoglobin accounts for approximately 70% of the bilirubin excreted in humans. All mammalian cells contain heme in the form of hemoproteins (e.g., cytochromes). With the notable exception of the liver, however, the tissue concentrations of these hemoproteins are so low, or their turnover rates so slow (e.g., myoglobin), that their overall contribution to bilirubin production is insignificant. Studies using the heme precursor glycine, isotopically labeled, show that production of the "early labeled bilirubin" (ELB) fraction begins within minutes of administration of the labeled precursor, reaches a peak within 1 to 3 hr, and then declines asymptotically over a period of several days.[21] The existence of two or more ELB components has been demonstrated using isotopically labeled δ-aminolevulinic acid (δ-ALA), which is preferentially incorporated into the heme of liver cells rather than into maturing erythroid cells in bone marrow.[22-24] The initial component, as well as most of the second component, appears to be derived predominantly from hepatic heme sources. Breakdown of hemoglobin heme resulting from the premature destruction of newly formed erythrocytes, either in the marrow or following their release into the circulation, constitutes a smaller portion of the second component. The hepatic contribution to total bilirubin production in normal man was initially estimated to be 10% to 20%,[25] but recent estimates tend to be higher, ranging from 23% to 37%.[20,26,27] Although the initial ELB component itself may consist of several distinct phases, these have not yet been assigned to specific hepatic heme or hemoprotein compounds. The major contribution could be expected from cytochrome P-450, since this hemoprotein incorporates at least 70% of the total heme synthesized in the liver,[28] and treatment with xenobiotics, which accelerate hepatic cytochrome P-450 synthesis, significantly alters the magnitude and shape of the ELB peak.[29,30] Analysis of the early phase of the ELB peak reveals that the liver[31] and developing erythroid cells[32,33] contain a small "free" heme pool that has a turnover rate (60 to 90 min) exceeding that of any known hemoproteins.[34,35] This pool may represent heme, newly synthesized in mitochondria, in transit to the subcellular sites of hemoprotein synthesis.[36]

Enhanced formation of ELB derived from turnover of hepatic heme and hemoproteins has been demonstrated experimentally after partial hepatectomy and following release of bile duct obstruction.[31] The normally small erythropoietic contribution to the later ELB fraction may increase when erythropoiesis is accelerated or abnormal. In fact, 30% to 80% of total fecal bile pigments may originate from the premature destruction of developing or young erythroid cells ("ineffective erythropoiesis") in clinical disorders such as iron deficiency anemia, megaloblastic anemia, sideroblastic anemia, thalassemia minor, congenital erythropoietic porphyria, and lead poisoning.[37,38] A decreased erythropoietic contribution to the ELB peak has been observed in patients with aplastic anemia.[39] Hemolytic disorders cause an earlier and augmented "late-labeled" bilirubin peak.[24]

Senescent erythrocytes are normally sequestered and degraded to hemoglobin in the mononuclear phagocytic cells of the spleen, liver, or bone marrow.[40] However, the heme moiety of methemoglobin, methemalbumin, hemin, heme-hemopexin, free hemoglobin, and haptoglobin-bound hemoglobin resulting from intravascular hemolysis is taken up and catabolized predominantly by hepatic parenchymal cells.[41-44] It is not established whether bilirubin formed in hepatocytes, following the removal of circulating heme, is directly excreted into bile or first refluxes back into the plasma bilirubin pool, as occurs for the initial component of ELB[20,45] or subsequent to infusion of biliverdin.[46]

The heme-cleaving enzyme, microsomal heme oxygenase,[47] exhibits a high degree of substrate specificity, is most active on free heme or heme loosely associated with protein (e.g., methemalbumin), and is most abundant in those tissues normally involved in heme degradation. Activity of the enzyme may be stimulated three- to fivefold by substrate-mediated induction with heme or hemoglobin,[48-50] thus providing an efficient adaptive response to the increased amounts of heme released in hemolytic disorders or internal hemorrhage. Microsomal heme oxygenase has recently been purified to apparent homogeneity from pig spleen[51] and partially purified from rat liver.[52] Despite earlier controversy, the enzyme appears to be distinct from cytochrome P-450 and other terminal oxidases of the microsomal electron-transport system.[51] The activity of heme oxygenase is rate-limiting in the overall conversion of heme to bilirubin and is dependent on molecular O_2 and NADPH, which is regenerated by NADPH-cytochrome c reductase.[53] Cleavage of the protoporphyrin ring requires the presence of a central iron atom,[54] although cobalt protoporphyrin IX is also a substrate for heme oxygenase.[55]

Although some details remain unclear, recent concepts of the heme oxygenase reaction have been developed largely from in vitro model systems[56] and animal studies using$^{18}O_2$ combined with mass spectrometric analysis.[57,58] The heme is postulated to be dissociated from its apoprotein (e.g., globin) and bound to heme oxygenase in the membrane of the endoplasmic reticulum in such a manner that oxidation is prevented at the non-α carbon bridges.[59] The enzyme-bound heme is reduced to its ferrous form by NADPH and then binds a molecule of molecular O_2 activated by the transfer of electrons from the apoprotein. The activated oxygen attacks the α-methene carbon bridge of the heme group, forming α-hydroxyheme, so that heme actually mediates its own destruction. This unstable intermediate reacts spontaneously at the hydroxylated α-bridge with oxygen to produce CO and a biliverdin-iron complex. The latter is hydrolyzed to biliverdin IXα and iron, which is incorporated into ferritin or reutilized for heme synthesis. In birds, amphibia, and most other nonmammalian vertebrates the process of heme degradation terminates at this step and unconjugated biliverdin is excreted in bile.

Why mammals find it necessary to reduce biliverdin to the less polar bilirubin, which requires the complex energy-consuming process of conjugation in order to achieve biliary excretion, remains an enigma. However, a clue may be provided by studies in the guinea pig which indicate that biliverdin, in contrast to bilirubin, is not readily transported across the placenta.[60] Biliverdin is hydrogenated to bilirubin by the NADPH-dependent enzyme biliverdin reductase,[61] which is present in abundance in the cell cytosol and again has a stereochemical preference for the IXα isomer.[62] The total time required in vivo for the chemical transformations involved in the formation of biliverdin, its reduction to bilirubin, and conjugation and excretion of the bilirubin is 1 to 2 min.[46,58]

BILIRUBIN TRANSPORT IN PLASMA

In plasma, unconjugated bilirubin is bound reversibly to albumin at a primary high-affinity site that has been reported to have a binding constant of 3×10^7 M^{-1} at 37°C.[63] Since this site presumably is relatively hydrophobic, bilirubin can be displaced by substances such as ethanol or methanol,[64,65] but not by low concentrations of polar organic anions that also bind to albumin.[66] Fluctuations of pH within the physiologic range also do not significantly influence bilirubin dissociation from this site.[67] At plasma concentrations beyond its molar equivalence with albumin (approximately 600 μmole/liter or 35 mg/dl), bilirubin binds to albumin on at least two low-affinity sites. Bilirubin can be displaced from these secondary sites by other organic anions or by small reductions in pH.[68] Free or unbound bilirubin in plasma has been of great interest, since it is widely presumed that this is the fraction available for transit across cell membranes, such as the blood-brain barrier. Analytical methods for direct determination of the unbound bilirubin fraction in plasma are not available,[69] and most studies have been performed with crystalline human albumin preparations, which may not reflect the binding of bilirubin in hyperbilirubinemic plasma.[70] Using the peroxidase method,[70] the plasma free bilirubin concentration in normal adults has been estimated to be 0.12 nmole/liter, and in neonates the level beyond which kernicterus may occur is about 50 nmole/liter.[69]

Within the physiologic concentration range, long-chain fatty acids are transported bound to albumin without interfering with bilirubin binding. When the concentration of free fatty acids is increased beyond a 4:1 molar ratio with regard to albumin, however, there is a progressive displacement of bilirubin from the primary site to the secondary sites, making it susceptible to subsequent displacement by organic anions. At fatty acid/albumin molar ratios greater than 4:1, direct competition occurs at the secondary sites.[71] Indeed, the elevated levels of plasma free fatty acids reported in breast-fed infants may result in the displacement of bilirubin from albumin in vivo.[72] Numerous compounds can competitively displace bilirubin from its binding site(s) on albumin and increase the risk of kernicterus in jaundiced neonates.[69] The list of drugs includes certain sulfonamides and other antibiotics, analgesics, food additives, diuretics, and x-ray contrast media for cholangiography.

The affinity of conjugated bilirubin for albumin in plasma appears to be somewhat less than that of the unconjugated pigment.[73] This is consistent with the observation that non-protein-bound conjugated bilirubin (which comprises less than 1% of plasma conjugated bilirubin in conjugated hyperbilirubinemia), is freely filtered by the glomeruli,[74] whereas unconjugated bilirubin is presumably filtered to a lesser extent or not at all. Most of this filtered conjugated bilirubin is reabsorbed by the renal tubules,[75] so that the bilirubinuria noted in cholestatic and hepatocellular jaundice represents the residual nonreabsorbed bilirubin fraction.

HEPATIC UPTAKE

The hepatic uptake of tightly protein-bound molecules such as bilirubin, BSP, and ICG presents physiologists with the following dilemma. The very high association constant between bilirubin and albumin implies that any individual bilirubin molecule, even if transiently dissociated from albumin, is unlikely to have enough time for free diffusion to travel to and across a cell membrane before binding to another albumin molecule.[64] Nonetheless, hepatocytes extract bilirubin from sinusoidal blood separately from albumin.[76-78] The peculiar anatomy of the hepatic microcirculation provides a clue to the mechanism by which this may occur; namely, fenestrations exist in the sinusoidal lining cells that are large enough to permit plasma proteins free access to the space of Disse and presumably direct contact with the hepatocyte membrane.[79] This serves to minimize the diffusion distance required of a dissociated bilirubin molecule and may even permit direct transfer of substances such as bilirubin from plasma proteins to membrane binding sites. The presence of these large fenestrations and the absence of a basement membrane between plasma and the sinusoidal surface of the hepatocyte[80] also offer a unique advantage to hepatic physiologists in that they allow direct study of transport phenomena across the sinusoidal membrane in vivo.[81]

Studies using the multiple indicator dilution technique or simple analysis of initial plasma disappearance rates (both techniques being subject to certain limitations in interpretation[82]) indicate that hepatic uptake of bilirubin and other organic anions shows the following characteristic features of carrier-mediated transport:[83,84] (1) Saturation: the hepatic uptake of bilirubin,[85-87] ICG,[85,88,89] and BSP[83,85,90,91] are saturable processes. (2) Competitive inhibition: bilirubin, ICG, and BSP show relatively selective, mutually competitive inhibition of uptake;[85] hepatic uptake of conjugated bilirubin is also inhibited by unconjugated bilirubin.[92] (3) Countertransport: i.e., reflux from liver to plasma against the apparent prevailing concentration gradient;[83,84] this phenomenon has been demonstrated for bilirubin, ICG,[85] and BSP.[85,93] (4) Accelerated hepatic uptake if the liver is preloaded with substrate: this has been demonstrated for bilirubin[85,87] and is analogous to the "preloading effect"[94] or "accelerative exchange diffusion,"[84] both of which were described in transport work in isolated cell systems.[84,95] These findings constitute sufficient evidence[84] to characterize the hepatic uptake mechanism as carrier-mediated, rather than simple diffusion, and indicate that several organic anions, including unconjugated and conjugated bilirubin, BSP, and ICG, share the same transport system(s). This carrier system appears to be generally distinct from that of bile acids,[85,86,89,96] although bile acids may compete with hepatic BSP uptake in dogs.[97] Preliminary evidence also suggests that unlike the carrier system for bile acids,[98] it is not sodium-dependent.[99] In addition, proteins capable of binding bilirubin and other organic anions have been isolated from liver plasma membrane preparations, and preliminary characterization of these proteins has been reported.[100,101] Together, these studies suggest that bilirubin is "stripped" from albumin in the space of Disse by binding proteins located on the cell membrane. Once bound to these "carriers," bilirubin is translocated to the interior surface of the cell membrane. Since continuous flow of albumin-bilirubin complexes past free, stationary membrane binding sites creates a nonequilibrium situation, uptake of bilirubin (and other organic anions) could occur even if the affinity of bilirubin for albumin exceeds that for the putative membrane carrier. Thus the rate of unidirectional flux into the hepatocyte of bilirubin and other organic anions depends on their plasma concentration as well as on the plasma concentration of potential inhibitors, the availability of membrane carriers, the affinity of these carriers for substrate and competitor relative to that of albumin, and the rate at which bilirubin bound to carrier or the free carrier translocates from one side of the membrane to the other. Net uptake reflects influx minus efflux, and the latter is dependent on the intrinsic capacity of the membrane transport system as well as on the subsequent intracellular fate of the bilirubin molecule as outlined below.

Once inside the liver cell, the hydrophobic bilirubin molecule, which by itself is poorly water soluble, binds to one of two cytoplasmic protein fractions designated Y protein, or ligandin, and Z protein[102] (see Chapter 11). Ligandin, which constitutes 5% of cytoplasmic protein in rat liver and is found to a lesser extent in kidney and intestine,[103] has a molecular weight of 46,000 daltons and a greater affinity but lesser capacity for bilirubin than Z protein. As its name would indicate, ligandin was originally considered important because of its ability to bind a variety of compounds, including steroids and aminoazo dyes as well as organic anions.[104] Ligandin is one of a family of glutathione S-transferases, enzymes that catalyze the conjugation of glutathione with many different electrophilic substrates.[105] Each of the five rat[106] and five human[107] glutathione S-transferases purified can bind bilirubin. Ligandin, or glutathione S-transferase B, thus binds organic anions that are (e.g., BSP) or are not (e.g., bilirubin, ICG) substrates, as well as substrates that are not organic anions (e.g., iodomethane).[105] It consists of two nonidentical monomeric subunits that may be responsible for different catalytic and binding functions.[108] Z protein,[102] which is probably identical with aminoazo-dye-binding protein A and fatty acid binding protein,[109] may be principally involved with fatty acid transport, since it has a high affinity for long-chain fatty acids; it is found in intestinal mucosa, myocardium, and other tissues that take up and metabolize fatty acids; and its concentration in rat intestine appears to be regulated by dietary lipid intake.[110]

The association constant between bilirubin and purified rat ligandin has been estimated, using circular dichroism,[111] fluorescence spectroscopy,[112] difference spectrophotometry,[113] and a competitive adsorption technique,[114] to be of the order of 10^6 M^{-1}, which is lower than that for rat albumin.[115] This observation, together with the finding that bilirubin fractionates with albumin rather than with ligandin by gel filtration,[78] has been considered evidence that ligandin is not important in hepatic uptake. By contrast, studies of ligandin in unfractionated rat liver cytosol, using moving boundary sedimentation (which prevents separation of ligandin from smaller cytoplasmic constituents), showed that bilirubin sediments with ligandin rather than albumin and indicated a ligandin-bilirubin association constant of 10^9 M^{-1}, which is greater than that for rat albumin.[115] These findings, which suggest that a cytoplasmic constituent, perhaps glutathione,[116] increases the affinity of ligandin for bilirubin, have been considered experimental support for the importance of ligandin in hepatic bilirubin uptake.[115] Such assessments of the physiologic importance of ligandin with respect to hepatic uptake based on its affinity for bilirubin (and other organic anions) relative to albumin are probably oversimplified in that they are more applicable to a diffusion equilibrium system than the actual situation in vivo, in which bilirubin entering the hepatocyte is continuously being conjugated and excreted. Rather, it is likely that any factor, including accelerated intracellular metabolism and binding to ligandin, that decreases the "effective" concentration of bilirubin inside the hepatocyte and hence its availability for transport back into plasma increases net uptake. Studies using the multiple indicator dilution technique, which allows independent quantitation of influx and efflux, support this hypothesis.[117] Because agents that alter hepatic ligandin levels may also alter the membrane transport system or the rate of intracellular metabolism, attempts to correlate hepatic ligandin content with net uptake rate are more difficult to interpret and have yielded both positive[118,119] and negative[120] results.

Patients with Gilbert's syndrome[121] and Rotor's syndrome[122] have been reported to show a reduced bilirubin storage capacity. Storage capacity, however, as calculated on the basis of tracer kinetic studies[121] or intravenous infusion of bilirubin or BSP,[123] probably reflects several steps in overall hepatic transport and therefore is difficult to translate into physiologic terms at the cellular level. Preliminary evidence suggests that the decreased storage in Gilbert's syndrome is not explainable by reduced hepatic ligandin levels.[124]

Patients with Gilbert's syndrome (Table 1) also have a moderately reduced rate of hepatic bilirubin uptake,[121] and some, but not all, of these patients have a similar reduction in BSP[125] and ICG[126] uptake rates. Since the intrinsic capacity of the uptake system enormously exceeds the normal net transport rate of bilirubin from blood to bile,[85,86] these findings do not necessarily imply that the moderate reduction in uptake rate is the cause of the syndrome. However, these defects in uptake of various organic anions, including ICG, which is not conjugated prior to excretion, suggest that patients with Gilbert's syndrome constitute a heterogeneous population with regard to their defects in organic anion transport, some of which do not appear to be related to impaired conjugation (see "Bilirubin Conjugation"). This heterogeneity is further demonstrated by studies in 5 patients undergoing splenectomy who had both Gilbert's syndrome (as defined by a reduced hepatic bilirubin clearance[127]) and increased bilirubin production as a result of hereditary spherocytosis.[128] Compared with preoperative measurements, hepatic bilirubin clearance increased an average of 75% following splenectomy, and in 2 patients, bilirubin clearance returned completely to normal. This suggests that some undefined step in the overall hepatic transport of bilirubin is more readily saturable in patients with Gilbert's syndrome than in normal subjects. Normal rates of bilirubin production may saturate this step in some patients, while in other patients with "latent" Gilbert's syndrome, decreased bilirubin clearance may be detectable only when bilirubin production is increased.[128]

BILIRUBIN CONJUGATION

A comprehensive review of the analysis and nature of bilirubin conjugates is presented in Chapter 12, Volume V of this series.[129] Bilirubin may be esterified with a variety of carbohydrate moieties on the carboxyl groups of one or both of the propionic acid side chains. Chromatographic separation of the dipyrrolic azo pigments[130] and more recently of the native tetrapyrroles[75,131,132] has shown that bilirubin β-D-diglucuronide constitutes the major pigment fraction in human bile[133,134] and that monoglucuronides represent a smaller fraction. Trace amounts of other conjugates, such as glucosides and xylosides, have been demonstrated also,[133] but these are of minor physiologic significance. Considerable species differences exist in the nature and relative distribution of bilirubin conjugates.[135] In dogs, a complex pattern of many different conjugates, mostly acyl glycosides, has been identified, including heterogeneous conjugates containing two different carbohydrate moieties.[136]

Esterification of the propionic acid side chains of bilirubin with glucuronic acid results in the formation of 1-o-acylglucuronides, which are present in vivo and in freshly collected bile. With storage of bile in vitro and presumably also with cholestasis, chromatographic separation of the azo pigments consistently reveals additional pigment bands.[133,137] These bands result from isomerization to non-C-1-glucuronides by sequential migration of the bilirubin acyl group from position 1 to positions 2, 3, and 4 of the glucuronic acid (forming 2-,3- and 4-o-acylglucuronides), and this acyl "shift" is accelerated at alkaline pH.[137] This intramolecular rearrangement may account for some of the complex bilirubin conjugates (e.g., aldobiouronides) previously isolated in small amounts from pooled human T-tube bile[138] and may complicate the interpretation of reported bile pigment studies based solely on the azo pigment analysis of stored bile samples.

Bilirubin monoglucuronide formation is mediated by uridine diphosphate glucuronate glucuronyl transferase (UDP-glucuronyl transferase) in the membranes of smooth and rough endoplasmic reticulum. Although the liver contains several glucuronyl transferases with overlapping substrate specificities for a variety of endogenous compounds and xenobiotics,[139,140] a specific conjugating form(s) of the enzyme exists that transfers the glucuronyl group from the cosubstrate UDP-glucuronic acid to bilirubin. Despite extensive study,[129,140] purification and characterization of this enzyme, like that of many other membrane-associated enzymes, has been only partially successful.[141,142] The in vitro activity of hepatic microsomal preparations may be enhanced or "activated" by agents such as detergents which alter the interaction between glucuronyl transferase and its membrane phospholipid environment. Indeed, digitonin is still widely utilized to activate microsomes and facilitate the measurement of glucuronyl transferase activity in vitro.[143] Such treatment influences the kinetics of the enzyme and raises doubt about the physiologic significance of glucuronyl transferase activity measured by this technique. Compared with normals, glucuronyl transferase activity by this assay is greatly decreased in Gilbert's syndrome,[144-146] is similarly decreased or absent in type II congenital nonhemolytic jaundice,[147-149] and is absent in type I congenital nonhemolytic jaundice[150,151] (Table 1). Since the mean plasma bilirubin concentration can be correlated with the mean glucuronyl transferase activity in groups of patients with these disorders,[152] it is tempting to ascribe the hyperbilirubinemia to the apparent enzyme deficiency. There is no correlation, however, between enzyme activity and bilirubin concentration within an individual group (e.g., Gilbert's syndrome).[144] Moreover, phenobarbital lowers bilirubin concentration in patients with Gilbert's syndrome[153,154] and type II congenital nonhemolytic jaundice[148-150] without an associated increase in glucuronyl transferase activity. Finally, decreased glucuronyl transferase activity is found in patients with a variety of acquired liver diseases, including Wilson's disease,[144] end-stage cirrhosis,[129] chronic persistent hepatitis,[155] noncirrhotic portal fibrosis,[156] portal vein thrombosis,[156] and granulomatous liver disease;[156] but some of these patients have no associated hyperbilirubinemia.[156] Thus, diminished glucuronyl transferase activity, at least as measured in vitro by the standard digitonin activation assay,[143] does not in itself satisfactorily explain the unconjugated hyperbilirubinemia found in these hereditary and acquired hepatic disorders. The factors controlling glucuronyl transferase activity in vivo are also unclear. For example, a twofold increase in activity is reported in patients with sickle cell disease and has been attributed to substrate (i.e., bilirubin) induction,[157] but such substrate induction apparently does not occur in patients with other types of hemolysis.[158]

The conversion of mono- to diglucuronide may not be catalyzed by microsomal glucuronyl transferase but by an enzyme system with a different pH optimum[159] and intracellular location.[160] This is consistent with the fact that the in vitro assay of glucuronyl transferase in rat liver measures exclusively formation of monoglucuronide, not diglucuronide[143] (this may not be true in man[135]), as well as with the observation that mono-, not diglucuronide, is normally found in the liver cell.[161] This latter finding supports the postulate[162] that conversion of mono- to diglucuronide is catalyzed by an enzyme located on the liver plasma membrane, and there is, in fact, a precedent for what thus might be a linked conjugation-transport process.[163] The observation that monoglucuronide is increased in the bile of patients with Gilbert's syndrome[164,165] and constitutes the predominant pigment in patients with type I and type II Crigler-Najjar syndrome[148,149,164] further suggests that the putative enzyme defects in these syndromes require reevaluation.

In the postulated transglucuronidation mechanism,[162] the glucuronic acid moiety of one bilirubin monoglucuronide molecule is transferred to another monoglucuronide, resulting in the equimolar formation of diglucuronide and unconjugated bilirubin; the metabolic fate of the latter remains undetermined. Both technical and conceptual questions have been raised with regard to this hypothesis,[6] including the apparent metabolic inefficiency of this postulated mechanism, which necessitates deconjugation of one-half of the monoglucuronide formed in order to produce diglucuronide. In addition, studies in intact rats infused with bilirubin monoglucuronide, isotopically labeled in the glucuronyl group, indicate that transglucuronidation is not responsible for the in vivo formation of bilirubin diglucuronide.[166] Further study is necessary to resolve these apparent ambiguities and clarify the mechanism and site of conversion of bilirubin monoglucuronide to diglucuronide in the liver cell.

BILIARY EXCRETION

The hepatic excretory mechanism for bilirubin and other organic anions has proved difficult to study. Unlike the case of sinusoidal uptake, examination of events occurring in plasma provides only indirect information about transport across the canalicular membrane, as "viewed" through the interposed steps of sinusoidal membrane transport and intracellular metabolism. Moreover, since canalicular bile cannot be sampled, neither electrical potential differences nor unidirectional solute flux rates across the canalicular membrane are known.

Nonetheless, important inferences can be drawn from the available information. First, virtually every organic anion studied, including bilirubin, has a definite maximum hepatic excretory rate or T_m. Since the observed T_m is less than the maximal uptake capacity for each of these anions,[82] even in the non-preloaded state, and since infusion rates greater than the T_m result in reflux of conjugated pigment into plasma,[167] these findings suggest that transport across the canalicular membrane is a saturable process that may be rate-limiting in the overall transport of bilirubin and other organic anions from blood to bile. Intrahepatic BSP concentration increases nonlinearly with increasing rates of BSP excretion, also suggesting a saturable process.[168] Second, various organic anions compete for excretion.[169,170] Together, these properties of saturation and competition suggest that canalicular excretion, like sinusoidal uptake, is a carrier-mediated process. There is also limited evidence that more than one carrier may be involved in the transport of various organic anions.[171,172]

Normal human bile contains only a small amount of unconjugated bilirubin (1.2% of total bilirubin in gallbladder bile), and this appears to be secreted rather than resulting from hydrolysis of conjugated bilirubin by β-glucuronidase.[173] The conjugating moiety, per se, may allow bilirubin to "fit" with a specific carrier. Alternatively, it is possible that conjugation may serve simply to disrupt the internal hydrogen bonding responsible for the hydrophobic properties of unconjugated bilirubin IXα, thereby allowing transport by a carrier system(s) showing broad specificity for a variety of hydrophilic anions.[6,174] Several observations support this latter hypothesis. First, unlike bilirubin, many hydrophilic organic anions are excreted into bile only partially conjugated (e.g., BSP) or in unconjugated form (ICG, rose bengal, and i-urobilin). Second, the unconjugated bilirubin isomers β, γ, and δ,[10,175] mixtures of biliverdin structural isomers,[176,177] and purified biliverdin IXα (J. L. Gollan, unpublished observations), also are excreted largely in unconjugated form. This hypothesis may also explain why phototherapy results in hepatic excretion of unconjugated bilirubin and reduction of plasma bilirubin concentration; namely, photoisomerization, like conjugation, appears to disrupt the internal hydrogen bonds of bilirubin IXα (Z-Z), thereby making it more suitable for secretion via the organic anion carrier system(s).[12-14,178]

Studies in mutant Corriedale sheep, an animal model that shows many features of the Dubin-Johnson syndrome, suggest that organic anions including bilirubin and bile acids are excreted via functionally distinct pathways.[179] This is consistent with the observation that the organic anions ICG and probenecid do not compete with bile acids for binding to bile acid receptors in isolated liver surface membranes enriched in bile canaliculi, although BSP did show some competition.[180] Despite this apparent functional separation between bile acid and organic anion excretion, bile acid infusion increased the T_m for bilirubin,[181] BSP,[182-184] ICG,[185] and iopanoic acid,[186] whereas substances that increase canalicular bile flow but not bile salt output did not increase T_m for most organic anions studied.[184,186,187] Infusion of bile acids has been postulated to saturate the capacity of periportal hepatocytes to extract bile acids from incoming sinusoidal blood, thereby leading to increased delivery of bile acids to centrolobular cells.[181,188] The resultant increase in bile acid secretion by centrolobular hepatocytes is further postulated to increase the capacity of these cells to excrete organic anions, causing an overall increase in T_m. This concept of functional separation of hepatocytes at opposite poles of the canaliculus has direct experimental support[189-191] and provides an appealing framework in which to visualize a link between bile acid and organic anion excretion, although it does not in itself explain the link. One possibility is that bile acids directly stimulate organic anion excretion or that the two membrane carrier systems are in some way coupled.[82,184,187] The observations that bile acid infusion (1) alters the appearance of bile canalicular membranes by scanning electron microscopy,[192,193] (2) alters bile canalicular membrane lipid composition and the activity of associated enzymes,[193] and (3) decreases the K_m (as defined by standard transport kinetics) for BSP excretion[168] are all consistent with a direct membrane effect. Another possibility is that bilirubin and other organic anions show a physicochemical association with bile salts and/or mixed micelles. Such an association might decrease the effective concentration of bilirubin in bile, thereby decreasing its availability for back diffusion across the canalicular membrane and thus increasing its net excretion.[82,181,185,187,188,194-196] Alternatively, if mixed micelles are formed within the hepatocyte or its organelles and excreted intact, physical association between organic anions and mixed micelles might actually increase the unidirectional efflux rate of organic anions. Although the functional importance of micellar sequestration has yet to be established, this general hypothesis is supported by ultracentrifugation and gel chromatography studies of normal bile or synthetic solutions, which indicate a physical association between BSP and taurocholate[195] and between bilirubin and mixed micelles or some other macromolecular complex in bile.[197-200] Quantitative studies established that compounds concentratively excreted in bile, including bilirubin and other organic anions for which T_m is increased by bile acid infusion, are associated with biliary mixed micelles.[201] In addition to their association with mixed micelles, these organic anions form self-aggregates, so that only a small percentage of these solutes (range, 0% to 5%) are present in bile in molecular form or as low-molecular-weight complexes.[201] These studies support the concept that physical association between organic anions and mixed micelles explains the observed link in their rates of excretion.

The question of whether the excretory mechanism is actively concentrative or merely equilibrative is also unresolved. Estimates of the bilirubin and BSP concentration ratios between bile and liver homogenate have ranged from 30:1 to 50:1.[87,170,202] With the reservation that measurement of whole liver homogenate ignores possible intracellular compartmentation,[20] these findings have been taken as evidence that a steep concentration gradient exists across the canalicular membrane.[83,182,203-205] Since binding to intracellular proteins presumably reduces the effective intracellular concentration and increases further the apparent concentration gradient, it is widely presumed that the excretory mechanism for organic anions is intrinsically concentrative, i.e., active and energy requiring.[83,182,203-205] Physical association of these anions with mixed micelles and other aggregates[201] serves to reduce their free concentration, however. The effective concentration of these substances in bile thus may equal that inside the hepatocyte and explain the apparent concentration gradient, without invoking an intrinsically concentrative transport process.

Dubin-Johnson syndrome and Rotor's syndrome are both characterized by conjugated hyperbilirubinemia that results from defective excretion of conjugated bilirubin and other organic anions, including BSP. Studies in Dubin-Johnson syndrome patients[206] and mutant Corriedale sheep[172] indicate that the excretion of unconjugated BSP is minimally impaired, while conjugated BSP excretion is profoundly depressed. In addition, these patients show a striking and diagnostic increase in urinary excretion of coproporphyrin isomer type I, whereas total urinary excretion of coproporphyrins is normal.[207-209] These findings suggest that Dubin-Johnson syndrome results from a genetically defective canalicular transport system for organic anions and perhaps specifically from a defect in the particular carrier system for conjugated bilirubin and BSP.[172] The relationship of this defect to the observed abnormalities in coproporphyrin excretion is unclear. However, the findings of normal uroporphyrinogen III cosynthetase activities in erythrocytes and liver of patients with the Dubin-Johnson syndrome suggest that the altered urinary coproporphyrin excretion is related to the hepatic excretory defect rather than to an abnormality in the relative production rates of porphyrinogen isomers I and III.[210] The existence of Rotor's syndrome as an entity distinct from the Dubin-Johnson syndrome[211] was established by the finding that patients with Rotor's syndrome show increased total urinary excretion of coproporphyrins as well as a relative increase in type I isomer, but a lesser increase than that seen in Dubin-Johnson syndrome.[212] This is a nonspecific pattern observed in many cholestatic disorders[212] and may therefore reflect impaired hepatic porphyrin excretion.

REFERENCES

1. Berk PD, Howe RB, Berlin NI: Disorders of bilirubin metabolism. Edited by PK Bondy and LE Rosenberg: Duncan's Diseases of Metabolism. Philadelphia, WB Saunders, 1974, pp 825–880

2. Berk PD, Wolkoff AW, Berlin NI: Inborn errors of bilirubin metabolism. Med Clin N Am 59:803–816, 1975

3. Billing BH: Bilirubin metabolism. Edited by L. Schiff: Diseases of the Liver (ed 4). Philadelphia, JB Lippincott, 1975, pp 287–313

4. Schmid R, McDonagh AF: Hyperbilirubinemia. Edited by JB Stanbury, JB Wyngaarden, and DS Fredrickson: The Metabolic Basis of Inherited Disease. New York, McGraw-Hill, 1978, pp 1221-1257

5. Fischer H, Plieninger H: Synthese des biliverdins (uteroverdins) and bilirubins, der biliverdine XIIIα and IIIα sowie der vinylneoxanthosäure. Hoppe Seylers Z Physiol Chem 274: 231-260, 1942

6. Schmid R: Bilirubin metabolism: State of the art. Gastroenterology, 74:1307–1312, 1978

7. Bonnett R, Davies JE, Hursthouse MB: Structure of bilirubin. Nature 262: 326–328, 1976

8. Manitto P, Monti D: Free-energy barrier of conformational inversion in bilirubin. JCS Chem Comm: 122-123, 1976

9. Brodersen R, Theilgaard J: Bilirubin colloid formation in neutral aqueous solution. Scand J Clin Lab Invest 24:395–398, 1969

10. Blanckaert N, Heirwegh KPM, Zaman Z: Comparison of the biliary excretion of the four isomers of bilirubin IX in Wistar and homozygous Gunn rats. Biochem J 164:229–236, 1977

11. Blumenthal SG, Taggart DB, Ikeda RM, Ruebner BH, Bergstrom DE: Conjugated and unconjugated bilirubins in bile of humans and rhesus monkeys. Structure of adult human and rhesus monkey bilirubins compared with dog bilirubins. Biochem J 167:535–548, 1977

12. McDonagh AF: Photochemistry and photometabolism of bilirubin IXα. Edited by D Bergsma and SH Blondheim: Bilirubin Metabolism in the Newborn. Vol. 11. New York, American Elsevier, 1976, pp 30–40

13. Zenone EA, Stoll MS, Ostrow JD: Mechanism of excretion of unconjugated bilirubin (UCB) during phototherapy. Gastroenterology 72: A-157/1180, 1977

14. Lightner DH: The photoreactivity of bili-

rubin and related pyrroles. Photochem Photobiol 26:427–436, 1977

15. Ostrow JD: Photocatabolism of labeled bilirubin in the congenitally jaundiced (Gunn) rat. J Clin Invest 50:707–718,1971

16. Lundh HT, Jacobsen J: Influence of phototherapy on unconjugated bilirubin in duodenal bile of newborn infants with hyperbilirubinemia. Acta Paediatr Scand 61:693–696, 1972

17. Berk PD, Howe RB, Bloomer JR, Berlin NI: Studies of bilirubin kinetics in normal adults. J Clin Invest 48:2176–2190, 1969

18. Landaw SA: Carbon monoxide production as a measurement of heme catabolism. Edited by CA Goresky and MM Fisher: Jaundice. New York, Plenum Press, 1975, pp 103–127

19. Berk PD, Rodkey FL, Blaschke TF, Collison HA, Waggoner JG: Comparison of plasma bilirubin turnover and carbon monoxide production in man. J Lab Clin Med 83:29–37, 1974

20. Kirshenbaum G, Shames DM, Schmid R: An expanded model of bilirubin kinetics: Effect of feeding, fasting, and phenobarbital in Gilbert's syndrome. J Pharmacokinet Biopharm 4:115–155, 1976

21. Robinson SH: Origins of the early-labeled peak. Edited by PD Berk and NI Berlin: Chemistry and Physiology of Bile Pigments. DHEW No (NIH) 77-1100. Washington, DC, US Government Printing Office, 1977, pp 175–188

22. Yamamoto T, Skanderberg J, Zipursky A, Israels LG: the early appearing bilirubin: Evidence for two components. J Clin Invest 44:31–41,1965

23. Robinson SH, Lester R, Crigler JF, Tsong M: Early-labeled peak of bile pigment in man. Studies with glycine-^{14}C and δ-aminolevulinic acid-^{3}H. N Engl J Med 277:1323–1329, 1967

24. Robinson SH: Formation of bilirubin from erythroid and nonerythroid sources. Semin Hematol 9:45–53, 1972

25. Robinson SH: The origins of bilirubin. N Engl J Med 279:143–149, 1968

26. Jones EA, Shrager R, Bloomer JR, Berk PD, Howe RB, Berlin NI: Quantitative studies of the delivery of hepatic-synthesized bilirubin to plasma utilizing δ-aminolevulinic acid-4-^{14}C and bilirubin-^{3}H in man. J Clin Invest 51:2450–2458, 1972

27. Berk PD, Blaschke TF, Scharschmidt BF, Waggoner JG, Berlin NI: A new approach to quantitation of the various sources of

bilirubin in man. J Lab Clin Med 87:767–780, 1976

28. Marver HS, Schmid R: The porphyrias. Edited by JB Stanbury, JB Wyngaarden and DS Fredrickson: The Metabolic Basis of Inherited Disease. New York, McGraw-Hill, 1972, pp 1087–1140

29. Schmid R, Marver HS, Hammaker L: Enhanced formation of rapidly labeled bilirubin by phenobarbital: Hepatic microsomal cytochromes as a possible source. Biochem Biophys Res Commun 24:319–328, 1966

30. Robinson SH, Tsong M, Brown BW, Schmid R: Sources of bile pigment in rat: Studies of "early-labeled" fraction. J Clin Invest 45:1569–1586, 1966

31. Levitt M, Schacter BA, Zipursky A, Israels LG: The nonerythropoietic component of early bilirubin. J Clin Invest 47:1281–1294, 1968

32. Yannoni CZ, Robinson SH: Early-labelled haem in erythroid and hepatic cells. Nature 258:330-331, 1975

33. Yannoni CZ, Robinson SH: Early labeled heme synthesis in normal rats and rats with iron deficiency anemia. Biochim Biophys Acta 428:533–549, 1976

34. Bissell DM, Hammaker LE: Cytochrome P-450 heme and the regulation of δ-aminolevulinic acid synthetase in the liver. Arch Biochem Biophys 176:103–112, 1976

35. Bissell DM, Hammaker LE: Effect of endotoxin in tryptophan pyrrolase and δ-aminolaevulinate synthetase: Evidence for an endogenous regulatory haem fraction in rat liver. Biochem J 166:301–304, 1977

36. Schmid R: Synthesis and degradation of microsomal hemoproteins. Drug Metab Dispos 1:256–258, 1973

37. Robinson SH, Tsong M: Hemolysis of "stress" reticulocytes: a source of erythropoietic bilirubin formation. J Clin Invest 49:1025–1034, 1970

38. Ostrow JD: Bilirubin and jaundice. Edited by FF Becker: The Liver. Normal and Abnormal Functions. New York, Marcel Dekker, 1974, pp 303–369

39. Barrett PVD, Cline MJ, Berlin NI: The association of the urobilin "early peak" and erythropoiesis in man. J Clin Invest 45:1657–1665, 1966

40. Harris JW, Kellermeyer RW: The Red Cell. Production; Metabolism; Destruction: Normal and Abnormal. Cambridge, Harvard University Press, 1970

41. Bissell DM, Hammaker L, Schmid R: Hemoglobin and erythrocyte catabolism in

rat liver: the separate roles of parenchymal and sinusoidal cells. Blood 40:812–822, 1972

42. Hershko C, Cook JD, Finch CA: Storage iron kinetics. II. The uptake of hemoglobin iron by hepatic parenchymal cells. J Lab Clin Med 80:624–634, 1972

43. Muller-Eberhard U, Liem HH: Hemopexin, the heme-binding serum β-glycoprotein. Edited by AC Allison: Structure and Function of Plasma Proteins. Vol. 1. London, Plenum Press, 1974, pp 35–53

44. Bissell DM: Formation and elimination of bilirubin. Gastroenterology 69:519–538, 1975

45. Bergan A, Östrem T, Gjelstad N: Conjugation of non-erythroid bilirubin in chronic experimental cholestasis in the dog. Scand J Gastroenterol 10:565–569, 1973

46. Gollan JL, McDonagh AF, Schmid R: Biliverdin IXα: A new probe of hepatic bilirubin metabolism. Gastroenterology 72:A-163/1186, 1977

47. Tenhunen R, Marver HS, Schmid R: The enzymatic conversion of heme to bilirubin by microsomal heme oxygenase. Proc Natl Acad Sci USA 61: 748–755, 1968

48. Tenhunen R, Marver HS, Schmid RG The enzymatic catabolism of hemoglobin: Stimulation of microsomal heme oxygenase by hemin. J Lab Clin Med 75:410–421, 1970

49. Pimstone NR, Engel P, Tenhunen R, Seitz P, Marver HS, Schmid R: Inducible heme oxygenase in the kidney: A model for the homeostatic control of hemoglobin catabolism. J Clin Invest 50:2042–2050, 1971

50. Gemsa D, Woo CH, Fudenberg HH, Schmid R: Erythrocyte catabolism by macrophages in vitro: The effect of hydrocortisone on erythrophagocytosis and on the induction of heme oxygenase. J Clin Invest 52:812–822, 1973

51. Yoshida T, Kikuchi G: Heme oxygenase purified to apparent homogeneity from pig spleen microsomes. J Biochem 81:265–268, 1977

52. Maines MD, Ibrahim NG, Kappas A: Solubilization and partial purification of heme oxygenase from rat liver. J Biol Chem 252:5900–5903, 1977

53. Tenhunen R, Marver HS, Schmid R: Microsomal heme oxygenase. Characterization of the enzyme. J Biol Chem 244:6388–6394, 1969

54. Brown SB, Grundy MS: The role of iron in haem degradation. Biochem Soc Trans 5:1017–1920, 1977

55. Maines MD, Kappas A: Enzymatic oxidation of cobalt protoporphyrin IX: Observations on the mechanism of heme oxygenase action. Biochemistry 16:419–423, 1977

56. Schmid R, McDonagh AF: The enzymatic formation of bilirubin. Ann NY Acad Sci 244:533–552, 1975

57. Brown SB, King RF: An [18]O double-labelling study of haemoglobin catabolism in the rat. Biochem J 150:565–567, 1975

58. Brown SB, King RF: The mechanism of haem catabolism. Bilirubin formation in living rats by [18O] oxygen labelling. Biochem J 170:297–311, 1978

59. Brown SB: Stereospecific haem cleavage. A model for the formation of bile-pigment isomers in vivo and in vitro. Biochem J 159:23-27, 1976

60. Palma L, McDonagh AF, Schmid R: Why mammals reduce biliverdin. Gastroenterology 73:A-40/1238, 1977

61. Tenhunen R, Ross ME, Marver HS, Schmid R: Reduced nicotinamide-adenine dinucleotide phosphate dependent biliverdin reductase: Partial purification and characterization. Biochemistry 9:298–303, 1970

62. Colleran E, O'Carra P: Enzymology and comparative physiology of biliverdin reduction. Edited by PD Berk and NI Berlin: Chemistry and Physiology of Bile Pigments. Washington DC, US Government Printing Office, 1977, pp 69–80

63. Jacobsen J: Binding of bilirubin to human serum albumin. Determination of the dissociation constants. FEBS Lett 5:112–114, 1969

64. Plotz PH, Berk PD, Scharschmidt BF, Gordon JK, Vergalla J: Removing substances from blood by affinity chromatography. I. Removing bilirubin and other albumin-bound substances from plasma and blood with albumin-conjugated agarose beads. J Clin Invest 53:778–785, 1974

65. Scharschmidt BF, Plotz PH, Berk PD, Waggoner JG, Vergalla J: Removing substances from blood by affinity chromatography. II. Removing bilirubin from the blood of jaundiced rats by hemoperfusion over albumin-conjugated agarose beads. J Clin Invest 53:786–795, 1974

66. Odell GB: The distribution of bilirubin between albumin and mitochondria. J Pediatr 68:164–180, 1966

67. Odell GB: Influence of pH on the distribution of bilirubin between albumin and mitochondria. Proc Soc Exp Biol Med 120:352–354, 1965

68. Nelson J, Jacobsen J, Wennberg RP: Effect

of pH on the interaction of bilirubin with albumin and tissue culture cells. Pediatr Res 8:963–967, 1974

69. Brodersen R: Prevention of kernicterus, based on recent progress in bilirubin chemistry. Acta Paediatr Scand 66:625–634, 1977

70. Jacobsen J, Wennberg RP: Determination of unbound bilirubin in the serum of newborns. Clin Chem 20:783–789, 1974

71. Odell GB, Cukier JO, Ostrea EM, Maglalang AC, Poland RL: The influence of fatty acids on the binding of bilirubin to albumin. J Lab Clin Med 89:295–307, 1977

72. Yong F-C, Cheah S-S: Breast milk jaundice: An in vitro study of the effect of free fatty acids on the bilirubin-serum albumin complex. Res Commun Chem Pathol Pharmacol 17:679–688, 1977

73. Jacobsen J: Dimerisation of bilirubin diglucuronide and formation of a complex of bilirubin and the diglucuronide. Scand J Clin Lab Invest 26:395–398, 1970

74. Fulop M, Sandson J, Brazeau P: Dialyzability, protein binding and renal excretion of plasma conjugated bilirubin. J Clin Invest 44:666–680, 1965

75. Gollan JL, Dallinger KJ, Billing BH: Excretion of conjugated bilirubin in the isolated perfused kidney. Clin Sci Mol Med 54:381–389, 1978

76. Bernstein LH, Ben-Ezzer J, Gartner L, Arias IM: Hepatic intracellular distribution of tritium-labeled unconjugated and conjugated bilirubin in normal and Gunn rats. J Clin Invest 45:1194–1201, 1966

77. Goresky CA: Bilirubin and sulfobromophthalein uptake by liver. Gastroenterology 60:194, 1971

78. Bloomer JR, Berk PD, Vergalla J, Berlin NI: Influence of albumin on the hepatic uptake of unconjugated bilirubin. Clin Sci Mol Med 45:505–516, 1973

79. Motta P: A scanning electron microscopic study of the rat liver sinusoid: Endothelial and Kupffer cells. Cell Tissue Res 164:371–385, 1975

80. Vracko R: Basal lamina scaffold — anatomy and significance for maintenance of orderly tissue structure. Am J Pathol 77:314–346, 1974

81. Goresky CA: Hepatic membrane carrier transport processes: Their involvement in bilirubin uptake. Edited by PD Berk and NI Berlin: Chemistry and Physiology of Bile Pigments. DHEW No (NIH) 77-1100. Washington DC, US Government Printing Office, 1977, pp 265–291

82. Forker EL: Mechanisms of hepatic bile formation. Annu Rev Physiol 39:323–347, 1977

83. Goresky CA: The hepatic uptake and excretion of sulfobromophthalein and bilirubin. Can Med Assoc J 92:851–857, 1965

84. Stein WD: The Movement of Molecules Across Cell Membranes. New York, Academic Press, 1967, pp 126–176

85. Scharschmidt BF, Waggoner JG, Berk PD: Hepatic organic anion uptake in the rat. J Clin Invest 56:1280–1292, 1975

86. Paumgartner G, Reichen J: Kinetics of hepatic uptake on unconjugated bilirubin. Clin Sci Mol Med 51:169–176, 1976

87. Bloomer JR, Zaccaria J: Effect of graded bilirubin loads on bilirubin transport by perfused rat liver. Am J Physiol 230:736–742, 1976

88. Leevy CM, Smith F, Longueville J, Paumgartner G, Howard MM: Indocyanine green clearance as a test for hepatic function. JAMA 200:236–240, 1967

89. Paumgartner G, Probst P, Kraines R, Leevy CM: Kinetics of indocyanine green removal from the blood. Ann NY Acad Sci 170:134–147, 1970

90. Goresky CA: Initial distribution and rate of uptake of sulfobromophthalein in the liver. Am J Physiol 207:13–26, 1964

91. Hunton DB, Bollman JL, Hoffman HN: II. The plasma removal of indocyanine green and sulfobromophthalein: effect of dosage and blocking agents. J Clin Invest 40:1648–1655, 1961

92. Shupeck M, Wolkoff AW, Scharschmidt BF, Waggoner JG, Berk PD: Studies of the kinetics of purified conjugated bilirubin-^{3}H in the rat. Am J Gastroenterology 70:259–264, 1978

93. Brauer RW: Paper presented to the American Association for the Study of Liver Diseases. Chicago, 1961

94. Silverman M, Goresky CA: A unified kinetic hypothesis of carrier mediated transport: its applications. Biophys J 5:487–509, 1965

95. Heinz E: Kinetic studies on the "influx" of glycine-1-C^{14} into the Ehrlich mouse ascites carcinoma cell. J Biol Chem 211:781–790, 1954

96. Paumgartner G, Reichen J: Different pathways for hepatic uptake of taurocholate and indocyanine green. Experientia 31:306–307, 1975

97. Delage Y, Erlinger S, Duval M, Benhamou J-P: Influence of dehydrocholate and taurocholate on the bromsulphthalein uptake,

storage, and excretion in the dog. Gut 16:105–108, 1975.

98. Reichen J, Paumgartner G: Uptake of bile acids by perfused rat liver. Am J Physiol 231:734–742, 1976

99. Mender E, Paumgartner G: Disparate Na$^+$-requirement of bile acids and indocyanine green uptake by isolated hepatocytes. Gastroenterology 73:A-37/1235, 1977

100. Reichen J, Berk PD: Isolation of an organic anionic dye (OAD) binding protein from rat liver plasma membrane (LPM). Gastroenterology 73:A-44/1242, 1977

101. Wolkoff AW, Arias IM: ^{35}S-BSP binding by purified rat liver cell plasma membrane subfractions. Gastroenterology 73: A-57/1255, 1977

102. Levi AJ, Gatmaitan Z, Arias IM: Two hepatic cytoplasmic protein fractions, Y and Z, and their role in the hepatic uptake of bilirubin, sulfobromophthalein, and other anions. J Clin Invest 48:2156–2167, 1969

103. Fleischner G, Robbins J, Arias IM: Immunological studies of Y protein: a major cytoplasmic organic anion binding protein in rat liver. J Clin Invest 51:677–684, 1972

104. Litwack G, Ketterer B, Arias IM: Ligandin: an abundant protein which binds steroids, bilirubin, carcinogens, and a number of exogenous organic anions. Nature 234:466–467, 1971

105. Habig WH, Pabst MJ, Fleischner G, Gatmaitan Z, Arias IM, Jakoby WB: The identity of glutathione S-transferase B with ligandin, a major binding protein of liver. Proc Natl Acad Sci USA 71: 3879–3882, 1974

106. Jakoby WB, Habig WH, Keen JH, Ketley JN, Pabst MJ: Glutathione S-transferases: catalytic aspects. Edited by IM Arias and WB Jakoby: Gluthathione: Metabolism and Function. New York, Raven Press, 1976, pp 189–211

107. Kamisaka K, Habig WH, Ketley JN, Arias IM, Jakoby WB: Multiple forms of human glutathione S-transferase and their affinity for bilirubin. Eur J Biochem 60:153–161, 1975

108. Bhargava M, Listowsky J, Arias IM: Ligandin: Subunits and function. Gastroenterology 73:A-15/1213, 1977.

109. Ockner RK, Manning JA, Poppenhausen RB, Ho WK: A binding protein for fatty acids in cytosol of intestinal mucosa, liver, myocardium, and other tissues. Science 177:56–58, 1972

110. Ockner RK, Manning JA: Fatty acid binding protein in small intestine: Identity, isolation, and evidence for its role in cellular fatty acid transport. J Clin Invest 54:326–338, 1974

111. Kamisaka K, Listowsky I, Arias IM: Circular dichroism studies of Y protein (ligandin), a major organic anion binding protein in liver, kidney, and small intestine. Ann NY Acad Sci 226:148–161, 1973

112. Ketley JN, Habig WH, Jakoby WB: Binding on non-substrate ligands to the glutathione S-transferases. J Biol Chem 250:8670–8673, 1975

113. Tipping E, Ketterer B, Christodoulides L, Enderby G: Spectroscopic studies of the binding of bilirubin by ligandin and aminoazo-dye-binding protein A. Biochem J 157:211–216, 1976

114. Meuwissen JATP, Heirwegh KPM: Transfer of adsorbed bilirubin to specific binding proteins. Biochem J 120:19P, 1970

115. Meuwissen JATP, Ketterer B, Heirwegh KPM: Role of soluble binding proteins in overall hepatic transport of bilirubin. Edited by PD Berk and NI Berlin: Chemistry and Physiology of Bile Pigments. DHEW No (NIH) 77-1100. Washington, DC, US Government Printing Office, 1977, pp 323–337

116. Meuwissen JATP, Zeegers M, Srai KS, Ketterer B: Effect of glutathione on the activity of bilirubin-binding proteins from rat liver cytosol. Biochem Soc Trans 5:1404–1407, 1977

117. Wolkoff AW, Sellin J, Gatmaitan Z, Goresky CA, Arias IM: Role of ligandin in the transfer of bilirubin from plasma into the liver. Gastroenterology 73:A-57/1255, 1977

118. Levi AJ, Gatmaitan Z, Arias IM: Deficiency of hepatic organic anion binding: A possible cause of "physiologic" jaundice in the newborn. Lancet 2:139–140, 1969

119. Reyes H, Levi AJ, Arias IM: Studies of Y and Z: Two hepatic cytoplasmic organic anion-binding proteins: Effect of drugs, chemicals, hormones, and cholestasis. J Clin Invest 50:2242–2252, 1971

120. McDevitt DG, Nies AS, Wilkinson GR: Influence of phenobarbital on factors responsible for hepatic clearance of indocyanine green in the rat: Relative contributions of induction and altered liver blood flow. Biochem Pharmacol 26: 1247–1250, 1977

121. Berk PD, Bloomer JR, Howe RB, Berlin

NI: Constitutional hepatic dysfunction (Gilbert's syndrome). A new definition based on kinetic studies with unconjugated radiobilirubin. Am J Med 49:296–305, 1970

122. Wolpert E, Wolkoff AW, Pascasio F, Arias IM: BSP metabolism and transport in Rotor's syndrome. Gastroenterology 68: A-210/1067, 1975

123. Bradley SF: Storage — concepts and implications. Edited by PD Berk and NI Berlin: Chemistry and Physiology of Bile Pigments. DHEW No (NIH) 77-1100. Washington, DC, US Government Printing Office, 1977, pp 300–305

124. Fleischner G, Kamisaka K, Habig W, Arias IM: Human ligandin: Characterization and quantitation. Gastroenterology 69:821, 1975

125. Berk PD, Blaschke TF, Waggoner JG: Defective BSP clearance in patients with constitutional hepatic dysfunction (Gilbert's syndrome). Gastroenterology 63:472–481, 1972

126. Martin JF, Vierling JM, Wolkoff AW, Scharschmidt BF, Vergalla J, Waggoner JG, Berk PD: Abnormal hepatic transport of indocyanine green in Gilbert's syndrome. Gastroenterology 70:385–391, 1976

127. Berk PD, Blaschke TF: Detection of Gilbert's syndrome in patients with hemolysis. Ann Intern Med 77:527–531, 1972

128. Berk PD, Scharschmidt BF, Martin JF, Vierling JM, Wolkoff AW, Blitzer BL, Chretien P: Diagnosis of Gilbert's syndrome (GS) in patient with hemolysis by studies of bilirubin (BR) kinetics: A fly in the radioactive ointment. Clin Res 24:431A, 1976

129. Fevery J, Blanckaert N, Heirwegh KPM, De Groote J: Bilirubin conjugates: Formation and detection. Edited by H Popper and F Schaffner: Progress in Liver Disease. Vol. V. New York, Grune & Stratton, 1976, pp 183–214

130. Heirwegh KPM, Van Hees GP, LeRoy P, Van Roy FP, Jansen FH: Heterogeneity of bile pigment conjugates as revealed by chromatography of their ethyl anthranilate azopigments. Biochem J 120:877–890, 1970

131. Thompson RPH, Hofmann AF: Free and conjugated bile pigments of body fluids: qualitative analysis by thin-layer chromatography. J Lab Clin Med 82:483–488, 1973

132. Gordon ER, Chan T-H, Samodai K, Goresky CA: The isolation and further char-acterization of the bilirubin tetrapyrroles in bile-containing human duodenal juice and dog gall-bladder bile. Biochem J 167:1–8, 1977

133. Fevery J, Van Damme B, Michiels R, De Groote J, Heirwegh KPM: Bilirubin conjugates in bile of man and rat in the normal state and in liver disease. J Clin Invest 51:2482–2492, 1972

134. Gordon ER, Goresky CA, Chang T-H, Perlin AS: The isolation and characterization of bilirubin diglucuronide, the major bilirubin conjugate in dog and human bile. Biochem J 155:477–486, 1976

135. Fevery J, Van De Vijver M, Michiels R, Heirwegh KPM: Comparison in different species of biliary bilirubin-IXα conjugates with the activities of hepatic and renal bilirubin-IXα-uridine diphosphate glycosyltransferases. Biochem J 164:737–746, 1977

136. Heirwegh KPM, Fevery J, Michiels R, Van Hees GP, Compernolle F: Separation by thin-layer chromatography and structure elucidation of bilirubin conjugates isolated from dog bile. Biochem J 145:185–199, 1975

137. Blanckaert N, Compernolle F, Leroy P, Van Houtte R, Fevery J, Heirwegh KPM: The fate of bilirubin-IXα glucuronide in cholestasis and during storage in vitro: Intramolecular rearrangement to positional isomers of glucuronic acid. Biochem J 171:203–214, 1978

138. Kuenzle CC: Bilirubin conjugates of human bile: The excretion of bilirubin as the acyl glycosides of aldobiouronic acid, with a branched-chain hexuronic acid as one of the components of the hexuronosylhexuronide. Biochem J 119:411–435, 1970

139. Dutton GJ: The biosynthesis of glucuronides. Edited by GJ Dutton: Glucuronic Acid, Free and Combined. New York, Academic Press, 1966, pp 185–299

140. Zakim D, Vessey DA: Techniques for the characterization of UDP-glucuronyltransferase, glucose-6-phosphatase, and other tightly-bound microsomal enzymes. Methods Biochem Anal 21:1–37, 1973

141. Burchell B: Studies on the purification of rat liver uridine diphosphate glucuronyltransferase. Biochem J 161:543–550, 1977

142. Gorski JP, Kasper CB: Purification and properties of microsomal UDP-glucuronyltransferase from rat liver. J Biol Chem 252:1336–1343, 1977

143. Heirwegh KPM, Van de Vijver M, Fevery J: Assay and properties of digitonin-acti-

vated bilirubin uridine diphosphate glucuronyltransferase from rat liver. Biochem J 129:605–618, 1972

144. Black M, Billing BH: Hepatic bilirubin UDP-glucuronyl transferase activity in liver disease and Gilbert's syndrome. N Engl J Med 280:1266–1271, 1969

145. Felsher BF, Craig JR, Carpio N: Hepatic bilirubin glucuronidation in Gilbert's syndrome. J Lab Clin Med 81:829–837, 1973

146. Gollan JL, Bateman C, Billing BH: Effect of dietary composition on the unconjugated hyperbilirubinaemia of Gilbert's syndrome. Gut 17:335–340, 1976

147. Black M, Fevery J, Parker D, Jacobsen J, Billing BH, Carbon ER: Effect of phenobarbitone on plasma ^{14}C-bilirubin clearance in patients with unconjugated hyperbilirubinemia. Clin Sci Mol Med 46:1–17, 1974

148. Gollan JL, Huang SN, Billing B, Sherlock S: Prolonged survival in three brothers with severe type 2 Crigler-Najjar syndrome. Gastroenterology 68:1543–1555, 1975

149. Gordon ER, Shaffer EA, Sass-Kortsak A: Bilirubin secretion and conjugation in the Crigler-Najjar syndrome Type II. Gastroenterology 70:761–765, 1976

150. Arias IM, Gartner LM, Cohen M, Ben Ezzer J, Levi A: Chronic nonhemolytic unconjugated hyperbilirubinemia with glucuronyl transferase deficiency. Am J Med 47:395–409, 1969

151. Blaschke TF, Berk PD, Scharschmidt BF, Guyther JR, Vergalla JM, Waggoner JG: Crigler-Najjar syndrome: An unusual course with development of neurologic damage at age eighteen. Pediatr Res 8:573–590, 1974

152. Berk PD, Martin JF, Blaschke TF, Scharschmidt BF, Plotz PH: Unconjugated hyperbilirubinemia. Physiologic evaluation and experimental approaches to therapy. Ann Intern Med 82:552–570, 1975

153. Black M, Sherlock S: Treatment of Gilbert's syndrome with phenobarbitone. Lancet 1:1359–1362, 1970

154. Blaschke TF, Berk PD, Rodkey FL, Scharschmidt BF, Collison HA, Waggoner JG: Drugs and the liver. I. Effects of glutethimide and phenobarbital on hepatic bilirubin clearance, plasma bilirubin turnover and carbon monoxide production in man. Biochem Pharmacol 23:2795–2806, 1974

155. Felsher BF, Carpio NM: Non-familial unconjugated hyperbilirubinemia and reduced hepatic bilirubin UDP-glucuronyl transferase activity in patients with chronic persistent hepatitis. Gastroenterology 73: A-22/1220, 1977

156. Datta DV, Nair R, Nair CR: Estimation of hepatic bilirubin UDP-glucuronyl transferase in patients with noncirrhotic portal fibrosis and liver disease: significance and limitations. Am J Dig Dis 20:961–967, 1975

157. Maddrey WC, Cukier JO, Magalang AC, Boitnolt JK, Odell GB: Hepatic bilirubin UDP-glucuronyltransferase in patients with sickle cell anemia. Gastroenterology 74:193–195, 1978

158. Auclair C, Feldmann G, Hakim J, Boivin P, Boucherot J, Troube H: Bilirubin and paranitrophenol glucuronyl transferase activities and ultrastructural aspect of the liver in patients with chronic hemolytic anemias. Biomedicine 25:61–65, 1976

159. Jansen PLM: The enzyme-catalyzed formation of bilirubin diglucuronide by a solubilized preparation from cat liver microsomes. Biochim BiophysActa 338: 170–182, 1974

160. Halac E, Dipiazza M, Detwiler P: The formation of bilirubin mono- and diglucuronide by rat liver microsomal fractions. Biochim BiophysActa 279:544–553, 1972

161. Wolkoff AW, Ketley JN, Waggoner JG, Berk PD, Jakoby WB: Hepatic accumulation and intracellular binding of conjugated bilirubin. J Clin Invest 61:142–149, 1978

162. Jansen PLM, Chowdhury JR, Fischberg EG, Arias IM: Enzymatic conversion of bilirubin monoglucuronide to diglucuronide by rat liver plasma membranes. J Biol Chem 252:2710–2716, 1977

163. Lin ECC: The molecular basis of membrane transport systems. Edited by LI Rothfield: Structure and Function of Biological Membranes. New York, Academic Press, 1971, pp 285–341

164. Fevery J, Blanckaert N, Heirwegh KPM, Préaux A-M, Berthelot P: Unconjugated bilirubin and an increased proportion of bilirubin monoconjugates in the bile of patients with Gilbert's syndrome and Crigler-Najjar disease. J Clin Invest 60:970–979, 1977

165. Goresky C, Gordon ER, Shaffer EA, Paré P, Carassavas D, Aronoff A: Definition of a conjugation dysfunction in Gilberts' syndrome: Studies of the handling of bilirubin

loads and of the pattern of bilirubin conjugates secreted in bile. Clin Sci Mol Med 55:63–71, 1978

166. Blanckaert N, Gollan JL, Schmid R: Is bilirubin diglucuronide formed in vivo by transglucuronidation of bilirubin monoglucuronide? Gastroenterology 74:1166, 1978

167. Schalm L, Weber APh: Jaundice with conjugated bilirubin in hyperhaemolysis. Acta Med Scand 176:549–553, 1964

168. Forker EL: Canalicular anion transport. Edited by PD Berk and NI Berlin: Chemistry and Physiology of Bile Pigments. DHEW Publication No (NIH) 77-1100. Washington, DC, US Government Printing Office, 1977, pp 383–389

169. Clarenberg R, Kao C-C: Shared and separate pathways for biliary excretion of bilirubin and BSP in rats. Am J Physiol 225:192–200, 1973

170. Whelan G, Combes B: Competition of unconjugated and conjugated sulfobromophthalein sodium (BSP) for a single excretory system. J Lab Clin Med 78:230–244, 1971

171. Mahu J-L, Duvaldestin P, Dhumeaux D, Berthelot P: Biliary transport of cholephilic dyes: evidence for the two different pathways. Am J Physiol 232:E445–450, 1977

172. Barnhart JL, Gronwall RR, Combes B: Selective defect in biliary excretion of conjugated BSP compounds in mutant Corriedale sheep: evidence for a second canalicular carrier. Gastroenterology 73:A-59/1257, 1977

173. Boonyapisit ST, Trotman BW, Ostrow JD: Unconjugated bilirubin, and the hydrolysis of conjugated bilirubin, in gallbladder bile of patients with cholelithiasis. Gastroenterology 74:70–74, 1978

174. Lester R, Klein PD: Bile pigment excretion: A comparison of the biliary excretion of bilirubin and bilirubin derivatives. J Clin Invest 45:1839–1846, 1966

175. Blanckaert N, Fevery J, Heirwegh KPM, Compernolle F: Characterization of the major diazo-positive pigments in bile of homozygous Gunn rats. Biochem J 164:237–249, 1977

176. Barrowman JA, Bonnett R, Bray PJ: Metabolism of biliverdin. Biliary excretion of bile pigments after intravenous injection of biliverdin isomers. Biochim BiophysActa 444:333–337, 1976

177. Colleran E, O'Carra P: Specificity of biliverdin reductase. Biochem J 119:16–17, 1970

178. McDonagh AF, Palma LA: Mechanism of bilirubin photodegradation. Edited by PD Berk and NI Berlin: Chemistry and Physiology of Bile Pigments. DHEW Publication No (NIH) 77-1100, Washington, DC, US Government Printing Office, 1977, pp 81–102

179. Arias IM: The excretion of conjugated bilirubin by the liver cell. Medicine 45:513–515, 1966

180. Accatino L, Simon FR: Identification and characterization of a bile acid receptor in isolated liver surface membranes. J Clin Invest 57:496–508, 1976

181. Goresky CA, Haddad HH, Kluger WS, Nadeau BE, Back GG: The enhancement of maximal bilirubin excretion with taurocholate-induced increments in bile flow. Can J Physiol Pharmacol 52:389–403, 1974

182. O'Maille ERL, Richards TG, Short AH: Factors determining the maximal rate of organic anion excretion by the liver and further evidence on the hepatic site of action of the hormone secretin. J Physiol (London) 186:424–438, 1966

183. Boyer JL, Scheig RL, Klatskin G: The effect of sodium taurocholate on the hepatic metabolism of sulfobromophthalein sodium (BSP). The role of bile flow. J Clin Invest 49:206–215, 1970

184. Barnhart J, Ritt D, WareA, Combes B: A comparison of the effects of taurocholate and theophylline on BSP excretion in dogs. Edited by G Paumgartner and R Preisig: The Liver. Quantitative Aspects of Structure and Function. Basel, Karger, 1973, pp 315–325

185. Vonk RJ, Veen Hvd, Prop G, Meijer DK: The influence of taurocholate and dehydrocholate choleresis on plasma disappearance and biliary excretion of indocyanine green in the rat. Naunyn Schmiedebergs Arch Pharmacol 282:401–410, 1974

186. Berk RN, Goldberger LE, Loeb P: The role of bile salts in the hepatic excretion of iopanoic acid. Invest Radiol 9:7–15, 1974

187. Gibson GE, Forker EL: Canalicular bile flow and bromsulphthalein transport maximum: the effect of a bile salt-independent choleretic, SC-2644. Gastroenterology 66:1046–1053, 1974

188. Goresky CA: The hepatic uptake process: its implications for bilirubin transport. Ed-

ited by CA Goresky and MM Fisher: Jaundice. Proceedings of the Second International Symposium of the Canadian Hepatic Foundation. New York, Plenum Press, 1975, pp 159–174

189. Jones AL, Schmucker DL, Adler RD, Ockner RK, Mooney JS: A quantitative analysis of hepatic ultrastructure in rats after selective biliary obstruction. Edited by R Preisig, J Bircher, and G Paumgartner: The Liver. Quantitative Aspects of Structure and Function. Aulendorf, Editio Cantor, 1976, pp 36–51

190. Layden TJ, Boyer JL: Influence of bile acids on bile canalicular membrane morphology and the lobular gradient in canalicular size. Lab Invest 39:110–119, 1978

191. Gumucio JJ, Balabaud C, Miller DL, De Mason LJ, Appleman HD, Stoecker TJ, Franzblau DR: Bile secretion and liver cell heterogeneity in the rat. J Lab Clin Med 91:350–362, 1978

192. Miyai K, Richardson AL, Mayr W, Javitt NB: Subcellular pathology of rat liver in cholestasis and choleresis induced by bile salts. I. Effects of lithocholic, 3β-hydroxy-5-cholenic, cholic, and dehydrocholic acids. Lab Invest 36:249–258, 1977

193. Nemchausky BA, Layden TJ, Boyer JL: Effects of chronic choleretic infusions of bile acids on the membrane of the bile canaliculus. Lab Invest 36:259–267, 1977

194. Bissell DM, Deal DR, Hammaker LE: Determinants of bilirubin transport into bile. Gastroenterology 69:A-9/809, 1975

195. Ware AJ, Carey MC, Combes B: Solution properties of sulfobromophthalein sodium (BSP) compounds alone and in association with sodium taurocholate (TC). J Lab Clin Med 87:443–456, 1976

196. Javitt NB: Bile salt regulation of hepatic excretory function. Gastroenterology 56:622–624, 1969

197. Vershure JCM, Mijnlieff PF: The dominating macromolecular complex of human gallbladder bile. Clin Chim Acta 1:154–166, 1956

198. Juniper K: Physiocochemical characteristics of bile and their relation to gallstone formation. Am J Med 39:98–107, 1965

199. Nakayama F: Nature of cholesterol-complexing macromolecular fractions in bile. Clin Chim Acta 13:212–220, 1966

200. Bouchier IAD, Cooperband SR: Isolation and characterization of a macromolecular aggregate associated with bilirubin. Clin Chim Acta 15:291–302

201. Scharschmidt BF, Schmid R: The micellar sink: A quantitative assessment of the association of organic anions with mixed micelles and other macromolecular aggregates in rat bile. J Clin Invest 62:1122–1132, 1978

202. Billing BH, Maggiore Q, Carter MA: Hepatic transport of bilirubin. Ann NY Acad Sci 111:319–324, 1963

203. Sperber I: Secretion of organic anions in the formation of urine and bile. Pharm Rev 11:109–134, 1959

204. Sperber I: Biliary secretion of organic anions and its influence on bile flow. Edited by W Taylor: The Biliary System. Oxford, Blackwell, 1965, pp 457–467

205. Fleischer G, Arias IM: Recent advances in bilirubin formation, transport, metabolism and excretion. Am J Med 49:576–589, 1970

206. Abe H, Okuda K: Biliary excretion of conjugated sulfobromophthalein (BSP) in constitutional hyperbilirubinemias. Digestion 13:272–283, 1975

207. Koskelo P, Toivonen I, Adlercreutz H: Urinary coproporphyrin isomer distribution in the Dubin-Johnson syndrome. Clin Chem 13:1006–1009, 1967

208. Ben Ezzer J, Rimington C, Shani M, Seligsohn U, Sheba CH, Szeinberg A: Abnormal excretion of the isomers of urinary coproporphyrin by patients with Dubin-Johnson syndrome in Israel. Clin Sci 40:17–30, 1971

209. Wolkoff AW, Cohen LE, Arias IM: The inheritance of the Dubin-Johnson syndrome. N Engl J Med 288:113–117, 1973

210. Shimizu Y, Konto T, Kuchiba K, Urata G: Uroporphyrinogen III cosynthetase in liver and blood in the Dubin-Johnson syndrome. J Lab Clin Med 89:517–523, 1977

211. Dubin IN: Rotor's syndrome and chronic idiopathic jaundice. Arch Intern Med 110:823–824, 1962

212. Wolkoff AW, Wolpert E, Pascasio FN, Arias IM: Rotor's syndrome. A distinct inheritable pathophysiologic entity. Am J Med 60:173–179, 1976

213. Dubin IN, Johnson FB: Chronic idiopathic jaundice with unidentified pigment in liver cells: New clinicopathologic entity with report of 12 cases. Medicine 33:155–197, 1954

214. Dubin IN: Chronic idiopathic jaundice: a review of 50 cases. Am J Med 24:268–292, 1958

215. Shani M, Seligsohn U, Gilon E, Sheba C,

Adam A: Dubin-Johnson syndrome in Israel. I. Clinical, laboratory, and genetic aspects of 101 cases. Q J Med 39:549–567, 1970

216. Shani M, Seligsohn U, Ben Ezzer J: Effect of phenobarbital on liver functions in patients with Dubin-Johnson syndrome. Gastroenterology 67:303–308, 1974

217. Owens D, Sherlock S: Diagnosis of Gilbert's syndrome: Role of reduced caloric intake test. Br Med J 3:559–563, 1973

218. Powell LW, Hemingway EH, Billing BH, Sherlock S: Idiopathic unconjugated hyperbilirubinemia (Gilbert's syndrome): A study of 42 families. N Engl J Med 227:1108–1112, 1967

219. Rotor AB, Manahan L, Florentin A: Familial non-hemolytic jaundice with direct van den Bergh reaction. Acta Med Phillipina 5:37–49, 1948

220. Owens D, Evans J: Population studies on Gilbert's syndrome. J Med Genet 12:152–156, 1975

221. Kornberg A: Latent liver disease in persons recovered from catarrhal jaundice and in otherwise normal medical students as revealed by the bilirubin excretion test. J Clin Invest 21:299–308, 1972

222. Alwall N, Laurell CB, Nilsby I: Studies on heredity in cases of ''non-hemolytic bilirubinemia without direct van den Bergh reaction'' (hereditary, non-hemolytic bilirubinemia). Acta Med Scand 124:114–125, 1946

223. Childs B, Sidbury JB, Migeon CJ: Glucuronide acid conjugation by patients with familial non-hemolytic jaundice and their relatives. Pediatrics 23:903–913, 1959

224. Crigler JF, Najjar VA: Congenital familial nonhemolytic jaundice with kernicterus. Pediatrics 10:169–180, 1952

225. Sleisenger MH, Kahn I, Barniville H, Rubin W, Ben Ezzer J, Arias IM: Nonhemolytic unconjugated hyperbilirubinemia with hepatic glucuronyl-transferase deficiency: A genetic study in four generations. Trans Assoc Am Physicians 80:259–266, 1967

226. Hunter JO, Thompson RPH, Dunn PM, Williams R: Inheritance of type 2 Crigler-Najjar hyperbilirubinemia. Gut 14:46–49, 1973

227. Edwards RH: Inheritance of the Dubin-Johnson-Sprinz syndrome. Gastroenterology 68:734–749, 1975

228. Foulk WT, Butt HR, Owen CA, Whitcomb FF, Mason HL: Constitutional hepatic dysfunction (Gilbert's disease): Its natural history and related syndromes. Medicine 38:25–46, 1959

229. Powell LW, Billing BH, Williams HS: The assessment of red cell survival in idiopathic unconjugated hyperbilirubinaemia (Gilbert's syndrome) by the use of radioactive diisopropylfluorophosphate and chromium. Aust Ann Med 16:221–225, 1967

230. Lima JEP, Utz E, Roisenberg I: Hereditary nonhemolytic conjugated hyperbilirubinemia without abnormal liver cell pigmentation. Am J Med 40:628–633, 1966

231. Schiff L, Billing BH, Oikawa Y: Familial nonhemolytic jaundice with conjugated bilirubin in the serum. N Engl J Med 260:1315–1319, 1959

232. Sprinz H, Nelson RS: Persistent non-hemolytic hyperbilirubinemia associated with lipochrome-like pigment in liver cells: report of 4 cases. Ann Intern Med 41:952–962, 1954

233. Barth RF, Grimley PM, Berk PD, Bloomer JR, Howe RB: Excess lipofuscin accumulation in constitutional hepatic dysfunction (Gilbert's syndrome). Light and electron microscopic observations. Arch Pathol 91:41–47, 1971

234. Felsher BF, Rickard D, Redeker AG: The reciprocal relation between caloric intake and the degree of hyperbilirubinemia in Gilbert's syndrome. N Engl J Med 283:170–172, 1970

235. Barrett PVD: Hyperbilirubinemia of fasting. JAMA 217:1349–1353, 1971

236. Fromke VL, Miller D: Constitutional hepatic dysfunction (CHD; Gilbert's disease); a review with special reference to a characteristic increase and prolongation of the hyperbilirubinemic response to nicotinic acid. Medicine 51:451–464, 1972

237. Blumenschein SD, Kallen RJ, Storey B, Natjscha JC, Odell GB, Childs B: Familial nonhemolytic jaundice with late onset of neurological damage. Pediatrics 42:786–792, 1968

Chapter 11

The Multiple Roles of the Glutathione Transferases (Ligandins)

By ALLAN W. WOLKOFF, RICHARD A. WEISIGER,
and WILLIAM B. JAKOBY

THE LAST DECADE revealed a remarkable group of proteins, the glutathione transferases, or ligandins, that have a multifunctional role as detoxifying agents in the liver and probably in other tissues as well. The initial description of these proteins is linked to their presumed activity in the liver, and it is their role in this organ about which we know the most. They have been nominated elsewhere[1] as a "triple threat" in detoxification, and the aim of this review is to enlarge that concept. We consider the manifold roles of the transferases as binding proteins, as catalysts for an extraordinary variety of reactions that utilize glutathione (GSH), as scavengers reacting covalently with highly electrophilic compounds including carcinogens, as possible intermediates in the transfer of bilirubin into the hepatocyte, and as intrahepatocellular storage proteins for compounds such as bilirubin.

The term "ligandin" was coined for a protein from rat liver that has been isolated by three different groups of investigators on the basis of seemingly distinct properties. One group isolated a protein (Y protein) and identified it by assaying affinity for bilirubin and sulfobromophthalein (BSP).[2] Another isolation resulted from purification of a protein with affinity for a metabolite of cortisol.[3] The third group, isolated the protein on the basis of the yellow color associated covalently with protein after rats were injected with the azo-dye carcinogen, butter yellow.[4] Once a monospecific antibody to the Y protein was obtained, the three groups recognized that they were working with the same entity, which they labeled "ligandin."[5]

Subsequent studies with glutathione transferase activity (EC 2.5.1.18) resulted in the isolation of several homogeneous proteins which, because of similar though nonidentical patterns of substrate specificity, were labeled glutathione transferases A, B, C, and so on.[6,7] When the appropriate comparisons were made, glutathione transferase B was established to be identical with ligandin.[8] Since the transferases had affinity for similar ligands, affinity for hydrophobic ligands was proposed to be an intrinsic feature of these enzymes.[9] Conversely, we may define a family, the *ligandins*, as proteins with both glutathione transferase activity and an avidity for hydrophobic compounds.

From the Liver Research Center and Department of Medicine, Albert Einstein College of Medicine, Bronx, New York, and Section on Enzymes and Cellular Biochemistry, Laboratory of Biochemistry and Metabolism, National Institute of Arthritis, Metabolism and Digestive Diseases, National Institutes of Health, Bethesda, Maryland.

TABLE 1.—*Physical Properties of Rat Glutathione Transferases**

Property	Transferase					
	AA	A	B	C	D	E
Molecular weight ($\times 10^3$)	45	46	47	47		40
Number of subunits	2	2	2	2		2
Reaction with antibody†	None	A,C	B	A,C		E
Isoelectric point	10	8.9	9.8	8.0		7.3
Relative concentration	0.14	0.22	1.0	0.52	0.02	0.1

*This table summarizes data from work on the specific enzymes.[21-23]

†The capital letters refer to IgG obtained as a response to a specific transferase, e.g., the letter A notes reaction with antibody produced after injection of homogeneous glutathione transferase A.

THE PROTEINS AND THEIR AFFINITY FOR LIGANDS

The glutathione transferases have been found in all the mammals tested[7,10,11] and within diverse tissues. Highly purified preparations are available from human liver,[12] human erythrocytes,[13] porcine liver,[14] and rat kidney,[15] and additions to this list are expected to continue. The work reviewed here is limited to the enzymes from rat liver because this tissue has been extensively studied at the level of purified, homogeneous proteins. Work with this same group of proteins from rat gastrointestinal tract has also received attention.[16]

The physical properties of the five liver glutathione transferases that have been purified to homogeneity are summarized in Table 1; the details have been reviewed recently.[7] This is a family of proteins of similar molecular weight, each consisting of two subunits. Transferase B has two subunits of unequal molecular weight, 23,000 and 25,000,[17,18] although it is not clear whether the smaller species arises by posttranscriptional modification.[17] Cyanogen bromide treatment of transferase C indicates that this protein has subunits that are identical.* Each transferase has a distinct amino acid composition and specific reactivity with antibody, except for transferases A and C, which resemble and cross-react with each other. All the enzymes listed have an isoelectric point in the alkaline pH range.

Transferase B constitutes 5% of the proteins extracted from rat liver cytosol.[19] From the ratio of the concentrations of the several transferases as estimated at the time of their elution from carboxymethylcellulose,[20] the major separation step, it is apparent that transferase B, the original ligandin, constitutes about half of all the glutathione transferases. It follows that these enzymes constitute 10% of the total protein present in extracts of rat liver[20] (and 3% of extracts of human liver[12]).

That these are all binding proteins, several with very high affinity for their ligands, is evident from Table 2. Hence the claim that transferase function, i.e., catalysis, and ligandin binding activity are intrinsically related.[9] As a rough approximation, these proteins could be considered to resemble serum albumin

---

*Unpublished data obtained by Albert Light and Jiri Vanecek from analysis of the cyanogen bromide peptides of transferase C.

TABLE 2.—*Binding of Certain Ligands to the Rat Glutathione Transferases*

| | K_D for transferases (μM) | | | | |
Ligand	AA	A	B	C	Reference
Bilirubin	100	15	2	2	9
Bilirubin monoglucuronide	4	2	3	6	24
Bilirubin diglucuronide	40	23	10	20	24
Hematin	4	2	0.1	7	9
Indocyanine green	100	3	3	1	9
3,6-Dibromosulfophthalein	200	100	15	80	9

with respect to binding. Although transferase B has been called an "anion binding protein," we now know that it has no specificity for anions as such; this is documented in the next section, where nonanions such as iodomethane are shown to be ligands. Equally pertinent is the observation that in many instances, ligands that are unable to serve as substrates for the transferases nevertheless inhibit catalytic activity in a strictly competitive fashion, i.e., they bind at the same site as substrate. For example, bilirubin, a nonsubstrate, binds to each of the transferases and does so in a competitive manner when 1-chloro-2,4-dinitrobenzene is used as substrate.[9]

The data in Table 2 require explanation in that they were obtained by measuring, after the addition of ligand, the decrease in the fluorescence of a tryptophan that forms part of each transferase molecule. Prior[25] and subsequent[26] studies have evaluated the binding of compounds such as bilirubin to ligandin B, i.e., transferase B, by an entirely different method, namely circular dichroism spectroscopy. The dissociation constants obtained by this method were of the order of 10^{-7} and 10^{-6} M, indicating even tighter binding than observed by the fluorescence technique. Although questions of interpretation of these measurements remain, two binding sites, one of high and one of relatively low affinity, could possibly be involved.[18] For bilirubin there is only one site for the dissociation constant noted in Table 2 per mole of transferase B.[9]

From both binding and substrate studies, we can say that the ligandins bind compounds that have only one feature in common: a sufficiently large hydrophobic domain. This is a central assumption for the mechanism of action of glutathione transferases and is discussed in the next section.

CATALYTIC FUNCTION

The study of catalysis by the glutathione transferases has proceeded in much the same fashion as one peels an onion. After removing the first few layers, we found additional layers beneath that were different but of equal simplicity. Although some of the strata have yet to be removed, we suspect that the system is not at all complex; it is just an onion and, at certain stages, can make one cry. Our present view of the catalytic mechanism is that the transferases are binding proteins much like albumin, but they differ in that they have a second, specific binding site for GSH. They are proteins that have catalytic activity only by reason of placing a compound with sufficient electrophilicity near the nucleophilic glutathione thiolate ion (GS⁻). The catalytic efficiency of the transferases results from a proximity effect, i.e., placing two substrates in close juxtaposition. This is an enzyme mechanism of such simplicity that its mechanical counterpart would be the wedge.

$$GSH + \text{[2,4-dinitrochlorobenzene]} \rightarrow \text{[2,4-dinitrophenyl-SG]} + HCl \tag{1}$$

The evidence for this mechanism has been developed in some detail[26,27] and has been reviewed.[7] Here we need only summarize the peeling of the onion, which began with the knowledge that many compounds were excreted in the form of mercapturic acids. We know of hundreds of compounds bearing an electrophilic carbon that react with GSH to form the corresponding glutathione thioether,[28] e.g., reaction 1. This conjugate may subsequently undergo trans-peptidation with loss of the γ-glutamyl group;[29] glycine is removed and the cysteine moiety is *N*-acetylated. The product is a mercapturic acid, an *N*-acetylcysteine thioether of the original electrophilic compound. Table 3 presents a few of the many substrates available for conjugation with GSH and notes the overlapping specificity of the several transferases from rat liver.

Since the specificity (if that is the proper word for these enzymes) is so broad, it is necessary to search for those properties that substrates have in common. The answer appears to be that a substrate must have a hydrophobic aspect and that it bear an electrophilic carbon. Because of the low specificity, it appeared that even the electrophilic carbon need not be required. Would other atoms that are sufficiently electrophilic suffice? This appears to be the case, and reactions 2 and 3 are examples of the target for nucleophilic attack by glutathione thiolate of an electrophilic nitrogen (in nitroglycerin) and sulfur

TABLE 3.—*Specific Activities of the Rat Glutathione Transferases with Selected Substrates that Undergo Conjugation*[a]

Substrate	Transferase				
	AA	A	B	C	E
	(μmol/min/mg protein)				
Benzo[a]pyrene-4,5-oxide	0.004	0.087	0.011	0.098	0.069
BSP	0.004	0.53	0.006	0.18	0[b]
1,Chloro-2,4-dinitrobenzene	14	62	11	10	0.01
1,2-Dichloro-4-nitrobenzene	0.008	4.3	0.003	2.0	0[b]
1,2-Epoxy-3-(*p*-nitrophenoxy) propane		0.1	0[b]	0[b]	6.7
Ethacrynic acid	0.3	0[b]	0.26	0.11	0[b]
Iodomethane	1.4	0[b]	0.59	0[b]	8.9
p-Nitrobenzyl chloride	0.09	11.4	0.1	10.2	4.1
2-Nitropropane	0.01	0.012	0.008	0.014	0
Prostaglandin A₁		0.013	0.005	0.021	

[a] Data based on material presented in references 21, 22, 23, 37, 38, and 39.
[b] No activity detected at the highest enzyme concentration tested.

(in ethyl thiocyanate), respectively.[26] When other possibilities were examined, the transferases were found to catalyze isomerization by nucleophilic attack of a double bond system followed by elimination as exemplified by the formation of several α,β-unsaturated Δ^4-3-ketosteroids from Δ^5-3-ketosteroids.[31] In addition, the transferases were observed to catalyze the reaction of GSH and p-nitrophenylacetate to form the thioester, S-acetylglutathione.[27] An enzyme in the liver, free of selenium, was found with glutathione peroxidase activity and was identified as a glutathione transferase; hydrogen peroxide is inactive, and only organic peroxides serve with GSH as substrates.[32]

$$2GSH + CH_2 (ONO_2)CH(ONO_2) CH_2ONO_2 \rightarrow$$
$$CH_2 (ONO_2) CH(OH)CH_2 ONO_2 + GSSG + HNO_2 \qquad (2)$$

$$GSH + CH_3CH_2SCN \rightarrow CH_3CH_2SSG + HCN \qquad (3)$$

This wealth of reactions with the nucleophilic GSH suggests that all such reactions should be catalyzed by the transferases. However, although maleic acid undergoes both spontaneous and enzymatic conversion to fumarate in the presence of thiols,[33] the reactions was not catalyzed by the transferases. Similarly, disulfide interchange, as exemplified by the reaction of cystine and GSH to form cysteine and the mixed disulfide of GSH and cysteine, was not catalyzed by the transferases. These obvious contradictions to the hypothesis for the mechanism of action of the transferases are resolved when the hydrophilic nature of the inactive substances are considered. That is, maleic acid would probably serve as substrate if it were bound to the enzyme at the active site. It does not do so, since it is not an inhibitor for other substrates.[27] Its more hydrophobic analogs do act as substrates; diethylmaleate is conjugated with GSH[34] and maleylacetone and maleylacetoacetic acid are both isomerized.[27] Similarly, when the hydrophilic cystine is esterified to form the more hydrophobic diacetylcystine, the transferases catalyze the formation of the mixed disulfide of N-acetylcysteine and GSH.[27]

Despite their versatility, this group of enzymes uses a very simple and weak method of catalysis. It is as though the design process of Nature sacrificed catalytic efficiency for the capacity to detoxify a wider variety of the noxious compounds that we inhale, ingest, and produce metabolically. Perhaps in compensation, the relative simplicity of the system results in the production by higher organisms of large amounts of these enzymes.

A SCAVENGER ROLE

A major research effort[35,36] has brought into focus the role that highly electrophilic compounds, e.g., the oxidation products of the mixed function oxidases of the cytochrome P-450 type, may play in carcinogenesis. Many compounds of this sort, e.g., reactive epoxides, are the substrates of the glutathione transferases.[37] That is, they bind to the enzyme and then react with GSH. Sufficiently reactive electrophiles have more than one option for reaction, however, in that other nucleophilic reactants are available on the enzyme surface, e.g., protein thiol groups. Indeed, in the absence of exogenous GSH, transferases A and B react with the best of the transferase substrates, 1-chloro-2,4-dinitrobenzene, to form a covalent bond with protein; 0.3 moles of reagent react per mole of transferase within 5 min.

Since they can detoxify by what amounts to a suicidal approach, we speculatively ascribe a scavenger function to the transferases. Some of the substrates are vigorous alkylating agents, and it is not surprising that when they interact with the transferases they inactivate them. This is not to identify the glutathione transferases as the only participating scavengers of strong electrophiles. Many proteins behave similarly,[36] including alcohol dehydrogenase (W. H. Habig and W. B. Jakoby, unpublished data), but by reason of their avid binding, the transferases are able to "come close" to reactive compounds and to provide the opportunity for reaction. As mentioned, one of the three isolations of ligandin was based on the yellow color resulting from its covalent linkage to a reactive species produced in vivo by oxidation of an azo-dye carcinogen.

ROLE IN TRANSPORT

Despite a high affinity for plasma albumin, organic anions such as bilirubin and BSP are rapidly removed from the circulation by the liver with a half-time of only a few minutes.[40,41] The specificity of the uptake process has been documented for these and related compounds;[40,42] they have been found to be mutually competitive with each other and not with other anions such as taurocholic acid.[40] Saturation of the uptake process has been described,[40,43] and the phenomenon of countertransport may occur.[40] All of these findings suggest that entrance into the hepatocyte involves facilitated transport, i.e., a carrier-mediated process.

The initial step requires that the ligand be extracted from albumin prior to entrance into the cell,[43-46] presumably by an appropriate component on the outer sinusoidal membrane. Despite the fact that the purified glutathione transferases may have a somewhat lower affinity than albumin for organic anions,[12,25] they are sufficiently avid binders to allow consideration of a possible role in hepatic anion uptake. More significant are the results of recent elegant work pointing to the loss of affinity of albumin for bilirubin in the presence of liver cytosol.[46]

Since the flux of ligands across plasma membrane depends not only on affinity but also on the concentration of carriers in each compartment, the transferases (ligandins), which are present in high concentrations, would be ideal candidates for such a role. Quantitation of the influence of ligandins on bilirubin uptake has been difficult to attain, however, because of the inability of determining the bound and free concentrations of ligand simultaneously in plasma and intracellularly. Hepatic ligandin B concentration has been correlated with differences in plasma disappearance of organic anions in various species,[11] ontogenetically in the monkey,[47] and after administration of drugs that alter hepatic ligandin B content.[2] These studies are indirect and are difficult to analyze kinetically because of differences in other physiologic parameters between experimental and control animals, e.g., cardiac output or regional blood flow. The influence of increased ligandin B concentration, after thyroidectomy or phenobarbital pretreatment, on hepatic bilirubin transport has been investigated in the isolated perfused rat liver.[48] This system allowed physiologic conditions to be maintained constant between animal groups, and no influence of ligandin on the uptake rate constant was noted. Ligandin correlated inversely with efflux from liver to plasma, however. Thus, since flux of bilirubin between plasma and liver cell is bidirectional, ligandin influences net hepatic uptake of organic anions by reducing the efflux component across the plasma membrane.

Study of interaction of isolated plasma membranes with organic anions represents a more direct approach for identification of a putative membrane-associated organic anion receptor. Efforts in this direction have been made with rat liver plasma membrane preparations interacting with BSP. Evidence for binding was readily obtained but with a surfeit of riches.[49] The magnitude of binding, about 200 nmole (or 0.1 mg) of BSP per milligram of membrane protein, is obviously outside of the physiologically expected range. Bilirubin, which is known to be competitive with BSP for uptake,[40] was not bound.[49] In another attempt to isolate a receptor, material of molecular weight 170,000 was obtained, but it has about 20 binding sites per mole of protein.[50] Despite much effort, the methods used to obtain the binding data remain open to criticism because the ligands bind strongly to those materials that are generally used in assessing binding, such as dialysis tubing, ultrafiltration membranes, gel filtration media, and detergent micelles.

We also have attempted to obtain binding data in our respective laboratories (A. W. Wolkoff, in preparation; R. A. Weisiger and W. B. Jakoby, unpublished data) with membranes from liver and other tissues, the results of which can be summarized. There are both high and lower affinity sites on plasma membranes obtained from isolated hepatocytes and from liver, as well as on turkey and human erythrocytes. From Scatchard plots of the binding data, dissociation constants for BSP of the order of $10^{-6}M$ can be identified with a capacity of about 8 nmoles/mg of plasma protein. Although binding is radically decreased after preincubation of membranes with either trypsin or phospholipase A_2, boiling the membranes does not reduce binding. In fact, human erythrocyte ghosts increase severalfold in their capacity for BSP after boiling and retain the high affinity. Furthermore, similar binding data given by linear Scatchard plots are attainable with liposomes, i.e., with synthetic ''organelles'' prepared from lecithin and cholesterol and completely free of protein (R. A. Weisiger and W. B. Jakoby, unpublished data).

The last observation suggests that the membrane lipids, rather than membrane protein, may serve as receptors; the results of heating could be reversible, leaving the lipid bilayer relatively intact. Work with synthetic bimolecular lipid membranes free of protein has shown that organic anions have a strong affinity for adsorption to the water-membrane interface and that the rate-limiting step for bulk transport of these molecules across the bilayer is deadsorption into the water phase on the far side of the membrane.[51,52] If a similar rate-limiting accumulation of organic anions occurs on the inner side of the plasma membrane during hepatic uptake, a binding protein could directly interact with the membrane-organic anion complex to speed the rate of readsorption and thus the overall rate of uptake. Glutathione transferases E and A, both associated with exhaustively washed isolated hepatic plasma membrane (R. A.

Weisiger and W. B. Jakoby, unpublished data), are candidates for this role.

The synthetic bimolecular lipid membranes[51,52] also display saturation effects at higher concentrations and allow the prediction of mutual competition of one organic anion for another. Both effects follow from an accumulation of negative charges on the membrane, thereby preventing further anions from binding. Thus, saturation kinetics and mutual competition for uptake by the liver in vivo, while consistent with a protein receptor or carrier, could be explained by interaction with membrane lipid.

This discussion of organic anion uptake and the possible role of the ligandins in that process is highly speculative and without biochemical evidence. Insight may be gained by methods that are independent of the high affinity for lipid of the organic anions and in which the most rigorous controls are applied. Animals with mutations in the uptake of bilirubin, e.g., the mutant Southdown sheep,[53] can be a useful source for comparison in view of the considerable hazard of generating artifacts in this area of research.

ROLE AS HEPATIC "STORAGE" PROTEIN

Included in the concept for bilirubin transport is the suggestion that bilirubin accumulates within the hepatocyte bound to ligandin and that, once conjugated as the glucuronide, affinity for the protein is lost, thereby facilitating excretion into bile.[54,55] Recent work[24] has shown that this hypothesis is only partially correct.

When tracer amounts of ^{3}H-bilirubin were injected intravenously into Sprague-Dawley rats, 36% of the injected dose was found in liver homogenates, and 20% in the cytosol, 1.5 min after injection. Between 3 and 15 min, the hepatic content of radioactive material declined from 37% to 23% of the injected dose and was similarly decreased in the cytosol.[24] That this represents storage of bilirubin by the liver is evident from comparison of plasma disappearance of ^{3}H-bilirubin with its accumulation in liver and appearance in bile. Plasma half-life of ^{3}H-bilirubin after intravenous injection is approximately 3 min. When bile is collected at 2-min intervals after injection, there is a 4-min lag before radioactive material appears (Fig. 1). Over the subsequent 15 min, cumulative appearance of radioactivity in bile is approximately linear (Fig. 1, insert) with about 3% of injected bilirubin excreted per minute. The relatively large amount of ^{3}H-bilirubin that accumulates during this period points to a pool of bilirubin retained in the liver after removal from plasma; the pool is slowly released into bile.

Analysis of the intrahepatic radioactive material revealed not only that bilirubin had accumulated but also that a large proportion, between 37% and 64%, was present as bilirubin conjugates (Fig. 2). Over the time period examined, the most predominant form was the monoconjugated derivative of bilirubin. Although the accumulation of bilirubin monoglucuronide could be due to the more rapid excretion of the diglucuronide immediately after the latter's formation, this does not appear to be the case. Analysis of bile samples collected at 2-min intervals discloses that only bilirubin monoglucuronide is excreted initially; diglucuronide appears in bile after a 6-min delay and does not reach a stable baseline level of excretion until 20 min after injection.[24]

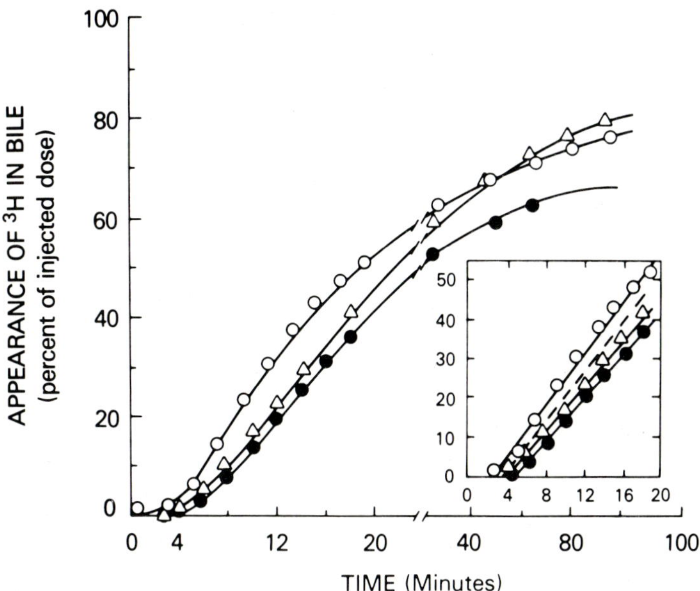

FIG. 1—Cumulative appearance of radioactivity in bile after injection of three rats with ³H-bilirubin. The insert presents the linear least-squares fit to the initial 20 min of study; the broken line illustrates the linear least-squares fit to all the data combined and has a slope of 3% of the injected dose per minute. (Modified from Wolkoff AW, Ketley JN, Waggoner JG, Berk PD, Jakoby WB: J Clin Invest 61:142–149, 1978, and reproduced by courtesy of the Journal of Clinical Investigation.)

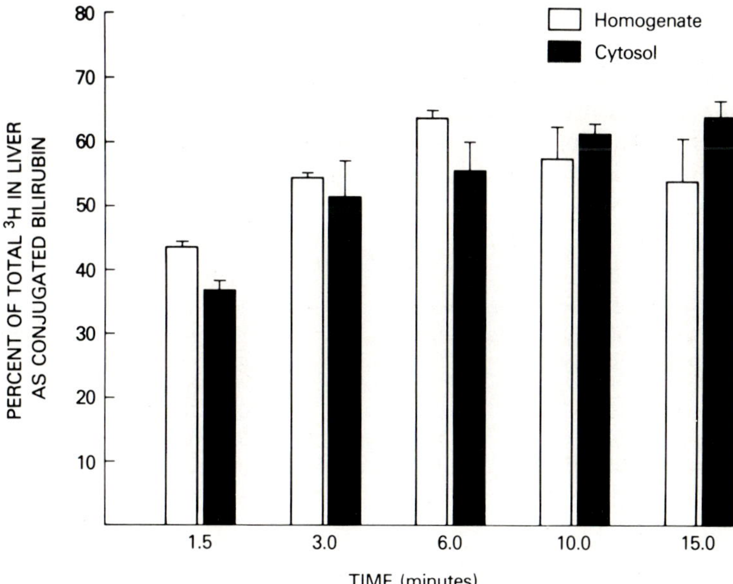

FIG. 2—Proportion of total hepatic content of ³H-bilirubin present in conjugated form. After intravenous injection of ³H-bilirubin into Sprague-Dawley rats, livers were removed at timed intervals and homogenized. The results are presented as the mean ± SEM. At all time periods, a large proportion of bilirubin that had accumulated within liver was identified as conjugated bilirubin.

The intrahepatic accumulation of both bilirubin and conjugated bilirubin is in accord with the capability for binding of these compounds to intracellular proteins, most likely ligandin and the other glutathione transferases. That these proteins are able to bind bilirubin and its conjugates with high affinity is shown in Table 2. Since the transferases also represent such a large proportion of all the soluble intrahepatic proteins, they appear to be more than reasonable candidates to account for hepatic accumulation, i.e., storage of bilirubin and its glucuronide.

On a more speculative level, these results may be related to the mode of excretion of bilirubin conjugates. Thus the formation of bilirubin monoglucuronide from bilirubin and UDP-glucuronate by a microsomal system is well established.[56] Evidence has been presented for the transesterification of 2 moles of bilirubin monoglucuronide to form bilirubin and bilirubin diglucuronide.[56] This last step is catalyzed by an enzyme preparation localized in the liver plasma membrane and found in highest concentration in the canalicular-enriched membrane fraction.[57] Localization of the last enzyme in the process at the exit gate, as it were, suggests the possibility of interaction of bilirubin monoglucuronide, perhaps bound to a ligandin, with the transesterification enzyme of the canalicular membrane thereby facilitating immediate excretion into the bile. Under such circumstances, the diglucuronide would not be expected to accumulate appreciably in the liver, which is in conformity with our observations.

The data for bilirubin and BSP should be taken as only an example of the physiologic binding function of these proteins. Many compounds that are ingested can be removed quickly from the circulation and stored while awaiting metabolic conversion to less toxic entities.

The glutathione transferases are a uniquely useful group of proteins in providing a detoxification system. Although some of the roles that have been outlined for them are speculative, any single function is an important one. These proteins are only primitive enzymes and nonspecific binding proteins, but we observe that it is precisely this simplistic design that allows such protean serviceability.

REFERENCES

1. Jakoby WB, Keen JH: A triple-threat in detoxification: The glutathione S-transferases. Trends Biochem Sci 2:229–231, 1977

2. Reyes H, Levi AJ, Arias IM: Studies of Y and Z: Two hepatic cytoplasmic organic anion-binding proteins. J Clin Invest 50:2242–2252, 1971

3. Morey KS, Litwack G: Isolation and properties of cortisol metabolite binding proteins of rat liver cytosol. Biochemistry 8:4813–4821, 1969

4. Ketterer B, Ross-Mansell P, Whitehead JK: The isolation of carcinogen-binding protein from livers of rats given 4-dimethyl-aminoazobenzene. Biochem J 103:316–324, 1967

5. Litwack G, Ketterer B, Arias, IM: Ligandin: A hepatic protein which binds steroids, bilirubin, carcinogens and a number of exogenous organic anions. Nature 234:466–467, 1971

6. Pabst MJ, Habig WH, Jakoby WB: Mercapturic acid formation: The several glutathione transferases of rat liver. Biochem Biophys Res Commun 52:1123–1128, 1973

7. Jakoby WB: The glutathione S-transferases A group of multifunctional detoxification proteins. Adv Enzymol 46:383–414, 1977

8. Habig, WH, Pabst MJ, Fleischner G, Gatmaitan Z, Arias IM, Jakoby WB: The identity of glutathione S-transferase B with ligandin, a major binding protein of liver.

Proc Natl Acad Sci USA 71:3879–3882, 1974

9. Ketley JN, Habig, WH, Jakoby WB: Rat liver glutathione S-transferases: A family of binding proteins. J Biol Chem 250: 8670–8673, 1975

10. Grover PL, Sims P: Conjugations with glutathione: Distribution of glutathione S-aryltransferase in vertebrate species. Biochem J 90:603–606, 1964

11. Levine RJ, Reyes, H, Levi AJ, Gatmaitan Z, Arias IM: Phylogenetic study of hepatic organic anion uptake mechanisms. Nature [New Biol] 231:277–279, 1971

12. Kamisaka K, Habig WH, Ketley JN, Arias, IM, Jakoby WB: Multiple forms of human glutathione S-transferase and their affinity for bilirubin. Eur J Biochem 60:153–161, 1975

13. Marcus CJ, Habig WH, Jakoby WB: Glutathione transferase from human erythrocytes: Non-identity with the enzymes from human liver. Arch Biochem Biophys 188:287–293, 1978

14. Graham A, Sjoholm I: The preparation of ligandin with glutathione S-transferase activity from porcine liver cytosol by affinity chromatography on bromosulphophthalein-Sepharose. Eur J Biochem 80:573–580, 1977

15. Kirsch R, Kamisaka K, Fleischner G, Arias IM: Structural and functional studies of ligandin, a major renal organic anion binding protein. J Clin Invest 55:1009–1019, 1975

16. Pinkus LM, Ketley JN, Jakoby WB: The glutathione S-transferases as a possible detoxification system of rat liver intestinal epithelium. Biochem Pharmacol 26:2359–2363, 1977

17. Daniel V, Smith GJ, Litwack G: Translation in vitro of rat liver messenger RNA coding for ligandin (glutathione S-transferase B). Proc Natl Acad Sci USA 74: 1899–1902, 1977

18. Bhargava MM, Listowsky I, Arias IM: Studies on subunit structure and evidence that ligandin is a heterodimer. J Biol Chem 253:4116–4119, 1978

19. Fleischner G, Robbins J, Arias IM: Immunological studies of Y protein. A major cytoplasmic organic anion-binding protein in rat liver. J Clin Invest 51:677–684, 1972

20. Jakoby WB, Ketley JN, Habig WH: Glutathione S-transferases: Binding and physical properties. Edited by IM Arias and WB Jakoby: Glutathione: Metabolism and Function. New York, Raven Press, 1976, pp 213–223

21. Habig WH, Pabst MJ, Jakoby WB: Glutathione S-transferases. The first enzymatic step in mercapturic acid formation. J Biol Chem 249:7130–7139, 1974

22. Pabst MJ, Habig WH, Jakoby WB: Glutathione S-transferase A: A novel kinetic mechanism in which the major reaction pathway depends on substrate concentration. J Biol Chem 249:7140–7148, 1974

23. Habig WH, Pabst MJ, Jakoby WB: Glutathione S-transferase AA from rat liver. Arch Biochem Biophys 175:710–716, 1976

24. Wolkoff AW, Ketley JN, Waggoner JG, Berk PD, Jakoby WB: Hepatic accumulation and intracellular binding of conjugated bilirubin. J Clin Invest 61:142–149, 1978

25. Kamisaka K, Listowsky I, Gatmaitan Z, Arias IM: Interactions of bilirubin and other ligands with ligandin. Biochemistry 14:2175–2180, 1975

26. Keen JH, Habig WH, Jakoby WB: A mechanism for the several activities of the glutathione S-transferases. J Biol Chem 251:6183–6188, 1976

27. Keen JH, Jakoby WB: Glutathione transferases: Catalysis of nucleophilic reactions of glutathione. J Biol Chem 253:5654–5657, 1978

28. Chasseaud LI: Conjugation with glutathione and mercapturic acid excretion. Edited by IM Arias and WB Jakoby: Glutathione: Metabolism and Function. New York, Raven Press, 1976, pp 77–113

29. Tate SS, Meister A: Interaction of γ-glutamyl transpeptidase with amino acids, dipeptides and derivatives and analogues of glutathione. J Biol Chem 249:7593–7602, 1974

30. Jakoby WB, Habig WH, Keen JH, Ketley JN, Pabst MJ: Glutathione S-transferases: Catalytic aspects. Edited by IM Arias and WB Jakoby: Glutathione: Metabolism and Function. New York, Raven Press, 1976, pp 189–211

31. Benson AM, Talalay P, Keen JH, Jakoby WB: Relationship between the soluble glutathione-dependent Δ^5-3-ketosteroid isomerase and the glutathione S-transferases of the liver. Proc Natl Acad Sci USA 74:158–162, 1977

32. Prohaska JR, Ganther HE: Glutathione peroxidase activity of glutathione-S-transferase purified from rat liver. Biochem Biophys Res Commun 76:437–445, 1977

33. Scher W, Jakoby WB: Maleate isomerase. J Biol Chem 244:1878–1882, 1969

34. Boyland E, Chasseaud LF: Enzyme catalyzed conjugations of glutathione with un-

saturated compounds. Biochem J 104:95–102, 1967

35. Miller EC, Miller JA: Biochemical mechanisms of chemical carcinogenesis. Edited by H Busch: Molecular Biology of Cancer. New York, Academic Press, 1974, pp 377–402

36. Sarrif AM, Heidelberg C: On the interactions of chemical carcinogens with soluble proteins of target tissues and in cell cultures. Edited by IM Arias and WB Jakoby: Glutathione: Metabolism and Function. New York, Raven Press, 1976, pp 317–338

37. Nemoto N, Gelboin HV, Habig WH, Ketley JN, Jakoby WB: K-Region benzo [a]-pyrene 4,5-oxide is conjugated by homogeneous glutathione S-transferase. Nature 255:512, 1975

38. Fjellstedt TA, Allen RH, Duncan BK, Jakoby WB: Enzymatic conjugation of alkyl epoxides with glutathione. J Biol Chem 248:3702–3707, 1973

39. Cagan LM, Pisano JJ, Ketley JN, Habig WH, Jakoby WB: The conjugation of prostaglandin A and glutathione catalyzed by homogeneous glutathione S-transferase from human and rat liver. Biochem Biophys Acta 398:205–208, 1975

40. Scarschmidt, BF, Waggoner JG, Berk PD: Hepatic organic anion uptake in the rat. J Clin Invest 56:1280–1292, 1975

41. Berk PD, Wolkoff AW, Scharschmidt BF, Shupeck M, Ketley JN, Waggoner JG, Jakoby WB: Recent studies of the metabolism of conjugated bilirubin. Edited by L Bianchi, W Gerok, and K Sickinger: Liver and Bile. Lancaster, MTP Press, 1977, pp 177–185

42. Alpert S, Mosher M, Shanske A, Arias IM: Multiplicity of hepatic excretory mechanisms for organic anions. J Gen Physiol 53:238–247, 1969

43. Paumgartner G, Reichen J: Kinetics of hepatic uptake of unconjugated bilirubin. Clin Sci Mol Med 51:169–176, 1976

44. Bloomer JR, Berk PD, Vergalla J, Berlin NI: Influence of albumin on the hepatic uptake of unconjugated bilirubin. Clin Sci Mol Med 45:505–516, 1973

45. Goresky CA: Initial distribution and rate of uptake of sulfobromophthalein in the liver. Am J Physiol 207:13–26, 1964

46. Listowsky I, Gatmaitan Z, Arias IM: Ligandin retains and albumin loses bilirubin binding capacity in liver cytosol. Proc Natl Acad Sci, USA 75:1213–1216, 1978

47. Levi AJ, Gatmaitan Z, Arias IM: Deficiency of hepatic anion binding protein, impaired organic anion uptake by liver and "physiological" jaundice in newborn monkeys. N Engl J Med 283:1136–1139, 1970

48. Wolkoff AW, Sellin J, Gatmaitan Z, Goresky CA, Arias IM: Role of ligandin in the transfer of bilirubin from plasma into the liver. Gastroenterology 73:1255, 1977

49. Cornelius CE, Ben-Ezzer J, Arias IM: Binding of sulfobromophthalein sodium (BSP) and other organic anions by isolated hepatic cell membranes in vitro. Proc Soc Exp Biol Med 124:665–667, 1967

50. Tiribelli C, Lunazzi G, Luciani M, Panfili E, Gazzin B, Liut G, Sandri G, Sottocasa G: Isolation of a sulfobromophthalein-binding protein from hepatocyte plasma membrane. Biochim Biophys Acta 532:105–112, 1978

51. Benz R, Lauger P, Janko K: Transport kinetics of hydrophobic ions in lipid bilayer membranes. Charge-pulse relaxation studies. Biochem Biophys Acta 455:701–720, 1976

52. Ketterer B, Neumcke B, Lauger P: Transport mechanism of hydrophobic ions through lipid bilayer membranes. J Membr Biol 5:225–245, 1971

53. Mia AS, Gronwall RR, Cornelius CE: Bilirubin-^{14}C turnover studies in normal and mutant Southdown sheep with congenital hyperbilirubinemia. Proc Soc Exp Biol Med 133:955–959, 1970

54. Erlinger S, Dhumeaux D, Desjeux JF, Benhamou JP: Hepatic handling of unconjugated dyes in the Dubin-Johnson syndrome. Gastroenterology 64:106–110, 1973

55. Bernstein LH, Ben-Ezzer J, Gartner L, Arias IM: Hepatic intracellular distribution of tritium labeled unconjugated and conjugated bilirubin in normal and Gunn rats. J Clin Invest 45:1194–1201, 1966

56. Jansen PLM, Chowdhury JR, Fischberg EB, Arias IM: An enzyme of liver plasma membrane which converts bilirubin monoglucuronide to bilirubin diglucuronide. J Biol Chem 252:2710–2716, 1977

57. Chowdhury JR, Jansen PLM, Fischberg EB, Daniller A, Arias IM: Hepatic conversion of bilirubin monoglucuronide to diglucuronide in uridine diphosphate-glucuronyl transferase-deficient man and rat by bilirubin glucuronoside glucuronsyltransferase. J Clin Invest 62:191–196, 1978

Chapter 12

BileAcid Metabolism in Health and Disease

By M. A. GOLDMAN, C. C. SCHWARTZ, L. SWELL,
and Z. R. VLAHCEVIC

THE RECENT SURGE of interest in various aspects of bile acid metabolism has been prompted by an extensive series of reports defining (1) the physico-chemical properties of bile acids, which account for their capacity to solubilize biliary cholesterol and dietary lipids; (2) the alteration of bile acid metabolism, which may be present in a number of diseases; and (3) the existence of an important relationship between cholesterol and bile acid metabolism. A better understanding of the basic concepts of bile acid metabolism, coupled with advances in methodology, has outlined the important role of bile acids in the pathogenesis of several diseases (i.e., cholesterol cholelithiasis, secretory diarrhea and/or steatorrhea associated with the diseases of the small bowel, etc.), which in turn has helped design effective forms of medical therapy for some of these conditions. A great deal of progress has also been made in defining the abnormalities of bile acid metabolism in parenchymal and cholestatic liver disease and in several rare diseases of inborn errors of bile acid synthesis. In view of these many new developments, a summary of current concepts of bile acid metabolism is timely, giving special emphasis to the role of bile acids in various disease states and simultaneously providing some insight into how the accrued knowledge of bile acid metabolism influences the clinician's approach to diagnosis and therapy.

BILE ACID METABOLISM IN HEALTH

Bile Acid Biosynthesis and Enterohepatic Circulation

Cholesterol is the obligatory precursor of bile acids in all species studied. The conversion of cholesterol to bile acids occurs exclusively in the liver in a series of sequential steps involving a number of intermediates (Fig. 1).[1,2] The process of conversion involves the addition of either one or two hydroxyl groups, epimerization of 3β-hydroxyl group, reduction of the double bond at C-5 and degradation of the C-27 side chain of cholesterol into a C-24 bile acid and propionic acid. In man, the major bile acids synthesized in the liver ("primary" bile acids) are cholic acid (CA) and chenodeoxycholic acid (CDCA).

From the Division of Gastroenterology, Department of Medicine, VeteransAdministration Hospital and Medical College of Virginia, Richmond, Virginia.

This work was supported in part by U.S. Public Health Service Research Grant 1R01-AM14668 from the National Institute of Arthritis and Metabolic Diseases, National Institutes of Health and the Veterans Administration.

Almost twice as much CA is synthesized daily as CDCA, but because CDCA is preserved more efficiently, about equal proportions of these two bile acids are in bile. The major synthetic pathway for CA and CDCA involves transformation of cholesterol to 7α-hydroxycholesterol, which is converted to 7α-hydroxy-4-cholesten-3-one. From this point, synthesis of CA and CDCA proceed separately (Fig. 1). The factors determining the absolute rate of CA versus CDCA synthesis are not well understood. Several alternate pathways to CA and CDCA exist in man, but their contribution to total bile acid synthesis is not known.[1,2]

The rate of bile acid synthesis is probably controlled by the magnitude, circulation rate, and composition of the bile acid pool. The mechanism by which bile acids control their own synthesis ('negative feedback') has not been clearly established in man. The rate-limiting enzyme for bile acid synthesis is cholesterol-7α-hydroxylase which catalyzes the conversion of cholesterol to 7α-hydroxycholesterol. Interruption of the enterohepatic circulation of bile

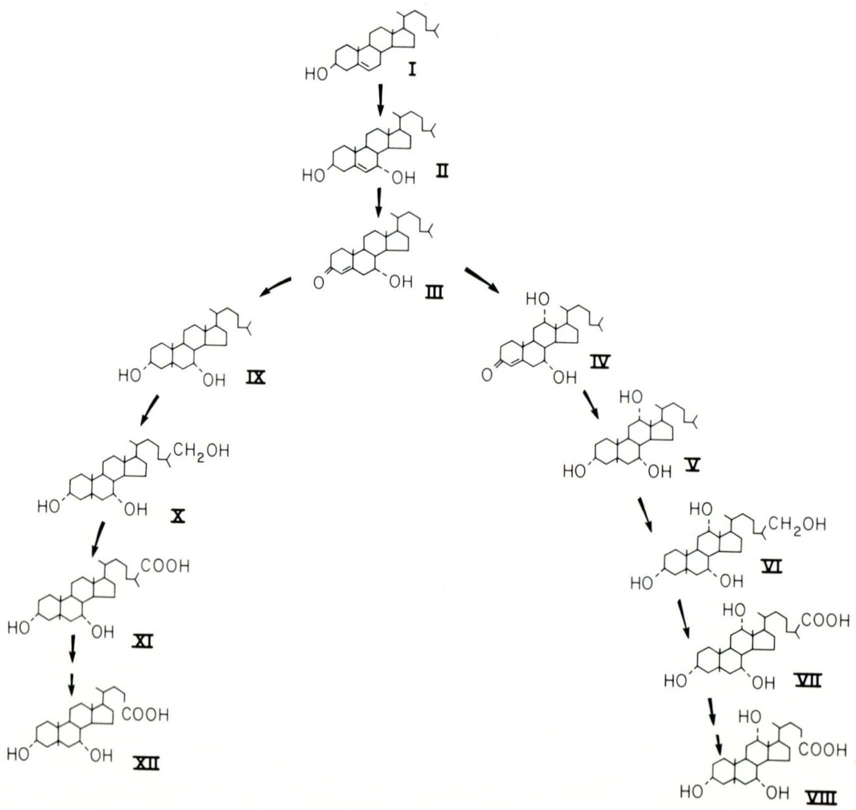

FIG. 1—Bile acid biosynthesis pathway. Cholesterol (I); 7α-hydroxycholesterol (II); 7α-hydroxy-4-cholesten-3-one (III); 7α,12α-dihydroxy-4-cholesten -3-one (IV); 5β-cholestane, 3α,7α,12α-triol (V); 5β-cholestane, 3α,7α,12α, 26-tetrol (VI); 3α,7α,12α-trihydroxy-cholestanoic acid (THCA) (VII); cholic acid (VIII); 5β-cholestane, 3α,7α-diol (IX); 5β-cholestane, 3α,7α, 26-triol (X); 3α,7α-dihydrocholestanoic acid (DHCA) (XI); chenodeoxycholic acid (XII). This schematic presentation of bile acid pathway does not include all intermediates and minor alternate pathways.

acids (total bile fistula, biliary diversion, ileal resection) or administration of cholestyramine increases hepatic 7α-hydroxylase activity and also increases bile acid synthesis severalfold. Conversely, bile acid feeding suppresses 7α-hydroxylase activity and reduces bile acid synthesis.[2]

Newly synthesized bile acids are conjugated in the liver with either glycine or taurine. The normal glycine/taurine ratio in man is about 3:1. The conjugated bile acids are not absorbed in the upper intestine in significant amounts, which enables them to participate in the process of small intestinal digestion of dietary fat. About 95% of bile acids are absorbed in the terminal ileum by an active transport mechanism, returned to the liver, reconjugated, and excreted into the biliary tree. Hepatic uptake of conjugated and free bile acids returning via portal blood is dependent on a saturable mechanism, and at physiologic levels the transport system operates far from saturation.[3] There is evidence for a bile acid receptor protein in liver surface membranes which may be responsible for the initial interaction in bile acid transport across the hepatic cell.[4] Normally, only negligible amounts of bile acids are found in the plasma. A small but significant rise in plasma bile acid concentration occurs after meals.[5] In the lower intestine, CA is dehydroxylated by the bacterial 7α-dehydroxylase enzyme to deoxycholic acid (DCA), while CDCA is converted by the same enzyme into lithocholic acid (LCA). These two bile acids are also called "secondary" bile acids. About one-third to one-half of DCA is reabsorbed in the colon and incorporated into the bile acid pool. On the average, DCA represents about 20% of the total bile acids in bile. About 20% of newly formed LCA is also absorbed. In man the absorbed LCA is not only conjugated with glycine or taurine but is also partially sulfated in the liver at the C-3 position to form sulfolithocholylglycine and sulfolithocholyltaurine. These two compounds are not well absorbed from the intestine, resulting in their rapid excretion in the feces. Consequently, the proportion of lithocholate in bile and the lithocholate pool in man remains very small.[6] LCA is known to be hepatotoxic in several animal species but not in man. It appears that effective sulfation of LCA by the liver protects man from hepatotoxic effects of this bile acid.

Studies in man have revealed the presence of small amounts of ursodeoxycholic acid (UDCA) (a 7β epimer of CDCA) in bile. This compound is considered a "tertiary" bile acid, since its formation requires both hepatic and bacterial events.[7]

The total amount of bile acids circulating in the enterohepatic circulation can be quantitatively determined by the isotope dilution technique. This method enables the calculation of individual and total bile acid pool sizes, daily bile acid synthesis, and the daily turnover rates of bile acids. Normal values for the bile acid pool sizes (individual and total), CA and CDCA synthesis, and fractional daily turnovers in man were described[8] and are shown in Table 1.

Bile is an aqueous solution in which the major solids are three biliary lipids: cholesterol, bile acids, and phospholipid (lecithin). Cholesterol, a water-insoluble compound is solubilized in bile in mixed micelles of bile salts and lecithin. Bile acid micelles are formed spontaneously above a certain level of bile acid concentration (critical micellar concentration, CMC). When lecithin is present in the solution, however, the amount of cholesterol solubilized increases about

stones secrete a bile supersaturated with cholesterol (lithogenic bile).[16] Third, formation of lithogenic bile could be caused by a decrease in the cholesterol solubilizing substances in bile (bile acid, lecithin), an excess of biliary cholesterol, or a combination of both factors.

Isotope dilution studies using labeled CA and CDCA demonstrated that Caucasian males[17] and American Indians (males and females) with cholesterol gallstones[18,19] have a significantly diminished bile acid pool size. The diminished bile acid pool in these patients may lead to a decrease in bile acid and lecithin secretion, which in turn could result in the formation of lithogenic bile and gallstones. An increase in the fractional daily turnover of bile acids (increase in bile acid loss relative to the pool size), coupled with an inappropriately low bile acid synthesis, is the most plausible explanation for the diminution of the bile acid pool size. Lithogenic bile in American Indian and Caucasian females with cholesterol gallstones is caused by an increase in biliary cholesterol secretion, which, in these individuals, is coupled with a less impressive decrease in bile acid secretion.[20,21] The mechanism responsible for the observed increase in cholesterol secretion is not known but could be related to an increase in dietary intake of cholesterol,[22] an increase in endogenous cholesterol synthesis,[23] or an increase in fluxes of plasma free cholesterol and/or newly synthesized cholesterol into a hepatic cholesterol precursor compartment associated with the excretion of biliary cholesterol.[12]

Data from nonobese patients with cholesterol gallstones and obese subjects without stones provided a unifying concept between these seemingly discrepant hypotheses.[24] These very thorough studies clearly demonstrated that cholesterol gallstone formation in nonobese patients is due to a defect in bile acid metabolism, as we postulated.[15-17] Conversely, in obese patients the predominant defect responsible for cholesterol gallstone formation seems to be related to a pronounced increase in biliary cholesterol secretion. Thus the formation of cholesterol gallstones may be associated with a spectrum of changes of biliary lipid metabolism ranging from a predominantly abnormal bile acid and phospholipid metabolism in one group of patients to a predominantly abnormal cholesterol metabolism in another group of patients. Present concepts of pathogenesis of gallstone formation in man are presented in Fig. 3.

A better understanding of the role of bile acid and lecithin in solubilization of biliary cholesterol and the presence of a conceivably correctable defect of bile acid and cholesterol metabolism in patients with cholelithiasis inevitably led to attempts of gallstone prevention and in situ stone dissolution. The initial hypothesis was that exogenously administered bile acids enlarge the bile acid pool, which in turn enhances biliary bile acid and lecithin secretion and consequently decrease lithogenicity of bile. Cholesterol stones can be dissolved if they are continuously bathed with bile unsaturated with cholesterol.[25] This hypothesis was put to the test by the demonstration that gallstone dissolution can be achieved by the prolonged exogenous administration of CDCA but not CA.[26] Several large-scale clinical trials have confirmed the effectiveness of CDCA therapy in gallstone dissolution.[27,28] Also, UDCA has been shown to be an effective and safe agent for gallstone dissolution.[29,30]

CDCA desaturates bile by decreasing biliary cholesterol secretion.[31,32] Tau-

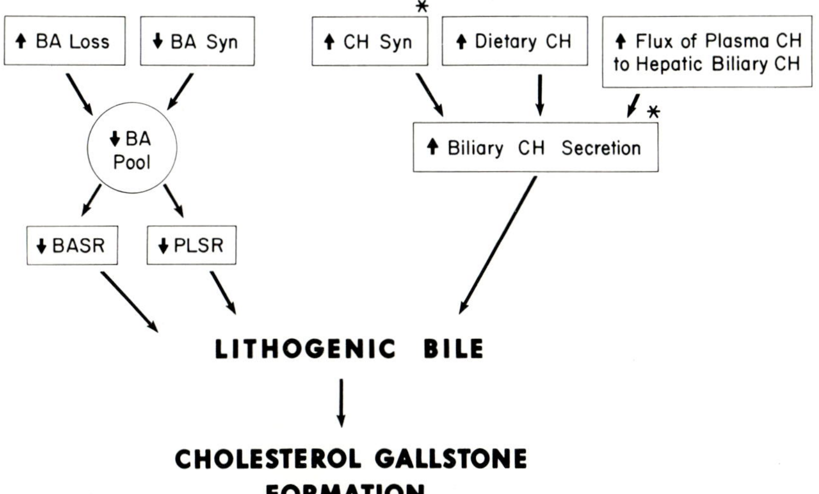

FIG. 3—Present concept of cholesterol gallstone formation in man. BA (bile acid), CH (cholesterol), BASR (bile acid secretion rate), PLSR (phospholipid secretion rate). The role of bile acid in the pathogenesis of gallstone formation was experimentally confirmed (left side of figure).[17-19,24] The asterisks designate the observations regarding CH metabolism in man which were experimentally confirmed.[20,21,31,32]

rochenodeoxycholate suppresses HMG-CoAR but has much less effect on 7α-hydroxylase enzyme, while taurocholate inhibits both enzymes similarly.[33] These studies were supported in man by several investigators[23,34] who showed inhibition of HMG-CoAR by the CDCA feeding. In view of CDCA depression of HMG-CoAR activity, the observed decrease in biliary cholesterol secretion may be secondary to a decrease in cholesterol synthesis. This hypothesis, however, has not been universally accepted, and additional studies are necessary to clarify the specific effect of CDCA on hepatic cholesterol metabolism. Several studies[31,32] demonstrated that the effectiveness of CDCA and the lack of effectiveness of CA in dissolving gallstones are related to their differential effects on biliary cholesterol secretion rather than to enlargement of the bile acid pool size or an increase in bile acid and phospholipid secretion rates. No significant correlation was found between cholesterol secretion and HMG-CoAR activity during CDCA therapy, in contrast to that found in patients with cholesterol gallstones on no therapy.[35] This observation therefore suggests that factors other than a decrease in cholesterol synthesis may be responsible for a decrease in biliary cholesterol secretion after administration of CDCA. UDCA desaturates bile probably in a manner similar to that of CDCA, i.e., by decreasing biliary cholesterol secretion.[36]

The potential side effects of long-term CDCA administration to man have been carefully studied. First, an increased production and absorption of LCA in the colon could lead to hepatotoxicity, since this bile acid has uniformly caused liver injury in every animal species tested.[37] In nonhuman primates (rhesus monkey and baboons) CDCA feeding results in unequivocal liver injury.[38,39] Rhesus monkey sulfates LCA quite poorly, as most of the LCA in bile is nonsulfated.[40] Because hepatic necrosis and cirrhosis in rabbits are proportional to the dose of LCA and CDCA[41] and antibiotics decrease liver injury after CDCA feeding,[42] liver injury after CDCA in animals is probably related to the amount of LCA formed in the intestine. Many liver biopsies were carried out in man during long-term CDCA therapy. The evidence suggests that CDCA therapy has not been associated with significant liver damage.[43] Elevations of amino transferase activity occur in 25% of patients, but they are transient and are not associated with morphologic abnormalities. The lack of LCA toxicity in man is attributed to effective sulfation of this bile acid by the liver.[44] Second, CDCA could both enhance cholesterol absorption and suppress 7α-hydroxylase activity; these effects could result in an increase of total body cholesterol. The long-term studies, however, have not shown a significant increase in serum cholesterol[43] or an increase in the exchangeable cholesterol mass.[45] Long-term studies determining the effect of CDCA on cholesterol absorption and metabolism in man have not been carried out; occasional diarrhea appears to be the only major complication associated with CDCA therapy.

By contrast with CDCA, the administration of UDCA to rhesus monkeys did not result in abnormal findings in liver function tests or in structural changes in the liver. Biliary LCA did not change appreciably. Therefore, UDCA may be safer than CDCA in the medical therapy of cholelithiasis.[46]

The long-term usefulness of CDCA or UDCA for gallstone dissolution is not fully evaluated. Dissolution of gallstones requires 6 to 12 months of continuous therapy, but the bile becomes lithogenic shortly after these bile acids are stopped, and recurrent stones have been documented in about 20% of patients after a 6- to 43-month follow-up.[43]

Bile Acid Metabolism in Hyperlipoproteinemia

Hyperlipoproteinemic states are associated with abnormalities in bile acid metabolism. Type IIa hyperlipoproteinemia is characterized by a subnormal synthesis of CA, a defect compensated by a higher CDCA synthesis so that total primary bile acid synthesis is normal. The reason for a specific reduction of CA synthesis in this disease is not known.[47] In type IV hyperlipoproteinemia an abnormally high incidence of cholesterol cholelithiasis was observed. Despite the increased incidence of cholesterol gallstones in type IV, the bile acid pool size in these patients is similar to normal subjects.[47] Thus the major underlying reason for gallstone development in these patients is not in altered bile acid metabolism but more likely in a poorly defined abnormality of cholesterol metabolism resulting in enhanced biliary cholesterol secretion.

Bile Acid Metabolism in Intestinal Diseases

The small intestine plays a central role in the preservation of the enterohepatic circuit. Consequently, in diseases of the small bowel, some abnormality of bile acid metabolism is to be expected. Loss of the ileal surface following ileitis, ileal resection, or ileal bypass results in an increased loss of bile acids to the colon and subsequent diarrhea or steatorrhea. Clinical implications of these events were described in a series of articles.[48-50] If the degree of ileal loss is not severe (e.g., < 100 cm of ileum resected or < 20 g of fat excreted in stool per day), patients had watery diarrhea that responded to cholestyramine administration, suggesting that diarrhea is secondary to bile acid malabsorption. Bile acid concentration in the small intestine in this group of patients is not significantly decreased. These patients had an increase in bile acid synthesis which increased still further after cholestyramine. In vivo and in vitro, DCA and CDCA (but not CA) induced active sodium and water secretion in the colon.[51,52] Further studies support the contention that bile acids stimulate colonic electrolyte secretion by increasing mucosal cyclic AMP.[53] When ileal loss is more extensive (> 100 cm of ileum resected and steatorrhea > 20 g/ day) fat malabsorption and subsequent steatorrhea result. Bile acid concentration in the upper small intestine is decreased, which results in an inadequate micellar solubilization of fat. Diarrhea in these patients does not respond to cholestyramine treatment. Removal of the long-chain triglyceride from the diet and administration of MCT, the absorption of which is not dependent on micellar solubilization, are indicated in these patients.[49] Findings from these studies could probably be extrapolated to subjects with regional ileitis without ileal resection.

Regional ileitis and other diseases with abnormal bowel motility (blind loops, jejunal diverticulosis, scleroderma, diabetes) are frequently associated with bacterial overgrowth in the small intestine, which in turn results in enhanced deconjugation of bile acids, rapid absorption of free bile acids in the proximal jejunum, and subsequently fat maldigestion and steatorrhea (contaminated small bowel syndrome, CSBS). Under these circumstances steatorrhea may be alleviated with the use of appropriate antibiotics. Chronic intractable diarrhea in children under 5 years of age, frequently a major health problem in developing countries, is associated with a striking alteration of bacterial microflora and subsequent steatorrhea. These malnourished children have decreased intestinal bile acid concentrations, elevation of intestinal free bile acid to conjugated bile acid ratios, and incomplete micellar solubilization of fat after a standard lipid meal.[54] Moreover, long-lasting perturbations of bile acid metabolism were observed in the setting of malnutrition even in children recovering from the diarrhea.

A bile acid breath test was developed as an aid in the diagnosis of ileal dysfunction and/or bacterial overgrowth syndromes.[55] The rationale for the test is based on the observation that in cases of bacterial overgrowth in the small intestine the deconjugation of bile acids increases and that the labeled amino acid moiety of conjugated bile acid is exhaled as $^{14}CO_2$. In all patients with stasis and bacterial overgrowth and in most patients with ileal resection and bile acid malabsorption, $^{14}CO_2$ specific activity is significantly higher than in matched controls. The combined measurement of $^{14}CO_2$ in breath and ^{14}C in stool after administration of ^{14}C cholylglycine is quite specific and a sensitive test for the CSBS and bile acid malabsorption, respectively.[56]

Metabolism of bile acids is also altered in adult celiac disease. The bile acid pool is large, bile acid synthesis is normal, and bile acid half-life is prolonged in these patients.[57] These findings were attributed to reduced gallbladder contractability presumably secondary to defective release of cholecystokinin from the abnormal small bowel mucosa. The observed increase in bile acid pool size presumably was a result of a decreased loss of bile acids via feces due to less frequent recycling of EHC in the face of unchanged or increased bile acid synthesis.

A common problem in the practice of gastroenterology is chronic diarrhea without an obvious organic cause, which is frequently considered to be a part of the clinical presentation of functional bowel disease. Diarrhea in at least some of these patients may be related to the selective malabsorption of bile acids in the ileum. Some patients with chronic diarrhea of no obvious etiology have increased fecal ^{14}C radioactivity after oral administration of ^{14}C cholylglycine coupled with an increase in fractional turnover rates of bile acids.[58] The latter findings and response of long-standing diarrhea to cholestyramine suggest that idiopathic bile acid malabsorption may be present in these patients.

Bile Acids in Gastric Ulcer, Gastritis and Esophageal Reflux

Bile has been implicated as a possible noxious agent in the pathogenesis of gastric ulcer. This hypothesis is supported by the observation that reflux of bile acids into the stomach of patients with gastric ulcers is higher than in normal controls.[59] The increase in bile reflux in these patients may be due to pyloric sphincter dysfunction, i.e., an inappropriate response to secretin and cholecystokinin.[60] The damaging agent to the gastric mucosa could be bile acids or lysolecithin, either of which could damage the gastric mucosal barrier.[61,62] Bile reflux has been implicated in the gastritis associated with the Billroth II gastrectomy procedure. Circumstantial evidence has implicated bile reflux in the pathogenesis of reflux esophagitis.[63] The effectiveness of cholestyramine in the therapy of these conditions has not been adequately tested.

Bile Acid Metabolism in Liver Disease

In considering the disturbances of bile acid metabolism produced by liver disease, the central role of the liver in almost all phases of bile acid metabolism must be appreciated. These include synthesis and conjugation of bile acids, maintenance of the integrity of the EHC, and control of the size and composition of the bile acid pool. Liver disease (parenchymal or cholestatic) should significantly alter bile acid metabolism.

Acute and Chronic Liver Disease

Impaired hepatocytic function and significant portal-systemic shunts in patients with acute and chronic liver disease alter the EHC by shunting bile acids away from the liver.[64] As a result of this shunting, serum and urinary bile acids are elevated in these patients. Significant proportions of the urinary bile acids are sulfated in patients with liver disease. Renal clearance of sulfated bile acids is 20 to 200 times greater than the clearance of nonsulfated bile acids.[65] A striking abnormality is found in primary bile acid metabolism in cirrhotic patients.[66] The size of the CA pool in these patients is greatly decreased owing to a large reduction in CA synthesis. By contrast, the CDCA pool and synthesis are not significantly altered. Decrease in CA synthesis correlates well with the advancement of liver disease. Despite a conspicuous decrease in the size of the total bile acid pool, cirrhotic patients show no significant propensity to cholesterol gallstone formation mainly because of a simultaneous decrease in cholesterol secretion, the net result of which is the formation of bile undersaturated with cholesterol.[67]

Patients with cirrhosis also have a defect in secondary bile acid metabolism, since they frequently lack DCA in bile and plasma.[68,69] Impaired absorption of DCA from the colon and rehydroxylation of DCA to CA are excluded as possible causes for the absence of DCA in the bile of these patients.[68] Oral feeding of CA does not result in enhanced DCA production, suggesting that reduced CA substrate is probably not a reason for the absence of DCA from bile.[68] Fecal extracts from cirrhotic patients convert CA to DCA less efficiently than do extracts from normal subjects, suggesting a big decrease in 7α-dehydroxylase activity possibly owing to subtle abnormalities in the colonic milieu of these patients.[69]

Very elevated serum bile acid levels have been noted in acute hepatitis which greatly exceed those observed in chronic hepatitis, cirrhosis, or extrahepatic obstruction. The postprandial serum bile acid level was reported to be as sensitive as SGOT in the detection of mild hepatic dysfunction.[71] Elevated serum bile acids have also been reported in chronic active hepatitis (CAH) and, to a lesser extent, in patients with chronic persistent hepatitis.[72] Fasting serum levels of cholyl conjugates obtained by radioimmunoassay may provide a more sensitive index for the presence of histologically active disease than do conventional "liver function" tests. Serum bile acid tests may also be a better predictor of relapse of CAH than SGOT activities. A study of bile acid metabolism in patients with Wilson's disease has revealed that serum CA and biliary bile acid composition in these patients is similar to that in a control group.[74] The clearance of intravenously administered glycine conjugate of CA is delayed in all patients with Wilson's disease, however.

Serum bile acids in alcoholic liver disease have been correlated with liver biopsy findings.[75] Patients with fatty livers did not have elevated serum bile acids. Alcoholic hepatitis and cirrhosis were accompanied by increased serum bile acids in 93%, while only 43% of these patients had increased serum bilirubin levels. The CA to CDCA ratio was reversed, and the levels of secondary bile acids were uniformly decreased in these patients.

Cholestasis

Profound disturbances of bile acid metabolism have also been noted in cholestasis.[76] Because of the impediment of bile acid flow from the liver, less bile acids reach the EHC with subsequent spillover into the systemic circulation, ascites, skin, etc. A variety of bile acids heretofore not known to exist in normal subjects have been described in patients with cholestasis. Many of these bile acids are present as sulfate esters or glucuronides.[77,78] The renal clearances of sulfated bile acids and glucuronides are approximately the same, suggesting that both represent important metabolic pathways in these patients. A number of bile acids in these patients still remain unidentified. Only a small amount of LCA has been found in the bile, serum, or urine of patients with severe cholestasis.[67,76] Since the EHC in these patients is efficiently interrupted, bacterial formation of LCA is decreased. Therefore, this bile acid in the urine may be formed de novo in the liver probably via an alternative pathway from cholesterol.[79] This hypothesis is strengthened by the finding of LCA in the urine but not the feces of patients with biliary atresia.[80]

Normal subjects excrete less than 1.5 mg/day of bile acids in the urine (5% to 15% sulfated). In cholestatic syndromes, as much as 150 mg of bile acids may be eliminated daily. More than 50% of the urinary bile acids are sulfated. Other polar metabolites, such as glucuronides, may account for 12% to 20% of urinary bile acids in cholestasis. No significant differences in the sulfation of bile acids can be detected between patients with extrahepatic obstruction, hepatitis, cirrhosis, and liver metatasis.[77]

One of the cardinal symptoms of cholestasis is pruritus. The evidence is conflicting concerning the role of bile acids in itching. In general, the serum bile acid level correlates with the presence or absence of itching. A high concentration of bile acids in the skin (particularly dihydroxy) has been suggested to cause itching.[81] By contrast, a consistent correlation was not observed between pruritus and either serum bile acid levels or the bile acid concentration in the skin.[82] This does not exclude the possibility that a less known bile acid may be responsible for pruritus in cholestasis. These findings are difficult to interpret in view of the known beneficial effect of cholestyramine in the therapy of pruritus.

Patients with primary biliary cirrhosis and cholestasis have 12% to 35% of monohydroxy bile acids in their serum. By contrast, these bile acids are not detectable in patients without cholestatic features. Cholestyramine causes a conspicuous reduction in serum bile acids but does not consistently relieve pruritus.[83] Serum bile acids are increased in a great majority of patients with advanced primary biliary cirrhosis.[84] Patients with an early clinical and histologic disease have normal serum bile acids. The response of pruritus and the serum bile acid pattern to cholestyramine may be used as a rough indicator to differentiate between surgical and nonsurgical jaundice.[85] In addition to cholestyramine, phenobarbital has been used with some success to relieve itching in patients with primary biliary cirrhosis, benign recurrent cholestasis, and intrahepatic biliary atresia. Phenobarbital relieves itching presumably by increasing biliary bile acid secretion, but the mechanism by which phenobarbital exerts this effect is not well understood.

Bile Acids and Colon Cancer

Epidemiologic studies have implicated dietary factors in the wide geographical variation in the incidence of colon cancer. Animal fat and protein provide 40% of the calories in the average diet in the United States, where the incidence of colon cancer is higher than in Japan. This westernized diet has been associated with an elevation of fecal neutral and acidic steroids as well as changes in the colonic microflora. Conversely, fecal steroid excretion falls to a lower level after 4 weeks on a meat-free diet.[86]

Some bile acids (DCA, LCA) are colonic tumor promoters in rats.[86] A population with a higher incidence of cancer has a higher fecal count of *Bacte-*

roides and a higher concentration of fecal sterols than a population with low incidence of cancer.[87,88] The correlation was good between the incidence of colonic cancer and DCA, suggesting that this bile acid may be a carcinogen or a cocarcinogen. There is a similarity between polycyclic aromatic carcinogens (e.g., 20-methylcholanthrene) and bile acids; i.e., DCA can be converted chemically into 20-methylcholanthrene. Conceivably, bacteria can facilitate this conversion in the colon. The concentration of dehydrogenating clostridia was also significantly elevated in cancer patients.[88] However, uniform agreement on the abnormality of bile acid metabolism in patients with colonic cancer is lacking.[89] Confirmation of a pathogenetic role for bile acids requires identification of putative carcinogens and/or prospective studies wherein individuals with altered colonic flora and abnormal metabolism of bile acids are shown to be at increased risk for colon cancer.

Inborn Errors of Bile Acid Synthesis

Several syndromes have been described in which there is a primary defect in bile acid synthesis. The best known is cerebrotendinous xanthomatosis (CTX), a disease characterized clinically by dementia, paresis, xanthomatosis, premature arteriosclerosis, and cataracts. Multiple abnormalities of sterol and bile acid metabolism have been described in this disease entity: (1) an increased deposition of cholestanol in the tissues associated with a low normal serum cholesterol, (2) an increase in cholesterol synthesis, (3) increased excretion of cholesterol precursors in bile, (4) a decreased proportion of CDCA and a virtual absence of secondary bile acids in bile, and (5) C-25 hydroxy bile alcohols in bile and feces.[90] 5β-Cholestane-$3\alpha,7\alpha,12\alpha$, 25-tetrol and the series of pentols were identified in these patients, which suggested impaired oxidation of the cholesterol side chain, resulting in the production of CA via an alternative pathway, i.e., 25-hydroxylation pathway. To inhibit enhanced cholesterol and cholestanol synthesis, CDCA was administered to these patients.[91] Cholesterol and cholestanol synthesis decreased during CDCA treatment, suggesting that this drug may arrest the progression of this rare disease.

Another inborn error of bile acid biosynthesis was described in 2 children with severe intrahepatic cholestasis.[92] They had a substantial increase of trihydroxy cholestanoic acid (THCA) in bile. This bile acid is an intermediate in CA synthesis (see Fig. 1) and is present in normal human bile in trace amounts only. The excessive amount of THCA in the bile of these patients results from a specific block in the process of side chain oxidation of CA.[93] Interestingly, the defect seems to be specific for CA synthesis, since CDCA synthesis appears to be normal.

Cystic Fibrosis

Fecal bile acids are significantly increased in children with untreated cystic fibrosis (CFP) and pancreatic insufficiency.[94] A strong correlation was found between fecal fat and bile acids in CFP in contrast to celiac disease. The mechanism responsible for the greater bile acid loss in these patients is unknown, but products of maldigestion may interfere with bile acid absorption. In 6 patients with cystic fibrosis studied before and during pancreatic enzyme supplementation, the bile acid pool was decreased prior to therapy, whereas bile acid synthesis, turnover rate, and fecal excretion were increased.[95] Pancreatic replacement therapy increased fat absorption and the bile acid pool size.

The progress in our understanding of bile acid metabolism in man in the last 10 years is truly remarkable. Because of space limitations, it is impossible to describe many other worthy achievements in this field. The major progress is to be expected from the basic studies aimed at a better understanding of cholesterol and bile acid interrelationships as they may hold a clue to at least some diseases of lipid metabolism.

REFERENCES

1. Mosbach EH, Salen G: Bile acid biosynthesis. Pathways and regulation. Am J Dig Dis 19:920–929, 1974
2. Danielsson H, Sjovall J: Bile acid metabolism. Annu Rev Biochem 44:233–253, 1975
3. Reichen J, Paumgartner G: Kinetics of taurocholate uptake by the perfused rat liver. Gastroenterology 68:132–136, 1975
4. Accatino L, Simon FR: Identification and characterization of a bile acid receptor in isolated liver surface membranes. J Clin Invest 57:496–508, 1976
5. LaRusso NF, Korman MG, Hoffman NE, Hofmann AF: Dynamics of the enterohepatic circulation of bile acids. N Engl J Med 291:689–692, 1974
6. Cowen AE, Korman MG, Hofmann AF, Cass OW, Coffin SB: Metabolism of lithocholate in healthy man. II. Enterohepatic circulation. Gastroenterology 69:67–76, 1975
7. Federowski T, Salen G, Colalillo A, Mosbach EH, Hall JC: Metabolism of ursodeoxycholic acid in man. Gastroenterology 73:1131–1137, 1977
8. Vlahcevic ZR, Miller JR, Farrar JT, Swell L: Kinetics and pool size of primary bile acids in man. Gastroenterology 61:85–90, 1971
9. Admirand WH, Small DM: The physicochemical basis of cholesterol gallstone formation in man. J Clin Invest 47: 1043–1052, 1968
10. Smith FR, Bell RB, Noble RP, Goodman DeW: Parameters of the three-pool model of the turnover of plasma cholesterol in normal and hyperlipidemic humans. J Clin Invest 57:137–148, 1976
11. Quarfordt SH, Greenfield MF: Estimation of cholesterol and bile acid turnover in man by kinetic analysis. J Clin Invest 52: 1937–1945, 1973
12. Schwartz CC, Berman M, Vlahcevic ZR, Halloran LG, Gregory DH, Swell L: Multicompartmental analysis of cholesterol metabolism in man. Characterization of the hepatic bile acid and biliary cholesterol precursor sites. J Clin Invest 61:408–423, 1978
13. Schwartz CC, Halloran LG, Vlahcevic ZR, Gregory DH, Swell L: Preferential utilization of free cholesterol from high-density lipoproteins for biliary cholesterol secretion in man. Science 200:62–64, 1978
14. Halloran LH, Schwartz CC, Vlahcevic ZR, Nisman RM, Swell L: Evidence for high-density lipoprotein-free cholesterol as the primary precursor for bile-acid synthesis in man. Surgery 84:1–7, 1978
15. Swell L, Gregory DH, Vlahcevic ZR: Current concepts of the pathogenesis of cholesterol gallstones. Med Clin North Am 58:1449–1471, 1974
16. Vlahcevic ZR, Bell CC Jr, Swell L: Significance of the liver in the production of lithogenic bile in man. Gastroenterology 59:62–68, 1970
17. Vlahcevic ZR, Bell CC Jr, Buhac I, Farrar JT, Swell L: Diminished bile acid pool size in patients with gallstones. Gastroenterology 59:165–173, 1970
18. Vlahcevic ZR, Bell CC Jr, Gregory DH, Buker G, Juttijudata P, Swell L: Relationship of bile acid pool size to the formation of lithogenic bile in female Indians of the Southwest. Gastroenterology 62:73–79, 1972
19. Bell CC Jr, McCormick WC, Gregory DH, Law DH, Vlahcevic ZR, Swell L: Relationship of bile acid pool size to the formation of lithogenic bile in the male Indians of the Southwest. Surg Gynecol Obstet 134: 473–478, 1972
20. Grundy SM, Metzger AL, Adler RD: Mechanisms of lithogenic bile formation in

American Indian women with cholesterol gallstones. J Clin Invest 51:3026–3043, 1972

21. Grundy SM, Duane WC, Adler RD, Aron JM, Metzger AL: Biliary lipid outputs in young women with cholesterol gallstones. Metabolism 23:67–73, 1974

22. Den Besten L, Connor WE, Bell S: The effect of dietary cholesterol on the composition of human bile. Surgery 73:266–273, 1973

23. Coyne MJ, Bonorris GG, Goldstein LT, Schoenfield LJ: Effect of chenodeoxycholic acid and phenobarbital on the rate-limiting enzymes of hepatic cholesterol and bile acid synthesis in patients with gallstones. J Lab Clin Med 87:281–291, 1976

24. Shaffer EA, Small DM: Biliary lipid secretion in cholesterol gallstone disease. The effect of cholecystectomy and obesity. J Clin Invest 59:828–840, 1977

25. Naunyn B: A Treatise on Cholelithiasis. New Sydenham Society 1896, p 22

26. Thistle JL, Hofmann AF: Efficacy and specificity of chenodeoxycholic acid for dissolving gallstones. N Engl J Med 289:655–659, 1973

27. Iser JH, Dowling RH, Mok YIH, Bell DG: Chenodeoxycholic acid treatment of gallstones. N Engl J Med 293:378–383, 1975

28. Coyne MJ, Bonorris GC, Chung A, Goldstein LI, Lahuna D, Schoenfield LJ: Treatment of gallstones with chenodeoxycholic acid and phenobarbital. N Engl J Med 292:604–607, 1975

29. Makino I, Shinozaki G, Yoshino K, Nakagawa S: Dissolution of cholesterol gallstones by ursodeoxycholic acid. Jpn J Gastroenterol 72:690–691, 1975

30. Thistle JL, Turcott J, Ott BY, Carlson GL, LaRusso NF, Hofmann AF: Ursodeoxycholic acid unsaturates bile at a lower dose than chenodeoxycholic acid. Gastroenterology 74:1103–1109, 1978

31. Northfield TC, LaRusso NF, Hofmann AF, Thistle JL: Biliary lipid output during three meals and an overnight fast. II. Effect of chenodeoxycholic acid treatment in gallstone subjects. Gut 16:12–17, 1975

32. LaRusso NF, Hoffman EN, Hofmann AF, Northfield CT, Thistle JL: Effect of primary bile acid ingestion in bile acid metabolism and biliary lipid secretion in gallstone subjects. Gastroenterology 69:1301–1314, 1975

33. Shefer S, Hauser S, Lapar V, Mosbach EH: Regulatory effects of sterols and bile acids on hepatic 3-hydroxy-3-methylglutaryl CoA reductase and cholesterol 7α hydroxylase in the rat. J Lipid Res 14:573–580, 1973

34. Salen G, Nicolau G, Shefer S: Chenodeoxycholic acid inhibits elevated hepatic HMG-CoA reductase activity in subjects with gallstones. Clin Res 21:523, 1973

35. Key PH, Bonorris GG, Marks JW, Schoenfield LJ: Mechanism of cholesterol desaturation of bile by chenodeoxycholic acid in gallstone patients. Gastroenterology 74:1161, 1978

36. Von Bergman K, Gutsfeld M, Schulze-Hogen K, von Vuruh G: Effect of ursodeoxycholic acid on biliary lipid secretion in patients with radiolucent gallstones. Adv Bile Acid Res. V. Bile Acid Meeting (in press)

37. Palmer RH: Bile acids, liver injury and liver disease. Arch Intern Med 130:606–617, 1972

38. Webster KH, Lancaster MC, Wease DF: Influence of primary bile acid feeding on cholesterol metabolism and hepatic function in the rhesus monkey. Mayo Clin Proc 50:134–138, 1975

39. Morrissey KP, McSherry CK, Swarm RL: Toxicity of chenodeoxycholic acid in the non-human primate. Surgery 77:851–860, 1975

40. Gadacz RT, Allan NR, Mach E, Hofmann AF: Impaired lithocholate sulfation in rhesus monkey. A possible mechanism for chenodeoxycholic toxicity. Gastroenterology 70:1125–1129, 1976

41. Fisher CD, Cooper SN, Rothschild AM, Mosbach EH: Effect of dietary chenodeoxycholic acid and lithocholic acid in the rabbit. Am J Dig Dis 19:877–886, 1974

42. Salen G, Dyrszka H, Chen T, Saltzwan HW, Mosbach EH: Prevention of chenodeoxycholic acid toxicity with lincomycin. Lancet 1:1082, 1975

43. Dowling RH: Chenodeoxycholic acid therapy of gallstones. Clin Gastroenterol 6:141–163, 1977

44. Allan RN, Thistle JL, Hofmann AF: Lithocholate metabolism during chenotherapy for gallstone dissolution. II. Absorption and sulfation. Gut 17:413–419, 1976

45. Pedersen L, Arnfred T, Thaysen HE: Cholesterol kinetics in patients with cholesterol gallstones before and during chenodeoxycholic acid treatment. Scand J Gastroenterol 9:787–791, 1974

Chapter 13

Lipoprotein Disturbances in Liver Disease

By SEYMOUR M. SABESIN, M.D., JAMES B. RAGLAND, Ph.D., *and*
MICHAEL R. FREEMAN, M.D.

THE MAIN FUNCTION of lipoproteins is the transport of lipids in the plasma. Except for the intestinal synthesis of chylomicrons, the liver is the major source of plasma lipoproteins. In addition to its function in lipoprotein biosynthesis, the liver subserves a central role in lipoprotein metabolism. As the complexities of normal plasma lipoprotein metabolism have been gradually elucidated, it has become apparent that the profound lipid and lipoprotein abnormalities of liver disease reflect derangements in the regulation of an exceedingly intricate process. This chapter provides a conceptual framework of lipoprotein metabolism, emphasizing the central role of the liver, and describes the disturbances of this process that occur in liver disease and in extrahepatic biliary obstruction.

GENERAL ASPECTS OF PLASMA LIPOPROTEIN METABOLISM

The lipoproteins normally found in fasting plasma represent the end products of the metabolism of lipoproteins secreted primarily by the liver and the intestine.[1-3] Preparative methods of separation using the ultracentrifuge led to the present-day system of nomenclature. The most commonly used procedure involves the sequential ultracentrifugation of plasma at increasing solution densities and isolation of each fraction within a predetermined density range. Each fraction has a characteristic electrophoretic mobility. Chylomicrons do not move during paper electrophoresis, while low-density lipoprotein (LDL) migrates with beta, very low density lipoprotein (VLDL) with pre-beta, and high-density lipoprotein (HDL) with alpha$_1$ globulins. Each of these lipoprotein classes has a characteristic lipid and protein composition.

Lipoproteins can also be recognized by their morphologic features when examined by electron microscopy using negatively stained preparations (Figs. 1, 2, and 3), and each lipoprotein class has a characteristic appearance and size range. These size ranges are indicated in Table 1.

The protein moieties of the various lipoprotein classes are very heterogeneous. The individual proteins are referred to as apoproteins or apolipoproteins and are written as the prefix, apo, with a letter designation for type. Each of

From the Division of Gastroenterology, Department of Medicine, University of Tennessee Center for the Health Sciences, Memphis, Tennessee.

The work from our division cited in this review was supported by grants from the National Institutes of Health AM-17398, the American Heart Association, the Tennessee Heart Association, and the Veterans Administration.

243

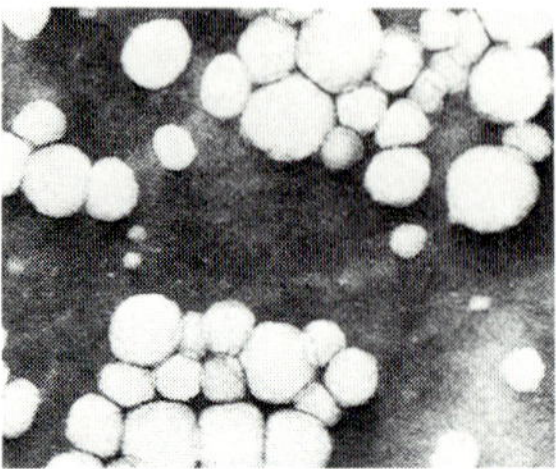

FIG. 1—Electron micrograph of isolated normal plasma VLDL negatively stained with 2% phosphotungstic acid ($\times$ 95,000).

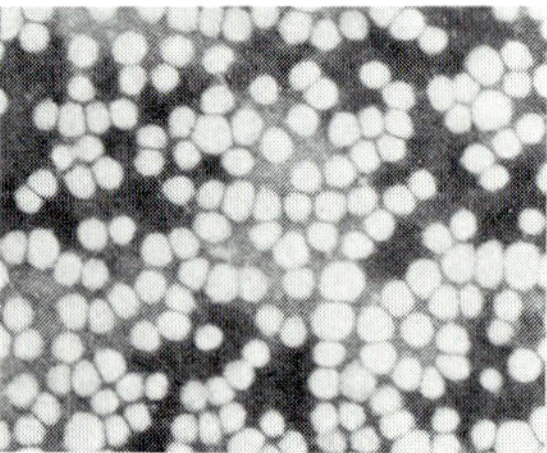

FIG. 2—Electron micrograph of isolated normal plasma LDL, stained as in Fig. 1 ($\times$ 95,000).

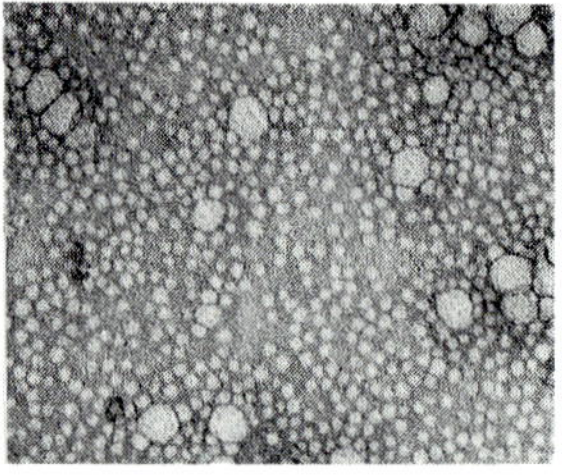

FIG. 3—Electron micrograph of isolated normal plasma HDL, stained as in Fig. 1 ($\times$ 95,000).

these apoproteins has a specific function either in transporting a particular type of lipid class or in acting as a cofactor for enzymes involved in lipoprotein metabolism. Table 1 summarizes data relative to the characterization of the various lipoprotein classes. This classification of lipoproteins represents a segregation based on the methods of separation rather than a reflection of functional or physiologic differences. Newer techniques of separation and characterization make it increasingly apparent that much more heterogeneity exists in lipoprotein types than previously thought and that the physiologic functions and metabolic interrelationships among these various classes overlap considerably.

Chylomicrons

Chylomicrons are involved primarily in the transport of triglycerides of exogenous origin which are absorbed from the gastrointestinal tract. In plasma, chylomicrons must acquire certain apoproteins of the C group by exchange with lipoproteins of liver origin before they can be metabolized.

VLDL

Most of the endogenously formed triglycerides in plasma are present in the VLDL, primarily synthesized in the liver, although some VLDL is made in the gut from endogenously synthesized triglycerides. Nascent or secretory VLDL is different in composition from circulating plasma VLDL. The extent to which

TABLE 1.—*Characterization of Plasma Lipoproteins*

Name	Density	Electrophoretic Mobility	Major* Lipids	Major Apoproteins	% Protein	Diameter Å
CM†	.95	origin	$\simeq$ 90% TG	CIII, B, CI, CII, AI	2	> 1000
VLDL	<1.006	alpha-2	$\simeq$ 60% TG	C, B, E	10	300–800
LDL	>1.006<1.063	beta	$\simeq$ 50% CE	B	25	170–250
HDL	>1.063<1.21	alpha-1	$\simeq$ 80% CE phospholipid 1:1	AI, AII, C	50	75–150

* TG, triglycerides; CE, cholesteryl esters
† CM, chylomicrons

the cholesterol and phospholipids of circulating VLDL represent those of nascent VLDL is not known. The apoprotein content of circulating VLDL includes apo C (55% to 60% of total protein), apo B (35% to 40%), and apo E as most of the remainder. The apoprotein composition of nascent VLDL, however, is different; most of the apo C is acquired during the metabolism of nascent VLDL to circulating VLDL. The one apoprotein that is essential for the formation and secretion of triglyceride-rich VLDL and also chylomicrons is apo B.[4]

Incorporation of labeled amino acids into lipoprotein apoproteins has been studied by liver perfusion.[5] The incorporation of labeled amino acids into the apo B of VLDL is much higher in proportion to that incorporated into apo C. Apo C is not detectable in lipoproteins isolated from Golgi cisternae of rat intestinal mucosa. However, apo C has been detected in hepatocytic Golgi complexes, which may also have nascent HDL known to contain apo C.[6] The VLDL, isolated from hepatocytic Golgi complexes are relatively poor activators of lipoprotein lipase, an enzyme that requires the presence of apo C. Nascent VLDL may contain little, if any, apo C.[4] Further evidence that nascent VLDL contains primarily apo B comes from our own studies of severe alcoholic hepatitis in which the VLDL found in fasting plasma, at the peak of the illness, contains more than 90% apo B, which may represent accumulation of nascent VLDL.[7]

HDL

The other type of lipoprotein synthesized and secreted by the liver is nascent HDL, which is different in structure and composition from the HDL found in fasting plasma. Nascent HDL, isolated from rat liver perfusates,[8] consists primarily of protein, high levels of phospholipid, and unesterified cholesterol. HDL obtained from liver perfusates, containing an lecithin/cholesterol acyltransferase (LCAT) inhibitor to prevent the rapid metabolism of nascent HDL, appears almost entirely as 45-Å thick and 200-Å diameter disk-shaped particles similar to those found in familial LCAT deficiency. This HDL fraction contains much apo E and relatively little apo AI, normally the major constituent (85%) of the protein of circulating HDL. When radiolabeled amino acids were added to rat liver perfusates,[9] the major labeled apoprotein in HDL was apo E and very little label was incorporated into apo AI of perfusate lipoproteins. Nascent HDL accumulating in hepatic perfusates in the presence of LCAT inhibitor are a preferred substrate for LCAT.[8] We found a similar nascent HDL accumulating in the plasma of patients with severe alcoholic hepatitis in whom LCAT

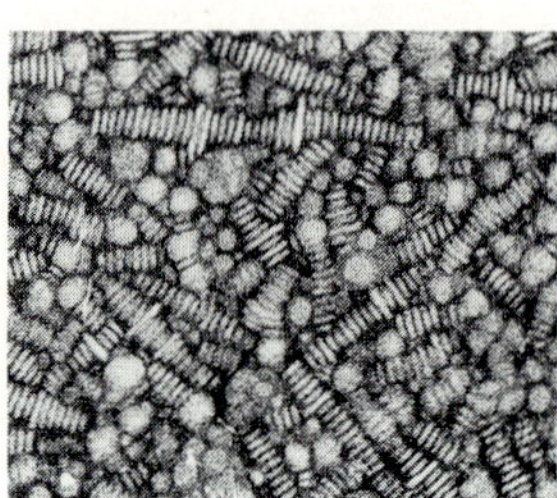

FIG. 4—Electron micrograph of isolated plasma HDL negatively stained with 2% phosphotungstic acid. HDL is from a patient with alcoholic hepatitis (× 95,000).

and cholesteryl esters may be almost absent in plasma.[10] The protein moiety of HDL consists of only apo E, apo C, and apo AII in these patients. Apo AI is not found in HDL until recovery begins. The human nascent HDL fraction is very similar in lipid composition to rat nascent HDL, is a preferred LCAT substrate, and also appears as stacked bilamellar disks (Fig. 4).

LDL

The major lipoprotein of human plasma, LDL, does not appear to be directly synthesized by the liver but is formed almost entirely in plasma from the metabolism of VLDL.[4] LDL contains almost only apo B. The principal lipid component of LDL is esterified cholesterol, which appears to be transferred from HDL after formation as a result of LCAT activity.[10,11]

LCAT

Of great significance in lipoprotein metabolism are the hepatic synthesis and secretion of LCAT. The manner in which LCAT is secreted is not known; most of the enzyme is derived from the liver, since it is almost absent in hepatectomized animals and is severely deficient in many types of liver disease. LCAT transfers a fatty acyl group (usually polyunsaturated) from the 2 position of lecithin to cholesterol to form cholesteryl esters. Indeed, LCAT appears to be responsible for all the cholesteryl esters found in plasma under normal conditions. Nascent HDL has been suggested to be the principal substrate for this enzyme, and as a result of its action, nascent HDL is converted to cholesteryl ester-rich normal HDL, rich in apo AI.[8,10] Most cholesteryl esters formed as a result of LCAT activity are transferred to the pathway leading from VLDL to LDL.[11] Apo AI is a required activator of this enzyme and is also the major apoprotein constituent of normal HDL, the product of the reaction. There is some question as to the source of apo AI in plasma. Although some apo AI is synthesized by the liver, it does not appear to be a principal secretory product when labeled amino acid precursors are used in perfusion systems.[9] Immunofluorescent studies have shown that apo AI is actively synthesized by rat small intestine during lipid absorption and that it is the major apoprotein of mesenteric lymph chylomicrons.[12] Rat intestine may also secrete a discoid-like high-density lipoprotein containing primarily apo AI.[13] Thus, a significant portion of plasma apo AI may be derived from intestinal sources.

Lipoprotein Lipase

The other major enzyme involved in the transformation and metabolism of plasma lipoproteins is lipoprotein lipase (LPL), an enzyme that hydrolyzes the triglycerides of both chylomicrons and VLDL. LPL is found principally in adipose tissue, heart and skeletal muscles, lactating mammary glands, and lung.[14] The liver is important in this reaction because it synthesizes and secretes nascent HDL, which contains the apo CII required for LPL activation. Chylomicrons and VLDL are apo-C-deficient when secreted and acquire these apoproteins after entering plasma. In addition, apo CIII secreted by the liver acts as an inhibitor of LPL, as does apo E, the principal constituent of nascent HDL.[15] Following metabolism of VLDL and chylomicrons by lipoprotein lipase and the associated transfer to these particles of cholesteryl esters derived from the action of LCAT, remnant lipoprotein particles are formed. VLDL remnants are metabolized to LDL by the further action of lipoprotein lipase, and most of the apoproteins, other than apo B, are lost. A significant portion of the remnants is metabolized by the liver which contains a heparin-releasable lipase attached to the hepatocytic plasma membrane designated hepatic triglyceride lipase (H-TGL).[16] H-TGL may be important in the final removal of triglyceride from the remnant particles during their catabolism by the liver.

Catabolism of Lipoproteins

Considerably less is known about the catabolism of plasma lipoproteins than is known about their synthesis and transformation within the plasma compartment. The major site of catabolism of chylomicron remnants and HDL appears to be the liver. These lipoproteins are taken up by the liver as intact particles and metabolized inside the hepatocyte.[16-21] These conclusions are based primarily on studies of clearance of lipoproteins in hepatectomized animals, lipoprotein uptake by perfused livers, and uptake and accumulation of isotopically labeled lipoproteins by the liver. To what extent LDL is catabolized by the liver is not clear, and peripheral tissues may be very important in the removal of LDL from the circulation.[22]

A study of hydrolysis of chylomicron cholesteryl esters by cell free preparations of rat liver, in which the activities of different cholesteryl ester hydrolases in liver cells were compared, led to the conclusion that a plasma membrane-bound enzyme was not necessary to hydrolyze chylomicron cholesteryl esters before their uptake by hepatocytes.[23] Cholesteryl esters could be hydrolyzed without the prior hydrolysis of triglyceride, and lysosomal enzymes could degrade both cholesteryl esters and triglycerides of chylomicron remnants taken up by endocytosis. Heparin stimulated the uptake of chylomicron remnants by hepatocyte monolayers, in contrast to its inhibition of receptor-mediated binding of LDL to fibroblasts.[24] The fact that the heparin concentrations used were high enough to release membrane-bound hepatic lipase from the cells mitigates against this enzyme being involved in binding of remnants during remnant degradation by the liver. The role of H-TGL in triglyceride hydrolysis of lipoproteins has recently been examined in intact rats and isolated perfused liver.[25] Using cycloheximide, a protein synthesis inhibitor, synthesis of H-TGL by hepatocytes was shown and its transport to the cell surface was inhibited by colchicine. Furthermore, chloroquine, known to inhibit lysosomal enzymes, decreased H-TGL degradation. From these results H-TGL was suggested to reside near a lipoprotein remnant receptor; it may be interiorized during remnant endocytosis and may play a role in triglyceride hydrolysis within the lysosome. The metabolism of VLDL remnants in rats is very similar to that of chylomicron remnants.[26]

The capacity of homogenates of human liver, rat parenchymal cells, and rat nonparenchymal cells in the degradation of human and rat HDL and LDL has been studied.[27] Parenchymal cells are unable to catabolize LDL. Nonparenchymal cells may do so to a limited extent, however. Parenchymal cells can metabolize HDL, and nonparenchymal cells possess a high capacity to degrade

HDL, accounting for more than 50% of the liver's capacity for HDL protein breakdown and cholesteryl ester hydrolysis. Thus, LDL is probably the main transport mechanism for cholesterol to extrahepatic tissue, while HDL represents the primary vehicle for transport of cholesterol to the liver for catabolism. HDL catabolism by the liver may involve a sequence of binding, uptake, and finally proteolytic degradation, and the hepatocyte membrane may have a specific receptor site for apo AI.[28] Liver lysosomes may be the principal site of HDL proteolytic degradation, just as they appear to be for chylomicron and VLDL remnants.[28]

Role of the Liver

The liver thus secretes two types of nascent lipoproteins: one is a nascent VLDL, rich in triglyceride and apo B, and the other is nascent HDL, rich in phospholipid, unesterified cholesterol, apo E, apo C, and apo AII. Following its entry into plasma, nascent HDL is acted upon by LCAT, an enzyme also secreted by the liver, and cholesterol is esterified and transferred to the pathway leading from nascent VLDL to remnant particles and LDL. Apo C is transferred to nascent VLDL and chylomicrons. Apparently, apo E, perhaps in association with esterified cholesterol, is also transferred to nascent VLDL.[10] As VLDL is degraded to LDL, cholesteryl esters accumulate as triglycerides are removed. Intermediates in this pathway are further metabolized to LDL with loss of apo E and apo C. Some of the apo C is transferred back to the apo AI-rich, normal HDL, which is the product of LCAT activity.

ULTRASTRUCTURAL ASPECTS OF HEPATIC LIPOPROTEIN ASSEMBLY AND SECRETION

Studies utilizing in vitro techniques, or isolated hepatic perfusion, have shown that the liver is the major site of VLDL biosynthesis. Recent concepts of the steps involved in lipoprotein synthesis indicate that the apoproteins are synthesized by ribosomes on the rough endoplasmic reticulum (RER) and subsequently translocated to RER cisternae. The enzymes involved in triglyceride and cholesterol synthesis are located in the smooth endoplasmic reticulum (SER). Association of the lipid and the apoprotein moieties probably occur at the junction of SER and RER. The final assembly, concentration, and glycosylation of the lipoproteins probably take place within the Golgi apparatus (Fig. 5). Secretory vesicles, derived from the Golgi apparatus, containing nascent VLDL then migrate to the cell surface and secrete their contents across the hepatocyte plasma membrane (Fig. 6) into the perisinusoidal space of Disse.[29]

LIPOPROTEIN ABNORMALITIES IN LIVER DISEASE

Because certain characteristic abnormalities arise secondary to impairment of hepatic parenchymal function and somewhat different lipid abnormalities are thought to be of cholestatic origin, we have divided this discussion into two sections. This is, in many respects, an arbitrary distinction, as parenchy-

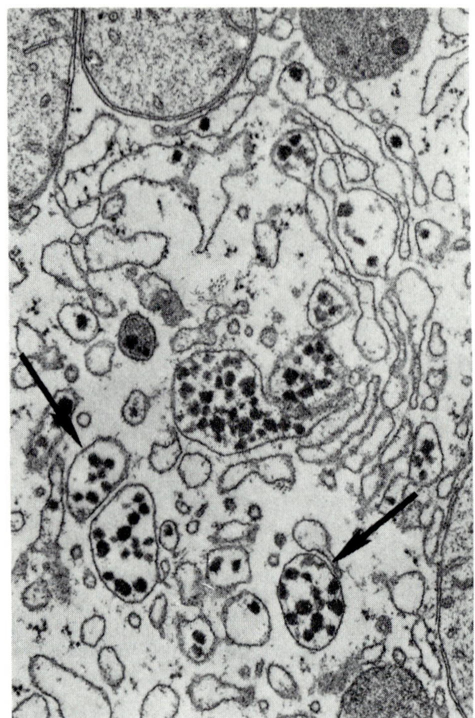

FIG. 5—Electron micrograph of rat liver demonstrating the accumulation of VLDL-size particles in the Golgi apparatus. Note the formation of secretory vesicles (arrows) containing VLDL ($\times$ 30,000).

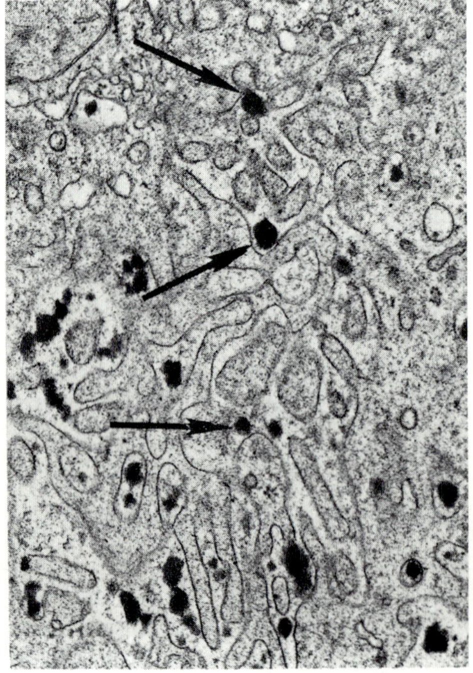

FIG. 6—Electron micrograph of rat liver showing secretion of VLDL-size particles into hepatic sinusoids (arrows) ($\times$ 27,000).

mal injury is frequently accompanied by intrahepatic cholestasis, and biliary obstruction, particularly if chronic, may produce secondary parenchymal disease. In an individual patient, therefore, the lipid and lipoprotein abnormalities may depend upon the relative predominance of parenchymal or cholestatic injury. Classification of the abnormalities into those secondary to impaired hepatocellular function and those of cholestatic origin is derived, to a certain extent, from animal studies and should be extrapolated to human liver disease cautiously.

Lipoprotein Disturbances in Parenchymal Liver Disease

On initial screening, patients with acute hepatocellular injury (e.g., alcoholic or viral hepatitis) have increased plasma triglycerides, decreased percentage of cholesteryl esters, and abnormal lipoprotein electrophoretic patterns (Fig. 7). Many of these abnormalities may be related to deficiencies of enzymes of hepatic origin such as LCAT[30] and H-TGL.[31,32] Correlation of the enzyme deficiencies with the composition of plasma lipoproteins acutely and then during recovery, when these parameters normalize, provides a means of understanding the in vivo role of the various hepatic factors that influence normal lipoprotein metabolism. Absence of alpha and pre-beta bands and a wide, densely staining beta band is a characteristic and reproducible feature of acute viral hepatitis[33] and other diffuse hepatic lesions such as alcoholic hepatitis (Fig. 7). These abnormalities gradually normalize with clinical recovery. The absence or presence of the alpha band in a series of 57 patients with viral hepatitis was a sensitive prognostic indicator.[34] Of 11 patients admitted with evidence of hepatic encephalopathy, 6 survivors showed evidence of a returning alpha band prior to recovery, while in 5 fatal cases the alpha band never returned. Traces of an alpha band returning prior to clinical improvement was frequently observed in sequential studies.[34]

The normal equivalence of alpha, beta, and pre-beta bands with HDL, LDL, and VLDL does not hold true in liver disease. Indeed, patients with acute hepatitis with an absent alpha band on electrophoresis have high-density li-

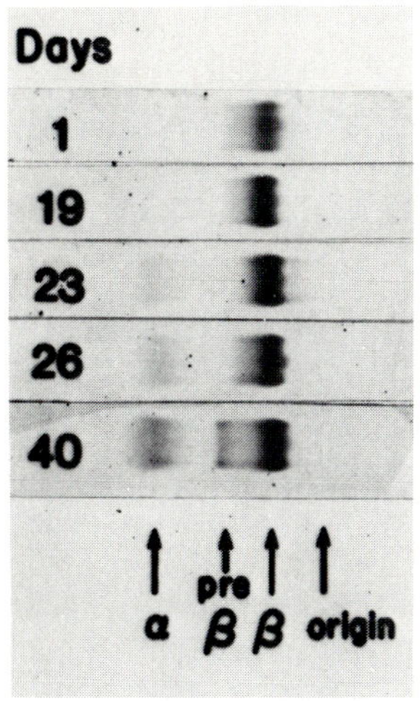

FIG. 7—Plasma lipoprotein electrophoretic pattern obtained during the course of illness and recovery in a patient with alcoholic hepatitis. Lipoprotein electrophoresis performed on agarose. Note the absence of an alpha band during the first 19 days of illness and the presence of a single abnormal band migrating between beta and pre-beta. These changes gradually returned to normal with clinical improvement.

poproteins of abnormal composition and morphology[35] which migrate as a component of the broad beta band.[36] VLDL can be isolated by ultracentrifugation even though pre-beta lipoproteins are absent on agarose electrophoresis in liver disease.[37]

Liver injury has been suggested to lead to the production of an apo AI with altered lipid binding ability to account for all the electrophoretic abnormalities.[37] However, support for this hypothesis is tenuous at best. A more plausible explanation is that the abnormal HDL of liver disease[35] represents a nascent HDL[10] that cannot be converted to "normal" HDL in an LCAT-deficient state. As nascent HDL contains predominantly apo E and lacks normal amounts of apo AI,[8] surface charge could be altered, leading to abnormal mobility.

A characteristic feature of acute hepatocellular injury is hypertriglyceridemia. Triglycerides are usually mildly elevated in most patients in the range of 150–300 mg/dl. Numerous studies have demonstrated hypertriglyceridemia in acute phases of hepatic injury which gradually returns to normal values with resolution of the disease.[34,36,38] Figure 8 demonstrates the initial elevation in serum triglycerides during acute phases of viral hepatitis and subsequent return toward normal with improvement in hepatic function. Unlike most conditions associated with hypertriglyceridemia in which the triglyceride is present in chylomicrons or VLDL, the excess triglycerides of liver disease are usually found in the LDL fraction.[31,36] Since LDL particles are too small to scatter light, the plasma may remain clear even in the presence of moderate hypertriglyceridemia. The triglyceride-rich LDL of acute hepatitis may represent the accumulation of lipoprotein remnants secondary to impaired hepatic remnant clearance.[31]

In 22 patients with hypertriglyceridemia and acute hepatitis, there was evidence of an abnormal triglyceride-rich LDL.[31] This lipoprotein, designated beta$_2$ lipoprotein, accounted in large measure for the elevated serum triglycerides and was thought to represent chylomicron remnants. Also present in

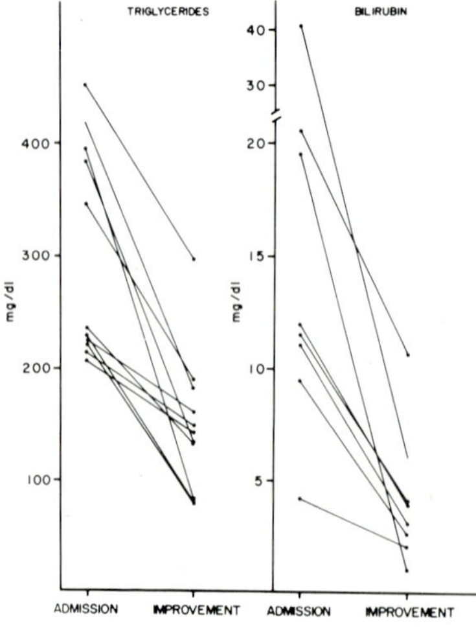

FIG. 8—Plasma triglycerides and bilirubin levels in patients with acute viral hepatitis determined on admission and at the time of clinical improvement.

the LDL class were "normal" LDL and lipoprotein-X, the characteristic lipoprotein of cholestasis (see below). Patients with normal serum triglycerides lacked evidence of beta[2] lipoprotein. Decreased H-TGL was found in two patients;[31] subsequently, decreased H-TGL and LPL in three similar patients was reported.[38] In a larger series,[32] we reported a decrease in H-TGL activity and found normal LPL in patients with acute liver disease. The discrepancy between the lipoprotein lipase values in these studies may reflect methodologic differences. Since the required cofactor for lipoprotein lipase, apo CII, is synthesized by the liver,[5] parenchymal liver injury may result in decreased or maldistributed circulating apo CII and thus reduced in vivo lipoprotein lipase activity.

Elevated LDL triglyceride in acute hepatitis may be secondary to a deficiency of H-TGL. The recent observation that H-TGL deficiency is associated with the appearance of a triglyceride-rich LDL in patients with chronic renal disease supports this hypothesis.[39] A definite physiologic role for H-TGL has not been established, however. Its location in the liver (site of remnant lipoprotein removal in animals), its wide spectrum of activity against lipid compounds, and its lack of required cofactors have led some investigators to infer that H-TGL is involved in remnant lipoprotein catabolism, although direct evidence for this is lacking. Indeed, in two conditions marked by the appearance of remnant-like lipoproteins (familial LCAT deficiency[40] and familial dysbetalipoproteinemia[41]), H-TGL levels are normal.[16,42] The H-TGL deficiency in liver disease may therefore not be related to the accumulation of the triglyceride-rich LDL. Nevertheless, the liver probably is involved in the final catabolism of remnant lipoproteins, and hepatocellular injury may lead to decreased clearance of these particles.

Abnormalities of cholesteryl esterification in hepatic disease received more attention than the hypertriglyceridemia and abnormal electrophoretic patterns. In 1932, Epstein made an important distinction between alterations associated with biliary obstruction and those due to parenchymal injury.[43] While the percentage of cholesterol present in the esterified form is decreased in both situations, the pathogenesis of the decreased cholesteryl esters is different. He observed that the concentration of cholesteryl esters in many obstructed patients may remain constant or even increase. With the larger increase in unesterified cholesterol, however, the percentage of cholesteryl esters is reduced. Conversely, in severe parenchymal injury, the total cholesterol was usually normal or decreased. Therefore, Epstein speculated that the decrease in the percentage of cholesteryl esters was due primarily to the inability of the damaged hepatocyte to produce cholesteryl esters, not because it could not produce LCAT. Thus the concept of hepatic synthesis of esterified cholesterol was the rationale for the utilization of the ester/free cholesterol ratio as a common clinical liver function test. The presence of the intracellular hepatic enzymes acyl-CoA/cholesterol acyltransferase (ACAT) and cholesteryl ester hydrolase in animals supported the idea that the liver produced cholesteryl esters. However, the repeated failure to demonstrate ACAT in human liver and the probable lysosomal location of cholesteryl ester hydrolase[44] argue against primary intrahepatic biosynthesis of cholesteryl ester in man.

Plasma LCAT activity is sufficient to account for all the plasma esterified cholesterol.[45,46] Furthermore, the rate of cholesteryl ester formation in vitro secondary to LCAT activity agrees with the estimated turnover rates of plasma cholesterol in vivo.[46] The importance of the liver in the production of this key enzyme, as well as its cofactor and principal substrate, provides a sufficient basis to explain the disturbances of cholesterol esterification that accompany liver injury. Plasma from patients with liver disease contains increased lecithin and unesterified cholesterol and decreased lysolecithin and cholesteryl ester, findings that are strikingly similar to those found in familial LCAT deficiency.[47] Familial LCAT deficiency is characterized by profound deficiency of cholesteryl esters in the absence of liver disease, confirming the negligible role of intrahepatic cholesteryl ester synthesis.

In vitro cholesterol esterification was studied in 254 patients with various forms of liver disease.[30] The 76 patients with viral hepatitis had decreased esterification activity, which gradually increased with clinical recovery. Subsequent investigators, utilizing more refined assay techniques, verified that LCAT activity is decreased in most patients with liver disease and that LCAT deficiency is the major, if not the only cause for the decreased plasma cholesteryl esters.[36,48-53] LCAT values and cholesteryl esters are closely related to the extent of liver damage and increase with clinical recovery[48,49,51,52,54,55] (Fig. 9). The prognostic significance of the severity of LCAT deficiency is emphasized by the protracted course of clinical recovery and decreased survival in patients with initially very low LCAT values.[30,56] The sometimes poor correlation of LCAT with results of standard liver functions tests[48,49,57] may reflect the limitations of these tests.

The mechanisms of the apparent LCAT deficiency have caused considerable controversy. Bile salts inhibit LCAT in vitro,[46] and elevation of serum bile salts has been suggested to explain the decreased LCAT activity of liver disease. However, the bile salt concentration, even in very severe liver disease, seems incapable of suppressing LCAT activity.[48,57] Mixed incubation studies have consistently failed to reveal LCAT inhibitors in plasma in liver disease.[47,49,51,52,57] A decrease in LCAT secondary to a deficiency of the re-

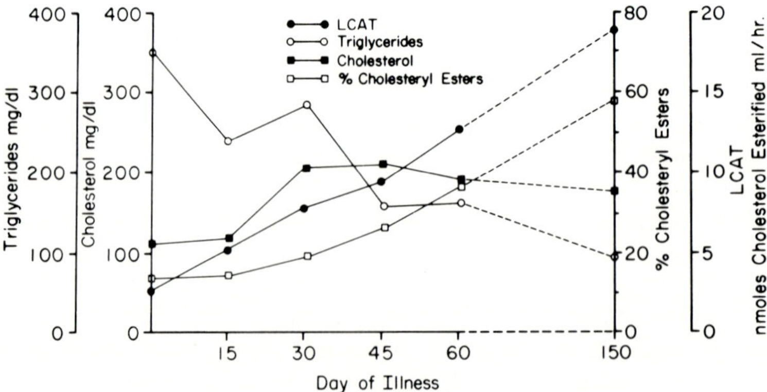

FIG. 9—Plasma lipids and lecithin/cholesterol acyltransferase (LCAT) activity obtained during the course of illness in a patient with alcoholic hepatitis.

quired cofactor or other activators has been largely excluded by similar experimental evidence.[48-50] Still another explanation for the decreased LCAT activity, accumulation of an abnormal unreactive substrate, is also excluded by mixed incubation experiments.[47-49,56] A decrease in plasma cholesterol esterification could result from the liberation of cholesteryl ester hydrolase from intracellular sites owing to disruption of the functional integrity of the hepatocyte plasma membrane.[44] It was proposed that the net cholesterol-esterifying ability of plasma is the end result of LCAT promoting and cholesteryl ester hydrolase opposing esterification.[57] However, a study utilizing a separate, independent assay for cholesteryl ester hydrolase failed to detect this enzyme in 13 patients.[56] "Cholesteryl-esterifying ability"[57] was closely correlated with independent assay of LCAT in a group of 25 patients, suggesting that "net cholesteryl esterification" can be equated with LCAT activity even in liver disease.[56] Similar LCAT deficiencies are found in hepatectomized animals.[58] LCAT deficiency and serum lipoprotein abnormalities similar to those seen in human acute hepatitis are found in hepatic parenchymal injury produced by ethionine,[59] carbon tetrachloride,[60] or galactosamine.[61] These data lead to the conclusion that LCAT deficiency is a primary result of decreased enzyme synthesis by the damaged liver. Until sufficient purification of human LCAT is achieved to permit immunologic quantitation of LCAT protein, a primary deficiency of LCAT cannot be proven absolutely.

Alterations in serum lipoproteins in chronic parenchymal liver disease are similar to those of acute liver injury but are usually less striking. Electrophoretic patterns generally show a trace of alpha, absent pre-beta, and normal to dense beta bands,[33] but they may be normal.[52] The cholesteryl esters have been reported as normal[54] to slightly decreased,[30,47,49,52] and LCAT is usually somewhat depressed.[30,49,50,52,54] As in acute liver disease, the determination of LCAT activity may be of prognostic importance. In 69 patients with cirrhosis, there were 11 deaths, all but 2 occurring in subjects with LCAT deficiency.[30] Two patients with normal LCAT activity died from ruptured esophageal varices, while the other 9 died of hepatic insufficiency, hemorrhage, or primary hepatic carcinoma. Lipoprotein abnormalities when seen in chronic liver disease probably reflect continuing hepatic injury.

Lipoprotein Disturbances in Cholestasis

Many of the lipid and lipoprotein abnormalities of parenchymal liver disease are also found in cholestasis. We feel that these abnormalities arise as a result of secondary hepatocellular dysfunction, and thus the pathogenesis of the abnormalities is similar or identical. One abnormality of cholestatic liver disease appears to be primarily the result of biliary stasis, however. The presence of an abnormal lipoprotein, lipoprotein-X (Lp-X), is a characteristic feature of cholestasis.

Lp-X, the circulating form of the increased phospholipid[62] and free cholesterol[63] seen in obstructive liver disease, was inferred by Russ et al.,[64] elucidated by Switzer,[65] and subsequently confirmed by a series of experiments by Seidel and co-workers.[66-69] In Lp-X, phospholipid and free cholesterol are complexed in roughly a 1:1 molar ratio with albumin, bile acids, and apoproteins of the

C group[46,73] to form a lipoprotein that floats at the density of LDL.[69,70] Only traces of cholesteryl ester and triglyceride are present, and apo B, the main component of normal LDL, is absent.[66,69] A minor degree of heterogeneity in protein composition has recently been discovered among subpopulations of Lp-X by Patsch et al.,[71] who have divided Lp-X into Lp-X$_1$, Lp-X$_2$, and Lp-X$_3$ on the basis of slight differences in buoyant densities. Initially the apo C component was mistakenly believed to be a unique new apoprotein, designated apo X, and therefore the total complex was designated lipoprotein-X (Lp-X). Lp-X appears as 400–600 Å diameter, 100-Å-thick disks with a tendency to form rouleaux.[70] Lp-X has the peculiar property of cathodal migration on agar gel electrophoresis that permits its ready qualitative and semiquantitative determination in whole plasma.

Lp-X has been suggested to be a highly sensitive and specific indicator of extrahepatic[54,65-68] and intrahepatic[47,54,68] cholestasis. One study concluded that the combined determination of LCAT and Lp-X could serve to differentiate between intrahepatic and extrahepatic cholestasis, a distinction of great clinical importance.[47] A subsequent study has concluded, however, that such assays are unable to discriminate between the two conditions.[54] The qualitative determination of Lp-X cannot differentiate between intrahepatic cholestasis and extrahepatic obstruction,[68] but quantitatively, patients with extrahepatic obstruction tend to have higher concentrations of Lp-X,[72,73] and this may serve to differentiate extrahepatic obstructive jaundice from that secondary to parenchymal injury.

An LDL fraction that accumulates in familial LCAT deficiency[74] appears similar to Lp-X in morphology,[35,70] lipid content, and cathodal migration in agar. However, the Lp-X-like LDL of familial LCAT deficiency is probably not identical to the Lp-X found in cholestasis.[75,76] Even though a lipoprotein of similar morphology and composition is found in familial LCAT deficiency and cholestasis, completely different pathogenetic mechanisms are present. The term "lipoprotein-X" should be reserved for the well-characterized low-density lipoprotein found in cholestasis and should not be applied to other conditions in which excess serum phospholipid leads to lipoproteins resembling Lp-X in some respects. Excess phospholipid in plasma, regardless of its origin (e.g., biliary source or accumulation secondary to LCAT deficiency), may lead to formation of phospholipid/cholesterol vesicles similar to Lp-X.

Although the origin of Lp-X is uncertain, the two most likely hypotheses are biliary regurgitation and substrate accumulation secondary to LCAT deficiency. Supporters of the latter hypothesis stress the presence of an Lp-X-like lipoprotein in sera from patients with familial LCAT deficiency and the fact that the composition of Lp-X from liver disease patients (free cholesterol and phospholipid in roughly an equimolar ratio) seems to represent an accumulation of LCAT substrate. Cholestatic plasma may indeed enchance LCAT activity,[47,49] inferring that Lp-X, directly or indirectly, is a preferred LCAT substrate. LCAT is decreased in many patients with biliary obstruction,[30,47-49,77] and an inverse relationship was observed between Lp-X and LCAT,[77] suggesting that LCAT deficiency leads to an accumulation of excess substrate that aggregates as Lp-X. The concept that cholestatic plasma, containing Lp-X, is a superior LCAT substrate has been challenged. One study showed that LCAT activity was decreased in cholestatic plasma,[50] while another showed that Lp-X had no effect on LCAT activity.[78] Highly purified Lp-X can inhibit LCAT, and Lp-X concentration remains constant even upon prolonged incubation with an LCAT source.[79] The decrease in LCAT is variable in obstructive jaundice, and LCAT may be normal, or even increased, in some patients.[54] The variation in LCAT activity is not accompanied by concomitant alterations in Lp-X which is consistently present in cholestasis. Numerous studies have documented normal LCAT activity in cholestasis, particularly when it is of short duration, as in acute cholelithiasis.[30,47,54] It appears that patients with decreased LCAT have a longer duration of cholestasis than do patients with normal LCAT,[30,47,50] suggesting that LCAT is decreased only after prolonged cholestasis causes secondary hepatocellular necrosis. Patients with primary biliary cirrhosis may have pronounced cholestasis but little hepatocellular destruction until late in the disease. Lp-X is consistently detected in these patients, but LCAT activity is usually in the upper normal range, particularly when autologous serum is utilized as the LCAT substrate.[48,49,52] This evidence indicates that the LCAT deficiency and Lp-X formation are independent events and that Lp-X results from biliary stasis, whereas LCAT reflects hepatocellular injury.

The bile regurgitation hypothesis of Lp-X formation in cholestasis is becoming widely accepted. Lp-X is thought to arise secondary to regurgitation of a biliary precursor into the plasma with subsequent plasma conversion into Lp-X at a rate sufficient to overcome normal removal mechanisms. Support for this hypothesis is as follows:

1. Electron microscopy of livers of bile-duct-ligated mice shows no evidence of Lp-X-like structures inside the hepatocyte, even though occasional particles similar to Lp-X are visualized in the space of Disse and in the plasma.[80]
2. Biliary lipid is complexed with albumin, and the lipid content of the biliary lipoprotein is almost identical to Lp-X.[81] Upon exposure to serum, biliary lipoprotein assumes the characteristic electrophoretic behavior and protein composition of Lp-X and can be converted back to biliary lipoprotein upon exposure to bile salts.
3. Anastomosis of the bile duct with the venous circulation results in the rapid appearance of Lp-X.[81]
4. When Lp-X is present following experimental bile duct ligation, the lecithin component contains fatty acyl moieties dissimilar to normal LDL and similar to biliary lecithin.[82]
5. With bile duct ligation, phospholipids increase in plasma, biliary lipids decrease, and labeled biliary lecithin appears rapidly in plasma.[82] With bile duct ligation in the rat, phospholipid and free cholesterol greatly increase in plasma (presumably Lp-X), while LCAT and cholesteryl ester are only initially increased.[83]
6. Phospholipid infused into animals results in increased serum cholesteryl ester levels, possibly due to leaching of membrane cholesterol.[84] Similar studies in man show an increase in cholesteryl esters predominantly in LDL as a result of lecithin infusion with transient elevations of phospholipid.[85]

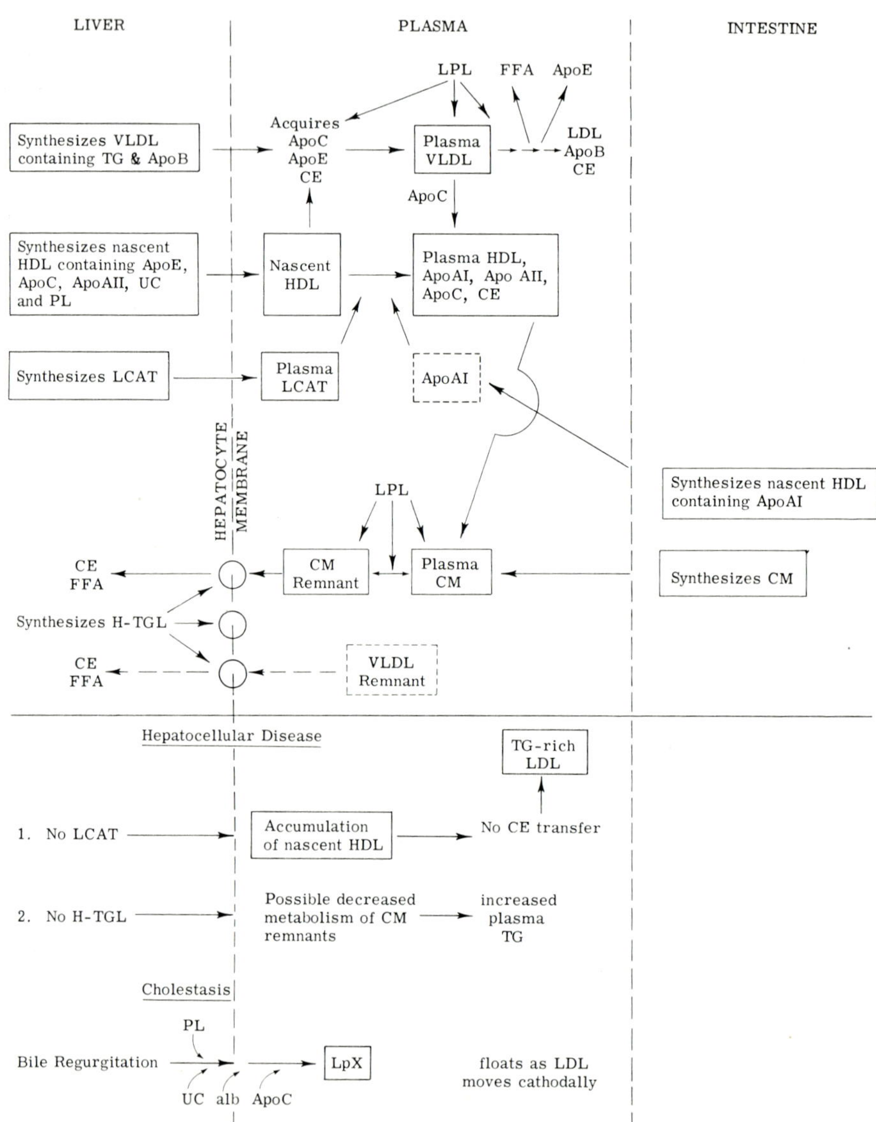

FIG. 10—Pathways of lipoprotein metabolsim and their possible derangements in liver disease.
Apo: apoprotein, such asAI, AII, B, etc. CE: cholesteryl ester. UC: unesterified cholesterol. TG:
triglycerides. CM: chylomicron. LpX: lipoprotein X. PL: phospholipid. FFA: unesterified fatty
acid. LPL: lipoprotein lipase. H-TGL: hepatic triglyceride lipase.

Accumulation of Lp-X in plasma probably depends upon the net results of
the regurgitation rate of biliary lipid and LCAT activity. When excess substrate
(lipoprotein-X) is available and LCAT is normal, free cholesterol is readily
converted into cholesteryl ester. At a higher rate of biliary regurgitation, however, as in clinical extrahepatic obstruction, excess substrate may appear as
Lp-X regardless of LCAT activity. At a lower rate of regurgitation, as in the
intrahepatic cholestasis of hepatitis, when LCAT is also deficient, Lp-X may

also appear. If this hypothesis is correct, use of the combined measurement of Lp-X and LCAT might not necessarily differentiate between intrahepatic and extrahepatic obstruction.

Figure 10 summarizes current concepts of the role of the liver in lipoprotein synthesis and metabolism and depicts the derangements in lipoprotein metabolism which accompany hepatocellular injury or cholestasis.

REFERENCES

1. Eisenberg S, Levy RI: Lipoprotein metabolism. Adv Lipid Res 13:1–89, 1975
2. Eisenberg S: Lipoprotein Metabolism and Hyperlipidemia. Edited by R Paoletti and AM Gotto: Atherosclerosis Reviews. New York, Raven Press, 1976, pp 23–60
3. Morrisett JD, Jackson RL, Gotto AM: Lipoproteins: Structure and function. Annu Rev Biochem 44:183–207, 1975
4. Berman M, Hall M, Levy RI, Eisenberg S, Bilheimer DW, Phair RD, Goebel RH: Metabolism of apo B and apo C lipoproteins in man: Kinetic studies in normal and hyperlipoproteinemic subjects. J Lipid Res 19:38–56, 1978
5. Windmueller HG, Herbert PN, Levy RI: Biosynthesis of lymph and plasma lipoprotein apoproteins by isolated perfusted rat liver and intestine. J Lipid Res 14:215–223, 1973
6. Mahley RW, Bennett BI, Morre DJ, Gray ME, Thistlewaite W, LeQuire VS: Lipoprotein associated with the Golgi apparatus isolated from epithelial cells of small intestine. Lab Invest 25:435–444, 1971
7. Ragland JB, Hawkins HL, Sabesin SM: Arginine-rich protein (ARP) in nascent high density lipoprotein of alcoholic hepatitis (AH). A model to study lipoprotein metabolism. Circulation 54(II):27, 1976
8. Hamilton RL, Williams MC, Fielding CJ, Havel RJ: Discoidal bilayer structure of nascent high density lipoproteins from perfused rat liver. J Clin Invest 58:667–680, 1976
9. Marsh J: Apoproteins of the lipoproteins in a nonrecirculating perfusate of rat liver. J Lipid Res 17:85–80, 1976
10. Ragland JB, Bertram PD, Sabesin SM: Identification of nascent high density lipoproteins containing arginine-rich protein in human plasma. Biochem Biophys Res Commun 80:81–88, 1978
11. Barter PJ, Conner WE: The transport of esterified cholesterol in plasma high density lipoproteins of human subjects: A mathematical model. J Lab Clin Med 88:627–639, 1976
12. Glickman RM, Green PHR: The intestine as a source of apolipoprotein A-I. Proc Natl Acad Sci USA 74:2569–2573, 1977
13. Green PHR, Tall AR, Glickman RM: Rat intestine secretes discoid high density lipoprotein. J Clin Invest 61:528–534, 1978
14. Fielding CJ, Havel RJ: Lipoprotein lipase. Arch Pathol Lab Med 101:225–299, 1977
15. Ganesan D, Bass HB, McConathy WJ, Alaupovic P: Is decreased activity of C-II activated lipoprotein lipase in type III hyperlipoproteinemia (broad-β-disease) a cause or an effect of increased apolipoprotein E levels? Metabolism 25:1189–1195, 1976
16. Krauss RM, Levy RI, Fredrickson DS: Selective measurement of two lipase activities in postheparin plasma from normal subjects and patients with hyperlipoproteinemia. J Clin Invest 54:1107–1124, 1974
17. Redgrave TC: Formation of cholesterol ester-rich particulate lipid during metabolism of chylomicrons. J Clin Invest 49:465–471, 1970
18. Eisenberg S, Rachmilewitz D: Metabolism of rat plasma very low density lipoprotein. II. Fate in circulation of apoprotein subunits. Biochim BiophysActa 326:391–405, 1973
19. Faergeman O, Sata T, Kane JP, Havel RJ: Metabolism of apo-lipoprotein B of plasma very low density lipoproteins in the rat. Circulation 50(III):114, 1974
20. Stein O, Rachmilewitz D, Sanger L, Eisenberg S, Stein Y: Metabolism of iodinated very low density lipoprotein in the rat: Autoradiographic localization in the liver. Biochim BiophysActa 360:205–216, 1974
21. Mjos OD, Faergeman O, Hamilton RL, Havel RJ: Characterization of remnants of lymph chylomicrons and lymph and plasma very low density lipoproteins in "supra-diaphragmatic" rats. Eur J Clin Invest 4:382–383, 1974

22. Sniderman AD, Carew TE, Chandler JG, Steinberg D: Paradoxical increase in rate of catabolism of low-density lipoproteins after hepatectomy. Science 183:526–528, 1974

23. Nilsson A: Hydrolysis of chyle cholesterol esters with cell-free preparations of rat liver. Biochim Biophys Acta 450:379–389, 1976

24. Floren CH, Nilsson A: Binding, interiorization and degradation of cholesteryl ester-labelled chylomicron-remnant particles by rat hepatocyte monolayers. Biochem J 168:483–494, 1977

25. Chajek T, Friedman G, Stein O, Stein Y: Effect of colchicine, cycloheximide and chloroquine on the hepatic triacylglycerol hydrolase in the intact rat and perfused liver. Biochim Biophys Acta 488:270–279, 1977

26. Faergeman O, Havel RJ: Metabolism of cholesteryl esters of rat very low density lipoproteins. J Clin Invest 55:1210–1218, 1975

27. VanBerkel TJC, Koster JF, Hulsmann WC: High density lipoprotein and low density lipoprotein catabolism by human liver and parenchymal and non-parenchymal cells from rat liver. Biochim Biophys Acta 486:586–589, 1977

28. Nakai T, Otto PS, Kennedy DL, Whayne TF: Rat high density lipoprotein subfraction (HDL$_3$) uptake and catabolism by isolated rat liver parenchymal cells. J Biol Chem 251:4914–4921, 1976

29. Stein O, Bar-on H, Stein Y: Lipoproteins and the liver. Edited by H Popper and F Schaffner: Progress in Liver Disease. Vol. IV New York, Grune & Stratton, 1972, pp 45–62

30. Turner KB, McCormack GH Jr, Richards A: The cholesterol esterifying enzyme of human serum. I. In liver disease. J Clin Invest 32:801–806, 1953

31. Müller P, Fellin R, Lambrecht J, Agostini B, Wieland H, Rost W, Seidel D: Hypertriglyceridemia secondary to liver disease. Eur J Clin Invest 4:419–428, 1974

32. Freeman M, Kuiken L, Ragland JB, Sabesin SM: Hepatic triglyceride lipase deficiency in liver disease. Lipids 12:443–445, 1977

33. Papadopoulos NM, Charles MA: Serum lipoprotein patterns in liver disease. Proc Soc Exp Biol Med 134:797–799, 1970

34. Thallasinos N, Hatzioannou J, Scliros P, Kanghinis T, Anastasiou C, Crocos P, Thomopoulos D, Gardikas C: Plasma alpha-lipoprotein pattern in acute viral hepatitis. Am J Dig Dis 20:148–155, 1975

35. Forte T, Nichols AV, Glomset J, Norum KR: The ultrastructure of plasma lipoproteins in lecithin:cholesterol acyltransferase deficiency. Scand J Clin Lab Invest 33(1370):121–132, 1974

36. Sabesin SM, Hawkins HL, Kuiken L, Ragland JB: Abnormal plasma lipoproteins and lecithin:cholesterol acyltransferase deficiency in alcoholic liver disease. Gastroenterology 72:510–518, 1977

37. Seidel D, Greten H, Geisen HP, Wengeler H, Wieland H: Further aspects on the characterization of high and very low density lipoproteins in patients with liver disease. Eur J Clin Invest 2:359–364, 1972

38. Sauar ZJ, Blomhoff JP, Gjone E: Triglyceride lipases in acute hepatitis. Clin Chim Acta 71:403–411, 1976

39. Mordasini R, Frey F, Flury W, Klose G, Greten H: Selective deficiency of hepatic triglyceride lipase in uremic patients. N Engl J Med 297:1362–1366, 1977

40. Glomset JA, Nichols AV, Norum KR, King W, Forte T: Plasma lipoproteins in familial lecithin:cholesterol acyltransferase deficiency. Further studies of very low and low density lipoprotein abnormalities. J Clin Invest 52:1078–1092, 1973

41. Bilheimer DW, Eisenberg S, Levy RI: Abnormal metabolism of very low density lipoproteins in type III hyperlipoproteinemia. Circulation 44(II):56, 1971

42. Greten H, Degrella R, Klose G, Rascher W, deGennes JL, Gjone E: Measurement of two plasma triglyceride lipases by an immunochemical method: Studies in patients with hypertriglyceridemia. J Lipid Res 17:203–210, 1976

43. Epstein EZ: Cholesterol of the blood in hepatic and biliary diseases. Arch Intern Med 50:203–222, 1932

44. Stokke KT: The existence of an acid cholesterol esterase in human liver. Biochim Biophys Acta 270:156–166, 1972

45. Glomset JA: The mechanisms of the plasma cholesterol esterification reaction: Plasma fatty acid transferase. Biochim Biophys Acta 65:128–135, 1962

46. Glomset JA: The plasma lecithin:cholesterol acyltransferase reaction. J Lipid Res 9:155–167, 1968

47. Norum KR, Gjone E: Familial plasma lecithin:cholesterol acyltransferase defi-

ciency. Biochemical study of a new inborn error of metabolism. Scand J Clin Lab Invest 20:231–243, 1967

48. Wengeler H, Greten H, Seidel D: Serum cholesterol esterification in liver disease. Combined determinations of lecithin:cholesterol acyltransferase and lipoprotein-X. Eur J Clin Invest 2:372–378, 1972

49. Calandra S, Martin MJ, McIntyre N: Plasma lecithin:cholesterol acyltransferase activity in liver disease. Eur J Clin Invest 1:352–360, 1971

50. Simon JB, Scheig R: Serum cholesterol esterification in liver disease. Importance of lecithin:cholesterol acyltransferase. N Engl J Med 283:841–846, 1970

51. Gjone E, Blomhoff IP: Plasma lecithin:cholesterol acyltransferase in obstructive jaundice. Scand J Gastroenterology 5:305–308, 1970

52. Gjone E, Blomhoff IP, Wienecke I: Plasma lecithin:cholesterol acyltransferase activity in acute hepatitis. Scand J Gastroenterology 6:161–168, 1971

53. Gjone E, Norum KR: Plasma lecithin cholesterol acyltransferase and erythrocyte lipids in liver disease. Acta Med Scand 187:153–161, 1970

54. Ritland S, Blomhoff JP, Gjone E: Lecithin:cholesterol acyltransferase and lipoprotein-X in liver disease. Clin Chim Acta 49:251–259, 1973

55. Blomhoff JP, Skrede S, Ritland S: Lecithin:cholesterol acyltransferase and plasma proteins in liver disease. Clin Chim Acta 53:197–207, 1974

56. Simon JB: Lecithin:cholesterol acyltransferase in human liver disease. Scand J Clin Lab Invest 33(137):107–113, 1974

57. Jones DP, Sosa FR, Shartsis J, Shah PT, Skromak E, Beher WT: Serum cholesterol esterifying and cholesterol ester hydrolyzing activity in liver diseases: Relationships to cholesterol, bilirubin, and bile salt concentration. J Clin Invest 50:259–265, 1971

58. Fex G, Wallinder L: Decreased esterification of (^{3}H) cholesterol by serum from partially hepatectomized rats in vitro. Biochim Biophys Acta 210:341–343, 1970

59. Lossow WJ, Shah SN, Brot N, Chaikoff IL: Effect of ethionine treatment on esterification in vitro of free (4-^{14}C) cholesterol by rat plasma. Biochim Biophys Acta 70:593–595, 1963

60. Sugano M, Hori K, Wada M: Hepatotoxicity and plasma cholesterol esterification by rats. Arch Biochem Biophys 129:588–596, 1969

61. Sabesin SM, Kuiken LB, Ragland JB: Lipoprotein and lecithin:cholesterol acyltransferase changes in glactosamine-induced rat liver injury. Science 190:1302–1304, 1975

62. Man EB, Kartin BL, Durlacher SH, Peters JP: The lipids of the serum and liver in patients with hepatic diseases. J Clin Invest 24:623–643, 1945

63. Widal F, Weil A, Laudat M: La Lipencie des brightiques:rapports de la retinite des brightiques avec l'azotemie et al cholesteremie. Semin Med 32:529–531, 1912

64. Russ EM, Raymunt J, Barr DP: Lipoproteins in primary biliary cirrhosis. J Clin Invest 35:133–144, 1956

65. Switzer S: Plasma lipoproteins in liver disease. I. Immunologically distinct low density lipoproteins in patients with biliary obstruction. J Clin Invest 46:1855–1866, 1967

66. Seidel D, Alaupovic P, Furman RH: A lipoprotein characterizing obstructive jaundice. I. Method for qualitative separation and identification of lipoproteins in jaundiced subjects. J Clin Invest 48:1211–1223, 1969

67. Seidel D: A new immunological technique for a rapid semiquantitative determination of the abnormal lipoprotein-X (Lp-X) characterizing cholestasis. Clin Chim Acta 31:225–229, 1971

68. Seidel D, Schmidt EA, Alaupovic P: An abnormal low density lipoprotein in obstructive jaundice. II. Its significance in the differential diagnosis of jaundice. Ser Med Mth 15:671–675, 1970

69. Seidel D, Alaupovic P, Furman RH, McConathy WJ: A lipoprotein characterizing obstructive jaundice. II. Isolation and partial characterization of the protein moieties of low density lipoproteins. J Clin Invest 49:2396–2407, 1970

70. Hamilton RL, Havel RJ, Kane JP, Blaurock AE, Sata T: Cholestasis: Lamellar structure of the abnormal human serum lipoprotein. Science 172:475–478, 1971

71. Patsch JR, Amme KC, Gotto AM, Morrisett JD: Isolation, chemical characterization and biophysical properties of these different abnormal lipoproteins: Lp-X$_2$ and Lp-X$_3$. J Biol Chem 252:2113–2120, 1977

72. Magnani HN, Alaupovic P: Utilization of the quantitative assay of lipoprotein X in the differential diagnosis of extrahepatic

and intrahepatic diseases. Gastroenterology 71:87–93, 1976

73. Ritland S, Gjone E: Quantitative studies of lipoprotein-X in familial lecithin:cholesterol acyltransferase deficiency and during cholesterol esterification. Clin Chim Acta 59:109–119, 1975

74. Torsvik H, Berg K, Magnani HN, McConathy WJ, Alaupovic P, Gjone E: Identification of the abnormal cholestatic lipoprotein (Lp-X) in familial lecithin: cholesterol acyltransferase deficiency. FEBS Lett 24:165–168, 1972

75. Seidel D, Gjone E, Blomhoff JP, Geisen HP. Edited by H Greten, R Levine, EF Pfeiffer, and RE Renold: Hormone and Metabolic Research. Stuttgart, Thieme-Verlag, Suppl 4, 1974, pp 6–11

76. Gjone E, Javitt NB, Blomhoff JP, Fausa O: Studies of lipoprotein-X (Lp-X) and bile acids in familial LCAT deficiency. Acta Med Scand 194:377–378, 1973

77. Ritland S, Gjone E: Quantitative studies of lipoprotein-X in familial lecithin:cholesterol acyltransferase deficiency and during cholesterol esterification. Clin Chim Acta 59:109–119, 1975

78. Wengeler H, Seidel D: Does lipoprotein-X (Lp-X) act as a substrate for the lecithin:cholesterol acyltransferase (LCAT)? Clin Chim Acta 45:429–432, 1973

79. Magnani HN: The influence of Lp-X and other lipoproteins associated with hepatic dysfunction of the activity of lecithin:cholesterol acyltransferase. Biochim Biophys Acta 450:390–401, 1976

80. Stein O, Aklan M, Stein V: Obstructive jaundice lipoprotein particles. Studies in ultrathin sections of livers of bile duct-ligated mice. Lab Invest 29:166–171, 1973

81. Manzato E, Fellin R, Baggio G, Walch S, Neubeck W, Seidel D: Formation of lipoprotein-X. Its relationship to bile compounds. J Clin Invest 57:1248–1260, 1976

82. Quarfordt SH, Oelschlager H, Krigbaum WR, Jakoi L, Davis R: Effect of biliary obstruction on canine plasma and biliary lipids. Lipids 8:522–530, 1973

83. Calandra S, Martin MJ, O'Shea MJ, McIntyre N: The effect of biliary obstruction on the structure and lipid content of rat erythrocytes. Biochim Biophys Acta 260:424–432, 1972

84. Byers SO, Friedman M: Probable sources of plasma cholesterol during phosphatide-induced hypercholesterolemia. Lipids 4:123–128, 1969

85. Thompson GR, Jadhov A, Nava M, Gotto AM Jr: Effects of intravenous phospholipid on low density lipoprotein turnover in man. Eur J Clin Invest 6:241–248, 1976

Chapter 14

Hepatic Microsomal Enzymes and Their Alterations in Pathologic Conditions

By H. DENK

THE ENDOPLASMIC RETICULUM of the hepatocyte (ER) is the site of oxidative metabolism and conjugation,[1] and liver disease is therefore likely to influence biotransformation and excretion of a variety of lipophilic endogenous and exogenous compounds. By contrast, malfunction of ER enzymes may itself cause or modify cell damage. The review focuses on the microsomal mixed function oxidase system and related enzymes in cholestasis, hepatitis and cirrhosis, primary hepatic neoplasia, porphyria, and some metabolic disorders of practical interest. It does not cover all possible alterations of microsomal enzymes associated with numerous disease states nor provide an exhaustive bibliography on the subject. For further detailed information on microsomal biotransformation under pathologic conditions the reader is referred to a recent review by Kato.[2]

TOPOGRAPHICAL AND FUNCTIONAL ASPECTS OF ER ENZYMES

The membranes of the ER harbor a variety of enzyme systems with specialized functions.[3] The enzymes hold different positions in the membrane, thus contributing to its longitudinal and transverse asymmetry.[3] The flavoprotein NADPH-cytochrome c(P-450) reductase, cytochrome b_5 (b_5), and part of the GDP-mannose transferase system are located on the cytoplasmic surface of the ER, whereas nucleoside diphosphatase, esterases, microsomal β-glucuronidase, and glucose-6-phosphatase are on the lumenal side. AMP-ase and UDP-glucuronyl transferases hold a position somewhere in the middle of the lipid bilayer.[3] Cytochrome P-450 (P-450), constituting a considerable portion of microsomal membrane protein, seems to be symmetrically and homogenously distributed.[3] Whether this applies to all P-450 species[4] or whether different members of the P-450 family are associated with different membrane domains is unknown.[3] The position of NADH-b_5-reductase is equivocal.[3] Microsomal proteins, including those with enzyme activity, are classified as integral or peripheral, depending on mode and force of interaction with the lipid bilayer. P-450, b_5, the flavoenzymes, and glucose-6-phosphatase are integral membrane constituents, being hydrophobic or amphipatic molecules, respectively.[3] The latter are anchored to the membrane by a hydrophobic peptide

---

From the Division of Gastroenterologic Pathology (Hans Popper Laboratory), Department of Pathology, University of Vienna School of Medicine, Vienna, Austria.

263

segment (see reference 3 for review). Some of the enzymes participate in distinct electron transfer pathways. One is concerned with the oxidative metabolism of lipophilic substances in a mixed function oxidase (MFO) reaction (MFO denotes the two electron reductive cleavage of molecular oxygen to yield one molecule of water with the second atom being incorporated into an organic substrate[5]) and consists of at least two components, the flavoprotein NADPH-cytochrome c (P-450) reductase and the hemoprotein P-450. The substrate binding site of P-450 is deeply buried in a hydrophobic membrane area.[6] Certain substrates, termed type I, bind to the lipoprotein moiety of P-450, and others, termed type II, affect the ligand of heme iron with formation of ferrihemochrome.[7,8] The active centers for type I and type II compounds are therefore associated with different hydrophobic zones in the microsomal membrane. Interaction of a substrate with P-450 is usually associated with a typical spectral shift.[7,8] The second pathway is involved in desaturation of fatty acids and consists of the flavoprotein NADH-b_5-reductase, b_5, and a cyanide-sensitive factor (desaturase).[9] The third electron transfer pathway, the lipid peroxidase, is responsible for the peroxidation of fatty acids, mainly arachidonate, and may cause membrane damage and degradation of heme.[10] NADPH-cytochrome c reductase is regarded as a component of this system.[11] The three pyridine nucleotide-dependent electron transfer chains utilize the same electron input enzymes, NADH-b_5 reductase and NADPH-cytochrome c reductase, and mutual interaction has been demonstrated.[12]

CHOLESTASIS

No convincing evidence exists for a causative role of ER and its enzymes in the initiation of cholestasis. ER alterations found in cholestasis are more likely to be consequences of cholestasis rather than its cause,[13,14] but knowledge of ER alterations in cholestasis is still valuable to predict drug effects under cholestatic conditions. Moreover, a functionally altered ER may be operative in amplifying cell damage and sustaining bile secretory failure by production of noxious and reactive metabolites.[13,14]

McLuen and Fouts[15] showed that hexobarbital and pentobarbital hypnosis is prolonged in cholestatic rats and rabbits, and competitive inhibition of ^{14}C-aminopyrine-N-demethylation was found in cholestatic rats by analysis of expired [14]CO_2.[16] Electron microscopy supplemented by morphometry and biochemical determinations disclosed an increase in ER in the hepatocytes[17-19] but the normal rough-to-smooth ER ratio was preserved.[19] The composition of ER membranes judged from the phospholipid-to-protein ratio remained unaltered,[17,19] although the lipid composition was slightly changed in that the phosphatidyl-choline-to-phosphatidyl-ethanolamine ratio decreased in microsomes from rats whose bile ducts were ligated for 8 days.[17] The prominent feature in cholestatic rat liver microsomes was the decrease of P-450 content and of P-450-dependent enzyme reactivity[17,19-22] (Table 1). Normally, P-450 in the rough ER is only about 50% of that in the smooth ER.[3] P-450 diminution in cholestasis was more pronounced in the rough than in the smooth membranes.[19] Thus, hypertrophic but P-450-deprived and enzymatically hypoactive membranes

TABLE 1.—*Liver Microsomal Enzymes in Bile-Duct-Ligated Rats (Duration of Cholestasis is 6 Days) Compared with Sham-operated Controls ($X \pm SE$, N= 7–9 rats)**

Microsomal Constituents	Ligation	Control
Protein (mg in liver/100 g body weight)	336 ± 53†	229 ± 20
Phospholipid (nmoles PLP/mg protein)	648 ± 83	623 ± 71
Glucose-6-phosphatase (μmoles P/mg protein/20 min)	4.82 ± 1.82†	9.21 ± 3.17
UDP-bilirubin glucuronyl transferase (μg bilirubin conjugated/mg protein/60 min)	28.41 ± 8.62	27.58 ± 8.37
P-450 (nmoles/mg protein)	0.47 ± 0.07†	0.80 ± 0.09
b_5 (nmoles/mg protein)	0.40 ± 0.08	0.45 ± 0.13
Aminopyrine-N-demethylase (K_m) (mM)	0.86 ± 0.15†	0.40 ± 0.22
Benzpyrene hydroxylase (nmoles 3-OH benzpyrene formed/mg protein/min)	0.076 ± 0.024†	0.413 ± 0.005
NADPH-cytochrome c reductase (nmoles/sec/mg protein)	0.98 ± 0.11†	1.36 ± 0.18
Lipid peroxidase (NADPH) (nmoles malondialdehyde formed/min/mg protein)	8.23 ± 0.56	10.61 ± 0.70
Stearyl-CoA desaturase (NADPH) (nmoles oleic acid formed/min/mg protein)	0.27 ± 0.14	0.27 ± 0.03

*For methodology, see reference 19.
†Significantly different from control, $P < 0.01$ (student's t-test).

arise in cholestasis, which may result from one or a combination of the following events: (1) impaired synthesis of heme or apoprotein, (2) destruction of P-450, and (3) "dilution" of P-450 by increased incorporation of non-P-450 membrane proteins. To solve this question, turnover studies were conducted with apparently conflicting results.[22,23] Mackinnon and Simon[22] observed a reduction of the relative degradation rate of P-450 apoprotein with an increase in half-life time from 24 hr to 50 hr in rats ligated for 3 days. Synthesis of higher molecular weight microsomal proteins was increased in addition, whereas synthesis of a protein suggestive of being P-450 apoprotein was depressed. Denk et al.[23] found neither decreased synthesis nor was increased breakdown of P-450 heme detected after radioactive labeling, and consequently, low microsomal P-450 was interpreted to result from "dilution" by non-P-450 membrane proteins. This assumption is certainly supported by the finding of increased synthesis of higher molecular weight microsomal proteins[22] and by the observation that total liver P-450 remained constant after bile duct ligation in young rats.[23] In older animals, however, impaired synthesis may still occur, since total P-450 was found to be decreased.[19] Cholestasis-associated impairment of P-450-dependent MFO was reversed by administration of inducing drugs.[21,24,25] Depressed in vivo drug metabolism[15,16] can be further characterized in vitro.

The metabolism of type I substrates by cholestatic liver microsomes was strongly inhibited in a mixed competitive-noncompetitive manner whereby the noncompetitive component roughly corresponded to the decreased P-450 level[17,19,20,26] (Fig. 1A). According to Gigon,[26] ethylmorphine and aminopyrine, both type I substrates, are handled differently by cholestatic rat liver microsomes in that aminopyrine-N-demethylation was competitively inhibited, whereas the K_m of ethylmorphine metabolism was almost unchanged. This may be explained by the existence of different enzymes with different susceptibility. Benzo(a) pyrene hydroxylation by cholestatic rat liver microsomes was also severely impaired[19] (Fig. 1D), indicating that the P-448 system may be particularly sensitive to cholestasis-linked cell alterations. Aniline hydroxylase paralleled microsomal P-450 content in its noncompetitive inhibition.[17] NADPH-cytochrome c (P-450) reductase was less affected in cholestasis than P-450 and was found to be 70% of control in rats 6 days after bile duct ligation[19] (Table 1), but a more pronounced decrease was reported by other authors.[21,24] Retained dihydroxylated (2-OH) bile salts are thought to be responsible by competition for the impairment of type I substrate metabolism.[17,27] Bile salt concentrations in the liver in cholestasis were indeed in the range where competitive inhibition occurs in vitro[28] (Figs. 1B and 1C). Trihydroxylated bile salts such as cholate which are no longer subject to microsomal hydroxylation did not interact with P-450 in lower concentrations and did not serve as competitive inhibitors[17,27] (Figs. 1B and 1C). Other substances retained in the liver in cholestasis, e.g., bilirubin, were ineffective.[17] With increasing bile salt concentrations (more than 1 mM for 2-OH bile salts and more than 2 mM for cholate) the P-450-dependent electron transfer system was severely affected, first by disturbance of the hydrophobic environment of the enzyme active site, then by solubilization of NADPH-cytochrome c (P-450) reductase, and finally by conversion of P-450 to its inactive form P-420.[27] Although bile salt levels sufficient for this detergent action were not found in the livers of cholestatic rats,[28] a detergent-active concentration is possible in human liver in single hepatocytes with feathery cytoplasmic degeneration[29] or in rat liver in certain compartments of the liver cell. P-420, increasing in amount with duration of cholestasis, was indeed observed,[26] but this was not confirmed by other authors.[17,19,20] Selective biliary obstruction (i.e., obstruction of one lobe of the liver with bile flow sustained by the others) mimics a situation occasionally occurring in man. In the obstructed lobe, P-450, NADPH-cytochrome c reductase, and glucose-6-phosphatase were greatly depressed.[19,30] Aminopyrine-N-demethylation was only slightly and noncompetitively inhibited,[19] supporting the concept of bile-salt-dependent inhibition of type I substrate metabolism in complete obstruction. Surprisingly, P-450 and NADPH-cytochrome c reductase were also diminished in the unobstructed lobes.[30] The reason is unknown. One possibility is again "dilution" of MFO components in the membrane by other proteins.

Besides the P-450-dependent MFO system, at least two other electron transfer systems are operative in liver microsomes. B$_5$, a constituent of the fatty acid desaturase system, remained unaffected in cholestasis, but the rate of b$_5$ reduction (measured by its ability to reduce an artificial electron acceptor,

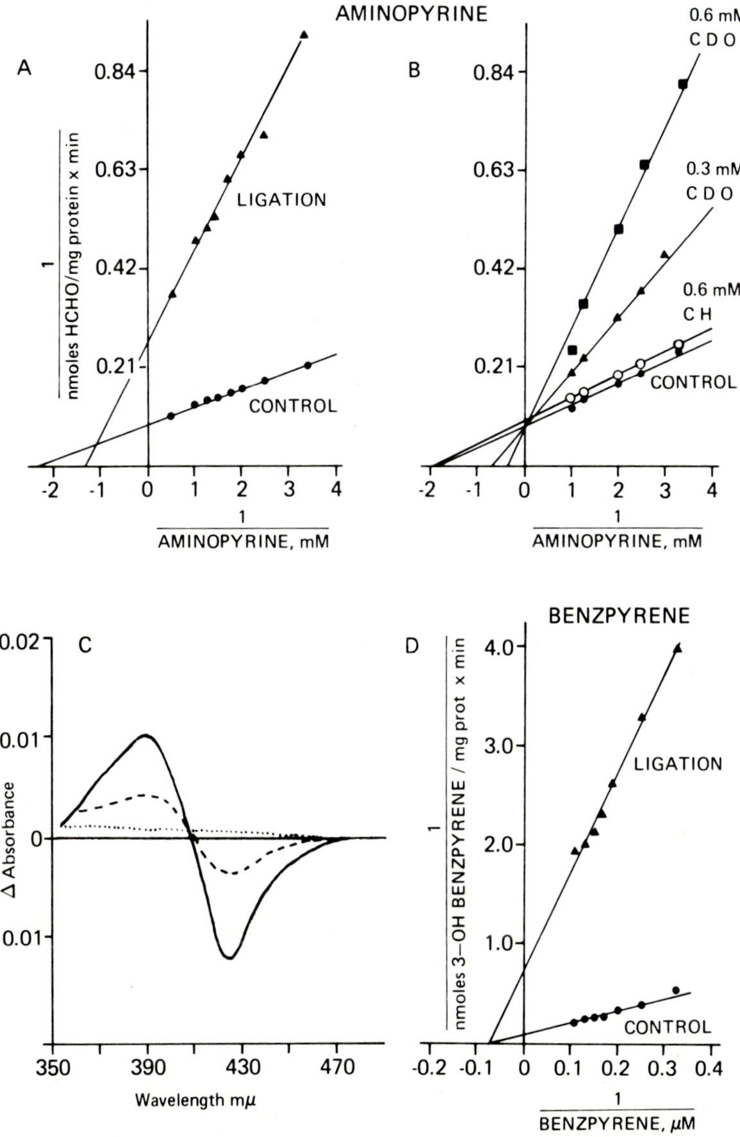

FIG. 1—(A) Aminopyrine-*N*-demethylation by liver microsomes derived from ligated and from sham-operated rats (duration of cholestasis, 6 days). Note mixed (competitive-noncompetitive) inhibition as the result of cholestasis. (B) Competitive inhibition of aminopyrine-*N*-demethylation by rat liver microsomes in vitro by chenodeoxycholic acid (CDO) in different concentrations. Cholic acid (CH) is not inhibitory in comparable concentrations. (C) Type I difference spectra after addition of taurochenodeoxycholic acid (———) and of chenodeoxycholic acid (----) to rat liver microsomes. Cholic acid (· · · · ·) does not induce a type I spectral shift. (D) Benzpyrene hydroxylation by liver microsomes in vitro. Strong noncompetitive inhibition as the result of cholestasis. (Methodology as described in references 17 and 19.)

such as ferricyanide) was reduced to only 50% of the sham-operated control without adverse influence on desaturase activity.[19] Lipid peroxidation, measured by estimation of malondialdehyde production, was at control levels in cholestatic liver microsomes in vitro[19] (Table 1).

Mechanical cholestasis had no effect on the conjugation of *p*-nitrophenol and bilirubin by liver microsomes in vitro or on the relative enzyme distribution in rough and smooth ER[19] (Table 1). In contrast to these in vitro observations using digitonin-activated microsomes, a shift in the ratio of conjugated to unconjugated bilirubin was shown in cholestatic rats,[26] pointing to impaired bilirubin glucuronyl transferase activity in vivo.

Glucose-6-phosphatase is a constitutive microsomal membrane component[3] and its activity is a good parameter for membrane integrity.[31] Cholestasis produced a significant drop in enzyme activity but apparently not as a result of lipid peroxidative destruction of the membrane[19] (Table 1). Since specific glucose-6-phosphatase activity in the microsomes paralleled P-450, speculation that "dilution" by other membrane proteins may again be responsible is tempting.

Alpha-naphthyl isothiocyanate (ANIT), ethinyl estradiol, norethandrolone, and lithocholate are the substances most commonly used for the experimental production of intrahepatic cholestasis.[14] The controversy concerning the mechanism of jaundice after ANIT administration has been resolved by the demonstration that organelle damage precedes bile stasis but that in the later stages, regurgitation of bile through damaged ducts, intrahepatic bile duct obstruction, and hemolysis contribute to jaundice.[32] Data obtained by several authors indicate that the precholestatic impairment of microsomal drug metabolism already seen 2 hr after ANIT administration is not associated with hypertrophic, hypoactive (P-450-deficient) ER.[14,20,32-35] In the later stages, P-450 diminution and impairment of hydroxylations may mainly result from bile stasis. By contrast with bile duct ligation, aniline hydroxylase in microsomes was already strongly and competitively inhibited 2 hr after ANIT administration.[17] This agrees with the observation of Drew and Priestly.[34] According to these authors, the precholestatic impairment of MFO is due to direct inhibition by ANIT and/ or a metabolite that is tightly bound to the microsomes. ANIT is a potent inhibitor of microsomal MFO if added in vitro,[20] the degree of inhibition depending on the type of substrate and the substrate concentration used in the test.

In norethandrolone cholestasis, P-450 declined within 3 days, but the diminution was less pronounced than after bile duct ligation.[20] Aminopyrine and aniline metabolism in vitro were inhibited to an extent comparable to bile duct obstruction.[20] Norethandrolone was also a potent competitive inhibitor of aminopyrine-*N*-demethylation in vitro.[20] Hence, as in the ANIT model, inhibition of microsomal MFO is not only a consequence of cholestasis but also results from direct drug action.[20]

Ethinyl estradiol treatment was also associated with a significant decrease of P-450, b_5, NADPH-cytochrome c reductase, and glucose-6-phosphatase.[24] If ethinyl estradiol and phenobarbital were administered simultaneously for 5 days, P-450 was raised even above control values, whereas b_5 and NADPH-cytochrome c reductase were only brought back to control levels.[24] With 3-methylcholanthrene as an inducer, only P-450 diminution was reversible, with b_5 and NADPH-cytochrome c reductase remaining unchanged.[24]

Pentobarbital elimination was decreased in patients with extrahepatic biliary obstruction. Pentobarbital hydroxylation by a 12,000 × g supernatant of human liver homogenate in vitro was significantly depressed to about 50% of control in those patients.[36] Hietanen et al.[37] reported a significant P-450 decrease in the 10,000 × g supernatant of liver homogenate derived from patients with obstructive jaundice as compared with patients with uncomplicated biliary tract disease. Hexobarbital hydroxylation by microsomes from cholestatic patients in vitro was approximately 40% lower than that from controls.[38] Glucose-6-phosphatase activity was also depressed in agreement with the experimental data.[38] O-aminophenol glucuronyl transferase in liver slices was raised in cholestatic patients[37] as a result either of the bilirubin effect, which agrees with the observation that microsomal glucuronidation of morphine and p-nitrophenol is enhanced by bilirubin in vitro,[39] or of membrane perturbation by bile salts, which agrees with the in vitro studies where latency of the enzyme was found to be relieved by membrane perturbing agents, e.g., bile salts.[40]

HEPATITIS AND CIRRHOSIS

Animal experiments on the effects of viral hepatitis on microsomal enzymes are lacking. Other models of hepatitis, e.g., murine hepatitis, are not readily comparable with the human disease and only are discussed briefly. Hexobarbital hydroxylase decreased to about 45% of the control, after initial stimulation, 48 to 60 hr after infection of mice with murine hepatitis virus (Buescher type).[41] Galactosamine-induced liver damage shows some morphologic similarities to human viral hepatitis[42] but differs in most other aspects. Hypertrophy of the ER[42] was not accompanied by an increase in enzyme activity. Alterations of microsomal enzymes and of their components in this model were species- and sex-dependent, and different results, i.e., unchanged or diminished levels, have been reported in the literature.[43-45] UDP-glucuronyl transferase activity was elevated, possibly resulting from membrane perturbation.[45]

Significantly prolonged half-life of hexobarbital has been found in patients with acute viral hepatitis apparently as a result of impaired metabolism by the liver[46] since hepatic blood flow is not significantly changed in hepatitis.[47] Clinical recovery was not readily accompanied by recovery of microsomal enzyme activity.[46] Phenobarbital disposition was not significantly impaired in patients with acute viral hepatitis, although intersubject variation was considerably greater than in the control group.[48] The activity of the MFO system in vitro decreased with the severity of cell damage[49]: in patients with severe hepatitis, P-450 and p-nitroanisole metabolism were decreased by 50%. From all these experiments, it is evident that the assessment of microsomal enzyme function in the patient has potential diagnostic and prognostic implications but that evaluation is difficult in individual cases. Determination of microsomal enzyme components and their function in biopsy material by refined techniques may be advantageous, particularly in patients with diffuse liver involvement.

synthesis or may reflect different affinities of the respective apoproteins for heme.[85]

The fungistatic antibiotic griseofulvin (GF) also interferes with heme formation by inhibiting ferrochelatase.[86] A transient decrease of P-450 occurs, followed by an elevation to 1.5- to 2-fold the control level after 48 hr of continuous feeding.[81] B_5 remained almost unchanged within the first 36 hr but was elevated after 48 hr. Azo-dye-N-demethylation roughly followed P-450 in its activity. P-450 decreased to about 50% of the control within 10 days of dietary GF administration; nevertheless, benzpyrene and benzphetamine metabolism by liver microsomes in vitro was stimulated.[87] A relationship between the development of porphyria and the GF effect on P-450 seemed to exist, since porphyria did not develop if GF was administered in a single daily dose,[88] and under these conditions, P-450 also remained unchanged.[87] This type of experiment may help to dissociate direct drug effects from those resulting from porphyria. Some of these findings[87] have been confirmed.[89] The metabolism of aminopyrine and aniline was slightly elevated after GF feeding for 12 days if related to microsomal protein, but it doubled if related to P-450 (Fig. 2A, Table 2). In addition, NADPH-cytochrome c reductase was increased in GF-fed mice to two to three times the control level (Table 2), which could account for the increased substrate metabolism despite P-450 diminution. B_5 was doubled within 12 days of GF feeding,[89] but total microsomal heme remained constant (Table 2). Thus, a shift occurred in the hemoprotein composition of the microsomes which may be caused by an alteration of apocytochrome P-450 synthesis or by the increased affinity of apocytochrome b_5 for heme provided in limiting amounts in the GF-treated animal. Turnover studies showed a stabi-

TABLE 2.—*Liver Microsomal Enzymes in Griseofulvin-treated, Protoporphyric Mice (Griseofulvin Treatment for 12 Days; Griseofulvin Was Administered in the Diet at a Concentration of 2.5%)* *

Microsomal Constituents	Griseofulvin	Control
Microsomal protein (mg/mouse liver)	129.57 ± 6.20	118.50 ± 14.00
Heme (nmoles/liver)	182.47 ± 20.79	190.21 ± 25.24
Heme (nmoles/mg microsomal protein)	1.49 ± 0.03	1.61 ± 0.09
P-450 (nmoles/mg microsomal protein)	0.57 ± 0.07†	1.10 ± 0.07
b_5 (nmoles/mg microsomal protein)	0.84 ± 0.03†	0.44 ± 0.04
NADH-ferricyanide (b_5) reductase (nmoles/sec/mg microsomal protein)	79.15 ± 3.70†	61.28 ± 2.23
NADH-cytochrome c reductase (nmoles/sec/mg microsomal protein	18.27 ± 0.58†	7.33 ± 0.74
NADPH-cytochrome c(P-450) reductase (nmoles/sec/mg microsomal protein)	3.41 ± 0.24†	0.91 ± 0.04

*For methodology, see reference 89. Each value is the mean ± SEM from four experiments each with the pooled livers of 7 to 8 mice.

†Significantly different from control, P <0.005 (student's t-test).

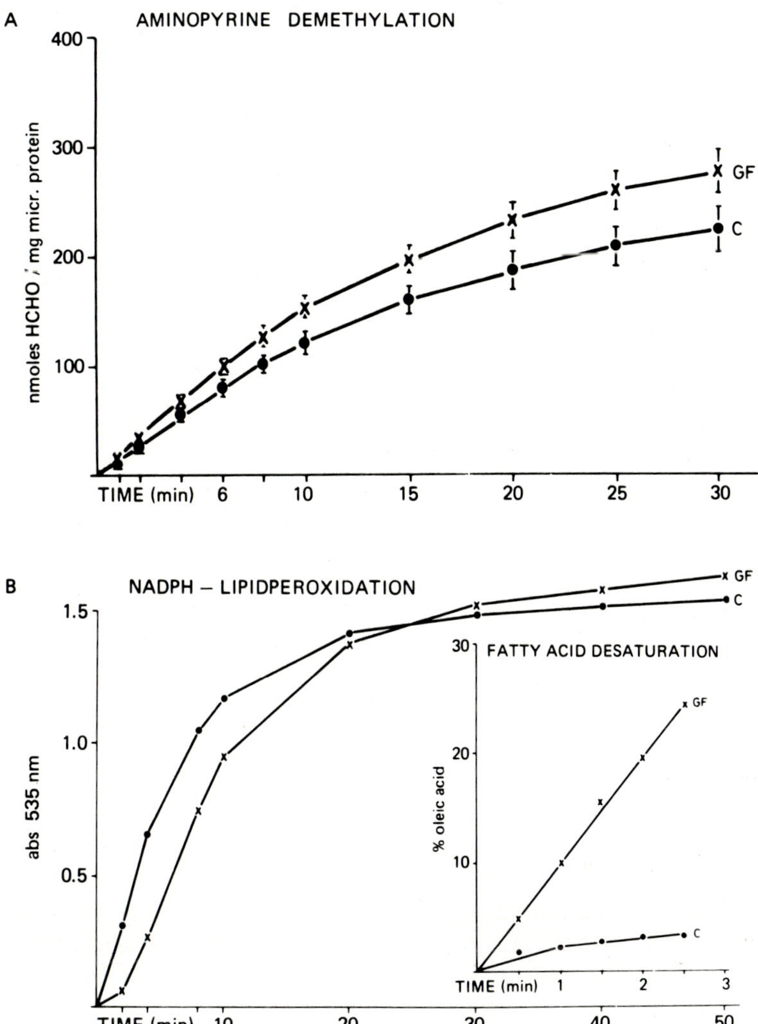

FIG 2—(A) Time course of aminopyrine-N-demethylation by microsomes of griseofulvin-treated and control mice in vitro. Duration of griseofulvin treatment was 12 days. Note increased demethylation by griseofulvin liver microsomes despite P-450 loss. (B) Time course of NADPH-supported lipid peroxidation by microsomes of griseofulvin-treated and control mice. Lipid peroxidation is measured by determination of malondialdehyde production. Inset shows increased stearyl-CoA desaturase activity in griseofulvin mouse liver microsomes. (Methodology as described in reference 89.)

lization of b_5 heme, which at least could contribute to b_5 elevation.[90] B_5 is an essential component of the desaturase system[9] and fortification of microsomes with external b_5 resulted in increased desaturase activity.[91] NADH-b_5 reductase was unaltered in the GF-treated animals, but NADH-cytochrome c reductase (which depends on b_5) was doubled. Desaturase activity was elevated by a factor of 12 and thus far exceeded the increase in b_5 level. It is possible but not proven that membrane lipid composition and fluidity are altered under these circumstances. NADPH- and NADH-supported lipid peroxidation remained almost unchanged[89] (Fig. 2B, Table 2). Glucose-6-phosphatase was unaffected in GF-treated mice and was slightly decreased under the same conditions in the rat.[92]

Lead interferes with several enzymes of the heme biosynthetic pathway,[93] and administration of this heavy metal indeed influenced P-450 formation negatively.[94] Similar effects of Zn^{2+}, Co^{2+}, and Mn^{2+} are known.[95]

Patients with intermittent acute porphyria (IAP) have a partial deficiency of uroporphyrinogen I synthetase catalyzing the conversion of porphobilinogen to uroporphyrinogen.[96] A similar situation is experimentally produced by lead administration.[94] In agreement with the experimental results,[94] impairment of hepatic hydroxylation of salicylamide in patients with IAP has been reported.[97] P-450, as well as microsomal biotransformation activities with aminopyrine and benzpyrene as test substrates, was determined in liver homogenates of patients with porphyria cutanea tarda, variegate porphyria, and protoporphyria.[98] A significant elevation of P-450 was only found in porphyria cutanea tarda, which agrees with the experimental results with HCB, without concomitant increase of smooth ER. No significant differences were found in the kinetics of benzpyrene hydroxylation and aminopyrine-N-demethylation between the porphyric and the control patient group, but considerable variation made the evaluation of these studies difficult. Difference spectroscopy, however, revealed a P-448-type hemoprotein. P-448 is the P-450 species that is preferentially induced by 3-methylcholanthrene and is characterized by increased maximal velocity with benzpyrene as substrate.[99] The P-448 in the livers of patients with porphyria cutanea tarda, however, did not show a similar behavior.[98]

In summary, no constant and regular relationship exists between altered heme synthesis and hemoprotein content in porphyria. Studies suggest that the heme pool is not rate-limiting in the formation of P-450, but apoprotein synthesis may control heme biosynthesis instead.[100] During restricted heme synthesis, however, the liver may not be able to readily adapt its hemoprotein concentration if increased enzyme activity is required.[94]

SELECTED NUTRITIONAL AND METABOLIC DISORDERS

Microsomal enzymes are intimately associated with the microsomal membrane, and changes in the membrane composition, such as those resulting from inadequate nutrition, probably alter enzyme activities, and particularly the ability of enzymes to bind substrate molecules.

The effect of starvation on microsomal enzyme activity is somewhat variable and seems to be sex- and species-dependent.[2] In the male rat, starvation mainly affects those drug-metabolizing enzymes that are sex-dependent in activity, such as hexobarbital hydroxylase, aminopyrine-N-demethylase, and pentobarbital oxidase, whereas aniline and zoxazolamine metabolism was decreased less or not at all, and N-demethylation of N-methylaniline and p-nitroanisole was only slightly decreased.[2] In female rats aminopyrine-N-demethylation was increased in proportion to P-450 (see reference 2 for review). P-450 was unchanged on a milligram microsomal protein basis in male Sprague-Dawley rats but was reduced if calculated per total liver.[101] Specific microsomal glucose-6-phosphatase activity was increased. There was no effect of starvation on P-450 and little depression of b_5, aminopyrine-N-demethylase, and NADPH-cytochrome c reductase, but a significant decrease of stearyl-CoA desaturase and a significant elevation of lipid peroxidase were found in male rats.[91] Sex differences in microsomal biotransformation did not occur in other species, including man.[2] In fasting male and female mice and rabbits, type I and type II substrate metabolism was increased;[102] in male guinea pigs, aminopyrine-N-demethylation, P-450, and b_5 were unaffected, but p-nitroanisol-O-demethylase was increased[103] or unchanged.[102] NADPH-cytochrome c reductase was elevated.[103] No consistent effect of fasting was found in man.[104] Glucuronyl transferase activity tended to be diminished during starvation.[2] Phenobarbital induction was clearly more pronounced in the fasting state.[101] P-450 heme is stabilized during fasting, and this may account for this effect.[105]

Protein deprivation led to a decrease in the activity and diminution of components of microsomal MFO.[106-108] Phenobarbital induction was impaired.[109] Conflicting results were reported with respect to conjugating enzymes which may be explained by inhomogeneity of the transferase family as well as by methodologic differences.[110-112]

Elevation of dietary carbohydrates decreased P-450, b_5, NADPH-cytochrome c reductase, NADH-b_5 reductase, as well as microsomal enzyme activities in vitro and in vivo.[2,91] The enzymes were less effectively inducible by phenobarbital.[2] Feeding a high-carbohydrate/fat-free diet to male rats reduced lipid peroxidation to almost zero, probably because of an increase of a cytosolic antioxidant,[113] whereas fatty acyl-CoA desaturase was considerably increased (1100% to 1500% of control).[91] Some of these enzyme changes may be related to deprivation of fat rather than to an increase in carbohydrate.

Phosphatidylcholine is an essential component of the microsomal MFO system.[114] Consequently, alterations of microsomal lipid composition may affect enzyme reactions. Essential fatty acid deficiency resulted in decreased and qualitatively changed P-450, as well as in depressed type I and type II substrate metabolism concomitant with decreased substrate binding.[115-117] Large amounts of unsaturated fatty acids may also be disadvantageous, however.[117] Supplementing the diet with large amounts of saturated fatty acids depressed P-450 and benzo(a)pyrene hydroxylase activity[118] but had no effect on hexobarbital metabolism.[119] Reports on aniline metabolism are contradictory.[118,119] Reduced response to phenobarbital was observed[115] if polyunsaturated fatty acids were absent from the diet; linoleic acid was particularly important in this respect.[120] The role of dietary lipid is equivocal.[115,120] Dietary sterols also seem to be essential for maximum activity of microsomal MFO.[120] Lipotropic factors, such as choline, play a role in phosphatidylcholine synthesis, and hence, lack of choline decreased MFO activity.[121] Stearyl-CoA desaturase was studied after dietary manipulation of microsomal membrane lipid composition.[122] Feeding a fat-free diet resulted in increased stearyl-CoA desaturase activity, a fat-free diet supplemented with tristearin or triolein gave intermediate values, and polyunsaturated fatty acids decreased desaturase activity. No significant change occurred in b_5 in contrast to other results.[91]

MFO enzyme reactions, as well as P-450 and substrate binding, were decreased in uremic rats, whereas other microsomal enzymes, such as glucose-6-phosphatase, glucuronyl transferase, b_5, and NADPH-cytochrome c reductase, remained unaltered.[123,124] P-450 was still inducible with phenobarbital.[123]

Vitamin deficiencies lead to impairment of microsomal enzyme activities in most instances in experimental animals and should therefore also be considered in man.

Prolongation of drug effects, a decrease in drug oxidation, in P-450, in b_5, and in flavoprotein levels, and reduced substrate binding were observed in ascorbic-acid-deficient guinea pigs[103,125-127] and were readily reversed by ascorbic acid administration.[103] Benzo(a)pyrene hydroxylase and epoxide hydrase, two enzymes important in carcinogen metabolism, were not adversely affected.[127] Induction of P-450 and related enzymes was not impaired.[103,127]

Vitamin E deficiency in rats is accompanied by decreased microsomal hydroxylations,[128,129] but reports on the behavior of P-450 and b_5 and on heme biosynthesis in deficient animals are contradictory.[128,130] In the Merino sheep, however, significant differences with respect to P-450 and type I and type II substrate metabolism by liver microsomes in vitro between vitamin-deficient and control animals were not detected.[131] Increased NADPH oxidation in the deficient animals probably reflected increased lipid peroxidation.[131]

Type I and type II substrate metabolism was impaired and P-450 depressed in vitamin-A-deficient rats.[132]

High-thiamine diets significantly depressed aniline and zoxazolamine metabolism by liver homogenates of male and female rats in vitro whereas aminopyrine metabolism was depressed in males but not in females. Hexobarbital metabolism was unaltered. In addition, P-450, b_5, and the flavoenzyme were decreased.[133]

Electron transport in P-450-dependent microsomal MFO occurs through a flavoenzyme (NADPH-cytochrome c reductase) and a heme protein (P-450). Therefore, flavin, as well as iron deficiency, may have an impact on biotransformation. No alterations, however, were found in the rates of metabolism of typical type I substrates, such as aminopyrine and hexobarbital, in old and young riboflavin-deficient mice. Aniline hydroxylation was increased. Benzpyrene metabolism was decreased in young and unchanged in old animals. P-450 and b_5 levels were consistently elevated in riboflavin-deficient mice, particularly in young animals.[134-136] Metabolism of most type I and type II substrates in rats was impaired,[137,138] and NADPH-cytochrome c reductase, P-450, and b_5 were reduced[137] or unchanged.[138] Chronic iron deficiency resulted in an increase in microsomal enzyme activities in mice[136] and rats,[139] but no significant P-450 changes occurred,[136,139] which is an indication that iron pools in the hepatocytes are not easily depleted in the iron deficient state.[136]

OUTLOOK

Transformation of lipid-soluble endogenous and exogenous compounds in order to render them suitable for excretion is an important function of the liver and is often, but not always, a detoxification process. Knowledge of the underlying mechanisms and the possible pathologic alterations is not only important for understanding the pathogenesis of disease processes but also for predicting drug effects and for therapeutic approaches. Clinical assessment of microsomal enzyme activity in the patient therefore serves as a valuable test of an essential partial function of the liver. This is particularly important in view of the poor correlation between the morphologic findings in the liver biopsy and results of tests of liver function.[140] Major emphasis has been placed on animal experimentation, but in relating results of animal studies directly to the patient, we must consider that the influence of liver disease on microsomal enzyme activity is often blurred by many variables, such as differences in nutrition, genetic factors, interference by other drugs, altered drug distribution volume, alterations in renal excretion, that are difficult to assess objectively in the individual patient.[53]

REFERENCES

1. Conney AH: Pharmacological implications of microsomal enzyme induction. Pharmacol Rev 19:317–366, 1967

2. Kato R: Drug metabolism under pathological and abnormal physiological states in animals and man. Xenobiotica 7:25–92, 1977

3. DePierre JW, Dallner G: Structural aspects of the membrane of the endoplasmic reticulum. Biochim Biophys Acta 415:411–472, 1975

4. Thomas PE, Lu AYH, Ryan D, West SB, Kawalek J, Levin W: Multiple forms of rat liver cytochrome P-450. Immunochemical evidence with antibody against cytochrome P-448. J Biol Chem 251:1385–1391, 1976

5. Gunsalus IC, Pederson TC, Sligar SG: Oxygenase-catalyzed biological hydroxylations. Annu Rev Biochem 44:377–407, 1975

6. Dean WL, Coon MJ: Immunochemical studies on two electrophoretically homogenous forms of rabbit liver microsomal cytochrome P-450: P-450 LM$_2$ and P-450 LM$_4$. J Biol Chem 252:3255–3261, 1977

7. Schenkman JB, Remmer H, Estabrook RW: Spectral studies of drug interaction with hepatic microsomal cytochrome. Mol Pharmacol 3:113–123, 1967

8. Remmer H, Schenkman JB, Estabrook RW, Sasame H, Gillette JR, Narasimhulu S, Cooper DY, Rosenthal O: Drug interaction with hepatic microsomal cytochrome. Mol Pharmacol 2:187–190, 1966

9. Oshino N, Imai Y, Sato R: Electron transfer mechanism associated with fatty acid desaturation catalyzed by liver microsomes. Biochim Biophys Acta 128:13–27, 1966

10. Bidlack WR, Tappel AL: Damage of microsomal membranes by lipid peroxidation. Lipids 8:177–182, 1973

11. Jansson I, Schenkman JB: Studies on three microsomal electron transfer enzyme systems. Specificity of electron flow pathways. Arch Biochem Biophys 178:89–107, 1977

12. Schenkman JB, Jansson I, Robie-Suh K: The many roles of cytochrome b$_5$ in hepatic microsomes. Life Sci 19:611–624, 1976

13. Popper H, Schaffner F, Denk H: Molecular pathology of cholestasis. Edited by W. Taylor: The Hepatobiliary System. New York, Plenum Press, 1976, pp 605–629

14. Plaa GL, Priestly BG: Intrahepatic cholestasis induced by drugs and chemicals. Pharmacol Rev 28:207–273, 1977

15. McLuen EF, Fouts JR: The effect of obstructive jaundice on drug metabolism in rabbit. J Pharmacol Exp Ther 131:7–11, 1961

16. Lauterburg BH, Bircher J: Expiratory measurement of maximal aminopyrine demethylation in vivo: Effect of phenobarbital, partial hepatectomy, porto-caval shunt and bile duct ligation in the rat. J Pharmacol Exp Ther 196:501–509, 1976

17. Denk H: Die chemische Struktur des endoplasmatischen Retikulums und die Funktion des mikrosomalen Biotransformationssytems der Leberzelle der Ratte bei experimenteller Cholestase. Pathol Eur 7:43–65, 1972

18. Schaffner F, Bacchin PG, Hutterer F, Scharnbeck HH, Sarkozi LL, Denk H, Popper H: Mechanism of cholestasis. 4. Structural and biochemical changes in the

67. Cameron R, Sweeney GD, Jones K, Lee G, Farber E: A relative deficiency of cytochrome P-450 and aryl hydrocarbon [benzo(a)pyrene] hydroxylase in hyperplastic nodules induced by 2-acetylaminofluorene in rat liver. Cancer Res 36:3888–3893, 1976

68. Saine SE, Strobel HW: Drug metabolism in liver tumors. Resolution of components and reconstitution of activity. Mol Pharmacol 12:649–657, 1976

69. Farber E, Parker S, Gruenstein M: The resistance of putative premalignant liver cell populations, hyperplastic nodules, to the acute cytotoxic effects of some hepatocarcinogens. Cancer Res 36:3879–3887, 1976

70. Sipes GI, Krishna G, Gillette JR: Bioactivation of carbon tetrachloride, chloroform and bromochloromethane: role of cytochrome P-450. Life Sci 20:1541–1548, 1977

71. Trams EG, Inscoe JK, Resnik RA: Liver enzymes during hepatic carcinogenesis, J Natl Cancer Inst 26:959–968, 1961

72. DeMatteis F, Stonard M: Experimental porphyrias as models for human hepatic porphyrias. Semin Hematol 14:187–192, 1977

73. Gschnait F, Konrad K, Hönigsmann H, Denk H, Wolff K: Mouse model for protoporphyria. I. The liver and hepatic protoporphyrin crystals. J Invest Dermatol 65:290–299, 1975

74. DeMatteis F: Rapid loss of cytochrome P-450 and haem caused in the liver microsomes by the porphyrogenic agent 2-allyl-2-isopropylacetamide. FEBS Lett 6:343–345, 1970

75. Levin W, Jacobson M, Kuntzman R: Incorporation of radioactive δ-aminolevulinic acid into microsomal cytochrome P-450: Selective breakdown of the hemoprotein by allylisopropylacetamide and carbon tetrachloride. Arch Biochem Biophys 148:262–269, 1972

76. Posalaki Z, Barka T: Alterations of hepatic endoplasmic reticulum in porphyric rats. J Histochem Cytochem 16:337–345, 1968

77. Sweeney GD, Rothwell JD: Spectroscopic evidence of interaction between 2-allyl-2-isopropylacetamide and cytochrome P-450 of rat liver microsomes. Biochem Biophys Res Comm 55:798–804, 1973

78. Baird MB, Birnbaum LS, Samis HU, Massie HR, Zimmerman JA: Allylisopropylacetamide preferentially interacts with the phenobarbital-inducible form of rat hepatic microsomal P-450. Biochem Pharmacol 25:2415–2417, 1976

79. Ioannides C, Parke DU: The effect of allyl compounds on hepatic microsomal mixed function oxidation and porphyrogenesis. Chem Biol Interact 14:241–249, 1976

80. Lui H, Sampson R, Sweeney GD: Hexachlorobenzene porphyria. Purity and metabolic fate of hexachlorobenzene. Edited by M Doss: Porphyrins in Human Diseases. Basel, Karger, 1976, pp 405–413

81. Wada O, Yano Y, Urata G, Nakao K: Behaviour of hepatic microsomal cytochromes after treatment of mice with drugs known to disturb porphyrin metabolism in liver. Biochem Pharmacol 17:595–603, 1968

82. Ivanov ED, Chernev K, Adjarov D, Krustev L, Georgiev G: The effect of different diets on porphyrin metabolism and microsomal liver enzyme induction in experimental hexachlorobenzene porphyria. Edited by M Doss: Porphyrins in Human Diseases. Basel, Karger, 1976, pp 438–444

83. San Martin de Viale LC, Tomio JM, Ferramola AM, Sancovich HA, Tigier HA: Experimental porphyria induced in rats by hexachlorobenzene. Studies on enzymes associated with haem pathway. Effect of 17β-oestradiol. Edited by M Doss: Porphyrins in Human Diseases. Basel, Karger, 1976, pp 453–458

84. DeMatteis F, Abbritti G, Gibbs AH: Decreased liver activity of porphyrin-metal chelatase in hepatic porphyria caused by 3,5-diethoxycarbonyl-1,4-dihydrocollidine. Studies in rats and mice. Biochem J 134:717–727, 1973

85. Sweeney GD: Hepatic catalase activity during states of altered heme synthesis. Edited by M Doss: Porphyrins in Human Diseases. Basel, Karger, 1976, pp 53–61

86. DeMatteis F, Gibbs AH: Stimulation of the pathway of porphyrin synthesis in the liver of rats and mice by griseofulvin, 3,5-diethoxycarbonyl-1,4-dihydrocollidine and related drugs: Evidence for two basically different mechanisms. Biochem J 146:285–287, 1975

87. Lin C, Chang R, Casmer C, Symchowicz S: Effects of phenobarbital, 3-methylcholanthrene, and griseofulvin on the O-demethylation of griseofulvin by liver microsomes of rats and mice. Drug Metab Disp 1:611–618, 1973

88. Weston Hurst E, Paget GE: Protoporphyrin, cirrhosis and hepatomata in the liv-

ers of mice given griseofulvin. Br J Dermatol 75:105–112, 1963

89. Denk H, Eckerstorfer R, Talcott RE, Schenkman JB: Alteration of hepatic microsomal enzymes by griseofulvin treatment of mice. Biochem Pharmacol 26:1125–1130, 1977

90. Denk H, Eckerstorfer R: Turnover of cytochrome P-450 and cytochrome b_5 hemes in griseofulvin-induced murine porphyria. FEBS Lett 76:67–70, 1977

91. Jansson I, Schenkman JB: Studies on three microsomal electron transfer enzyme systems; effects of in vivo and in vitro alteration of component enzyme levels. Mol Pharmacol 11:450–461, 1975

92. McIntosh DAO, Topham JC: A comparison of mouse and rat liver enzymes and their response to treatment with various compounds. Biochem Pharmacol 21:1025–1029, 1972

93. Campbell BC, Brodie MJ, Thompson GG, Meredith PA, Moore MR, Goldberg A: Alterations in the activity of enzymes of haem biosynthesis in lead poisoning and acute hepatic porphyria. Clin Sci Molec Med 53:335–340, 1977

94. Maxwell JD, Meyer UA: Effect of lead on hepatic δ-aminolaevulinic acid synthetase activity in the rat: A model for drug sensitivity in intermittent acute porphyria. Eur J Clin Invest 6:373–379, 1976

95. Wagner GS, Dinamarca ML, Tephly TR: Studies on ferrochelatase activity: Role in regulation of hepatic heme biosynthesis. Edited by M Doss: Porphyrins in Human Diseases. Basel, Karger, 1976, pp 111–122

96. Strand JL, Felsher BF, Redeker AG, Marver HS: Heme biosynthesis in intermittent acute porphyria: Decreased hepatic conversion of porphobilinogen to porphyrins and increased δ-aminolevulinic acid synthetase activity. Proc Natl Acad Sci USA 67:1315–1320, 1970

97. Song CS, Bonkowsky HL, Tschudy DP: Salicylamide metabolism in acute intermittent porphyria. J Lab Clin Med 15:431–435, 1974

98. Blekkenhorst G, Pimstone NR, Eales L: Porphyria cutanea tarda in South Africa. Metabolic basis of disordered haem biosynthesis. Edited by M Doss: Porphyrins in Human Diseases. Basel, Karger, 1976, pp 299–311

99. Alvares AP, Schilling G, Garbut A, Kuntzman R: Studies on the hydroxylation of 3, man R: Studies on the hydroxylation of 3, 4-benzpyrene by hepatic microsomes. Biochem Pharmacol 19:1449–1455, 1970

100. Correia MA, Meyer UA: Apocytochrome P-450: Reconstitution with hemin in vitro. Proc Natl Acad Sci USA 72:400–404, 1975

101. Bock KW, Fröhling W, Remmer H: Influence of fasting and hemin on microsomal cytochromes and enzymes. Biochem Pharmacol 22:1557–1564, 1973

102. Furner RL, Feller DD: The influence of starvation upon hepatic drug metabolism in rats, mice, and guinea pigs. Proc Soc Exp Biol Med 137:816–819, 1971

103. Zannoni VG, Flynn EJ, Lynch M: Ascorbic acid and drug metabolism. Biochem Pharmacol 21:1377–1392, 1972

104. Reidenberg MM: Obesity and fasting-effects on drug metabolism and drug action in man. Clin Pharmacol Ther 22:729–734, 1977

105. Greim H, Schenkman JB, Klotzbücher M, Remmer H: The influence of phenobarbital on the turnover of hepatic microsomal b_5 and cytochrome P-450 hemes in the rat. Biochim Biophys Acta 201:20–25, 1970

106. McLean AEM, McLean EK: The effect of diet and 1,1,1-trichloro-2,2-bis-(p-chlorophenyl) ethane (DDT) on microsomal hydroxylating enzymes and on sensitivity of rats to carbon tetrachloride poisoning. Biochem J 100:564–571, 1966

107. Paine AJ, McLean AEM: The effect of dietary protein and fat on the activity of aryl hydrocarbon hydroxylase in rat liver, kidney and lung. Biochem Pharmacol 22:2875–2830, 1973

108. Campbell TC: Nutrition and drug metabolizing enzymes. Clin Pharmacol Ther 22:699–706, 1977

109. Marshall WJ, McLean AEM: The effect of phenobarbitone on hepatic microsomal cytochrome P-450 and demethylation activity in rats fed normal and low protein diets. Biochem Pharmacol 18:153–157, 1969

110. Adlard BPF, Lester RG, Lathe GH: The effect of phenobarbitone treatment of rats and of protein deprivation on the capacity of liver slices to conjugate bilirubin. Biochem Pharmacol 18:59–63, 1969

111. Woodcock BG, Wood GC: Effect of protein-free diet on UDP-glucuronyltransferase and sulphotransferase activities in rat liver. Biochem Pharmacol 20:2703–2713, 1971

112. Smith JA, Butler TC, Poole DT: Effect of

protein depletion in guinea pigs on glucuronate conjugation of chloramphenicol by liver microsomes. Biochem Pharmacol 22:981–983, 1973

113. Talcott RE, Denk H, Eckerstorfer R, Schenkman JB: Inhibition of NADPH-driven microsomal lipid peroxidation by cytosol factor(s). Effect of a fat-free high carbohydrate diet. Chem Biol Interactions 12:355–361, 1976

114. Lu AYH, Levin W: The resolution and reconstitution of the liver microsomal hydroxylation system. Biochim Biophys Acta 344:205–240, 1974

115. Marshall WJ, McLean AEM: A requirement for dietary lipids for induction of cytochrome P-450 by phenobarbitone in rat liver microsomal fraction. Biochem J 122:569–573, 1971

116. Kaschnitz R: Aryl 4-hyroxylase, cytochrome P-450 and microsomal lipids in essential fatty acid deficiency. Z Physiol Chem 351:771–774, 1970

117. Norred WP, Wade AE: Dietary fatty acid-induced alterations of hepatic microsomal drug metabolism. Biochem Pharmacol 21:2887–2897, 1972

118. Agradi E, Spagnolo C, Galli: Cited by Kato R: Drug metabolism under pathological and abnormal physiological states in animals and man. Xenobiotica 7:25–92, 1977

119. Caster WO, Wade AE, Norred WP, Bargmann RE: A differential effect of dietary saturated fat on the metabolism of aniline and hexobarbital by the rat liver. Pharmacology 3:177–186, 1970

120. Lambert L, Wills ED: The effect of dietary lipid peroxides, sterols and oxidised sterols on cytochrome P-450 and oxidative demethylation in the endoplasmic reticulum. Biochem Pharmacol 26:1417–1421, 1977

121. Gallenkamp H, Brachtel D, Sundermann M, Grün J, Rietbrock J, Richter E: Ethylmorphine-N-demethylase activity and thiopentene half-life in rats fed a choline deficient diet. Nutr Metab 17:91–96, 1974

122. Holloway CT, Holloway PW: Stearyl CoenzymeA desaturase activity in mouse liver microsomes of varying lipid composition. Arch Biochem Biophys 167:486–504, 1975

123. Leber HW: Mechanismus der Aktivitätsabnahme mischfunktioneller Oxygenasen in Lebermikrosomen urämischer Ratten. Z Klin Chem Klin Biochem 10:543–547, 1972

124. Van Peer AF, Belpaire FM: Hepatic oxidative drug metabolism in rats with experimental renal failure. Arch Int Pharmacodyn 228:180–183, 1977

125. Degkwitz E, Luft D, Pfeiffer U, Staudinger HJ: Untersuchungen über mikrosomale Enzymaktivitäten (Cumarinhydroxylierung, NADPH Oxydation, Glucose-6-phosphatase und Esterase) und Cytochromgehalte (P-450 und b_5) bei normalen, skorbutischen und hungernden Meerschweinchen. Z Physiol Chem 349:465–471, 1968

126. Gundermann K, Degkwitz E, Staudinger HJ: Mischfunktionelle Oxygenierung von (+)- und (−)-Hexobarbital und spektrale Änderungen des Cytochroms P-450 in der Leber ascorbinsäurefrei ernährter Meerschweinchen. Z Physiol Chem 354:238–242, 1973

127. Kuenzig W, Tkaczevsky V, Kamm JJ, Conney AH, Burns JJ: The effect of ascorbic acid deficiency on extrahepatic microsomal metabolism of drugs and carcinogens in the guinea pig. J Pharmacol Exp Ther 201:527–533, 1977

128. Caygill CPJ, Diplock AT, Jeffery EH: Studies on selenium incorporation into, and electron-transfer function of, liver microsomal fractions from normal and vitamin E-deficient rats given phenobarbital. Biochem J 136:851–858, 1973

129. Giasuddin ASM, Caygill CPJ, Diplock AT, Jeffery EH: The dependence on vitamin E and selenium of drug demethylation in rat liver microsomal fractions. Biochem J 146:339–350, 1975

130. Murty HS, Caasi PI, Brooks SK, Nair PP: Biosynthesis of heme in the vitamin E-deficient rat. J Biol Chem 245:5498–5504, 1970

131. Gourlay GK, Savage JK, Stock BH: Hepatic drug metabolism in normal and vitamin E-deficient female merino sheep. Toxicol Appl Pharmacol 39:365–375, 1977

132. Becking GC: cited by Kato R: Drug metabolism under pathological and abnormal physiological states in animals and man. Xenobiotica 7:25–92, 1977

133. Grosse W, Wade AE: The effect of thiamine consumption on liver microsomal drug-metabolizing pathways. J Pharmacol Exp Ther 176:758–765, 1971

134. Rivlin RS, Menendez C, Langdon RG:

Biochemical similarities between hypothyroidism and riboflavin deficiency. Endocrinology 83:461–469, 1968

135. Chan PC, Okamoto T, Wynder EL: Possible role of riboflavin deficiency in epithelial neoplasia. III. Induction of microsomal aryl hydrocarbon hydroxylase. J Natl Cancer Inst 48:1341–1345, 1972

136. Catz CS, Juchau MR, Yaffe SJ: Effects of iron, riboflavin and iodide deficiencies on hepatic drug metabolizing enzyme systems. J Pharmacol Exp Ther 174:197–205, 1970

137. Patel JM, Pawar SS: Riboflavin and drug metabolism in adult male and female rats. Biochem Pharmacol 23:1467–1477, 1974

138. Shargel L, Mazel P: Effect of riboflavin deficiency on phenobarbital and 3-methylcholanthrene induction of microsomal drug-metabolizing enzymes of the rat. Biochem Pharmacol 22:2365–2373, 1973

139. Becking GC: Influence of dietary iron levels on hepatic drug metabolism in vivo and in vitro in the rat. Biochem Pharmacol 21:1585–1593, 1972

140. Popper H, Medline A: Die "Organellen-Pathologie". Ihre Bedeutung bei der Beurteilung von Leberfunktionsproben. Münch Med Wochenschr 111:1569–1574, 1969

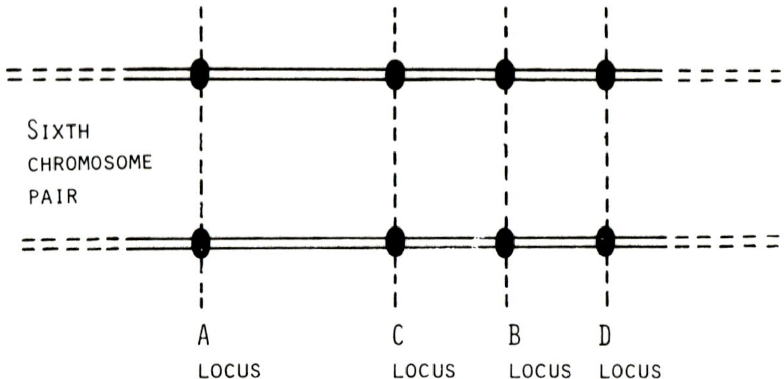

FIG. 1—The relative positions of the HL-A loci on the human sixth chromosome.

ologically detectable antigen, and since the chromosome is paired, there are potentially two A and two B antigens in each individual. Occasionally, only one A or B locus antigen can be detected, either because of homozygosity at one of the loci or as a result of the inheritance of an antigen that is not identifiable.

Further studies have identified two other loci, C and D, which lie close to the A and B sites on chromosome 6 (Fig. 1), but the detection of the associated antigens is not yet part of a routine analysis. Serologically identifiable D locus antigens (called Ia antigens) are restricted in their tissue distribution and found on B lymphocytes. The separation of these cells from the mixed peripheral blood populations of T and B cells is time-consuming and difficult, but it is essential in order to successfully test for these new antigens. Despite these problems, however, antisera that successfully detect the D locus products were identified at the 1977 Histocompatibility Workshop at Oxford, and preliminary results of the associations with some diseases were presented.[5]

THE LINK BETWEEN TRANSPLANTATION ANTIGENS AND IMMUNE RESPONSE GENES

Lilly's observations that resistance to established Gross virus leukemia in the mouse, which appeared to be transmitted as a mendelian dominant trait, was linked to certain alleles at the H2 locus[6] (the mouse equivalent of HL-A) prompted the first studies of HL-A and disease in man. The results in leukemia and lymphoma were disappointing, the few associations found being very weak. With some chronic inflammatory conditions, however, strong associations were evident, including the now well-recognized link between a second locus antigen, HLA-B27, and ankylosing spondylitis.[7] More than 90% of the patients were positive for HLA-B27, while its frequency in the general population was less than 10%.

One clue as to the possible mechanisms underlying such a strong association with inflammatory and autoimmune diseases came from further studies in the mouse where strict inbreeding reduced the background genetic noise to a level where links between particular H2 types and specific immune responses could be identified. Genes determining the intensity of the immune response to certain simple synthetic antigens were found to be closely associated with genes coding for the histocompatibility antigens,[8] and this led to the attractive concept that the association of certain HL-A with human chronic inflammatory diseases was due to the presence of similar immune response (IR) genes determining the intensity of the host response to a particular microorganism or its own tissue antigens. Experimentally, direct evidence for the operation of IR genes has been obtained in thyroid disease in animals, namely spontaneous autoimmune thyroiditis in chickens and the production of thyroid autoantibodies in the mouse.[9] Surprisingly, similar associations have not yet been detected in man. Indeed, Hashimoto's thyroiditis is one of the few putative autoimmune conditions that has not been shown to be associated with any particular HL-A type.[10] Although IR genes could be involved in liver disease susceptibility, they are almost certainly not responsible for the association with a particular HL-A antigen. A different mechanism seems to be responsible in each disease for the HL-A link and is, in each instance, just part of a complex polygenic pattern of inheritance of disease susceptibility.

IDIOPATHIC HEMOCHROMATOSIS

Idiopathic hemochromatosis has long been considered to be caused by an inborn error of metabolism.[11] The exact nature of the underlying defect(s) is not known, but in support of a genetic basis for the disease are the results of family studies in which first-degree relatives have been found to have abnormalities ranging from raised serum iron levels with only a minimal increase in iron stores to those with clinical abnormalities and gross excess iron in tissues.[12] Williams et al.[13] suggested that the disease develops in individuals homozygous for an abnormal autosomal gene, while the less severe abnormalities of iron metabolism are found in heterozygous carriers.[13]

An association between HLA-A3 and idiopathic hemochromatosis was reported from France,[14] and the same antigen was also found in 69% of our patients.[15] Similar results have been reported from the United States,[16] confirming the importance of the association by showing its presence in several different population groups. The most obvious explanation for this strong association of HLA-A3 with the disease was that the gene coding for this histocompatibility antigen was linked to the hypothetical gene controlling iron metabolism; to test this theory, we investigated the relationship between inheritance of HL-A types and abnormalities in iron metabolism in the relatives of some of our patients.

The propositus in the family shown in Fig. 2 presented at the age of 51 with an arthropathy and was found to have many of the clinical features of hemochromatosis. Iron overload was evident biochemically and histologically. One of his four brothers also had severe iron overload and hepatomegaly. On HL-A testing, the brother proved to be HL-A-identical to the propositus and both had inherited HLA-A3. Two subjects, another brother and the daughter of the propositus, had inherited the haplotype HLA-A3, B14, but contrary to the initial hypothesis, neither had an elevation in serum iron or increased trans-

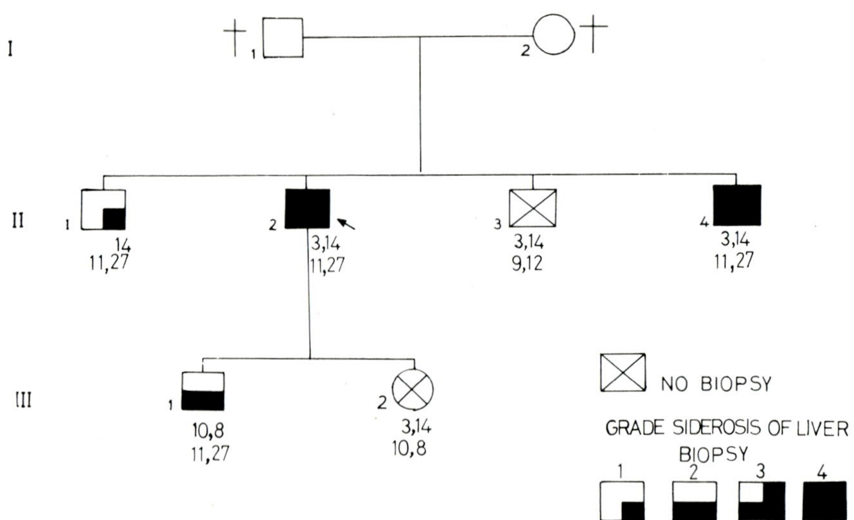

FIG. 2—The relationship between the segregation of HL-A haplotypes and the degree of iron overload on liver biopsy in a family in which two brothers were found to have idiopathic hemochromatotis. (Reproduced from Bomford A et al.: Histocompatibility antigens as markers of abnormal iron metabolism in patients with idiopathic haemochromatosis and their relatives. Lancet 1:327–329, 1977.)

ferrin saturation (Table 1). However, definite, though minor, abnormalities, including a small increase in hepatic storage iron, were present in two other subjects, another brother and the son of the propositus (Fig. 2, Table 1). Interestingly, they had both inherited the other haplotype found in the two subjects with massive iron overload, HLA-A11, B27. The inference was that this haplotype, although not generally associated with the disease, was carrying a gene responsible for increased iron absorption in this family. This abnormality alone, however, was insufficient to produce massive iron overload, and the additional influence of a gene inherited with the A3-associated haplotype was

TABLE 1.—*Serum Iron Levels and Estimates of Body Iron Stores in Propositus and First-Degree Relatives in Family 1*

Subject	Age (years)	Serum Fe (μmole/liter)	Transferrin (sat. %)	Chelatable Iron (μg/kg body weight)
II-1	54	39	78	344
II-2*	51	53	98	1657
II-3	48	21	43	232
II-4	43	52	95	1865
III-1	29		32	231
III-2	20	19	71	309
III-3	25	38	39	285
		23		
Normal Ranges		13–32	20–40	300

* Propositus.

required to develop the complete syndrome. This A3-associated gene did not lead to any increase in serum iron when operating on its own, and one possibility is that the defect it codes for is acting at a point in the iron distribution process distal to intestinal absorption, possibly at the stage of plasma to storage iron transfer. The serum ferritin level has been shown to be an accurate reflection of tissue iron content, and we have demonstrated that the inheritance of HLA-A3, both in this family and in others, is associated with elevated serum ferritin levels in the absence of an increase in serum iron, findings consistent with the postulated abnormality in plasma to storage iron exchange.

Other groups reported similar family studies, and in general the results support our hypothesis.[16] The French group, however, still considers that the HL-A identity of siblings with the severe disease argues in favor of autosomal recessive inheritance, the responsible genes being partially linked to HLA-A3.[17] However, the inheritance of either of the HL-A haplotypes in this case should confer the same metabolic abnormality, and our family data are not consistent with this view, the inheritance of each haplotype being associated with the presence of one of two quite distinct patterns of iron overload.

Thus the study of iron levels in blood and tissues in relation to the inheritance of HL-A types has clearly refuted the existing hypothesis of autosomal recessive inheritance of hemochromatosis, and our results strongly suggested that there are two loci on the sixth chromosome (one close to the HL-A region) that control iron absorption and distribution. The concordant presence of hemochromatotic alleles at both these loci leads to the full clinical disease.

CHRONIC ACTIVE HEPATITIS

Although the characteristic histologic picture in chronic active hepatitis is a chronic inflammatory process centered in and around the portal tracts with necrosis of periportal hepatocytes (chronic aggressive hepatitis), many subgroups probably exist, differing in their etiologic, genetic, and racial background. A common link seems to be the presence of an antibody directed against a liver-specific membrane lipoprotein,[18] which, in cooperation with cytotoxic lymphocytes,[19] may play an important role in the ongoing damage to the periportal hepatocytes.[20] The membrane lipoprotein is species cross-reactive and can induce the histologic lesion characteristic of the disease when injected repeatedly into rabbits[21] (see Chapter 22).

The two most easily defined subgroups of the disease are classified according to the presence or absence of the hepatitis B surface antigen (HBsAg) in the circulation. Each subgroup has quite different HL-A associations.

HBsAg-negative Chronic Active Hepatitis

A genetic factor may underlie the development of this variety of chronic active hepatitis. One family study from Scandinavia revealed hypergammaglobulinemia and antinuclear antibodies in some maternal relatives of a girl with ''lupoid'' hepatitis.[22] Raised immunoglobulins and an increased incidence of antinuclear antibodies, rheumatoid factor, and thyroid antibodies were found in families of patients with cirrhosis in whom the tests were positive.[23] Occasionally, overt disease may affect several family members,[24] but this is unusual. A study from our own unit in collaboration with Professor Deborah Doniach showed a remarkably high frequency of seroimmunologic abnormalities, including tissue autoantibodies, in the healthy relatives of patients with HBsAg-negative chronic active hepatitis.[25] Conceivably, some of these familial abnormalities could reflect powerful environmental influences, but the discovery by Mackay and Morris[26] of a strong association with inheritance of the histocompatibility antigen HLA-B8 was convincing evidence of a true genetic component. Several reports have now confirmed this observation.[27] The association is strongest in those cases with high titer antinuclear and smooth muscle autoantibodies, and as the original report stressed, there may be a particularly strong link with the lupus erythematosus (LE) cell phenomenon.

Any theory that attempts to explain the association between HLA-B8 and HBsAg-negative chronic active hepatitis must also be applicable to the many other diseases that are associated with B8 (Table 2). One common factor among these conditions is a tendency for excessive antibody production either to an extrinsic antigen or an autoantigen, and it is tempting to regard HLA-B8 as linked to an immune response gene. The wide range of target antigens involved, however, from the acetyl choline receptor in myasthenia gravis[35] to gluten in celiac disease, must make such an antigen-specific mechanism extremely unlikely. One alternative is that a different IR gene is associated with HLA-B8 in each disease. One of our patients, however, a young woman with chronic active hepatitis, had inherited the haplotype A1, B8 from her mother who had been treated for thyrotoxicosis. Thus the development of two of the B8-associated diseases was here associated with the inheritance of the same haplotype and hence the same hypothetical IR gene. Studies of the distribution of D-locus antigens and B-lymphocyte alloantigens in the various HLA-B8-associated conditions should give a definitive answer, but if, as seems likely, the relevant HL-A-associated genes prove to be identical in these diseases, then a B8-linked gene is more likely to be responsible in some way for an antigen-nonspecific increase in immune responsiveness and disease specificity resides in some other, non-HL-A-linked genetic or environmental influence.

Several additional pieces of evidence also point to this conclusion. Thus, HLA-B8 is associated with a high graft rejection rate in recipients of parental kidney grafts[36] and confers an increased ability to eliminate the hepatitis B virus in patients whose immune responsiveness has been impaired by chronic renal failure.[37] Furthermore, by using a standardized preparation of stimulating cells in a mixed lymphocyte reaction, HLA-B8-positive lymphocytes showed increased responsiveness in vitro.[38]

HLA-B8 and Antibody Levels

Many patients with chronic active hepatitis have antibodies to measles and rubella viruses in high titer without evidence of recent infection,[39] and this might be the result of a defect in the control of antibody production. We therefore examined the relation between particular histocompatibility antigens and the titer of antibodies to several antigens in patients with HBsAg-negative chronic active hepatitis and in the family members of some of these patients.

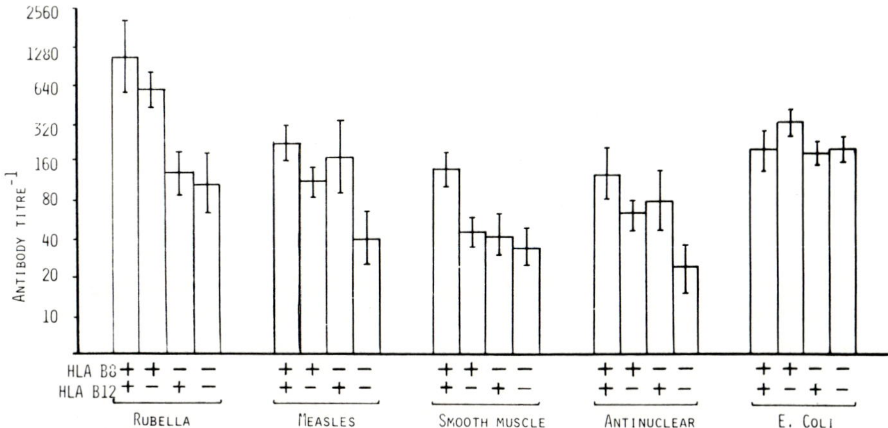

FIG.3—The relation between the geometric mean titers (± 1 SEM) of antibodies to various antigens and the presence of the histocompatibility antigens HLA-B8 and B12 patients with HBsAg-negative chronic active hepatitis. (Reproduced from Eddleston ALWF: Genetically determined immune hyperactivity in human liver disease. Proc R Soc Med 70:525–529, 1977.)

The first significant finding was a close association between HLA-B8 and the titer of rubella antibodies.[40] This was not a specific effect, however, for the mean titers of antibodies reacting with measles, smooth muscle, and nuclei were all higher in serum from HLA-B8-positive patients. Also, one other B-locus antigen, HLA-B12, was associated with a similar increase in antibody titers, particularly measles and antinuclear antibodies. The mechanism of this hyperreactivity seemed to be different for the two histocompatibility antigens, for a synergistic effect on antibody titers was noted when both were inherited together (Fig. 3). By contrast, *E. coli* antibody titers were not significantly related to any of the histocompatibility antigens but were influenced by the degree of portal-systemic shunting, a significant positive correlation being found between the *E. coli* antibody titer and the peak count rate over the spleen on a technetium sulfur colloid scintiscan.[40] This adds support to the concept that, in cirrhosis, increased antibody responses to gut-derived antigens, like *E. coli*, are caused by increased antigen delivery to the spleen and other sites of antibody production consequent to a defect in sequestration of antigen by Kupffer cells[41] (see Chapter 17).

Family studies of 17 first-degree relatives, 7 second-degree relatives, and 6 spouses revealed the mean titer of rubella antibodies to be significantly higher in the first-degree relatives than in the genetically unrelated spouses, but these high antibody levels were not related to the presence of HLA-B8 (Fig. 4). This is further evidence against the simple inheritance of an IR gene linked to HLA-B8 but is consistent with the polygenic inheritance of a more generalized nonspecific increase in immune responsiveness. The patients would have a full complement of the relevant genes, and in this setting the effects of HLA-B8 and B12 would be most evident. The genes in the family members would be split up, and the effect of B8 or B12 to increase antibody levels in some of the individuals might be similar in magnitude to the effect of other genes, not HL-A-linked, which other family members had inherited. The overall effect would

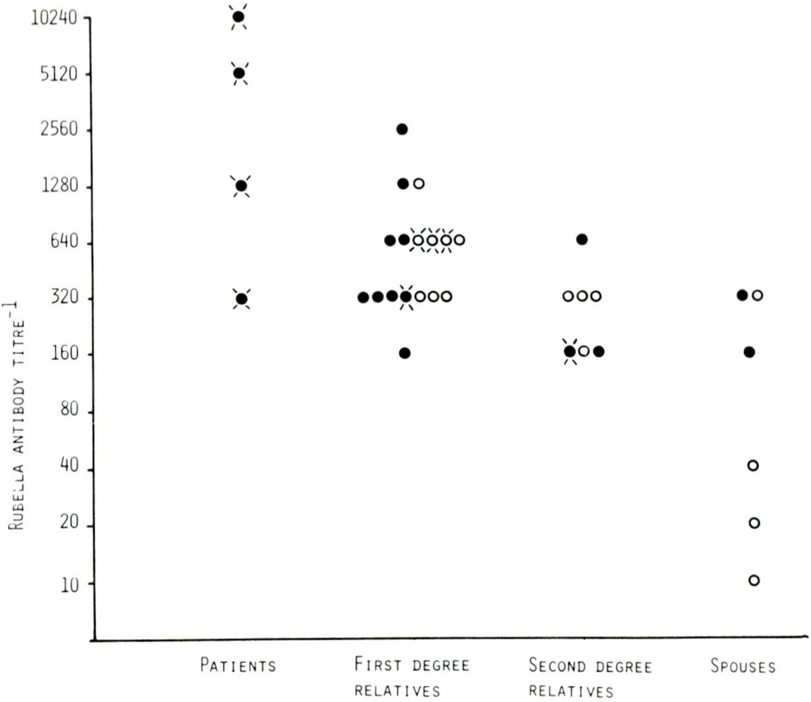

FIG. 4—Rubella antibody titers in 4 patients with chronic active hepatitis, 17 first-degree relatives, 7 second-degree relatives, and 6 genetically unrelated spouses. ●, HLA-B8-positive; ○, B8-negative; ⋈, smooth muscle and/or antinuclear antibodies detected. (Reproduced from Eddleston ALWF: Genetically determined immune hyperreactivity in human liver disease. Proc R Soc Med 70:525–529, 1977.)

be to produce, on the average, antibody levels in the first-degree relatives that were less than those in the patients but greater than those in the unrelated spouses. This is well illustrated in Fig. 4, which also demonstrates that the antibody levels in the few second-degree relatives tested were intermediate between those in the first-degree relatives and the spouses, further supporting the concept of polygenic control of antibody levels. A comparable animal model was described[42] in which mice were selectively bred for high and low antibody response to erythrocyte antigens. High and low responders differed genetically at approximately ten loci, at least one of which was histocompatibility-linked. The phenotypic expression of some of these genes has been identified in the mice where, for example, macrophage handling of antigen is different in the high and low line animals[42] The mechanisms in man responsible for the increased antibody levels are almost completely unknown, however. In our own family study, the inheritance of the tendency to acquire circulating antibodies that react with smooth muscle and nuclear antigens was clearly independent of both HLA-B8 and the height of the antibody response to rubella (Fig. 4) but was probably another of the genetic ingredients of HBsAg-negative chronic active hepatitis.

TABLE 2—*Diseases Associated with an
Increased Frequency of HLA-B8*

Chronic active hepatitis[26]
Gluten sensitive enteropathy[28]
Dermatitis herpetiformis[29]
Myasthenia gravis[30]
Diabetes mellitus[31]
Coombs' test positivity[32]
Addison's disease[33]
Thyrotoxicosis[34]

HLA-B8 and Immune Control Mechanisms

We have postulated that HLA-B8 might be associated with a gene promoting a defect in the activity of suppressor T cells, resulting in a loss of control of immune responses[20] and that this is the link between the many different B8-associated diseases listed in Table 2. Such a suppressor T-cell defect would result in a failure to adequately switch off immune responses, but only when combined with a powerful switch-on mechanism would it lead to very high antibody levels. The findings in the patients with chronic active hepatitis and their relatives are remarkably close to this predicted behavior. Furthermore, initial findings using techniques that can apparently measure suppressor T-cell function in man confirmed the presence of a defect in chronic active hepatitis,[43] although a link between B8 and suppressor cell activity has not been explored. Clinical evidence offers additional support for this concept of the B8-associated defect. In patients with juvenile-onset diabetes mellitus, HLA-B8 has been associated, not so much with the presence of antibodies reacting with pancreatic islet cells, but with the persistence of these antibodies for many years after the onset of the disease,[44] and the same effect probably occurs in thyrotoxicosis, in which HLA-B8 is associated with a high relapse rate after a full course of medical treatment.[45] A synergistic effect of HLA-B8 with other histocompatibility antigens is also found in diabetes in relation to titers of antibody to coxsackie viruses.[46]

The recognition that "turn off" and "turn on" of immune responses may be under independent genetic control implies that the predisposition to autoimmunity may be inherited quite separately from the genetic factors determining the severity and pattern of the autoimmune assault. The case summarized in Table 3 exemplifies this point. This patient has multiple immune-mediated disorders but has an extremely easily controlled disease. His liver biopsy on treatment continues to show no evidence of piecemeal necrosis of periportal hepatocytes and no cirrhosis, but two attempts to withdraw steroids have led to relapses with biochemical and histologic changes typical of chronic active hepatitis. Histocompatibility testing showed the presence of HLA-A1 and B8 only, but the titers of rubella and measles antibody were both very low at less than 1/20, smooth muscle antibody was only just detected at a titer of 1/10, and serum samples have been consistently negative for antinuclear antibodies. Thus, if the hypothesis outlined earlier is correct, he has inherited very poor "switch-off" mechanisms but, fortunately, has also been endowed with a poor

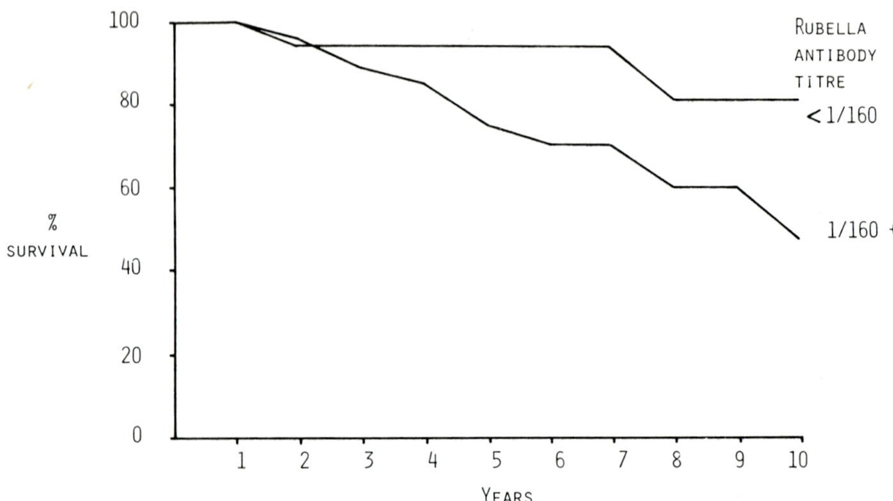

FIG. 5.—Survival curves for patients with HBsAg-negative chronic active hepatitis treated with conventional immunosuppressive therapy. The cases have been divided into two groups according to the titer of antibodies to rubella virus.[40]

"switch-on" mechanism. This combination would explain both the multisystem involvement with frequent relapses and the ease of control by steroids. A further inference from this case may be that the rubella and measles antibody titers reflect the intensity of the autoimmune assault against hepatocytes. This is supported by the finding of a correlation between length of survival and the rubella antibody titer in patients with HBsAg-negative chronic active hepatitis (Fig. 5).

While HLA-B8 and B12 may be associated with heightened immune responses, circumstantial evidence is accumulating suggesting that HLA-B7 may be linked with some degree of immunodeficiency. For example, B7 is

TABLE 3.—*Summarized Case History of Man with Multiple Immune-mediated Disorders but Very Easily Controlled Disease.**

Age (years)	Diagnosis	Treatment	Result
11	Nephrotic syndrome	Steroids	Remission
25	Chronic active hepatitis (CAH) (prolonged hepatitic illness with biopsy showing mildly active CAH)	Steroids	Remission
26	Myxedema		
27	Henoch-Schonlein purpura	Steroids	Remission
27	Epididymitis	Steroids	Remission
34 (now)	CAH continues	Steroids	Well controlled (withdrawal of steroids produces relapse)

*The only detectable histocompatibility antigens were HLA-A1 and HLA-B8, but titers of the various antibodies tested were all very low.

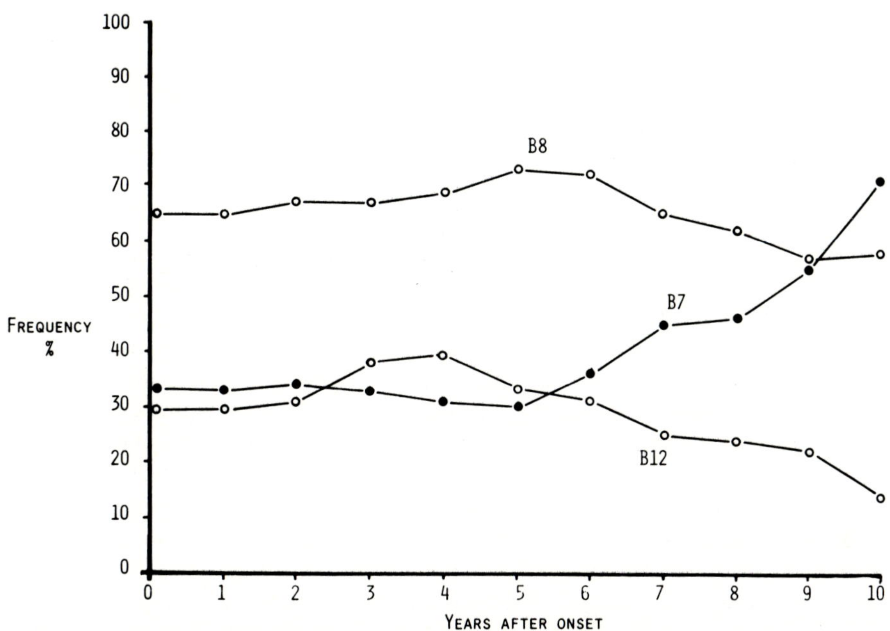

FIG. 6.—Changes in the frequency of HLA-B8, B12, and B7 related to survival time after onset of the disease in patients with HBsAg-negative chronic active hepatitis.

related to hyporesponsiveness to tuberculin.[47] The incidence of HLA-B7 in chronic active hepatitis does not differ from that in a control population, but analysis of our data showed that the presence of this histocompatibility antigen does alter immune responsiveness.[48] These reduced antibody responses in HL A-B7-positive chronic active hepatitis may also reflect a reduced intensity of autoimmune liver damage, for analysis of the frequencies of HL-A in patients with chronic active hepatitis in relation to length of survival clearly shows a deficit in HLA-B12 and a striking increase in HLA-B7 in those surviving up to 10 years after diagnosis (Fig. 6).

HBsAg-Positive Chronic Active Hepatitis

The HLA-B8 frequency in patients with HBsAg-positive chronic active hepatitis is very low, but it is also very low in unaffected members of the communities in which these patients live (i.e., Southern Europe, Middle East, etc). Few studies have been done in areas with a high prevalence of the disease but suggestions are that BW15 may be associated with long-term carriage of HBsAg,[49] and BW35, with HBsAg-positive chronic active hepatitis.[50] In our own small series of 17 patients with HBsAg-positive chronic active hepatitis, BW35 is increased to 35% (control population 17%), but with these small numbers the differences is not significant.

A series of American cases of chronic active hepatitis were reported in the Seventh Histocompatibility Workshop at Oxford.[5] All were HBsAg-negative and the frequency of HLA-B8 was only slightly increased, but there was an increase of BW35. This HBsAg-positive type of HL-A phenotype in the absence of HBsAg raises the possibility of persisting virus infection, possibly non-A, non-B in some of these patients. Infection with this agent(s) can progress to chronic liver disease, including chronic active hepatitis.[51]

One important conclusion from all these studies is that chronic active hepatitis is almost certainly multifactorial in its etiology although identical in its histopathology and probably in its final pathogenetic pathway.[20]

ALCOHOLIC LIVER DISEASE

The variability in the clinical response to high alcohol intake has intensified the search for genetic factors that could determine the type and/or severity of the alcohol-associated liver damage. Interest has been increasing in the immunologic reactions associated with alcoholic liver injury, particularly alcoholic hepatitis. Using lymphocyte transformation and leukocyte migration tests, sensitization to alcohol, acetaldehyde, homogenates of autologous liver, and a purified extract of alcoholic hyaline has been shown in patients with alcoholic hepatitis but not in those with steatosis or inactive alcoholic cirrhosis.[52] Autoimmunity may also play a part in the tissue damage. Sensitization to homogenates of normal liver[53] and the presence in peripheral blood of lymphocytes that are cytotoxic for isolated rabbit hepatocytes in patients with alcoholic hepatitis but not in those with steatosis or inactive cirrhosis were also reported.[54]

Against this background, many centers embarked on an analysis of the influence of the HL-A system on the pattern of alcoholic liver disease. Considering all cases with some evidence of alcoholic liver injury, no major disturbances in HL-A frequencies were found although HLA-B8 was slightly increased in many of the series.[55] Analysis of our cases in more detail showed that the frequency of B8 was significantly greater in those cases with alcoholic cirrhosis when compared to those with fatty liver or fibrosis only.[56] Even so, the B8 frequency of 45% in those with cirrhosis was not as high as in chronic active hepatitis, and this antigen is more likely to modify the expression of alcoholic injury rather than to directly determine the toxicity of alcohol. HL A-BW40, however, is present in a high proportion of patients with alcoholic hepatitis or cirrhosis in Oslo.[57] Further studies are needed to confirm this association and explore its disease specificity, but such a strong association would suggest a more direct link between this genetic marker and the toxic effect of ethanol on the liver. One possibility is that BW40 is linked to an IR gene that controls the presence or absence of an immune reaction to an alcohol-altered liver membrane antigen. The intensity of the immune responses to this neoantigen and thus perhaps the rate of progression to cirrhosis might then be modified by genes linked to other B-locus antigens such as HLA-B8.

HL-A AND DISEASE SUSCEPTIBILITY

In this review, we have emphasized the many ways in which histocompatibility antigens could be linked to genes controlling susceptibility to disease. The mechanisms involved in the association of HLA-A3 with idiopathic hemochromatosis are probably completely different from those involved in linking HLA-B8 with HBsAg-negative chronic active hepatitis. Family studies in both situations have been of crucial importance in identifying the genetic contribution to which the particular histocompatibility antigen is linked and have also emphasized the complex pattern of inheritance. Several genetic components seem to interact with each other and with the environment in any one individual to produce the full clinical expression of the disease. A further clinical consequence of the polygenic regulation of immune responses is that the histocompatibility antigen profile may be an important determinant of the clinical course and prognosis of diseases where immune reactions are implicated in pathogenesis. This not only applies to chronic active hepatitis but may also be relevant to alcohol-induced liver damage where both autoimmunity and direct toxicity of alcohol may be involved in the progression to cirrhosis.

REFERENCES

1. Medewar PB: Immunity to homologous grafted skin; relationship between antigens of blood and skin. Br J Exp Pathol 27:15–24, 1946

2. Dausset J, Tang Un, Y: Leucocyte and platelet groups and their practical significance. Vox Sang 10:641–659, 1965

3. Mittal KK, Mickey MR, Singal DP, Terasaki PI: Serotyping for homotransplantation. 18. Refinement of microdroplet lymphocyte cytotoxicity test. Transplantation 6:913–927, 1968

4. Mann DL, Rogentine GN, Fahey JL, Natherson SG: Human lymphocyte membrane (HL-A) alloantigens: Isolation, purification and properties. J Immunol 103:282–292, 1969

5. Bodmer WF, Batchelor JR, Morris PJ, Festenstein H (eds): Histocompatibility Testing. Copenhagen, Munksgaard, 1979 (in press)

6. Lilly F, Pincus T: Genetic control of immune viral leukemogenesis. Edited by G Klein, S Weinhouse, and A Haddosi. Adv Cancer Res 17:231–277, 1973

7. Brewerton DA, Laffrey M, Hart FD, James DCO, Nicholls A, Sturrock RD: Ankylosing spondylitis and HLA 27. Lancet 1:904–907, 1973

8. Benacerraf B, Katz DH: The nature and function of histocompatibility-linked immune response genes. Edited by B Benacerraf: Immunogenetics and Immunodeficiency. Lancaster, MTP Press, 1975, pp 117–143

9. Rose NR, Kite JH, Vladutiu AO, Tomazie V, Bacon LD: Genetic aspects of autoimmune thyroiditis. Int Arch Allergy Appl Immunol 45:138–149, 1973

10. Mays WR, Schernthanum L, Mehdi SQ, Hofer R: Missing evidence of a correlation between Hashimoto thyroiditis and HLA antigens. HLA and Disease. Paris, Editions INSERM, 1976, pp 137

11. Sheldon JH: Haemochromatosis. New York, Oxford University Press, 1935

12. Grace ND, Powell LW: Iron storage disorders of the liver. Gastroenterology 67:1257–1283, 1974

13. Williams R, Scheuer PJ, Sherlock S: The inheritance of idiopathic haemochromatosis. Q J Med 31:249–255, 1962

14. Simon M, Bourel M, Fauchet R, Genetet B: Association of HLA-A3 and HLA-B14 antigens with idiopathic haemochromatosis. Gut 17:332–334, 1976

15. Bomford A, Eddleston ALWF, Kennedy LA, Batchelor JR, Williams R: Histocompatibility antigens as markers of abnormal iron metabolism in patients with idiopathic haemochromatosis and their relatives. Lancet 1:327–329, 1977

16. Amos DB, Johnson AH, Cartwright G, Edwards C, Scolnick M: HLA and B cell antigens in haemochromatosis. Tissue-Antigens 10:206, 1977

17. Simon M, Bourel M, Genetet B, Fauchet R: Idiopathic haemochromatosis: Demonstration of recessive transmission and early detection by family HLA typing. N Engl J Med 297:1017–1020, 1977

18. Jensen DM, McFarlane IG, Portmann B, Eddleston ALWF, Williams R: The detection of antibodies directed against a liver-

specific membrane lipoprotein (LSP) in patients with acute and chronic active hepatitis. N Engl J Med 299:1–7, 1978

19. Cochrane AMG, Thomson AD, Moussouros A, Eddleston ALWF, Williams R: Antibody-dependent, cell-mediated (K cell) cytotoxicity against isolated rabbit hepatocytes in chronic active hepatitis. Lancet 1:441–444, 1976

20. Eddleston ALWF, Williams R: Inadequate antibody response to HB Ag or suppressor T-cell defect in development of active chronic hepatitis. Lancet 2:1543–1545, 1974

21. Meyer zum Buschenfelde KH, Kossling FK, Meischer PA: Experimental chronic active hepatitis in rabbits following immunisation with human liver proteins. Clin Exp Immunol 11:99–108, 1972

22. Cavell B, Leonhardt ETG: Hereditary hypergammaglobulinaemia and lupoid hepatitis. Acta Med Scand 177:751–759, 1965

23. Elling D, Panlov P, Bildsoe P: A genetic approach to the pathogenesis of hepatic cirrhosis. A clinical and serological study. Acta Med Scand 179:527–533, 1966

24. Joske RA, Laurence BH: Familial cirrhosis with autoimmune features and raised immunoglobulin levels. Gastroenterology 59:546–552, 1970

25. Galbraith RM, Smith MGM, Mackenzie RM, Tee DE, Doniach D, Williams R: High prevalence of seroimmunologic abnormalities in relatives of patients with active chronic hepatitis or primary biliary cirrhosis. N Engl J Med 290:63–69, 1974

26. Mackay IR, Morris PJ: Association of autoimmune active chronic hepatitis with HL-A1, 8. Lancet 2:793–795, 1972

27. Galbraith RM, Eddleston ALWF, Smith MGM, Williams R, MacSween RNM, Watkinson G, Dick H, Kennedy LA, Batchelor JR: Histocompatibility antigen in active chronic hepatitis and primary biliary cirrhosis. Bri Med J 3:604–605, 1974

28. Stokes PL, Asquith P, Holmes GKT, Mackintosh P, Cooke WT: Histocompability antigens associated with adult coeliac disease. Lancet 2:162–164, 1972

29. Gebhard RL, Katz SI, Marks J, Shuster S, Trapani RJ, Rogentine GN, Strober W: HL-A antigen type and small-intestinal disease in dermatitis herpetiformis. Lancet 2:760–762, 1973

30. Pirskanen R, Tulikairen A, Hokkaren E: Histocompatibility (HL-A) antigens associated with myasthenia gravis. Ann Clin Res 4:304–306, 1972

31. Cudworth AG, Woodrow JC: HL-A system and diabetes mellitus. Diabetes 24:345–349, 1975

32. DaCosta JAG, White AG, Parker AC, Grigor GB: Increased incidence of HL-A 1 and 8 in patients showing IgG or complement coating on their red cells. J Clin Pathol 27:353–355, 1974

33. Platz P, Ryder L, Staub Nielsen L, Svejgaard A, Thomson M, Nerup J, Christy M: HL-A and idiopathicAddison's disease. Lancet 2:289, 1974

34. Grumet C, Konishi J, Payne R, Kriss JP: Association of Graves' disease with HL-A8. Clin Res 21:493–495, 1973

35. Richman DP, Patrick J, Arnsson BGW: Cellular immunity in myasthenia gravis. Response to purified acetylcholine receptor and autologus thymocytes. N Engl J Med 294:694–698, 1976

36. Mickey MR, Kreisler M, Albert ED, Tanaka N, Terasaki PI: Analysis of HL-A incompatibility in human renal transplants. TissueAntigens 1:57–67, 1971

37. Bach JF, Zingraff J, Descamps B, Naret C, Jungen P: HL-A, 1.8 phenotype and HBs antigenaemia in haemodialysis patients. Lancet 2:707, 1975

38. Osaba D, Falk J: HLA genes regulating the magnitude of the mixed leukocyte reaction (MLR). HLA and Disease. Paris, Editions INSERM, 1976, p 280

39. Triger DR, MacCallum FO, Kurtz JB, Wright R: Raised antibody titres to measles and rubella viruses in chronic active hepatitis. Lancet 1:665–667, 1972

40. Galbraith RM, Eddleston ALWF, Williams R, Webster ADB, Pattison J, Doniach D, Kennedy LA, Batchelor JR: Enhanced antibody responses in active chronic hepatitis: Relation to HLA-B8 and HLA-B12 and portosystemic shunting. Lancet 1:930–934, 1976

41. Bjørneboe M, Prytz H: The mononuclear phagocytic functions of the liver. Edited by A Ferguson and RNM MacSween: Immunological Aspects of the Liver and Gastrointestinal Tract. Lancaster, MTP Press Ltd, 1976, pp 251–290.

42. Stiffel C, Mouton D, Bouthillier Y, Heumann AM, Decreuseford C, Mevel JC, Biozzi G: Polygenic regulation of general antibody synthesis in the mouse. Edited by L Brent and J Holborow: Progress in Immunology. Vol. 2. Amsterdam, North-Holland, 1974, pp 203–212

43. Hodgson HJF, Wands JR, Isselbacher KJ:

Suppressor lymphocytes: Their role in modulating the immune response in acute and chronic active hepatitis. Gastroenterology, 72:1070, 1977

44. Morris PJ, Vaughan H, Irvine WJ, Gray RS, McCallum CJ, Campbell CJ, Duncan LJP: HLA and pancreatic islet cell antibodies in diabetes. Lancet 2:652–653, 1976

45. Irvine WJ, Gray RS, Morris PJ, Ting A: Correlation of HLA and thyroid antibodies with clinical course of thyrotoxicosis treated with antithyroid drugs. Lancet 2:898–900, 1977

46. Cudworth AG, Gamble DR, White GBB, Lendrum R, Woodrow JC, Bloom A: Aetiology of juvenile-onset diabetes. Lancet 1:385–388, 1977

47. Buckley CE, White DH, Siegler HF: HLA-B7 associated tuberculin hyporesponsiveness in BCG treated patients. HLA and Disease. Paris, Editions INSERM, 1976, p 175

48. Eddleston ALWF, Galbraith RM, Batchelor JR, Pattison J, Doniach D, Williams R: Histocompatibility antigens and immune responses. Edited by ALWF Eddleston, JCP Weber and R Williams: Immune Reactions in Liver Disease. Tunbridge Wells, England, Pitman Medical and Philadelphia, J.B. Lippincott, 1979, pp 96–103

49. Chiaramonte M: HLA and persistent HBs antigenaemia. Edited by ALWF Eddleston, JCP Weber and R Williams: Immune Reactions in Liver Disease. Tunbridge Wells, England, Pitman Medical and Philadelphia, J.B. Lippincott, 1979, p 113

50. Mazzilli MC, Trabace S, Raimondo FD, Gandini E, Visco G: HLA and chronic active hepatitis. Digestion 15:278–285, 1977

51. Galbraith RM, Portmann B, Eddleston ALWF, Williams R, Gower PE: Chronic liver disease developing after outbreak of HBsAg-negative hepatitis in haemodialysis unit. Lancet 2:886–889, 1975

52. Zetterman RK, Luisada-Opper A, Leevy CM: Alcoholic hepatitis, cell-mediated immunological response to alcoholic hyaline. Gastroenterology 70:382–384, 1976

53. Mihas AA, Bull DM, Davidson CS: Cell-mediated immunity to liver in patients with alcoholic hepatitis. Lancet 1:951–953, 1975

54. Cochrane AMG, Moussouros A, Portmann B, McFarlane IG, Thomson AD, Eddleston ALWF, Williams R: Lymphocyte cytotoxicity for isolated hepatocytes in alcoholic liver disease. Gastroenterology 72:918–923, 1977

55. Eddleston ALWF, Weber JCP, Williams R: Immune Reactions in Liver Disease. Tunbridge Wells, England, Pitman Medical and Philadelphia, J.B. Lippincott, 1979, pp 225–226

56. Bailey RJ, Krasner N, Eddleston ALWF, Williams R, Tee DEH, Doniach D, Kennedy LA, Batchelor JR: Histocompatibility antigens, autoantibodies and immunoglobulins in alcoholic liver disease. Br Med J 2:727–729, 1976

57. Bell H, Nordhagen R: An association between HLA-BW 40 and alcoholic liver disease. Br Med J 1:822–824, 1978

58. Eddleston ALWF: Genetically determined immune hyperreactivity in human liver disease. Proc R Soc Med 70:525–529, 1977

Chapter 16

Clotting Abnormalities in Liver Disease

By P.T. FLUTE, M.D.

DETERMINATION of the primary structure of many of the coagulation factors has removed some of the previous uncertainties regarding the mechanisms of coagulation. A sequence of proenzyme to enzyme transformations, each depending on the product of the former, gives, in succession, a number of proteases each with the amino acid serine at the active site (Fig. 1). Thrombin (factor IIa), the final serine protease of the sequence, converts fibrinogen to fibrin, activates fibrin-stabilizing factor (factor XIII), induces fundamental changes in platelets, and has complex feedback effects on the earlier changes of coagulation.[1] The rate of the changes is increased by the ability of many of the constituents to complex with each other, with phospholipid, and with protein cofactors (factor V and factor VIII).

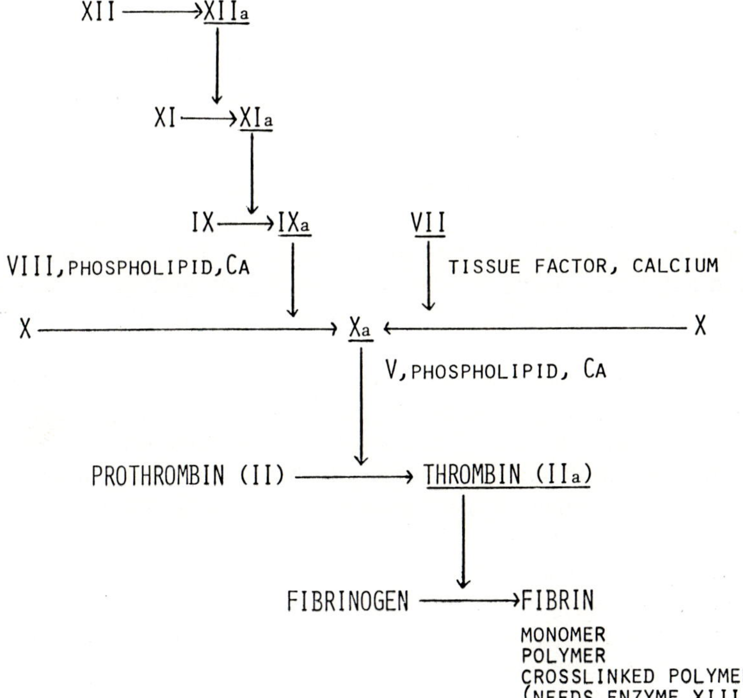

FIG. 1—The blood coagulation mechanism in outline (serine proteases underlined).

From the Department of Haemotology, St. George's Hospital Medical School, London, England.

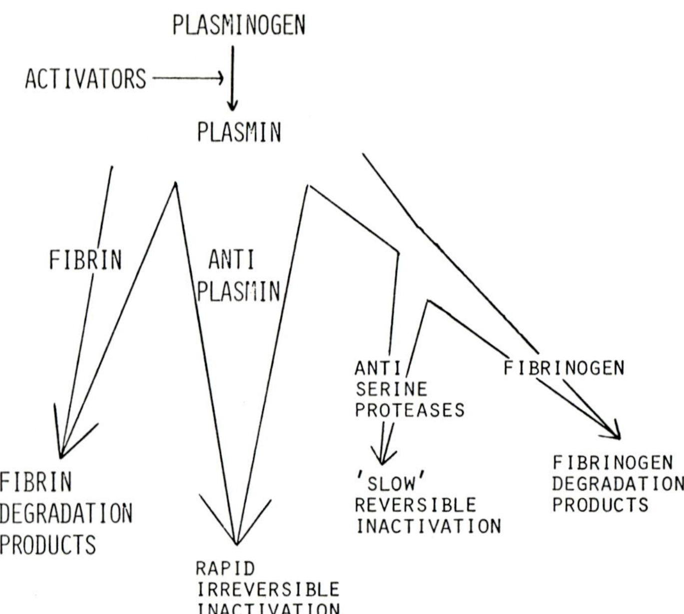

FIG. 2—The fibrinolytic enzyme system.

A particular liver-produced protein, variously referred to as antithrombin III, heparin cofactor, or factor-Xa inhibitor, opposes the action of each of the serine proteases concerned with coagulation. Its action is greatly accelerated by heparin,[2] which has no effect on the other protease inhibitors of blood. These, including alpha-2-macroglobulin, alpha-1-antitrypsin, inter-alpha trypsin inhibitor, Cl esterase inhibitor, or fast antiplasmin, may bind any traces of active enzyme not complexed by antithrombin III. Enzyme-inhibitor complexes and any free enzyme are cleared from the circulation by cells of the reticuloendothelial (mononuclear-phagocyte) system, especially their representatives in the liver.

Thus, considerable conceptual advances have been made. Many problems, however, remain all-important to the further understanding of the many changes found in liver disease. What is the effective stimulus to coagulation? How do the activation systems intrinsic to blood and those dependent on extrinsic materials interact? What regulates the synthesis of zymogens, cofactors, and inhibitors?

The fibrinolytic enzyme system shows many comparable features (Fig. 2).[3] Digestion of fibrin depends on another serine protease, plasmin, which is derived from its precursor plasminogen by the action of the plasminogen activators. The action of the enzymes is again regulated by a series of inhibitors and by reticuloendothelial clearance of complexes and active enzymes. The plasmin inhibitor of greatest biologic importance is the recently discovered alpha globulin now called fast antiplasmin or alpha-2-antiplasmin. This is synthesized by the liver[4,5] and is present in plasma at around 1 μM concentration, sufficient to neutralize only about half of the total potential plasmin. The special biologic relationship of plasmin to fibrin appears to depend on complex formation of the various enzymes and substrates and on the virtually instantaneous action of this α_2-antiplasmin compared with the slower action of the other serine protease inhibitors of blood.

In liver disease, derangements may involve quantitative or qualitative changes in hepatic synthesis of coagulation or fibrinolytic enzyme precursors or of the inhibitors. Reticuloendothelial clearance of these enzymes or their products may also become deranged. Defects of hepatic synthesis form the largest and most important group, but an increased catabolism of coagulation factors is also demonstrable in many patients, thus exaggerating the frequent deficiencies of the various plasma components.

No patient with serious liver disease is likely to be free of at least one of these defects. Subtle interrelationships of vessel and platelet function and more obvious anatomic changes in vessels, such as those associated with portal hypertension, must also be taken into account when considering the reasons for bleeding in hepatic disorders. Before turning to practical considerations of prognosis and therapy, however, this review will examine current ideas on hepatic synthesis, biologic turnover of clotting factors, and the pattern of these disorders seen in various forms of liver disease.

HEPATIC SYNTHESIS

The liver is thought to synthesize fibrinogen, the zymogen factors II, VII, IX, X, XI,XII, XIII, the cofactor, factor V, and the inhibitors of both coagulation and fibrinolysis. The liver may also be a site of plasminogen synthesis. Synthesis may be quantitatively deficient or qualitatively abnormal. The derangements are characteristically multiple.

Fibrinogen

Biosynthetic studies of liver slices[6] and suspensions of hepatocytes[7] confirm that the hepatocyte is the main and probably the only source of plasma fibrinogen. Fibrinogen synthesized by platelets does not appear to contribute to plasma levels.[8] The fibrinogen molecule consists of three pairs of polypeptide chains (aα, Bβ, and γ) covalently linked by disulfide bonds, and the polysome complexes involved have been isolated from hepatocytes.[9] Any tendency to increased catabolism of fibrinogen is rapidly compensated, and usually overcompensated, by increased synthesis. Fibrinogen is one of the acute-phase reactants whose concentration increases dramatically in response to inflammation anywhere in the body.[10] In liver disease the output of fibrinogen is maintained until a very late stage; low plasma levels of this protein are found in terminal hepatic coma.

Many patients with liver disease have abnormal molecules of fibrinogen in their plasma, which causes a delay in fibrin monomer polymerization. This is easily recognizable from the prolonged clotting time of their plasma with thrombin and also with extracts of the venoms of the snakes *Bothrops jararaca* or *Agkistrodon rhodostoma*. Unlike the thrombin time, the clotting times with these venoms are not affected by heparin. Other causes of a long thrombin time, such as a plasma fibrinogen level of less than 1 g/liter, very high levels of fibrin (ogen) degradation products of fibrinolysis (FDP), or the nonspecific inhibitory effects of paraproteins, can usually be excluded. While a defect of fibrinogen synthesis is postulated, damage to the preformed molecule by mechanical stress or proteolytic attack in the circulation has yet to be eliminated. The original observations were made by Fanconi in 1941 in a child with congenital syphilis, jaundice, and hepatomegaly, but such dysfibrinogenemia has been found in many cases of hepatic coma, uncompensated cirrhosis, and with primary hepatic carcinoma.[11,12]

Eleven patients with various liver diseases and long thrombin times have recently been investigated in detail.[13] They showed normal electrophoretic patterns of the isolated fibrinogen, its constituent chains, and its plasmin degradation products. Fibrin monomers prepared from the fibrinogen showed delayed polymerization, however. The change has been compared with the unusual production of alpha-fetoprotein in liver disease, but no clearly recognizable fetal fibrinogen has yet been isolated, and the defects are clearly heterogeneous.

Vitamin-K-dependent Factors

The liver is the main source of the vitamin-K-dependent coagulation factors II, VII, IX, and X, although it may not be the only one.[14] Immunologically similar but functionally inactive proteins appear in the plasma of subjects deficient in vitamin K or treated with one of the coumarin anticoagulants.[15] The Ca^{2+}-binding ability and absorption to $BaSO_4$ of these PIVKAs (protein induced by vitamin K absence or antagonists) were reduced as compared with the normal proteins. The explanation of all these attributes came with the discovery[16] of the γ-carboxy glutamic acid residues of the normal molecules. The new amino acid arises from a vitamin-K-dependent, postribosomal carboxylation reaction affecting several glutamic acid residues close to the NH_2-terminal end of the molecules. In addition to the vitamin-K-dependent coagulation factors, γ-carboxy glutamic acid residues necessary for the Ca^{2+} binding have been found in two bovine plasma proteins of uncertain function and in Ca^{2+}-binding proteins in animal and human bone.[17]

Thus, if the fat-soluble vitamin K is deficient, as in obstructive jaundice, or is antagonized by one of the coumarin anticoagulants, coagulation factors are synthesized at the normal rate, but they lack some or all of the necessary γ-carboxy glutamic acid residues necessary for Ca^{2+} binding to phospholipid and thus lack their procoagulant function. This is easily detected by a prolongation of the prothrombin time of plasma. The defect can be characterized by showing an excess of the inactive protein by immunologic methods using specific antisera and also by suitable modifications of the prothrombin time or thrombotest that demonstrate the PIVKA effect.

Other Zymogens

The synthesis of the ''contact factors'' (factors XI and XII of the coagulation system, prekallikrein and high-molecular-weight kininogen of the kinin system) is thought to occur in the liver, since hepatocellular necrosis is associated with decreased plasma levels. There is, however, no conclusive evidence. Similarly, plasminogen levels are decreased in hepatocellular disease, but liver perfusion studies have failed to provide positive support for its synthesis.[18]

Factor XIII is found in plasma as a tetramer of two alpha chains and two beta chains. The active form catalyzes γ-glutamyl-ε-lysyl cross-links in fibrin polymer; the active site is on the alpha chains. Both alpha and beta chains are formed by hepatocytes,[19] the latter at the faster rate. Platelets also form alpha chains, but their contribution to plasma factor XIII is uncertain. Plasma factor XIII levels have sometimes been reported as low in hepatocellular disease states.[20,21]

Cofactors

Perfusion of isolated rat liver suggests that factor V is synthesized by hepatocytes.[22] Since this is independent of vitamin K, the demonstration of a low factor V helps to differentiate between a vitamin-K-responsive disorder and reduced synthesis owing to hepatocyte loss. The molecule of factor V is notoriously unstable and has yet to be fully characterized. It appears to form a complex with prothrombin and, in the presence of phospholipid and Ca^{2+}, enhances its activation by factor Xa, a reaction that proceeds very slowly in its absence. The action of factor V is greatly enhanced in the presence of thrombin.

Factor VIII is a glycoprotein of immense size and complicated structure that binds with factor X to enhance its activation by IXa, again with phospholipid and Ca^{2+} as part of the complex. Thrombin enhances this nonenzymatic function.

Inherited deficiency of factor VIII occurs in classical hemophilia and in von Willebrand's disease. The procoagulant activity (FVIIIC) is reduced in both diseases, but factor VIII, recognized by heterologous precipitating antisera (FVIII-related antigen, FVIIIRA), is increased in the former and is reduced, or abnormal in the latter. The ability of factor VIII to support platelet aggregation by ristocetin (FVIIIRWF) is another defect found in von Willebrand's disease. FVIIIRA is probably synthesized by vascular endothelial cells,[23] and while this includes the endothelium of the liver, nothing suggests that the hepatocyte is involved in this synthesis.

Considerable controversy surrounds the relation of the other attributes of FVIIIC and FVIIIRWF to the FVIIIRA. Separate molecular components have been suggested.[24] Many physiologic and pathologic stimuli cause a parallel increase in FVIIIC and FVIIIRA, and FVIII may be one of the "acute phase reactants." During normal pregnancy a sustained increase of both suggests an increased rate of synthesis.[25] In states of intravascular coagulation, however, FVIIIC may be consumed at a faster rate than normal, and since FVIIIRA is detectable in equal amounts in serum as in plasma, a reduction in FVIIIC relative to FVIIIRA may result. Such a finding is common in hepatocellular disease.

Inhibitors

The protease inhibitors of plasma are probably synthesized by the hepatocyte.[26] Reduced plasma concentration of antithrombin III and alpha-2-antiplasmin are characteristic of hepatocellular disease.

INCREASED CATABOLISM

Normally, approximately 20±8% of the circulating fibrinogen is lost each day, and this fractional catabolic rate is remarkably constant and independent of the plasma concentration of fibrinogen. The fractional loss is increased in many liver diseases, particularly in fulminant hepatic failure[27] and cirrhosis[28] but also in severe acute viral hepatitis and chronic active hepatitis.[29] The increased catabolism is almost always counterbalanced by increased synthesis, giving normal or even increased plasma fibrinogen concentrations.

Turnover studies of labeled prothrombin and labeled plasminogen in patients with cirrhosis showed that increased fractional catabolic rate and decreased synthetic rate accounted for the low plasma levels.[30]

Physiologic losses of fibrinogen normally occur by an unknown route but are largely independent of coagulation and fibrinolysis. The increase in the fractional catabolic rate for fibrinogen that occurs in liver disease suggests that an unusual route of loss is involved. The association of many other changes suggests that this route may, at least in part, be via accelerated intravascular coagulation. This is supported by finding microthrombi in the organs at autopsy,[31] by excessive deposition of isotopically labeled fibrinogen in the organs of animals subjected to experimental hepatic necrosis,[32,33] by discrepancy between FVIIIC and FVIIIRA levels typical of intravascular coagulation,[34] by associated thrombocytopenia, by increase of circulating FDP, and by circulating soluble fibrin.[35] Also to be considered as possible routes of increased loss are bleeding, loss into extravascular compartments (e.g., ascites, areas of liver necrosis), intravascular proteolysis by enzymes other than thrombin (e.g., plasmin), and accelerated removal by the reticuloendothelial system (possibly the normal route). Heparin has no effect on the rate of fibrinogen loss in normal subjects but slows the rate of loss in liver disease, which is further evidence to support the role of intravascular coagulation.[36] Stimuli to coagulation would be expected to arise from necrotic hepatocytes or from defective clearance of intestinal endotoxin (see Chapter 17). Defective hepatic clearance of activated enzymes, soluble fibrin, and FDP could accentuate the tendency.

FIBRINOLYSIS

The blood of many patients with cirrhosis has increased plasminogen activator and decreased plasminogen concentration,[37] possibly owing to impaired clearance of activator by the liver[38] and perhaps accentuated by defective hepatic synthesis of normal plasma inhibitors. In fulminant hepatic failure[35] and after hepatic transplantation,[38] plasma plasminogen is often low, with normal or decreased plasminogen activator and a mild increase in FDP. However, none of these changes is greater than similar changes frequently found in response to mild physiologic stimuli (such as pregnancy), and their biologic significance is uncertain. Recent observations suggest that low levels of alpha-2-antiplasmin are found in severe liver disease.

COAGULATION PATTERNS
IN LIVER DISEASE

Despite considerable overlap, patterns characteristic of three main features of hepatic disorder can be identified: portal hypertension, cholestasis, and hepatocellular disease. Patients with portal hypertension tend to have extensive new collateral blood vessels of varying anatomic distribution which pose a severe hemostatic hazard to the surgeon and cause thrombocytopenia and defective clearance of plasminogen activator from the blood, resulting in short lysis times of blood clots. In the absence of associated hepatocellular necrosis, hepatic synthesis is well preserved and results of blood coagulation tests are therefore normal.

Patients with cholestasis ultimately develop a deficiency of blood-clotting factors limited to those that are vitamin-K-dependent, since the absorption of this fat-soluble vitamin is impaired. Prothrombin time is prolonged (deficiency of factors II, VII, and X), partial thromboplastin time becomes prolonged (deficiency of factors II, IX, and X), and immunologic determinations of these factors give higher values than do the corresponding procoagulant assays. Specific assays show normal factor V concentration. There is often an acute phase reaction with increased levels of fibrinogen and FVIIIRA, proportional increases of FVIIIC, and little evidence of increased catabolism in this group.

With acute or chronic hepatocellular disease, the predominant finding is deficient or defective hepatic synthesis. These changes may occur in acute hepatitis of any type, in chronic active hepatitis, or in uncompensated necrosis and are maximal in fulminant hepatic failure. The multiple deficiencies separate this from the isolated deficiencies of the congenital states. The actual level of a factor represents the balance between synthesis and catabolism, and the latter is often increased, tending to exaggerate the defect of synthesis. Fibrinogen synthesis is enough to maintain the plasma level in all but the most severe examples of hepatic coma. Factor VIIIRA is spared, since the hepatocyte is not concerned with its synthesis, which is often greatly increased. FVIIIC may be lower than FVIIIRA possibly as a result of intravascular consumption by coagulation. Platelets may also be reduced and show defective function.[40] Plasminogen activator is usually decreased in the blood, plasminogen levels are low, and serum FDP is slightly increased, a nonspecific pattern of changes common to many disorders. Inhibitors of coagulation and fibrinolysis are decreased, and this may represent a combination of decreased synthesis and increased removal owing to intravascular coagulation. Prothrombin time and partial thromboplastin time are prolonged by the coagulation factor deficiencies, and unusual inhibitors have been postulated but never clearly identified. Plasma thrombin or ''reptilase'' times are prolonged if abnormal fibrinogen molecules are formed.

While detailed assays are of considerable research interest, in clinical medicine frequently repeated simple screening tests, such as platelet count, prothrombin time, partial thromboplastin time, and thrombin time, give all the information needed for practical management. Thrombotest or normotest may be useful in place of the one-stage prothrombin time whose reliability depends on the availability of a standardized reagent such as the British comparative thromboplastin.[41]

The synthesis of abnormal proteins of other types may also play a role in the pathogenesis of the clinical manifestations of liver disease. While abnormal fibrinogen synthesis may be of little clinical significance and related congenital disorders are often symptom-free,[42] synthesis of abnormal regulatory proteins may have to await discovery. In this respect the abnormal acarboxy (PIVKA) forms of coagulation factors synthesized in vitamin K deficiency exert normal feedback regulation of their own synthesis.

PRACTICAL IMPLICATIONS

Prognosis

Severe liver disease leads to multiple coagulation factor defects that are easily demonstrated by simple screening tests of blood coagulation, which are therefore among the most sensitive of laboratory tests of liver function. Many authors, however, have noted the dissociation between the results of these tests and the incidence of clinical bleeding. This is not surprising, since the incidence of bleeding must depend both on the efficiency of the hemostatic mechanism and the level of challenge to which it is subjected.

Hemostasis depends on the interaction of blood vessels, platelets, blood coagulation, and fibrinolysis. Liver disease may affect any one or more of these in any combination and thus compromise hemostasis without direct involvement of blood coagulation. Even more important is the challenge to hemostasis. There are many examples in all clinical fields of patients with defective hemostasis who show no tendency to bleed unless and until blood vessels are damaged. Thus the pregnant mother whose dead fetus is retained in utero may show no sign of bleeding even when the resulting intravascular coagulation has largely removed fibrinogen, factor VIII, other clotting factors, and platelets from her blood. Caesarean section in such a patient causes torrential bleeding. Similarly, the severe multiple defects of fulminant hepatic failure may cause no bleeding unless vessels are damaged, for example, by ill-advised needle punctures, by surgery, or by more natural processes often related to gastric acidity.

One study of 105 deaths among 132 consecutive admissions for fulminant hepatic failure showed major bleeding as the cause of death in 28 patients.[43] Bleeding was usually from the gastrointestinal tract. The incidence of bleeding was not related to the coagulation screening tests, to the presence of renal failure, or to the etiology of the hepatic failure. Esophageal and gastric erosions were often noted, however. The same group later reported a prospective study in which H_2-receptor antagonists were given to patients in hepatic coma in sufficient amounts to maintain intragastric pH above 5.[44] In the 26 patients receiving these drugs, only 1 patient bled compared with 54% of the controls. Thus the reduction of gastric acidity and prevention of gastric erosions must take precedence over any prophylaxis directed at the correction of hemostatic efficiency. The survival of those who did not bleed differed strikingly from those who did.

In determining overall prognosis in terms of survival in other forms of liver disease the coagulation factor levels are of little importance compared with the presence or absence of significant bleeding. Once bleeding has occurred, however, for example, from esophageal varices, the prognosis is better in those patients with normal results of coagulation tests than in those with abnormal findings indicating associated hepatocellular dysfunction.

Used as a "liver function" test the prothrombin time has proved of some value in predicting the outcome for patients suffering from an overdose of acetaminophen (paracetamol).[35] There is a characteristic latent interval of 3 to 4 days between ingestion of the drug and maximum abnormalities in results of coagulation tests. Only those patients whose prothrombin time ratio of patient's result to normal was greater than 2.2 before the fourth day developed hepatic coma. However, the level of serum bilirubin is of greater predictive value for the outcome than the prothrombin time.

Specific assay of factor VII shares with less specific tests this lack of ability to predict survival. Determination of factor VII is a useful test of synthetic function of the liver, however, since this factor has a biologic half-life of only a few hours, so that changes develop rapidly and it is little affected by intravascular fibrinolysis.

Therapy

Patients with coagulation factor deficiencies who are not bleeding and who do not face an identifiable challenge to hemostasis need no special treatment for these deficiencies. This includes many patients with uncompensated chronic liver disease. Vitamin K should be given, however, when the clinical circumstances and laboratory tests indicate the need, and it is usually given routinely to patients with fulminant hepatic failure. Prophylaxis against bleeding in these patients should protect blood vessels, and this includes the use of H_2-receptor antagonists to abolish gastric acidity.

Replacement of missing coagulation factors by transfusion is neither easy to accomplish nor free from hazard but should be attempted in those who are bleeding or in those who face a definite hemostatic challenge (including liver biopsy). Fresh-frozen plasma supplies all the coagulation factors and may also be used after the cryoprecipitate fraction (rich in fibrinogen and factor VIII) has been removed. Large volumes are needed, however, because of the accelerated loss of coagulation factors, and the prothrombin time is difficult to correct completely. The short biologic survival of factor VII makes frequent administration necessary; 300 ml every 6 hr approaches the limits of tolerance for continuous administration to patients in hepatic coma and carries with it the risk of overloading the circulation or causing electrolyte imbalance; there is no convincing evidence of prophylactic benefit. However, fresh-frozen plasma is the mainstay of treatment in any patient actually bleeding, when larger amounts may be given rapidly.

Concentrates of the vitamin-K-dependent coagulation factors are available, but their place in therapeutics remains undecided. They carry the risk of transmitting hepatitis; some, but not all, lack factor VII. The factors concerned may be partially in their active form and thus precipitate intravascular microthrombosis. This risk is greatest in patients with fulminant hepatic failure already predisposed to intravascular coagulation. Thus, in a controlled trial[46] of one such concentrate in fulminant hepatic failure, clinical evidence of intravascular coagulation appeared in 2 patients and laboratory evidence progressed in others, even in those given simultaneous heparin. The magnitude of this risk is uncertain, however, and further controlled trials in different types of liver disease are in progress.

Similar arguments suggest that in the presence of severe hepatocellular necrosis the use of inhibitors of fibrinolysis, 6-aminohexanoic acid (EACA), tranexamic acid, or Trasylol may predispose to microthrombi.[32] The value of these inhibitors has yet to be tested by controlled trials in other forms of liver disease where the risk of associated intravascular coagulation seems less.

Heparin has been used by several groups in an attempt to restrict the increased loss of coagulation factors. Heparin elimination is reduced in patients with cirrhosis,[47] and dose regulation is critical. The only controlled human trial[48] showed no benefit. EACA increased the incidence of microthrombi in animals with experimental galactosamine-induced hepatitis,[33] while heparin prevented their formation, but heparin did not prolong the survival time of the animals nor reduce liver cell damage.

Platelet transfusions are being used with increasing frequency in the treatment of bleeding associated with thrombocytopenia, giving emphasis, if such is needed, for the importance of considering all aspects of hemostasis. Undoubtedly the most important seems to be the condition of the blood vessels themselves; challenges to hemostasis should be scrupulously avoided.

REFERENCES

1. Baugh RF, Hougie C: Biochemistry of blood coagulation. Poller L (ed) Recent Advances in Blood Coagulation. Vol. 2. Edinburgh, London, and New York, Churchill Livingstone, 1977, pp 1–34
2. Rosenberg RD: Biologic actions of heparin. Semin Hematol 14:427–440, 1977
3. Davidson JF: Recent advances in fibrinolysis. Poller L (ed) Recent Advances in Blood Coagulation. Vol. 2. Edinburgh, London, and New York, Churchill Livingstone, 1977, pp 91–122
4. Collen D: Identification and some properties of a new fast-reacting plasmin inhibitor in human plasma. Eur J Biochem 69:209–216, 1976
5. Aoki N, Moroi M, Tachiya K: Effects of α_2-plasmin inhibitor on fibrin clot lysis. Its comparison with α_2-macroglobulin. Thromb Haemostasis (Stuttg) 39:22–31, 1978
6. Pickart LR, Thaler MM: Free fatty acids and albumin as mediators of thrombin-stimulated fibrinogen synthesis. Am J Physiol 230:996–1002, 1976
7. Jeejeebhoy KN, Ho J, Greenberg GR, Philips MJ, Bruce-Robertson A, Sodtke V: Albumin, fibrinogen and transferrin synthesis in isolated rat hepatocyte suspensions: A model for the study of plasma protein synthesis. Biochem J 146:141–155, 1976
8. Plow EF, Edgington TS: Unique immunochemical features and intracellular stability of platelet fibrinogen. Thromb Res 7:729–742, 1975
9. Bouma H III, Kwan SW, Fuller GM: Radioimmunological identification of polysomes synthesizing fibrinogen polypeptide chains. Biochemistry 14:4787–4792, 1975
10. Reeve EB, Franks JJ: Fibrinogen synthesis, distribution and degradation. Semin Thromb Hemostasis 1:129–183, 1974
11. Soria J, Soria C, Samama M, Coupier J, Girard ML, Bousser J, Bilski-pasquier G: Dysfibrinogénémies acquises dans les atteintes hépatiques sévères. Coagulation 3:37–44, 1970
12. Verhaeghe R, Verstraete M, Vermylen J, Vermylen C: Fibrinogen 'Leuven' another genetic variant. Br J Haematol 26:421–433, 1974
13. Lane DA, Scully MF, Thomas DP, Kakkar VV, Woolf IL, Williams R: Acquired dysfibrinogenaemia in acute and chronic liver disease. Br J Haematol 35:301–308, 1977

14. Suttie JW, Jackson CM: Prothrombin structure, activation, and biosynthesis. Physiol Rev 57:1–70, 1977

15. Hemker HC, Veltkamp JJ, Hensen A, Loeliger EA: Nature of prothrombin biosynthesis: Preprothrombinaemia in vitamin K deficiency. Nature 200:589–590, 1963

16. Stenflo J, Fernlund P, Egan W, Roepstorff P: Vitamin K-dependent modifications of glutamic acid residues in prothrombin. Proc Natl Acad Sci USA 71:2730–2733, 1974

17. Prydz H: Vitamin K-dependent clotting factors. Semin Thromb Hemostasis 4, 1–14, 1977

18. Mattii R, Ambrus JL, Sokal JE, Munk I: Production of members of the blood coagulation and fibrinolysin systems by the isolated perfused liver. Proc Soc Exp Biol Med 116:69–72, 1964

19. Lee SY, Chung SI: Biosynthesis and degradation of plasma protransglutaminase (factor XIII). Fed Proc 35:1486, 1976

20. Walls WD, Losowsky MS: Plasma fibrin stabilizing factor (FSF) activity in normal subjects and patients with chronic liver disease. Thromb Diath Haemorrh 21:134–143, 1969

21. Lechner K, Niessner H, Thaler E: Coagulation abnormalities in liver disease. Semin Thromb Hemostasis 4:40–56, 1977

22. Giddings JC, Shaw E, Tiddenhaus EGD, Bloom AL: The synthesis of factor V in tissue culture and isolated organ perfusion. Thromb Diath Haemorrh 34:321, 1975

23. Bloom AL, Peake IR, Giddings JC, Shearn SAM, Tuddenham EGD: Endothelial cells and factor-VIII-related protein. Lancet 1:46, 1976

24. Bloom AL, Peake IR: Molecular genetics of factor VIII and its disorders. Semin Hematol 14:319–339, 1977

25. Bennett B, Ratnoff OD: Changes in anti hemophilic factor (AHF, factor VIII) procoagulant activity and AHF-like antigen in normal pregnancy, and following exercise and pneumoencephalography. J Lab Clin Med 80:256–263, 1972

26. Harpel PC, Rosenberg RD: α_2-Macroglobulin and antithrombin-heparin cofactor: Modulators of hemostatic and inflammatory reactions. Prog Hemostasis Thromb 3:145–189, 1976

27. Rake MO, Flute PT, Pannell G, Williams R: Intravascular coagulation in acute hepatic necrosis. Lancet 1:533–537, 1970

28. Tytgat GN, Collen D, Verstraete M: Metabolism of fibrinogen in cirrhosis of the liver. J Clin Invest 50:1690–1701, 1971

29. Clark RD, Gazzard BG, Lewis ML, Flute PT, Williams R: Fibrinogen metabolism in acute hepatitis and active chronic hepatitis. Br J Haematol 30:95–102, 1975

30. Verstraete M, Vermylen J, Collen D: Intravascular coagulation in liver disease. Annu Rev Med 25:447–455, 1974

31. Hillenbrand P, Parbhoo SP, Jedrychowski A, Sherlock S: Significance of intravascular coagulation and fibrinolysis in acute hepatic failure. Gut 15:83–88, 1974

32. Rake MO, Flute PT, Pannell G, Shilkin KB, Williams R: Experimental hepatic necrosis: Studies on coagulation abnormalities, plasma clearance, and organ distribution of ^{125}I-labelled fibrinogen. Gut 14:574–580, 1973

33. Müller-Berghaus G, Reuter C, Bleyl U: Experimental galactosamine-induced hepatitis. Am J Pathol 82:393–404, 1976

34. Baele G, Matthus E, Barbier F: Antihaemophilic factor A activity, FVIII-related antigen and von Willebrand factor in hepatic cirrhosis. Acta Haematol 57:290–297, 1977

35. Clark R, Rake MO, Flute PT, Williams R: Coagulation abnormalities in acute liver failure; pathogenetic and therapeutic implications. Scand J Gastroenterol 8 (Suppl 19):63–70, 1973

36. Coleman M, Finlayson N, Bettigole RE, Sadula D, Cohn M, Pasmantier M: Fibrinogen survival in cirrhosis: improvement by "low-dose" heparin. Ann Intern Med 83:79–81, 1975

37. Mowat NAG, Brunt PW, Ogston D: The fibrinolytic enzyme system in acute and chronic liver injury. Acta Haematol 52:289–293, 1974

38. Fletcher AP, Biederman O, Moore D, Alkjaersig N, Sherry S: Abnormal plasminogen-plasmin system activity (fibrinolysis) in patients with hepatic cirrhosis: Its cause and consequences. J Clin Invest 43:681–695, 1964

39. Flute PT, Rake MO, Williams R, Seaman MJ, Calne RY: Liver transplantation in man: IV. Haemorrhage and thrombosis. Br Med J 3:20–23, 1969

40. Rubin MH, Weston MJ, Bullock G, Roberts J, Langley PG, White YS, Williams R: Abnormal platelet function and ultrastructure in fulminant hepatic failure. Q J Med 44:339–352, 1977

41. Dymock IW, Tucker JS, Woolf IL, Poller L, Thomson JM: Coagulation studies as a prognostic index in acute liver failure. Br J Haematol 29:385–395, 1975

42. Flute PT: Disorders of plasma fibrinogen synthesis. Br Med Bull 33:253–259, 1977

43. Gazzard BG, Portmann B, Murray-Lyon IM, Williams R: Causes of death in fulminant hepatic failure and relationship to quantitative histological assessment of parenchymal damage. Q J Med 44:615–626, 1975

44. Macdougall BRD, Bailey RJ, Williams R: H$_2$-receptor antagonists and antacids in the prevention of acute gastrointestinal haemorrhage in fulminant hepatic failure. Two controlled trials. Lancet 1:617–619, 1977

45. Gazzard BG, Henderson JM, Williams R: Factor VII levels as a guide to prognosis in fulminant hepatic failure. Gut 17:489–491, 1976

46. Gazzard BG, Lewis ML, Ash G, Rizza CR, Bidwell E, Williams R: Coagulation factor concentrate in the treatment of the haemorrhagic diathesis of fulminant hepatic failure. Gut 15:993–998, 1974

47. Teien AN: Heparin elimination in patients with liver cirrhosis. Thromb Haemostasis (Stuttg) 38:701–706, 1977

48. Gazzard BG, Clark R, Borirakchanyavat V, Williams R: A controlled trial of heparin therapy in the coagulation defect of paracetamol-induced hepatic necrosis. Gut 15:89–93, 1974

Chapter 17

Endotoxins in Liver Disease

By HEINRICH LIEHR *and* MARTIN GRÜN

THE FIRST EVIDENCE that endotoxins of intestinal bacteria are significant in the pathogenesis of liver diseases was the prevention of choline deficiency by neomycin administration.[1] The reversal of this protection by orally fed endotoxin suggested that absorption of intraluminal endotoxin contributes to the development of fibrosis and cirrhosis.[2] The complexity of these problems can be seen by the fact that "*Salmonella typhosa* endotoxin in the drinking water of choline-deficient rats negates the protection against cirrhosis usually afforded by neomycin" was the subtitle of an article in *Nutrition Reviews*[3] but no final explanation could be given. Further information on the problem was provided by animal experiments demonstrating that endotoxin toxicity is enhanced in animals with early changes of choline deficiency and in combination with alcohol administration.[4,5] The explanation offered was that pretreatment impaired the clearance mechanism for endotoxins. Thus, amounts of endotoxins rendered innocuous by a healthy liver became toxic for an injured organ.

A test system that allows the detection of endotoxins in human blood is based on the observation that a protein of the amebocytes of the *Limulus polyphemus* is clottable by endotoxins and that the product of endotoxin action is a gel.[6,7] The specificity of the test was a matter of dispute,[8] but nonspecificity was ruled out by recent investigations.[9-11] Clinical investigations became possible to test the hypothesis that endotoxins are also of pathogenic significance in human liver disease.

BIOLOGY OF ENDOTOXINS

Chemical Characterization

Endotoxins are products of gram-negative bacteria including *E. coli*. Chemically, endotoxins are lipopolysaccharides (LPS) and are part of the cell wall of bacteria. The molecule consists of three different parts: a basal core that is linked with a polysaccharide chain, the determinant of the O-antigenicity, and a lipid component (lipid A), which is responsible for biologic activities other than immunologic effects.[12,13] In viable bacteria the polysaccharide part only has contact with the outer part of the cell membrane, whereas lipid A may be liberated after bacterial death from either natural causes or antibiotic action.

Biologic Activities

The biologic activities of LPS are numerous, and reference is made to three reviews.[13-15] Endotoxins alter the systemic circulation into a hyperdynamic state by opening arteriovenous shunts in the vascular periphery, activate the

313

coagulation system, and provoke a pyrogen reaction. Small doses lead to leukocytosis, but high doses cause leukopenia. Endotoxins affect carbohydrate metabolism, activate the complement system, and provoke a humoral immune response.

Administration to human volunteers of highly purified *Salmonella abortus equi* LPS preparations in a total dose of 0.1 μg led to pyrexia and an initial decrease of leukocyte counts with subsequent leukocytosis. EEG records registered before and during the febrile reaction displayed dysrhythmia of 6–7 per second.[16] Increase of fibrinolytic activity was observed during the initial phase of pyrexia by using a dose of 0.5 μg given intravenously.[17] These reactions could be produced by the lipid A component of LPS alone if a 10- to 100-fold higher dose was administered intravenously.[18,19] Thus the complete LPS molecule is much more toxic. In using an *E. coli* LPS preparation (1μg/kg intravenously), differences in host reactivity were found[20]: the responding subjects had a shaking chill accompanied by a fall in both white cell counts and phagocytosis of *E. coli* by granulocytes. Repeated doses resulted in tolerance, accompanied by increased phagocytic activity. Vasoconstriction disappeared with tolerance, as did drops in platelet counts and hypercoagulability after endotoxin administration.

Wolff[21] reviewed the literature in 1973 and added his own results. He stated that "the human being is the most sensitive animal to bacterial endotoxins." Granulocytosis is the most sensitive parameter, fever is next, increase in plasma cortisol is third, and the induction of the reproducible growth hormone response is the least sensitive. Endotoxins of *Salmonella abortus equi* and *Salmonella typhosa* were used in these studies, and differences in susceptibility between these preparations were observed both in man and rabbits.

Clearance of Endotoxins

The reticuloendothelial system (RES) is incriminated as the main clearance organ.[22,23] Platelets may have an additional function; a platelet endotoxin interaction seems to be necessary for the final detoxification of endotoxins by the RES, since a carrier function of these cells was found.[24] Most of the RES, i.e., 80% to 90%, is represented by the Kupffer cells of the liver.[25] Diseases of the liver may interfere with their clearance properties in choline deficiency,[26] after alcohol administration,[27] and in carbon-tetrachloride-induced cirrhosis.[28] The behavior is biphasic, since the RES phagocytic capacity initially decreases, followed by increased activity,[29] as shown in galactosamine hepatitis and ANIT-induced cholestasis.

RES phagocytic function in man is low when compared with other species such as mouse, guinea pig, and rabbit.[25] In addition to these species-dependent differences, the hepatic sinusoidal blood flow has an important physiologic significance, especially in cirrhosis.[25] Sinusoidal blood flow is seriously reduced, supposedly as a result of intrahepatic venous shunts, which may account for 50% of the blood flowing through the liver.[30] Wolter et al.[31] evaluated experimentally portal-sinusoidal blood flow in normal minipigs and found endotoxin clearance much more efficient when those substances are presented to Kupffer cells via the portal-venous route rather than the hepatic arterial route. Differences in bloodstream velocity, also found by others,[25,32,33] are probably responsible. The portal-sinusoidal bloodstream is reduced in cirrhosis because of portacaval collateral circulation. The differences in the amount of portacaval collateral circulation between one patient with cirrhosis and another may explain the normal and decreased values of RES phagocytic capacity observed in other studies.[25,28,34] Phagocytic activity increased in acute liver disease such as hepatitis 3 weeks after onset of icterus.[34] Normal and increased values were reported in another study, but no definition of stage was given.[28] Factor VIII antigen (VIII$_{AGN}$) is probably cleared by Kupffer cells in early stages of viral hepatitis and cirrhosis in man, which is indirect evidence for an early decreased phagocytic capacity.[35] One report indicates decreased RES phagocytic capacity in cholestasis in man.[36]

Thus, RES phagocytic activity in human liver disease seems to be ill defined and further evaluation is mandatory. The few data available indicate preferentially suppressed RES function especially in cirrhosis, probably due to hemodynamic disorders. Age, hormones, and stress also have some influence. Viruses as well as toxic agents, especially alcohol, may also decrease RES function.[27,37]

Thus, in liver disease the clearance system for endotoxins is insufficient to eliminate them from the bloodstream when they enter the general and/or the portal circulation.

ENDOTOXEMIA IN LIVER DISEASE

Frequency of Endotoxemia

Endotoxemia is frequent in both experimental liver injury and human liver diseases (Tables 1 and 2). Endotoxemia was first described by Cardis et al.[38] in human liver disease such as cirrhosis. The authors interpreted their observations to result from functional failure of the RES. Endotoxemia usually was accompanied by hepatic injury, bleeding (especially from the gastrointestinal tract), hemorrhagic and septic pneumonitis, a failing peripheral circulation, and a high mortality. There is convincing evidence[39-45] that endotoxemia is frequent in many liver diseases (Table 2).

TABLE 1.—*Frequency of Endotoxemia in Experimental Liver Diseases of Rats*

Model	n	Limulus Gelation Test* (Percentage of Test Result)		
		+++/++	+	Negative
Normal controls	21	–	5.0	95.0
GalN$^+$-hepatitis (1 g/kg i.p.)	142	27.5	50.0	22.5‡
PCA^{++}	34	44.1	44.1	11.8
CCl$_4$-Cirrhosis				
Plasma	30	46.7	33.3	20.0
Ascites	24	41.7	45.8	12.5
ANIT^{+++}-Cholestasis	10	70.0	30.0	–
Common bile duct ligation	14	21.5	57.1	21.4

$^+$ Galactosamine; $^{++}$ portacaval anastomosis; $^{+++}$ α-Naphthyl-iso-thiocyanate

* By +++/++ (= gel formation in test tube), and + (= gel granula)

‡ Mainly between 0 and 6 hr following GalN administration.

TABLE 2.—*Frequency of Endotoxemia Reported in Various Liver Diseases*

	Viral Hepatitis	FHF	Cirrhosis	Ascites	Alcohol Hepatitis	Chronic Active Hepatitis	Obstructive Jaundice	Cholangitis	PBC	Colitis Ulcer	Crohn's Disease
Cardis et al., 1972[38]	—	1/1*	2/2	—	—	—	—	—	—	—	—
Wardle, 1974[39]	—	3/3	2/10	—	—	—	4/16	4/4	—	—	—
Wilkinson et al. 1976[40]	—	16/24	—	—	—	—	—	—	—	—	—
Wilkinson et al., 1974[41]	—	—	14/18	—	—	4/4	6/12	—	1/1	2/4	7/11
Tarao et al., 1976[42]	—	—	16/36	16/20	—	—	—	—	—	—	—
Prytz et al., 1976[43]	—	—	15/31	—	—	—	—	—	—	—	—
Liehr and Grün 1977[44]	13/35	3/3	135/170	29/39	6/6	6/12	—	—	—	2/4	7/11
Clemente et al., 1977[45]	—	—	9/43	18/21	—	—	—	—	—	—	—
Jacob et al., 1977[46]	—	—	—	—	—	—	—	—	—	1/1	—

* Figures indicate number of patients positive for endotoxemia per total number of patients investigated.

Mechanisms of Endotoxemia

Three different routes permit intestinal endotoxins to enter the general circulation: absorption into the portal blood, escape into intestinal lymphatics, and transmural escape into the peritoneal cavity, the last displaying Michaelis-Menton kinetics.[47] Absorption of endotoxin into the portal blood in man was first described in subjects without liver disease[43] and was also found in patients with diseases of the intestine.[46] Endotoxin escape into the lymphatic circulation was seen experimentally.[48,49] The transmural escape of endotoxins from the colon is enhanced by edema of the colon wall,[50] and this possibility was demonstrated in man by detection of endotoxins in ascitic fluid.[42,44,45] Experimental data may be a further support (Table 1). Whatever the mechanism, endotoxemia in liver disease would have remained a mere epiphenomenon until data provided evidence for pathogenic significance.

Pathogenic Role of Endotoxin in Liver Disease

The role of endotoxins in the pathogenesis of liver disease can be demonstrated both by clinical and experimental investigations.

Experimental Studies

Liver injury induced by galactosamine was originally considered to be the result of chemical alterations of hepatocytes secondary to the metabolism of this amino sugar,[51] and a membrane defect was assumed to be of major significance.[52] Other investigations suggest the importance of extrahepatic extracellular mechanisms, since stimulation of RES function prevented liver cell death and inflammation in rats given galactosamine, and RES depression led to fulminant hepatic failure.[53] An explanation for the phenomena was provided by the observation that endotoxemia commonly develops in this model, and differences in the functional state of the RES modify endotoxin toxicity.[54] For example, colectomized rats were refractory to galactosamine-induced liver cell injury and inflammation,[54] although biochemical changes were present.[55] The mechanism by which endotoxemia develops in this model is via histaminemia, since galactosamine degranulates mast cells.[55] The subsequent histaminemia induces edema of the colon wall, allowing transmural escape of endotoxins.[50] Endotoxins activate the complement system[56] which in galactosamine hepatitis can be demonstrated by decreased hemolytic activity paralleling the degree of endotoxemia.[55] Biochemically, injury of the hepatocytic membranes may be produced by cytolytic complement activity, resulting in liver cell death. Soon after galactosamine administration the third component of complement was found by immunofluorescence fixed in a linear pattern on liver parenchymal cell membranes,[57] and necrotic liver cells accumulated C_3 later.[55] Animals genetically deficient in complement do not show signs of liver cell necrosis and inflammation after galactosamine administration, although they develop endotoxemia[55] and the biochemical response of hepatocytes to galactosamine (Reutter and Seelig, personal communication). If low doses of galactosamine are given to rats in order to induce membrane lesions only,[58] with the complement system being activated simultaneously by sublethal amounts of endotoxin administered intravenously, fulminant hepatic failure develops secondary to total liver necrosis.[57]

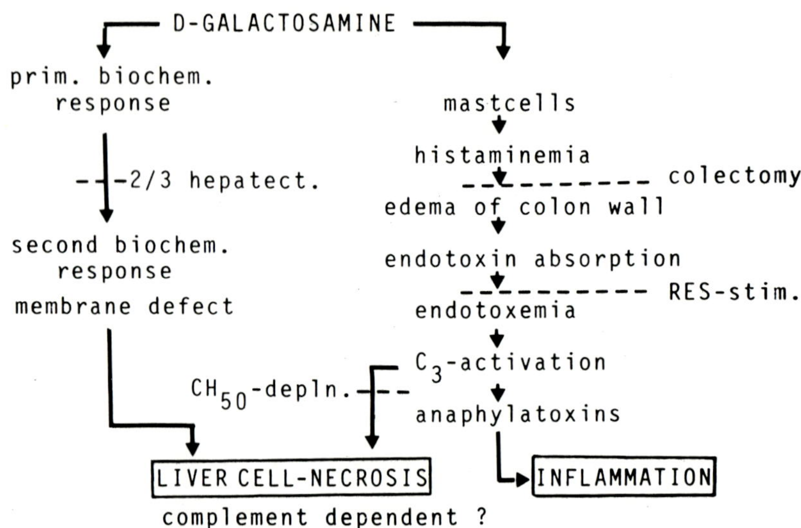

FIG. 1—Scheme of events occurring sequentially in galactosamine hepatitis of rats. Broken lines indicate means by which liver cell death and inflammation are prevented. Two-thirds (2/3) hepatectomy refers to investigations of Reutter et al.[52] For other items, see text. (Reproduced with permission of Springer-Verlag from Liehr H, Grün M, Seelig HP, Seelig R, Reutter W, Heine WD: On the pathogenesis of galactosamine hepatitis. Virchows Arch [Zellpathol] 26:331–344, 1978.)

Figure 1 is a scheme coordinating the mechanisms that cooperate to produce the liver lesion induced by galactosamine and illustrating the mediating role of endotoxins. This scheme explains an experimental model of acute liver disease.

With respect to chronic liver diseases, experiments in the rat with a portacaval shunt are of interest. These rats develop endotoxemia (Table 1) as a result of hemodynamic disorders. They are highly sensitive to endotoxin toxicity, since a normally sublethal dose of endotoxin administered intravenously led to a Shwartzman-like phenomenon associated with total to subtotal hepatic necrosis.[59] Thus, portacaval collateral circulation has the same biologic effect as a priming dose of endotoxin for a general Shwartzman reaction.

Extrahepatic events were observed in these models, such as consumption coagulopathy,[60,61] functional renal failure,[62] and a hyperdynamic circulation.[63] Supposedly, they are caused by circulating endotoxins, since in animals without liver injury, such disorders develop after endotoxin administration.[59,62] Because neurotoxicity of endotoxins is known,[64] the question arose whether encephalopathy may also be linked to endotoxemia. The hypothesis[65] was that endotoxins may act indirectly, predominantly via disorders in glucose metabolism.[66-68] Thus, experimental observations provide evidence of pathogenetic significance of endogenous endotoxemia for the course of both liver disease itself and extrahepatic disorders.

Clinical Investigation

Fulminant hepatic failure (FHF) in man resulting from viral hepatitis or toxic liver damage frequently was associated with endotoxemia, and death occurred only when persisting endotoxemia was present. Consumption coagulopathy and renal failure were observed in patients with endotoxemia. Thus, endotoxemia was felt to be a determining factor. This suggestion seems reasonable, since the mechanisms proposed in galactosamine hepatitis[55] may also be of significance in FHF. Elevated histamine levels were found in viral hepatitis and massive hepatic necrosis.[69,70] This may have contributed to endotoxin escape from the intestine. The complement system is involved in FHF,[71] and the values of complement hemolytic activity reported indicate complement depletion. Since disorders of synthesis largely can be excluded,[55] consumption of complement seems more reasonable. Supposedly, the system is activated by circulating endotoxins,[56] and the resulting cytolytic activity may be responsible for hepatocytic necrosis;[55] this mechanism may also explain the hemolysis frequently observed.[34] Disorders in glucose homeostasis such as hypoglycemia are accounted for by decreased metabolic activity of the hepatic parenchymal cells, since data were presented[68] that endotoxins block gluconeogenesis[72] and provoke hyperinsulinism. The resulting hypoglycemia depresses the RES,[68] which is involved in both endotoxin clearance and insulin catabolism. Thus, a vicious circle may act in addition to the original liver disease. Since hyperinsulinism also was held responsible for edema of the brain,[67] the neurologic effect in fulminant hepatic failure may be influenced, too. Thus, several biologic mechanisms activated by endotoxins interact, and FHF should be considered as an endotoxin shock syndrome subsequent to Kupffer cell failure and hepatic necrosis in addition to a metabolic disorder alone. Some extrahepatic events frequently occurring in FHF fit this concept well, such as hypotension due to peripheral vasodilation, functional renal failure, consumption coagulopathy, gastrointestinal bleeding, and acute pancreatitis.[39,40,45,73-76] All these disorders may either be caused directly or be mediated by endotoxins.[77] Consequently, support may be derived from some positive results of extracorporeal perfusion of the liver if they are interpreted as showing extracorporeal RES perfusion as a means of extracorporeal endotoxin detoxification.

Several mechanisms have been proposed to explain the pathogenesis of alcoholic hepatitis.[78] Alcohol has a "blocking" effect on the RES,[27] promoting spillover of endotoxins. This explains the observation that endotoxemia in alcoholic hepatitis was present in all the patients studied.[44] This may also explain the increase in the stimulation index of lymphocytes.[79] All these patients had symptoms that fit the definition of Zieve's syndrome,[80] such as pyrexia, leukocytosis, hemolysis, and disorders in fat metabolism. These symptoms subsided simultaneously with disappearance of endotoxemia. Thus the hypothesis was put forward that alcoholic hepatitis may be mediated if not even provoked by systemic endotoxemia.[44]

Endotoxemia also occurs in chronic active hepatitis (Table 2). Since endotoxins activate the complement system,[56] disorders in this system may be related, and the possible role in necrosis of hepatocytes was mentioned.[57]

Endotoxemia was found in 79% of 170 patients with cirrhosis.[44] The acute mortality within 7 days was 25% in cirrhotic patients who had endotoxemia as contrasted to 5% in patients without endotoxemia.[42,45] It is found sporadically in sequential examinations, and the frequency with which it occurs depends on the amount of the portacaval collateral circulation.[44] Clotting disorders, functional renal failure, pyrogen reactions, and humoral immune responses closely correlated with endotoxemia.[39,41,43,45,82]

Polymyxin B is an antibiotic with an antiendotoxin effect[83] on a molecular basis.[84] This drug was administered intravenously over 3 days (1.1 mg/kg/24 hr) to 10 cirrhotic patients.[85,86] Nine other patients received levulose as control. In the experimental group, clotting disorders that were thought to be most sensitive improved significantly. Functional renal failure, present in 4 patients of the experimental group, improved, but no improvement occurred in 2 patients of the control group. One patient treated twice responded twice to polymyxin B treatment[86] without complete recovery. Similar observations were made by other authors.[41] Since antiendotoxin treatment improves disorders that were thought to be due to endotoxin action, they are probably pathogenetically connected.

No correlation was found between encephalopathy and increase of the plasma ammonia level in children with Reyes' syndrome.[87] When the accompanying endotoxemia was compared with alterations of EEG records, however, a strong correlation was found.[88] These alterations in EEG were comparable to those found in man after LPS administration.[16]

Spillover of endotoxins is also important in the humoral immune response,[89] since the liver is an immune organ[90] controlling the immunogenicity of commensal bacteria in the gut.[91] Production of immunoglobulins is commonly increased in chronic liver diseases, and the antibodies are directed mainly against intestinal antigens.[92] The increase in antibody production correlated with destruction of the hepatic architecture[92] and with surgical portacaval anastomosis.[94] Increases of immunoglobulin classes A, M, and G parallel endotoxemia in cirrhosis, and patients positive for endotoxins had a higher titer of *E. coli* antibodies than did endotoxin-negative subjects.[43]

Endotoxins (*Salmonella abortus equi*) raised sulfobromophtalein reflux from the liver to plasma and to a decrease of storage capacity in man[95] and in experimental animals.[96,97] Activity of alkaline phosphatase increases, supposedly reflecting the cholestatic effect of endotoxins.[98] The role of endotoxemia in obstructive cholestasis is not entirely settled. Clotting disorders, acute renal failure, and respiratory distress were thought to be sequelae of endotoxemia,[36] and a close relation of renal failure to endotoxemia was found in another study of obstructive jaundice.[41] Unfortunately, increase of bile acids interferes with the *Limulus* gelation test,[82] so that correlations are difficult to elicit in cholestasis.

Endotoxemia has been observed in ulcerative colitis and in Crohn's disease (Table 2), and nonspecific reactive hepatitis[99,100] may be pathogenetically related, since such lesions can be produced by endotoxin injections to normal rats.[26,54,59]

Therapeutic Aspects

The accumulating evidence for the pathogenetic significance of endotoxins in various liver diseases has therapeutic implications. Several regimens could be considered. One action is elimination of the source of endotoxin, namely the intestinal flora, by means of nonabsorbable antibiotics. This may kill intestinal bacteria and actually liberate endotoxins with an undesired effect. In chronic liver disease associated with portal-systemic encephalopathy, such treatment is of benefit. No data can be offered to determine whether this benefit is caused by an antiendotoxin effect. Another approach is RES stimulation to increase the clearance of endotoxin. This approach in acute liver disease may have prophylatic value to prevent fulminant hepatic failure. RES is usually the stated answer to RES "blockade."[37] Nevertheless, such treatment has been tried using aluminium hydroxide,[101] and severe hepatitis and fulminant hepatic failure were said to be prevented. In chronic liver diseases with portacaval collateral circulation, this regimen seems to be of doubtful value, since Kupffer cells display their clearance properties most efficiently when in contact with portal blood.[31]

The use of drugs with antiendotoxin properties is thought to be most promising. Such drugs can be given either orally or systemically. Experimentally, Nolan and Ali[102] demonstrated the benefit of cholestyramine on both endotoxin toxicity and absorption. Polymyxin B has antiendotoxin properties.[83,84] Experimentally this drug protected animals against the lethal effects of CCl_4 and significantly modified hepatic injury.[103] In man, polymyxin B was beneficial in cirrhosis,[85,86] especially in functional renal failure,[41,86] but any value seems unlikely once tubular necrosis develops.[41,76]

Other regimens should be mentioned, such as peritoneal lavage if transmural escape of endotoxins from the colon is significant. This was shown to be beneficial in experimental pancreatitis[104] thought to be mediated by systemic endotoxemia.[105] Extracorporeal perfusion of blood through columns equipped with endotoxin-absorbing substances[106] is another means of treating systemic endotoxemia.

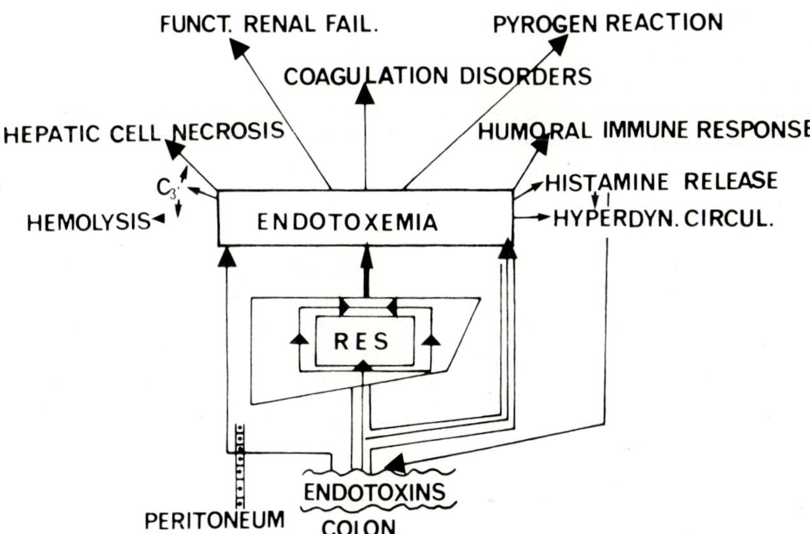

FIG. 2—Scheme of mechanisms responsible for the escape of bacterial endotoxins from the intestine and proposed events occurring as a sequel of systemic endotoxemia (Reproduced with permission of Elsevier, North-Holland Biomedical Press, from Liehr H, Grün M: Clinical aspects of Kupffer cell failure in liver diseases. Edited by E Wisse and DL Knook: Kupffer Cells and Other Sinusoidal Cells. Amsterdam, Elsevier, North-Holland, 1977, pp 427–436.)

PERSPECTIVE

The question of whether endotoxins of intestinal bacteria are of general pathogenetic significance is not new. In 1897, a report in *The Lancet* stated that certain symptoms following portacaval anastomosis were caused by intestinal toxins,[107] and much work was done both experimentally and clinically to evaluate endotoxemia subsequent to Kupffer cell failure in liver diseases. Figure 2 summarizes suggested endotoxin-dependent events,[108] and reference is made to a comparable scheme presented by Nolan.[26] We feel that the hypothesis initially formulated may be helpful in understanding the pathogenesis of liver diseases. Furthermore, a basis for more effective therapeutic regimens than those currently used is offered.

REFERENCES

1. Rutenburg A, Sonnenblick E, Koven J, Aprahamian HA, Reiner L, Fine J: The role of intestinal bacteria in the development of dietary cirrhosis in rats. J Exp Med 106:1–13, 1957
2. Broitman SA, Gottlieb LS, Zamcheck N: Influence of neomycin and ingested endotoxin in the pathogenesis of choline deficiency cirrhosis in the adult rat. J Exp Med 119:633–640, 1964
3. Endotoxin and cirrhosis. Nutr Rev 22:284–286, 1964
4. Nolan JP, Ali MV: Endotoxin and the liver. I. Toxicity in rats with choline deficient fatty livers. Proc Soc Exp Biol Med 129:29–31, 1968
5. Ali MV, Nolan JP: Unpublished data cited in Nolan JP: The role of endotoxin in liver injury. Gastroenterology 69:1346–1356, 1975
6. Levin J, Bang FB: Clottable protein in *Limulus*: Its localization and kinetics of its coagulation by endotoxin. Thromb Diath Haemorrh 19:186–197, 1968
7. Levin J, Tomasola PA, Oser RS: Detection of endotoxin in human blood and demonstration of an inhibitor. J Lab Clin Med 25:903–911, 1970
8. Elin RJ, Robinson RA, Levine AS, Wolff SM: Lack of clinical usefulness of the Limulus test in the diagnosis of endotoxemia. N Engl J Med 293:521–524, 1975
9. Yin ET: Endotoxin, thrombin, and the Limulus amebocyte lysate. J Lab Clin Med 86:430–434, 1975
10. Fumarola D, Jirillo E: Limulus test, parenteral drugs and biological products: An approach. Batteriol Virol Immunol 69: N 1–6, 1976
11. Elin RJ, Sandberg L, Rosenstreich DL: Comparison of the pyrogenicity, *Limulus* activity, mitogenicity and complement reactivity of several bacterial endotoxins and related compounds. J Immunol 117:1238–1242, 1976
12. Lüderitz O, Westphal O, Staub AM, Nikaido H: Isolation and chemical and immunological characterization of bacterial lipopolysaccharides. Edited by G Weinbaum, S Kadis, and SJ Ajl: Microbiol Toxins. Vol. IV. New York, Academic Press, 1971, pp 145–233
13. Endotoxin Conference. J Infect Dis Suppl 128:1–305, 1973
14. Zweifach BW, Janoff A: Bacterial endotoxemia. Annu Rev Med 16:201–220, 1965
15. Weinbaum J, Kadis S, Ajl SJ (eds): Microbial Toxins. Vols. IV and V. Academic Press, New York, 1971
16. Berg G, Brichzy W, Braunhofer J, Schricker KT: Vorläufige Erfahrungen mit pyrogenen Lipopolysacchariden. Dtsch Med Wochenschr 81:1156–1160, 1956
17. Hörder MH, Kickhöfen B: Vergleichende Untersuchungen über den Nachweis der Fibrinolyse nach Injektion eines bakteriellen Lipopolysaccharids (Pyrexal). Acta Haematol 17:321–332, 1957
18. Argenton H, Becker H, Fischer H, Otto J, Thiel R, Westphal O: Ober die resistenzsteigernde Wirkung von Lipoid A beim Menschen. Dtsch Med Wochenschr 86:774–781, 1961
19. Liehr, H.: Die Antwortreaktionen des menschlichen Organismus nachparenteraler Applikation von *Escherichia coli* 08. Dissertation (medicine), Hamburg, 1962
20. Ollodart RM, Hawthone J, Attar S: Studies in experimental endotoxemia in man. Am J Surg 113:599–607, 1967
21. Wolff SM: Biological effects of bacterial endotoxins in man. J Infect Dis Suppl 128: S259–264, 1973

22. Wiznitzer T, Better N, Rachlin W, Atkins N, Frank ED, Fine J: In vivo detoxification of endotoxin by the reticulo-endothelial system. J Exp Med 112:1157–1166, 1960

23. Rutenberg S, Skarnes R, Palmerio C, Fine J: Detoxification of endotoxin by perfusion of liver and spleen. Proc Soc Exp Biol Med 125:455–459, 1967

24. Das J, Schwartz AA, Folkman J: Clearance of endotoxin by platelets: Role in increasing the accuracy of the Limulus gelation test and in combating experimental endotoxemia. Surgery 74:235–240, 1973

25. Biozzi G, Stiffel C: The physiopathology of the reticuloendothelial cells of the liver and the spleen. Edited by H Popper and F Schaffner: Progress in Liver Disease. Vol. II. New York, Grune & Stratton, 1965, pp 166–191

26. Nolan JP: The role of endotoxin in liver injury. Gastroenterology 69:1346–1356, 1975

27. Ali MV, Nolan JP: Alcohol induced depression of reticuloendothelial function in the rat. J Lab Clin Med 70:295–301, 1967

28. Paumgartner G, Longueville J, Leevy CM: Determinations of phagocytosis in liver injury. Edited by J De Groote: Liver Research. Brügge, St. Catherine Press Ltd, 1967, pp 469–477

29. Grün M, Liehr H: Biological significance of altered Kupffer cell function in experimental liver disease. Edited by E Wisse and DL Knook: Kupffer Cells and Other Liver Sinusoidal Cells. Amsterdam, Elsevier, North-Holland, 1977, pp 437–446

30. Halpern BN, Biozzi G, Pequinot G, Delaloje G, Stiffel B, Monton D: Mesure de la circulation sanguine du foi et de l'activité phagocytaire du S.R.E. chez le suget normal et chez le suget cirrhotique. Pathol Biol 7:1637, 1959

31. Wolter J, Liehr H, Grün M: Hepatic clearance of endotoxins: Differences in arterial and portal venous infusion. J Reticuloendothel Soc 23:145–152 1978

32. Dobson EL: Factors controlling phagocytosis. Edited by BN Halpern: Physiopathology of the Reticuloendothelial System. Springfield, Ill, Charles C Thomas, 1957, pp 1–88

33. Brauer RW, Leong GF, Mc Ellroy RF: Circulatory pathways in the rat liver as revealed by P^{32} chromium phosphate colloid uptake in the isolated perfused liver preparation. Am J Physiol 184:593–598, 1956

34. Cooksley WGE, Powell LW, Halliday JW: Reticuloendothelial phagocytic function in human liver diseases and its relationship to haemolysis. Br J Haematol 25:147–164, 1973

35. Brunswig D, Liehr H, Grün M, Thiel H: Zur klinischen Bedeutung des antihämophilen Globulin A. Inn Med 3:245–253, 1976

36. Drivas G, James O, Wardle N: Study of reticuloendothelial phagocytic capacity in patients with cholestasis. Br J Med 1:1568–1569, 1976

37. Saba TM: Physiology and physiopathology of the reticuloendothelial system. Arch Intern Med 126:1031–1052, 1970

38. Caridis DT, Woodruff PWH, Reinhold RB, Fine J: Endotaxaemia in man. Lancet 1:1381–1386, 1972

39. Wardle NE: Fibrinogen in liver disease. Am J Surg 109:741–746, 1974

40. Wilkinson SP, Arroyo V, Gazzard BG, Moodie H, Williams R: Relation of renal impairment and haemorrhagic diathesis to endotoxemia in fulminant hepatic failure. Lancet 1:521–524, 1974

41. Wilkinson SP, Moodie H, Stammatakis JD, Kakkar VV, Williams R: Endotoxaemia and renal failure in cirrhosis and obstructive jaundice. Br Med J 2:1415–1418, 1976

42. Tarao K, Endo O, Ikeudi T, So K, Moroi T, Fukushima K: Endotoxin in ascitic fluid of liver cirrhosis in man. Jpn J Gastroenterol 37:1366–1372, 1976

43. Prytz H, Holst-Christenssen J, Korner B, Liehr H: Portal venous and systemic endotoxaemia in patients without liver disease and systemic endotoxemia in patients with cirrhosis. Scand J Gastroenterol 11:857–863, 1976

44. Liehr H, Grün M: Clinical aspects of Kupffer cell failure in liver diseases. Edited by E Wisse and DL Knook: Kupffer Cells and Other Sinusoidal Cells. Amsterdam, Elsevier, North-Holland, 1977, pp 427–436

45. Clemente C, Bosch J, Rodes J, Arroyo V, MasA, Maragall S: Functional renal failure and haemorrhagic gastritis associated with endotoxaemia in cirrhosis. Gut 18:556–560, 1977

46. Jacob AI, Goldberg PK, Bloom N, Degenschein GA, Kozim PJ: Endotoxin and bacteria in portal blood. Gastroenterology 72:1268–1270, 1977

47. Nolan JP, Hare DK, Mc Devitt JJ, Ali MV: In vitro studies of intestinal endotoxin absorption. I. Kinetics of absorption in the isolated everted gut sac. Gastroenterology 72:434–439, 1977

48. Daniele R, Singh H, Appert HE, Pairent FW, Howard JH: Lymphatic absorption of

Gastroenterology 71:A161/1184, 1977
104. Lankisch PG, Koop H, Winckler K, Schmidt H: Continous peritoneal dialysis in the treatment of acute experimental pancreatitis in the rat. Biol Gastroenterol (Paris) 8:251, 1975
105. Liehr H, Seelig R, Grün M, Seelig HP: Endotoxemia and complement activation in acute pancreatitis. Proc XIVth International Congress Internal Medicine, Rome, 1978 (in press)
106. Leibowitz Ai, Cerra FB, Mc Devitt JJ, Nolan JP: Charcoal hemoperfusion in endotoxemia. Gastroenterology 24:114A, 1976
107. Lancet, Paris correspondent: The antiendotoxic function of the liver. Lancet 2:1092, 1893
108. Liehr H, Grün M: Clinical aspects of Kupffer cell failure in liver diseases. Edited by E Wisse and DL Knook: Kupffer Cells and Other Liver Sinusoidal Cells. Amsterdam, Elsevier/North-Holland, 1977, pp 427–436

Chapter 18

Hepatic Encephalopathy: Summary of Present Knowledge with an Elaboration on Recent Developments

By LESLIE ZIEVE, M.D.

WITHIN THE PAST 4 years, three reviews[1-3] on hepatic encephalopathy have been written which are recommended, along with the invaluable review by Gabuzda[4] in 1962, as background for the summary information presented in this chapter. Most of the detailed data on which the present summary is based have been presented in two previous reviews[5,6] on the pathogenesis of hepatic coma published in 1966 and 1975. What follows are two sections which, although printed consecutively, are in fact presented in parallel. The first section provides a concise summary of the present knowledge on hepatic encephalopathy, including the recent developments. Numbers in parentheses refer to the material in the second section which provides an elaboration of recent developments. The first section should be read through once in its entirety before trying to fit the elaborations on recent developments into their appropriate places in the summary.

SUMMARY OF PRESENT KNOWLEDGE

Pathogenesis and Diagnosis

Hepatic encephalopathy is a syndrome of mental and neuromuscular abnormalities primarily associated with biochemical alterations resulting from hepatic failure. It may be endogenous (spontaneous) in origin or exogenous and can be induced by various precipitating factors, such as gastrointestinal bleeding; excess ingestion of protein, amino acids, ammonia-producing substances; sedatives, or tranquilizers; paracentesis or excessive use of diuretics; electrolyte depletion; shock and hypoxia; infections; or surgical procedures. The earliest evidence of encephalopathy may be limited to psychomotor abnormalities detected on psychometric tests (1). With progression, a whole spectrum of mental and neuromuscular signs become evident. The end point is coma and death. The soluble brain proteins are reduced, particularly in the gray matter, within 24 hr of death (2). As coma progresses the blood-brain barrier probably becomes more permeable to substances that usually do not get into the brain from the circulation (3).

From the Department of Medicine, Hennepin County Medical Center, University of Minnesota, Minneapolis, Minnesota.

327

The pathogenesis of hepatic encephalopathy can best be understood in relation to the following known metabolic abnormalities, none of which is pathognomonic:

The affinity of hemoglobin for oxygen is reduced.

Brain oxygen and glucose utilization are decreased, but the balance between the production and utilization of energy is maintained.

Ammonia is increased in blood, muscle, brain, and spinal fluid.

Glutamine and α-ketoglutaramate are increased in muscle, brain, and spinal fluid.

Pyruvate, lactate, citrate, and α-ketoglutarate are increased in blood and muscle. α-Ketoglutarate, fumarate, malate, and oxaloacetate are decreased in brain.

Ketone production is decreased.

Fatty acids are increased in blood.

Amino acid patterns are altered in blood, brain, spinal fluid, and urine.

Neurotransmitters are decreased in brain and muscle.

Neurotransmitter metabolites are increased in brain and spinal fluid.

False neurotransmitters are increased in blood, brain, muscle, and urine.

Mercaptans are increased in blood, brain, breath, and urine.

The shift to the right in the in vivo oxyhemoglobin dissociation curve is reversible as the encephalopathy improves. Utilization of brain oxygen and glucose is decreased by half if coma persists for at least 24 hr. During the first 24 hr of acute coma, however, such utilization is normal. Therefore, depression of brain energy metabolism cannot be the cause of acute hepatic encephalopathy. Studies of brain adenine nucleotides in rats verify that the energy state of the tissue is unchanged until the animals are near death (4,5).

Disturbed ammonia metabolism is in some way basic to the syndrome of hepatic encephalopathy, though not its only cause. Experimentally, in the presence of a portacaval shunt, ammonia may depress cerebral blood flow and oxygen consumption (6). After chronic exposure to ammonia or injections of methionine sulfoximine the rat brain ammonia exceeds what would be expected from the concentrations in the blood or spinal fluid (7). The lack of good correlation between blood ammonia and degree of encephalopathy in man and the occurrence of experimental hepatic encephalopathy in the germfree or the eviscerated (8) animal have been a source of confusion regarding the role of ammonia. No parameter has correlated better with clinical severity than the spinal fluid glutamine, which accumulates as a result of the excess of brain ammonia. Any explanation of hepatic encephalopathy must take this into account. A metabolic product of glutamine, α-ketoglutaramate, probably has the same significance as glutamine.[3]

The increased blood levels of pyruvate, lactate, citrate, and α-ketoglutarate reflect severe hepatic damage, not encephalopathy. They become abnormal promptly in the hepatectomized dog long before coma ensues. The alterations in cerebral glucose metabolism, including the Krebs cycle substrates, are similar to those produced by external agents that result in sedation or anesthesia (9). Thus the effects on cellular oxidative metabolism are nonspecific.

The reduction in blood ketones also reflects the severity of hepatic dysfunction rather than encephalopathy per se.

In vitro, very low concentrations of fatty acids depress a variety of enzymes, including glycolytic enzymes and membrane (Na^+, K^+)-ATPase. In pathologic concentrations, they interfere with the disposition of ammonia and augment the coma potential of NH_4^+ and mercaptans (10). A close relationship has been found in at least one instance between slow-wave electrical activity on the EEG and the concentration of fatty acid in the spinal fluid (11). Plasma concentrations of short-, medium-, and long-chain fatty acids increase in chronic hepatic failure in patients. Incomplete beta oxidation of long-chain fatty acids is probably the predominant source of the shorter-chain fatty acids (12). Except for the initial observations of Muto, attempts to show a relationship clinically between fatty acidemia and hepatic encephalopathy have not been successful (13). The free fatty acids have potential pathogenetic significance because of their intrinsic toxicity, their relation to the possible toxicity of tryptophan, and their augmentation of the toxic effects of ammonia and mercaptans.

Tryptophan is the most toxic amino acid (AA), in terms of lethality in animals, and the branched-chain amino acids are the least toxic. Lethal doses of individual AA in rats resulting in more than 300-fold elevations in plasma and 36-fold to more than 300-fold (in the case of tryptophan) elevations in brain do not cause coma up to the moment of death (14). Ingestion of large amounts of tryptophan by patients results in neurologic manifestations that are different from, but have been confused with, hepatic coma. Particular attention has been given to tryptophan because it increases in the brain and spinal fluid in hepatic coma and is the precursor of serotonin (15). Mixtures of essential AA deficient in arginine cause lethargy and coma in animals and man that are associated with hyperammonemia and can be prevented by supplying arginine. The house cat is particularly susceptible to ammonia intoxication in the absence of arginine (16).

In hepatic failure of chronic liver disease, plasma straight-chain AA increase and branched-chain AA decrease. Glutamine predominates overwhelmingly in the brain and spinal fluid, although methionine, phenylalanine, tyrosine, and tryptophan increase three- to fivefold. The molar ratio of the plasma branched-chain AA to phenylalanine + tyrosine decreases from a normal of 3–4 to approximately 1 or less. Associated with these changes and the development of encephalopathy are an approximately 50% increase in serum insulin and a 400% increase in serum glucagon, resulting in a decrease in the insulin/glucagon ratio to one-third the normal value. This probably reflects the catabolic state that is present. A synthetic mixture of AA low in methionine, phenylalanine, and tryptophan and high in branched-chain AA has successfully reversed hepatic encephalopathy produced in dogs by portacaval shunt or observed in cirrhotics requiring parenteral nutrition but intolerant to available standard AA solutions. While the improvement in mentation has been attributed to the use of larger amounts of branched-chain AA, the results observed may be simply caused by a combination of decreased generation and enhanced processing of ammonia since the content of glycine as well as the aromatic AA was greatly reduced while the amount of arginine was doubled in the mixture (17).

Fulminant hepatic failure with extensive acute hepatic necrosis presents a different pattern of AA abnormalities (18). All the AA in plasma are increased more strikingly, particularly methionine, phenylalanine, tyrosine, and free tryptophan. The branched-chain AA are normal or slightly depressed, but the molar ratio of (Leu + Isoleu + Val)/(Phe + Tyr) remains low. Brain aspartate and glutamate are also increased in contrast to the depressed values observed in the encephalopathy following hepatectomy or acute ischemic hepatic necrosis in experimental animals (19). Methionine in brain and spinal fluid increases more than 30-fold, and phenylalanine and tyrosine increase approximately 8- to 10-fold; in contrast glutamine only increases 3- to 6-fold, although its absolute amount is 15 to 20 times that of methionine, phenylalanine, or tyrosine. Taurine is not increased. The branched-chain AA are increased about 15-fold in the brain and 2-fold in the spinal fluid, being the only AA for which an increased brain-to-plasma ratio could be demonstrated. For the straight-chain AA the plasma concentration appears to be the main factor controlling brain concentration.

Brain concentrations of some neurotransmitters (aspartate, glutamate, norepinephrine) may be decreased, and others (e.g., serotonin) may be normal or increased. Since most studies have measured whole brain, variable results may be related to differences among regions of the brain and compartmentation effects. Thus, in a study of experimental hepatic coma in rats the greatest increases in serotonin and 5-hydroxyindolacetic acid were found in the midbrain, pons, and medulla (15). Neurotransmitter metabolites (asparagine, glutamine, homovanillic acid, and 5-hydroxyindolacetic acid) are increased in spinal fluid of patients with hepatic encephalopathy, but the only evidence available indicates no change in the synthesis of dopamine or serotonin (20). Tyramine, a derivative of tyrosine and a precursor of dopamine and octopamine, is increased in the blood (21). The false neurotransmitter octopamine is increased in brain, muscle, blood, and urine, and the correlation of severity of hepatic encephalopathy with serum octopamine is at least as good as that with blood ammonia (22). The extent to which platelets failed to take up octopamine (but not norepinephrine) was also significantly related to severity of encephalopathy (23). Such correlations, however, do not necessarily reflect cause and effect. By direct infusion of octopamine into the lateral cerebral ventricle of the rat, brain octopamine was raised over 200,000 times normal without causing coma, even though the brain dopamine and norepinephrine concentrations dropped to about 10% of control, far below any reductions observed in hepatic coma (24). By contrast, a small dose of NH_4^+ (0.5 mg) instilled in similar fashion results in convulsions and coma within 1 min. These results seem incompatible with the hypothesis that reduction of brain catecholamines is the cause of hepatic coma.

Methyl mercaptan (methanethiol) has been isolated from the urine of a patient in hepatic coma and is found in the breath along with dimethylsulfide and probably dimethyldisulfide. The combination of all three is probably responsible for fetor hepaticus, although this has never been established by measurements. Mercaptans cause reversible coma in animals and enhance the toxicity of ammonia and fatty acids. Methanethiol in low concentrations inhibits brain microsomal (Na^+, K^+)-ATPase and protects erythrocytes against hemolysis, supporting the idea of a direct membrane effect (25). Blood mercaptans are elevated in patients with liver failure and correlate better than the blood ammonia with the presence and severity of hepatic encephalopathy (26). The combination of both measurements is better than either alone in reflecting hepatic encephalopathy or abnormality after a protein load. Thus the blood mercaptan measurements has promise as a valuable adjunct to the ammonia determination in hepatic failure.

The coma-producing potential of toxic substances may be multiplied severalfold when they are present together as a result of their interdependent metabolism or interrelated effects. This synergism has been demonstrated experimentally with ammonia, fatty acids and mercaptans (27). In combination, much smaller doses and lower blood levels are required to produce coma. Fatty acids and mercaptans greatly increase the blood level of ammonia resulting from the injection of a subcoma dose of NH_4^+. Normal rats become comatose when they are given doses of NH_4^+, fatty acid, and mercaptan, which result in blood levels in the range of those observed in rats with acute experimental hepatic coma due to massive ischemic hepatic necrosis. Thus the encephalopathy that occurs following experimental acute massive necrosis can be explained by the synergistic interaction of these toxic substances without invoking other toxic factors.

Alterations in several toxic as well as protective factors appear to be involved in the pathogenesis of hepatic encephalopathy. Among the protective factors are substances such as sodium, potassium, and albumin whose depletion intensifies or augments the encephalopathy-generating effects of primary toxins when they are present in small amounts. The presence and severity of encephalopathy in a patient with severe liver disease depends upon a balance between the toxic and the protective substances. The relative significance of any single substance varies from case to case, but the net result depends upon a variable quantitative balance between the combined effects of coma producers and coma preventers. The precise locus of action in the brain of the coma producers is unknown; however, it seems likely that in terms of brain mechanisms the coma of hepatic failure will be found to have much in common with ordinary anesthesia.

Treatment

Except for the approaches to elimination of gut bacteria and the nitrogenous substances that they utilize, there is no specific therapy for hepatic encephalopathy. Good general care with careful monitoring of various bodily functions and attention to details has reduced mortality as well as any of the more dramatic forms of therapy (28). The spectrum of cases with hepatic encephalopathy varies widely both with respect to the severity of the underlying liver disease and the acuteness or chronicity of its course. In all instances the initial step is elimination or correction of precipitating factors. Thereafter, the intensiveness of care required will depend upon the extent and rapidity of hepatic destruction.

Fulminant hepatic failure presents the supreme challenge because such patients are most difficult to sustain and yet often have good potential for liver regeneration with ultimate recovery. Special liver units focusing on the intensive care of such patients have achieved survival rates of 30% to 40% by careful attention to acid-base and electrolyte abnormalities; cardiac, pulmonary, gastrointestinal, and renal complications; clotting abnormalities; and infections, in addition to details of personal nursing care (29). Special procedures such as charcoal hemoperfusion (30), polyacrylonitrile membrane hemodialysis (31), and exchange transfusion (32) have not yielded higher recovery rates, although they can clearly reverse the comatose state.

In chronic liver disease with acute or chronic recurrent hepatic encephalopathy, other substances such as arginine, L-dopa, and bromocriptine (33), and a special amino acid mixture high in branched-chain amino acids (17) have been shown to have arousal properties with respect to the encephalopathy but have not been shown to influence the outcome of the patient. The mechanisms of arousal in the latter three instances may not be those originally stimulating the use of the substances (34,17). The administration of lactulose or neomycin in chronic liver disease with chronic recurrent encephalopathy may result in improvement. The use of ketoanalogs of essential amino acids or of a vegetable protein diet in such patients has been reported; however, these intriguing theoretical possibilities have not yet had adequate trials (35).

Future Directions of Research

The occurrence of hepatic encephalopathy is determined by the balance that exists between toxic and protective factors and whatever interdependent or synergistic interactions that may occur among them. While there are many biochemical and physiologic alterations taking place in liver failure, our goal is to identify those that have etiologic significance for the production of encephalopathy. Delay in progress has resulted from the confusion between correlations and causes. While avoiding this pitfall, further work is needed on the identification and clarification of the role of toxic factors having a high probability of direct relevance to the occurrence of encephalopathy. Possible synergistic interactions among them must be identified, and the intensification of their effects by abnormalities, such as hypoxia and electrolyte depletion, that are indirect correlates of hepatic failure must be delineated. The ongoing work on amino acid abnormalities in hepatic encephalopathy is a good example of such research. Another is the work on mercaptans. A clarification of the role in pathogenesis in each of these instances may be expected within the next few years. The same may be anticipated with false neurotransmitters.

In addition to the identification of the important toxic factors and their interactions, a greater effort is desirable in the study of brain mechanisms of hepatic encephalopathy. Studies are needed regarding the effects of the various putative toxic factors on membrane function (e.g., effects on Na^+, K^+-ATPase) and neuronal function (e.g., inhibition and disinhibition).

Fulminant hepatic failure provides a particular and fascinating challenge to those interested in treating hepatic encephalopathy. Much effort has already been invested in the development of systems for removal of toxic substances, and significant progress has been made with hemoperfusion and medium-pore hemodialysis. Further work along the same lines is desirable. Improved adsorbents must be developed that are more selective in action (36). So far, toxicity has resulted from the all-encompassing nature of the adsorbents used with removal of essential substances. Special adsorbents acting only on specific kinds of compounds are needed. Once complications from the use of these procedures per se are eliminated, consideration may be given to their use earlier in the course of the development of encephalopathy to avoid irreversible cerebral changes and possibly to demonstrate significant improvement in survival statistics. Even though methods for sustaining patients with fulminant liver failure improve, progress toward improved survival will be limited by the capacity for regeneration of the liver in any given patient following massive necrosis. Knowledge concerning factors affecting liver regeneration is meager and the identification of conditions or substances that will promote regeneration is important and must be pursued (see Chapter 6).

ELABORATION ON RECENT DEVELOPMENTS

1. Rehnstrom and co-workers[7] found that *psychometric testing* was more sensitive than clinical judgment in detecting intellectual defects in 41 patients with advanced cirrhosis and suspected encephalopathy. This was primarily due to the fact that verbal ability was maintained, while psychomotor performance deteriorated. The cirrhotics' performance on the psychomotor tests was poorer than that of matched alcoholics without cirrhosis. No differences were detectable between 18 patients with alcoholic cirrhosis and 19 patients with nonalcoholic cirrhosis. Fairly severe intellectual impairment would have gone undetected in several patients without the psychomotor tests.

Smith and Smith[8] corroborated these observations in 20 patients with alcoholic cirrhosis who were compared to 20 alcoholics without cirrhosis. There were no differences between the groups on vocabulary and information tests. The cirrhotics scored more poorly on the performance tests, however, particularly on a Picture Arrangement Test and an Object Assembly Test. The noncirrhotic alcoholics had significantly poorer scores than did a corresponding group of normal subjects.

2. Brun and co-workers[9] analyzed *brain proteins* in 6 patients dying of hepatic failure, comparing them to 6 patients dying of nonliver disease. The brain was grossly normal in every patient. Hepatic coma was associated with a striking reduction of soluble brain protein, particularly in the gray matter of the frontal cortex and the thalamus, suggesting that the protein loss was largely neuronal.

3. Livingstone and co-workers[10] evaluated the *blood-brain barrier* in hepatectomized rats in deep hepatic coma, which occurred approximately 18 hr after the removal of the liver. At this time the barrier became permeable to D-sucrose, inulin, and L-glucose, as well as to trypan blue. Cerebral edema was

uniformly seen and was apparently associated with the break in the barrier.

4. Holmin[11] observed a *decrease in brain glutamate* 3 hr after total hepatectomy in the rat, while the intracellular pH and the adenylate energy charge remained unchanged. Derr and Zieve[12] demonstrated a normal adenylate energy charge in hepatic coma following massive hepatic necrosis resulting from ischemia.

5. Hindfelt and co-workers[13] observed that cerebral dysfunction occurred before any evidence of *primary energy failure* in portacaval-shunted rats that received a coma-producing dose of ammonium acetate. During the precoma phase, brain aspartate and glutamate decreased, while adenine nucleotides remained normal. After an hour when deep coma ensued, the ATP concentration decreased in all regions of the brain, especially the brain stem.

6. Gjedde and co-workers[14] found a reduction of approximately 50% in *cerebral blood flow and oxygen consumption* after injection of a coma-producing dose of ammonium acetate into rats with portacaval shunts of 8 weeks' duration. The NH_4^+ injection had no such effect in rats with portacaval shunts of only 4 weeks' duration.

7. Hindfelt[15] observed the *brain ammonia concentration* to be above what could be predicted from the CSF ammonia concentration and the pH gradient in rats exposed chronically to ammonia in the respired air. The concentration gradient between arterial plasma and the CSF could not be explained by pH-dependent nonionic diffusion of ammonia. He[16] also observed that after injection of methionine sulfoximine, the brain ammonia greatly exceeded what might be expected from the ammonia content of CSF or blood.

8. Degos and co-workers[17] observed similar *EEG alterations* in hepatectomized rats and in hepatectomized and eviscerated rats that were sustained with intravenous glucose while developing hepatic encephalopathy. The average plasma ammonia concentration in the hepatectomized and eviscerated rats were only two-fifths that of the simply hepatectomized rats 15 hr after the surgical procedure.

9. Zieve et al.[18] looked for, but did not find, a unique abnormality in *cerebral glucose metabolism* in the hepatectomized dog. The brain glycolytic substrates were normal and Krebs cycle substrates were depressed, but no differently than was observed with sedation or anesthesia.

10. Derr and Zieve[19] found approximately 50% inhibition of acetylglutamate-catalyzed *urea synthesis* by 9.5 mM octanoate in a rat liver homogenate system and 100% inhibition with 45 mM octanoate. Citrulline synthesis was similarly inhibited 28% and 86%, respectively. The longer the fatty acid chain, the greater was the inhibitory effect on the utilization of NH_4^+. Inhibition of carbamylphosphate synthetase was the critical step in this interference with the urea cycle. Glutamate dehydrogenase was similarly inhibited 83% in liver and 43% in brain by 13 mM octanoate, while glutamine synthetase was unaffected. These effects of fatty acids could account in large measure for the in vivo interference of fatty acids with the utilization of ammonia.[6]

11. Teychenne and co-workers[20] produced coma in rabbits by intravenous injection of *valeric* and *isovaleric acids*. The increase in concentration of these acids in a CSF perfusate correlated closely with an increase in slow-wave electrical activity in the EEG.

12. Rabinowitz et al.[21] found *serum octanoate levels* in 25 patients with alcoholic cirrhosis and hepatic encephalopathy to be 3 to 15 times normal. Using [^{14}C]-labeled palmitate, stearate, and oleate, they demonstrated that in these patients, 60% to 80% of the octanoate in the serum came from incomplete beta oxidation of long-chain fatty acids.

13. In 1966, Muto[22] reported elevations in *short-chain fatty acids*, particularly C_4 to C_6, in hepatic coma resulting from nonfulminant disease. Lai, Silk, and Williams[23] measured the short-chain fatty acids through C_7 in comatose patients with fulminant hepatic failure and found no correlation between initial or final plasma levels and the clinical outcome of the disease.

14. Doizaki and Zieve[24] injected *lethal doses of methionine* (40–45 mmole/ kg), *phenylalanine* (50–80 mmole/kg), and *tryptophan* (25–38 mmole/kg) into normal rats, producing dyspnea, dehydration (hematocrit values > 60%), prostration, and death without an intervening phase of coma. Plasma concentrations of the amino acids injected were increased more than 300-fold and brain concentrations were 141-fold for methionine, 36-fold for phenylalanine, and more than 300-fold for tryptophan.

15. Cummings et al.[25] found that *tryptophan* was increased in *all* parts of the *brain* in rats in hepatic precoma, while increases in serotonin and 5HIAA were predominatly found in the midbrain and the medulla and pons. They observed a correlation of 0.96 between plasma free tryptophan and cortical tryptophan. Curzon and co-workers[26] had previously established the correlation between plasma free tryptophan and brain tryptophan and concluded that a high plasma free tryptophan leads to high brain tryptophan in a variety of circumstances, not just hepatic failure. Under nonpathologic conditions in rats, Madras et al.[27] found no relation between plasma free tryptophan and brain tryptophan. Ono and co-workers[28] found that free plasma tryptophan increased 3.5-fold in 10 cirrhotics in hepatic coma as compared to 10 cirrhotics without evidence of encephalopathy. The CSF tryptophan was correspondingly increased by 57% and was the only amino acid of those measured (including methionine, phenylalanine, tyrosine, leucine, isoleucine, and valine) that was significantly elevated.

16. Morris and Rogers[29] observed that cats given a single meal of a complete *amino acid diet* without arginine had about a sixfold rise in blood ammonia and showed clinical signs of ammonia toxicity within 2 hr.

17. Fischer and co-workers[30] found that Freamine II, a *synthetic amino acid mixture* introduced for hyperalimentation, caused progression of the encephalopathy in dogs following portacaval shunts, leading to death. Replacement of the Freamine II with F080, a modified mixture of the amino acids in which the branched-chain amino acids leucine, isoleucine, and valine were increased by approximately 50%, resulted in reversal of the encephalopathy and improvement in the dogs. The improvement was attributed to the normalization of the ratio of the molar sum of the branched-chain amino acids to the molar sum of phenylalanine and tyrosine. The normal ratio is 3–4. After Freamine II it had dropped to 1.13, and after F080 it had risen to 3.74. In addition to the increase in branched-chain amino acids when Freamine II was replaced by F080, methionine and phenylalanine were decreased by approximately 78%, glycine was decreased by about 50%, and arginine was increased by almost

100%. The reduction in glycine was particularly important because it alone comprised 30% of the total amino acids in Freamine II. All three of the branched-chain amino acids together comprised 20% of the total amino acids. The change from Freamine II to F080 resulted in both a large reduction in the total amount of ammonia-generating amino acids and, simultaneously a doubling of the ammonia-processing amino acid arginine, in addition to the increase in branched-chain amino acids. Thus from these experiments, we cannot tell which of these changes was responsible for the improvement observed with F080.

Fisher and colleagues[31] also used F080 successfully in improving hepatic encephalopathy in 8 cirrhotics with superimposed gastrointestinal hemorrhage or alcoholic hepatitis. They found an inverse correlation between the molar ratio (branched-chain amino acids: phenylalanine + tyrosine) and an encephalopathic score. However, the patient in one case that was presented in detail (RJW in Fig. 10 of Fisher's report) had a ratio of 0.77 before use of F080, when he was unconscious, and a ratio of 0.71 just after cessation of F080, when he was alert. While the patient was receiving F080, his molar ratio went up to 3.22. Thus, a low ratio is compatible with absence of encephalopathy. Soeters and associates[32] measured plasma insulin and glucagon levels in dogs becoming encephalopathic following portacaval shunts and found that the average insulin level rose from a preshunt value of 8.6 to 13.0 μU/ml, while glucagon rose from 74 to 401 pg/ml. The net molar ratio of insulin/glucagon fell from 3.13 to 1.09.

18. Record and colleagues[33] are the only ones to have reported on plasma, spinal fluid, and brain *amino acids* in a large number of patients with hepatic coma following *fulminant hepatic failure*. Their results were reported in the preceding summary section. Rosen et al.[34] contrasted the plasma amino acid alterations in 5 patients with fulminant hepatic failure and in 13 patients with chronic hepatic failure. The 5 patients with fulminant failure followed, more or less, the pattern observed by Record et al.,[33] and in these patients, they observed a correlation of 0.95 between plasma tyrosine and the serum transaminase.

19. Biebuyck and co-workers[35] verified previous observations that *brain aspartate and glutamate* are depressed. They studied rats in early hepatic coma that followed acute ischemic massive hepatic necrosis. No significant alterations in cyclicAMP or gamma aminobutyric acid concentrations were observed.

20. Lal and co-workers[36] used probenecid to block *transport of homovanillic acid and 5HIAA from CSF to blood* as a means of assessing the rates of synthesis of brain dopamine and serotonin; they found no change in synthesis of these compounds in cirrhotics when in hepatic coma.

21. Faraj and colleagues[37] found *plasma tyramine* significantly higher in 7 cirrhotics with hepatic encephalopathy than in 6 cirrhotics without encephalopathy (average of 6.4 ng/ml compared to 2.7 ng/ml). The correlation between plasma tyramine and tyrosine was 0.84.

22. Rossi-Fanelli et al.[38] reassessed the relationship between *plasma octopamine* and severity of encephalopathy in 26 cirrhotics with clinically evident

encephalopathy. They found a significant association but could not distinguish effectively between grade 3 and grade 4 encephalopathy. In another study,[39] this group found no relationship between arterial ammonia and octopamine concentrations and found a correlation of only 0.5 in venous blood. These two substances seemed to vary independently, particularly in patients with portacaval shunts. As in the previous reports relating plasma or serum octopamine to hepatic encephalopathy, when the variability at each grade of encephalopathy is taken into account, the correlation is about the same low order of magnitude as that between blood ammonia and encephalopathy and is not comparable to the fairly good correlation between CSF glutamine and encephalopathy.

23. Morelli, Frintzelas, and Zimmon[40] observed that *uptake of octopamine and norepinephrine by platelets* of patients with hepatic encephalopathy was decreased. The extent of the decrease in octopamine uptake correlated significantly, but not strikingly, with the grade of encephalopathy. No such correlation was observed with norepinephrine. Plasma from patients with hepatic encephalopathy inhibited norepinephrine uptake by normal platelets.

24. Zieve and Olsen[41] depressed brain dopamine content by 92% and norepinephrine content by 86% in normal rats using *intraventricular infusions of octopamine* without affecting the alertness of the rats. Extremely high levels of brain octopamine were reached, levels higher than 847,000 ng/g in some rats. Corresponding values in normal rats are about 4 ng/g and are less than 15 ng/g in moribund rats in deep hepatic coma.[42] They found no reduction in brain dopamine or norepinephrine in 6 rats in hepatic coma following acute massive ischemic hepatic necrosis.

25. Quarfoth, Ahmed, and colleagues[43] found that *methanethiol* is a potent inhibitor of microsomal (Na^+, K^+)-ATPase activity, and its action occurs at several sites on the enzyme system. These effects are freely reversible. Methanethiol, like anesthetics, also stabilizes the erythrocyte membrane against hypotonic hemolysis, and the concentrations that give 50% protection against hemolysis are of the same order as those that produce 50% inhibition of the brain (Na^+, K^+)-ATPase.

26. Doizaki and Zieve[44] described an improved method for measuring *mercaptans* that enabled the measurement of methanethiol in blood of patients for the first time. They found striking elevations in patients with hepatic coma. McClain, Zieve, and co-workers[45] observed an increase of 56% in the average blood methanethiol of 52 cirrhotics and an increase of 139% in 42 patients with alcoholic liver disease (mostly cirrhotics) and hepatic encephalopathy. Elevation of blood methanethiol was observed in 93%, and both methanethiol and ammonia were elevated in 98% of the cases with hepatic encephalopathy. In 85% of the patients followed serially, blood methanethiol correlated with change in mental status. Using the method of Doizaki and Zieve, Brunner and Siehoff[46] verified that methanethiol was strikingly elevated in 13 cases of hepatic coma. McClain and co-workers[47] found that blood methanethiol was substantially better than blood ammonia in detecting abnormality in 17 cirrhotics after a single protein load but that both measurements were required to completely separate cirrhotics from normals.

27. Merino and co-workers[48] verified in dogs that *methionine* in large dosage causes coma in the presence of shunts and that synergism exists between the product formed in the gut from methionine (presumably methanethiol) and ammonia in the production of coma.

28. Maddrey and Weber[49] and Scharschmidt[50] have provided useful reviews of *management* of chronic hepatic encephalopathy and fulminant hepatic failure, respectively.

29. Ward and colleagues[51] reviewed their experience with 137 patients in a *special care unit for acute hepatic failure*, pointing out how all major organ systems are involved and the high standard of patient monitoring and intensive care that is required to optimize survival. Cerebral edema was the single most common cause of death. The vigorous approach of this group provides a useful reference standard for present-day care of patients with acute failure. Auslander and Gitnick[52] achieved 40% survival among 20 patients with fulminant hepatic failure resulting from viral hepatitis by utilizing an aggressive medical approach. Presumably the therapy and survival rate were related.

30. There have been no controlled studies with *charcoal hemoperfusion* in hepatic coma. The original report[53] from the Kings College Hospital in London was encouraging, with 10 of 22 patients in fulminant hepatic failure with grade IV coma surviving. The subsequent experience of this group was quite the contrary as a result of platelet aggregation[54] and hypotension, there being no survivors in the last 18 patients run.[51] Gelfand and co-workers[55] reported successful application of the technique to a cirrhotic patient in deep hepatic coma, providing another interesting but uncontrolled observation. Chirito et al.[56] studied the effects of albumin-collodion microencapsulated activated charcoal hemoperfusion in rats with galactosamine-induced acute hepatic necrosis; survival improved from 30% to 71% with hemoperfusion initiated 48 hr after the injection of the toxin but before the onset of hepatic encephalopathy.

31. Ordinary *hemodialysis* has no effect on hepatic coma. From the experimental studies of cross-hemodialysis[57,58] the procedure of direct polyacrylonitrile membrane hemodialysis has evolved which permits passage of compounds with molecular weights up to 15,000. Opolon and co-workers[59] applied this procedure to 22 patients in coma with fulminant viral hepatitis and observed recovery of consciousness in 59% but survival in only 22%. Silk and colleagues[60] also used this procedure in 24 patients with fulminant hepatic failure and grade IV coma, and 33% survived. In 81% of the failures, cerebral edema was present at autopsy. None of the foregoing work was controlled.

32. Controlled studies with *exchange transfusion* in patients are meager. Lewis and colleagues[61] observed a response to exchange transfusion in 42% of 19 patients (12 with hepatitis) with stage IV hepatic coma, but only 21% survived, which is what one would expect without the procedure. Cooper and co-workers[62] applied the technique of total body washout in 12 patients, achieving a reponse in 5 and survival in 3.

33. L-*dopa* appears to have arousal properties in hepatic coma, although a controlled trial is lacking. Fischer and co-workers[63] treated 35 patients with severe liver disease, 63% cirrhotics and 89% in grade IV coma. While 63% seemed to respond to the L-dopa, only 14% survived. The latter were treated

within 2 days of the onset of coma, while the nonresponders were not treated until an average of 9.5 days of coma. Morgan et al.[64] found bromocriptine of value in a patient with severe chronic hepatic encephalopathy, as they had previously[65] observed with L-dopa.

34. Zieve[66] demonstrated that L-*dopa* would prevent ammonia coma *in rats*. The presence or absence of coma was correlated with changes in blood and brain ammonia but not with brain dopamine, and the changes in blood (and brain) ammonia were related to increased renal excretion of ammonia and urea under the influence of L-dopa.

35. Maddrey and co-workers[67] gave *keto analogs of five essential amino acids* to 11 cirrhotics with chronic hepatic encephalopathy and observed improvement in 8. Plasma concentrations of the amino acids corresponding to the analogs increased significantly. At least 1 patient had a progressive fall in arterial ammonia. Greenberger and colleagues[68] showed in 3 patients with chronic hepatic encephalopathy that a vegetable protein diet resulted in clinical and intellectual improvement that was enhanced by the simultaneous use of lactulose.

36. Brunner and Jaworeck[69] purified rabbit *UDP-glucuronyl transferase* and then bound it covalently to an artificial carrier such as acrylamide and used this preparation in vitro to glucuronidate free phenols in blood from patients with liver failure. They propose to use this principle to selectively eliminate toxic substances from the blood by extracorporeal hemoperfusion.

REFERENCES

1. Schenker S, Breen KJ, Hoyumpa AM: Hepatic encephalopathy—current status. Gastroenterology 66:121–151, 1974

2. Fischer JE, Baldessarini RJ: Pathogenesis and therapy of hepatic coma. Edited by H Popper and F Schaffner: Progress in Liver Diseases. Vol. V. New York, Grune & Stratton, 1975, pp 363–397

3. Plum F, Hindfelt B: The neurological complications of liver disease. Edited by PJ Vinken, GW Brnyn, and HL Klawans: Handbook of Clinical Neurology (XXVII: Metabolic and Deficiency Diseases of the Nervous System). New York, American Elsevier, 1976, pp 349–377

4. Gabuzda GJ: Hepatic coma—clinical considerations, pathogenesis and management. Adv Intern Med 11:11–73, 1962

5. Zieve L: Pathogenesis of hepatic coma. Arch Intern Med 118:211–223, 1966

6. Zieve L, Nicoloff DM: Pathogenesis of hepatic coma. Annu Rev Med 26:143–157, 1975

7. Rehnstrom S, Simert G, Hansson JA, et al: Chronic hepatic encephalopathy. A psychometrical study. Scand J Gastroenterol 12:305–311, 1977

8. Smith HH, Jr, Smith LS: WAIS functioning of cirrhotic and non-cirrhotic alcoholics. J Clin Psychol 33:309–313, 1977

9. Brun A, Dawiskiba S, Hindfelt B, et al: Brain proteins in hepatic encephalopathy. Acta Neurol Scand 55:213–225, 1977

10. Livingstone AS, Potvin M, Goresky CA, et al: Changes in the blood-brain barrier in hepatic coma after hepatectomy in the rat. Gastroenterology 73:697–704, 1977

11. Holmin T: The effect of hepatectomy on the energy state and on acid-base variables of the rat brain. Scand J Clin Lab Invest 36:423–429, 1976

12. Derr RF, Zieve L: Decreased cerebral uptake of oxygen in coma—a consequence of decreased utilization of ATP. J Neurochem 21:1555–1557, 1973

13. Hindfelt B, Plum F, Duffy TE: Effect of acute ammonia intoxication on cerebral metabolism in rats with portacaval shunts. J Clin Invest 59:386–396, 1977

14. Gjedde A, Lockwood A, Duffy TE, et al: Effect of ammonia on cerebral metabolism of rats with portacaval shunts. Trans Am Neurol Assoc 101:180–181, 1976

15. Hindfelt B: The distribution of ammonia

between extracellular and intracellular compartments of the rat brain. Clin Sci Mol Med 48:33–37, 1975

16. Hindfelt B: L-methionine DL-sulphoximine (MSO) and ammonia distribution between extra- and intra-cellular compartments of the rat brain. J Neurol Sci 25:499–506, 1975

17. Degos F, Degos JD, Bourdiace D, et al: Experimental acute hepatic encephalopathy—comparison of the electroencephalographic changes in the liverless and in the eviscerated rat. Clin Sci Mol Med 47:599–608, 1974

18. Zieve L, Nicoloff D, Doizaki W: Effect of total hepatectomy on selected cerebral substrates and enzymes of the glycolytic pathway and Krebs cycle. Surgery 78:414–423, 1975

19. Derr RF, Zieve L: Effect of fatty acids on the disposition of ammonia. J Pharmacol Exp Ther 197:675–680, 1976

20. Teychenne PF, Walters I, Claveria LE, et al: The encephalopathic action of five-carbon-atom fatty acids in the rabbit. Clin Sci Mol Med 50:463–472, 1976

21. Rabinowitz JL, Staeffen J, Blauquet P, et al: Sources of serum [^{14}C]-octanoate in cirrhosis of the liver and hepatic encephalopathy. J Lab Clin Med 91:223–227, 1978

22. Muto Y: Clinical study on the relationship of short-chain fatty acids and hepatic encephalopathy. Jpn J Gastroenterol 63:19–32, 1966

23. Lai JCK, Silk DBA, Williams R: Plasma short-chain fatty acids in fulminant hepatic failure. Clin Chim Acta 78:305–310, 1977

24. Doizaki WM, Zieve L: Lethal doses of methionine, phenylalamine and tryptophan do not cause coma before death in normal rats. (unpublished observations)

25. Cummings MG, James JH, Soeters PB, et al: Regional brain study of indoleamine metabolism in the rat in acute hepatic failure. J Neurochem 27:741–746, 1976

26. Curzon G, Knott PJ, Murray-Lyon IM, et al: Disturbed brain tryptophan metabolism in hepatic coma. Lancet 1:1092–1093, 1975

27. Madras BK, Cohen EL, Munro HN, et al: Elevation of serum free tryptophan, but not brain tryptophan, by serum nonesterified fatty acids. Adv Biochem Psychopharmacol 11:143–151, 1974

28. Ono J, Hutson DG, Dombro RS, et al: Tryptophan and hepatic coma. Gastroenterology 74:196–200, 1978

29. Morris JG, Rogers QR: Ammonia intoxication in the near-adult cat as a result of a dietary deficiency of arginine. Science 199:431–432, 1978

30. Fischer JE, Funovics JM, Aguirre A, et al: The role of plasma amino acids in hepatic encephalopathy. Surgery 78:276–288, 1975

31. Fischer JE, Rosen HM, Ebeid AM, et al: The effect of normalization of plasma amino acids on hepatic encephalopathy in man. Surgery 80:77–90, 1976

32. Soeters PB, Weir G, Ebeid AM, et al: Insulin, glucagon, portal systemic shunting, and hepatic failure in the dog. J Surg Res 23:183–188, 1977

33. Record CO, Buxton B, Chase, RA, et al: Plasma and brain amino acids in fulminant hepatic failure and their relationship to hepatic encephalopathy. Eur J Clin Invest 6:387–394, 1976

34. Rosen HM, Yoshimura N, Hodgman JM, et al: Plasma amino acid patterns in hepatic encephalopathy of differing etiology. Gastroenterology 72:483–487, 1977

35. Biebuyck JF, Funovics J, Dedrick DF, et al: Neurochemistry of hepatic coma: alterations in putative transmitter amino acids. Edited by R Williams and IM Murray-Lyon: Artificial Liver Support. London, Pitman Medical, 1975, pp 51–56

36. Lal S, Aronoff A, Garelis E, et al: Cerebrospinal fluid homovanillic acid, 5-hydroxyindoleacetic acid, lactic acid, and pH before and after probenecid in hepatic coma. Clin Neurol Neurosurg 77:142–154, 1974

37. Faraj BA, Bowen PA, Isaacs JW, et al: Hypertyraminemia in cirrhotic patients. N Engl J Med 294:1360–1364, 1976

38. Rossi-Fanelli F, Cangiano C, Attili A, et al: Octopamine plasma levels and hepatic encephalopathy: a re-appraisal of the problem. Clin Chim Acta 67:255–261, 1976

39. Capocaccia L, Cangiano C, Attili AF, et al: Octopamine and ammonia plasma levels in hepatic encephalopathy. Clin Chim Acta 75:99–105, 1977

40. Morelli A, Frintzilas M, Zimmon DS: Platelet uptake of octopamine and norepinephrine in hepatic encephalopathy. Gastroenterology 73:560–564, 1977

41. Zieve L, Olsen RL: Can hepatic coma be caused by a reduction of brain noradrenaline or dopamine? Gut 18:688–691, 1977

42. Dodsworth JM, James JH, Cummings MC, et al: Depletion of brain norepinephrine in acute hepatic coma. Surgery 75:811–820, 1974

43. Quarfoth G, Ahmed K, Foster D, et al:

Action of methanethiol on membrane (Na^+, K^+)-ATPase of rat brain. Biochem Pharmacol 25:1039–1044, 1976

44. Doizaki WM, Zieve L: An improved method for measuring blood mercaptans. J Lab Clin Med 90:849–855, 1977

45. McClain CJ, Zieve L, Doizaki W, et al: Mercaptans in portal systemic encephalopathy (PSE) due to alcoholic liver disease. Gastroenterology 74:1064, 1978

46. Brunner G, Siehoff A: Untersuchungen uber die bedeutung von endogenen toxinen bei der entstehung des coma hepaticum. Verh Dtsch Ges Inn Med 82:445–447, 1976

47. McClain CJ, Kromhout J, Zieve L, et al: Blood mercaptan and ammonia concentrations in cirrhotics after a protein load. Gastroenterology 74:1064, 1978

48. Merino GE, Jetzer T, Doizaki WM, et al: Methionine-induced hepatic coma in dogs. Am J Surg 130:41–46, 1975

49. Maddrey WC, Weber FL, Jr: Chronic hepatic encephalopathy. Med Clin North Am 59:937–944, 1975

50. Scharschmidt BF: Approaches to the management of fulminant hepatic failure. Med Clin North Am 59:927–935, 1975

51. Ward ME, Trewby PN, Williams R, et al: Acute liver failure. Experience in a special unit. Anesthesia 32:228–239, 1977

52. Auslander MO, Gitnick GL: Vigorous medical management of acute fulminant hepatitis. Arch Intern Med 137:599–601, 1977

53. Gazzard BG, Weston MJ, Murray-Lyon IM, et al: Charcoal haemoperfusion in the treatment of fulminant hepatic failure. Lancet 1:1301–1307, 1974

54. Weston MJ, Langley PG, Rubin MH, et al: Platelet function in fulminant hepatic failure and effect of charcoal haemoperfusion. Gut 18:897–902, 1977

55. Gelfand MC, Knepshield JH, Cohan S, et al: Treatment of hepatic coma with haemoperfusion through polyacrylamide hydrogel-coated charcoal. Kidney Int 10 (Suppl 7):S239–S243, 1976

56. Chirito E, Reiter B, Lister C, et al: Artificial liver: The effect of ACAC microencapsulated charcoal haemoperfusion on fulminant hepatic failure. Artif Organ 1:76–83, 1977

57. Santiago-Delpin EA, Callender C, Kjellstrand CM, et al: Cross-dialysis in the treatment of experimental fulminant hepatic coma. J Surg Res 19:175–182, 1975

58. Opolon P, Lavallard MC, Huguet C, et al: Hemodialysis versus cross hemodialysis in experimental hepatic coma. Surg Gynecol Obstet 142:845–854, 1976

59. Opolon P, Rapin J-R, Huguet C, et al: Hepatic failure coma (HFC) treated by polyacrylonitrile membrane (PAN) hemodialysis (HD). Trans Am Soc Artif Intern Organs 22:701–710, 1976

60. Silk DBA, Trewby PN, Chase RA, et al: Treatment of fulminant hepatic failure by polyacrylonitrile-membrane haemodialysis. Lancet 2:1–3, 1977

61. Lewis JD, Hussey CV, Varma RR, et al: Exchange transfusion in hepatic coma. Factors affecting results with long-term followup data. Am J Surg 129:125–129, 1975

62. Cooper GN, Jr., Karlson KE, Clowes GHA, et al: Total blood washout and exchange. A valuable tool in acute hepatic coma and Reye's syndrome. Am J Surg 133:522–529, 1977

63. Fischer JE, Funovics JM, Falcao HA, et al: L-dopa in hepatic coma. Ann Surg 183:386–391, 1976

64. Morgan MY, Jakobovits A, Elithorn A, et al: Successful use of bromocriptine in the treatment of a patient with chronic portasystemic encephalopathy. N Engl J Med 296:793–794, 1977

65. Lunzer M, James IM, Weinman J, et al: Treatment of chronic hepatic encephalopathy with levodopa. Gut 15:555–561, 1974

66. Zieve L: Reversal of ammonia coma by L-dopa: A peripheral effect. Gastroenterology 73:1256, 1977

67. Maddrey WC, Weber FL, Jr., Coulter AW, et al: Effects of keto analogues of essential amino acids in portal-systemic encephalopathy. Gastroenterology 71:190–195, 1976

68. Greenberger NJ, Carley J, Schenker S, et al: Effect of vegetable and animal protein diets in chronic hepatic encephalopathy. Dig Dis 22:845–855, 1977

69. Brunner G, Jaworeck D: A new approach towards an extracorporeal management in liver failure. Diseases of the Liver and Biliary Tract. Fifth Quadrennial Meeting of the International Association for the Study of the Liver. Basel, Karger, 1976 pp 39–41

Chapter 19

Hepatitis A Virus: Identification, Characterization, and Epidemiologic Investigations

By JULES L. DIENSTAG, M.D.

WHEN THE LAST VOLUME of *Progress in Liver Diseases* was being prepared, new information about hepatitis A virus (HAV) was in an embryonic state, and in anticipation of future advances, the editors chose to defer review of the subject to the present volume. The wisdom of their decision and the accuracy of their prediction have been borne out by the logarithmic expansion of hepatitis A research during the last several years. Despite the fact that HAV remains refractory to in vitro culture, a progressive, unrelenting assault on the secrets of its identity, characteristics, epidemiology, and immunology has taken place.

If the study of hepatitis A reinforces any lesson learned from the study of hepatitis B, it is that progress depends on the availability of immunologic markers of infection. Epidemiologic investigations, studies in volunteers, and transmission of infection to marmoset monkeys were the mainstays of HAV research until 1973 and provided both a wealth of information and valuable reagents for subsequent work. Reviewed extensively in these volumes[1-3] and elsewhere,[4-6] these early studies will not be described in detail here. Suffice it to say that data generated in these studies characterized HAV as a small virus resistant to acid, ether, and heat, present in feces and blood during the late incubation period and acute phase of illness, and immunologically distinct from hepatitis B virus (HBV). Type A hepatitis was found to have a short incubation period (2 to 6 weeks), to be spread predominantly by the fecal-oral route, and to occur in large outbreaks; because it was considered highly infectious, it was designated ''infectious hepatitis.'' In light of the fact, however, that epidemiologic and clinical features do not discriminate adequately between infection with HAV and other hepatitis viruses, the term ''infectious hepatitis'' has been abandoned and replaced by the more accurate etiologic label, viral hepatitis type A.

Of the work preceding the new era of hepatitis A research heralded by the visualization of HAV, studies of the MS-1 strain at the Willowbrook State School by Krugman and colleagues,[7] successful transmission of HAV in mar-

From Medical Services (Gastrointestinal Unit), Massachusetts General Hospital, and the Department of Medicine, Harvard Medical School, Boston, Massachusetts.

Dr. Dienstag is the recipient of Clinical Investigator Award AM00458 from the National Institutes of Health.

343

mosets by Deinhardt and co-workers,[8] and extensive characterization of the CR326 strain in marmosets by Mascoli and Provost and colleagues[9,10] proved to have the greatest impact on more recent advances.

VISUALIZATION OF HAV

In 1973, Feinstone, Kapikian, and Purcell[11] reported the visualization by immune electron microscopy of viruslike particles associated with acute HAV infection. These investigators reasoned that antibody to HAV, which was known to be present in convalescent serum and gamma globulin, would bind to and surround or aggregate HAV, which had been shown in earlier transmission studies to be present in feces of patients with acute illness. Fecal and serum specimens were obtained from material collected in the late 1960s from volunteers at the State Prison in Joliet, Illinois, who had been inoculated with the MS-1 strain of HAV derived from studies at Willowbrook.[12] Viruslike particles measuring 27 nm and aggregated by antibody were visualized in filtrates of these acute phase (but not preinoculation) stool specimens incubated with convalescent serum or gamma globulin, and immunologic specificity was established by demonstrating serologic responses to the virus antigen (hepatitis A antigen, HA Ag) in patients with experimentally induced and naturally acquired type A hepatitis but not in patients with hepatitis B or viral gastroenteritis. An association between these HA Ag particles and HAV was confirmed quite early in studies of natural outbreaks in Arizona,[13] Melbourne, Australia,[14] and California.[15]

Almost simultaneously, a morphologically similar particle was visualized in homogenates of liver, in thin-section electron micrographs of liver cytoplasm, and in concentrated serum of marmosets infected experimentally with the CR326 strain of HAV,[16] derived from a naturally infected child in Costa Rica.[9,10] Preliminary studies had shown that the infectivity titer of acute phase marmoset liver was higher than that of serum. Therefore, the liver was a natural place to look for virus particles and turned out to be an excellent source of virus antigen for serologic tests. The discovery of HAV particles in stools of infected persons and in livers of infected marmosets revolutionized hepatitis A research, leading to the development of new sophisticated assays to detect HAV antigen and antibody, the demonstration of new animal models, the characterization of the virus, and an exhaustive definition of its seroepidemiology. The World Health Organization Expert Committee on Viral Hepatitis recognized the 27-nm particle as HAV and replaced the earlier nomenclature HA Ag and anti-HA with HAV and anti-HAV.[17]

CHARACTERIZATION OF HAV

Morphologically, HAV is a nonenveloped 27-nm particle with cubic symmetry that may appear either ''full'' (unpenetrated by stain) or ''empty'' (penetrated by stain) under the electron microscope (Fig. 1). Although empty particles probably represent virions devoid of nucleic acid and are found more commonly at low buoyant densities, the full and empty particles are immu-

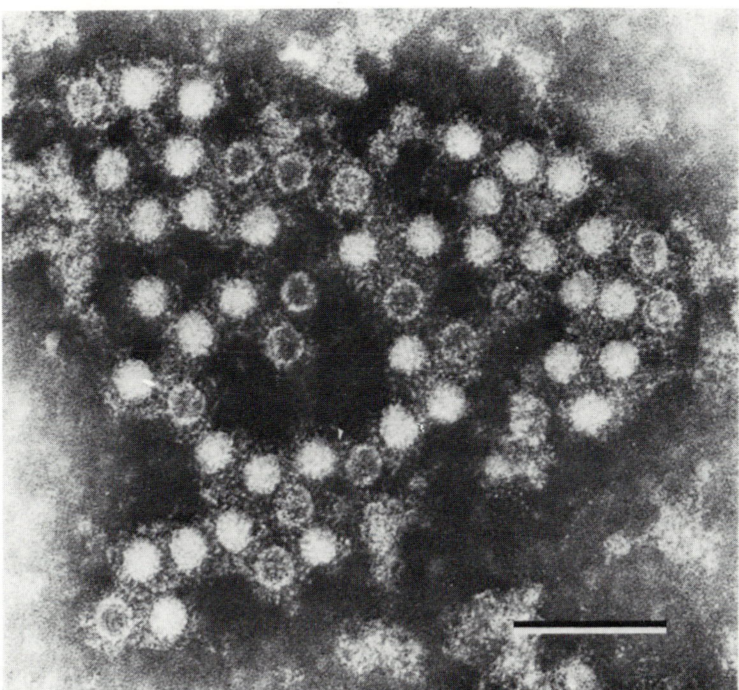

FIG. 1—Electron micrograph of 27-nm hepatitis A virus (HAV) particles aggregated by anti-body. Both "full" (unpenetrated by stain) and "empty" (penetrated by stain) particles are seen in this preparation derived from the liver of a marmoset infected experimentally with HAV. The bar represents 100 nm. Original magnification × 198,000. Two percent phosphotungstic acid neg-ative stain. (Reproduced with permission of CRC Press, Inc. from Dienstag JL, Purcell RH: Hepatitis A virus. CRC Handbook of Clinical Laboratory Science, in press. Copyright The Chemical Rubber Co., CRC Press, Inc.)

nologically indistinguishable. No excess virus coat material has been found, and there is no evidence to substantiate a distinct virus core. What has been described by some as a dense core[18] probably represents greater electron density at the center of the particle than at its periphery. Whether derived from stool, bile, liver, or serum, whether from man or nonhuman primate, all HAV particles are immunologically indistinguishable.[16,19-21]

Hepatitis A virus can be inactivated by ultraviolet light, formalin, chlorine, or heating for 1 min at 98°C. However, the virus maintains infectivity after heating for 1 hr at 60°C, freezing and thawing, or exposure to acid or ether.[4] Its resistance to ether inactivation and its recovery in aqueous phase after chloroform extraction[22,23] provide evidence that lipid is not an integral component of the virus. A multiplicity of buoyant densities ranging from approximately 1.23 to 1.48 g/cm^3 in cesium chloride have been described for HAV, but the principal density is 1.34 g/cm^3.[16,19-21,23-36,45,46] Particles detected in stool with a density of 1.40 g/cm^3 or greater are relatively unstable, and particles with densities < 1.30 g/cm^3 are generally empty and devoid of nucleic acid, but particles of different densities are immunologically indistinguishable.[19,32] Infectivity is not confined to particles of one density, but it is maximal at 1.34

g/cm³.[16] Although the less stable, high-density ($<$ 1.40 g/cm³) particles and the empty, low-density ($<$ 1.30 g/cm³) particles have lower sedimentation coefficients in sucrose, the major density particles (1.34 g/cm³) have a sedimentation coefficient of 160S.[35] The multiplicity of densities and heat stability of HAV is reminiscent of small single-stranded DNA parvoviruses; however, the 27-nm size, major density of 1.34 g/cm³, and S value of 160 are most consistent with classification of HAV among the enterovirus subgroup of picornaviruses. Moreover, several other enteroviruses also have a high-density component.[37] In support of classification as an RNA-containing enterovirus, acridine orange staining, partial inactivation with RNase, and cytoplasmic localization of the virus in the liver suggested an RNA genome.[16] More recently the nucleic acid and polypeptide composition of HAV have been determined definitively and support the contention that HAV is an enterovirus. Highly purified, concentrated preparations of HAV derived from human stools have been subjected to discontinuous SDS polyacrylamide gel electrophoresis,[34] and three polypeptides were distinguished. These peptides with molecular weights of 34,000, 25,500, and 23,000 daltons are similar to three of the four major polypeptides of the enterovirus poliovirus. Nucleic acid extracted from these purified particles by phenol-SDS and treated with diphenylamine or orcinol yielded a colorimetric reaction consistent with RNA (Coulepis, et al., unpublished observations). The most convincing evidence that HAV has an RNA genome comes from the demonstration that in the presence of urea and formamide, purified preparations of HAV released linear single-stranded nucleic acid which, like RNA genomes from other RNA viruses, was readily hydrolyzed under alkaline conditions (pH 12.9).[38] Similarly treated DNA virus nucleic acid, though denatured by these conditions, resisted hydrolysis. The genome extracted from HAV had two major-size peaks, 1.2 μ and 1.7 μ, a mean molecular weight of 1.9 $\times$ 10⁶ daltons, and was smaller than the genome of poliovirus type 2. These nucleic acid and polypeptide studies have been confirmed (Y. Moritsugu et al., unpublished observations) and, with immunofluorescence and immunoperoxidase localization of HAV exclusively to the cytoplasm,[39,40] confirm that HAV is enteroviruslike.

Many strains of HAV have been identified in countries all over the world.[11-16,36,41-46] Although each is designated by a different name, immunologic comparisons among isolates have failed to define any strain differences, suggesting that strains of HAV from all over the world are antigenically similar, if not identical.

DETECTION OF HAV AND ANTI-HAV

Before HAV was identified and before in vitro tests were developed for the detection of HAV and anti-HAV, the only method for documenting HAV infection was the demonstration of *infectivity* of acute phase clinical specimens (HAV) or *neutralization* of infectivity by convalescent serum (anti-HAV) in experimental animals.[10,47] These in vivo tests were described after the susceptibility of *Saguinus* marmosets to HAV was reported,[8] but practical applications were limited. *Immune electron microscopy* (IEM) was the first in vitro technique described to identify both HAV and anti-HAV.[11] The presence of

HAV in stool or liver homogenates is determined by incubation with a known anti-HAV-positive serum, and the presence of anti-HAV in serum is determined by incubating the serum with a HAV-positive stool filtrate or with purified HAV. Based on the immunologic specificity of the reaction between HAV and anti-HAV and on the quantitative rises in anti-HAV ratings[48] detectable with this technique, IEM proved a valuable research tool and, despite requirements for experienced personnel and specialized equipment, remains a basic reference technique.

More simple, practical, and quantitative assays followed. HAV antigen derived from liver homogenates of infected *Saguinus mystax* marmosets was used to develop *complement fixation* (CF)[49] and *immune adherence hemagglutination* (IAHA)[50] tests for anti-HAV. More sensitive and reliable than CF,[51] IAHA has enjoyed popularity as both a screening and a quantitative assay for anti-HAV. It is based on the fact that primate erythrocytes bear surface receptors for the third component of complement (C3). The immune complex formed by incubating HAV with anti-HAV is exposed to a fresh complement source, and the antigen-antibody-complement complex that forms agglutinates indicator red blood cells. This versatile assay is used in a number of research laboratories and works well with HAV purified from either marmoset liver[50] or human stool.[29]

Shortly after the description of IEM, CF, and IAHA, several groups reported adaptation of *radioimmunoassay* techniques to the detection of HAV and anti-HAV.[28,30] Both microtiter solid-phase[28,30] and competitive inhibition[52] assays have been described and provide "third-generation" sensitivity to the repertoire of serologic tests used to identify HAV infection. In addition, a variety of radioimmunoassay modifications have been described to identify acute phase anti-HAV of the IgM class, providing a tool for serologic diagnosis with a single serum specimen obtained during acute illness (discussed later in this Chapter). HAV has been demonstrated in hepatocyte cytoplasm by *immunofluorescence,*[39] and the newest addition to the ever-growing list of test methods applied to the detection of HAV and anti-HAV is the *enzyme-linked immunosorbent assay* (ELISA).[53] Entirely analogous and of comparable sensitivity with solid-phase radioimmunoassay, ELISA substitutes an enzyme label for radionuclide-labeled second antibody, the binding of which is reflected by hydrolysis of an enzyme substrate and quantitated colorimetrically.

Supplies of HAV-containing material are limited, and these test methods are performed in a handful of laboratories around the world. Still, sufficient quantities of HAV have been generated so that commercial availability of reagents for anti-HAV testing is imminent. Additional details of HAV antigen purification, test performance, and determinations of specificity, as well as advantages and disadvantages of each test method, have been reviewed.[54]

ANIMAL MODELS

The absence of successful in vitro cultivation of HAV gives its propagation in experimental animals special importance. Unlike the development of in vitro serologic tests that followed visualization of HAV, discovery of a susceptible nonhuman model predated visualization of the virus by almost a decade. After a series of fruitless attempts by many investigators to transmit HAV to a variety of laboratory animals and nonhuman primates, Deinhardt and colleagues[55] reported serial transmission of human hepatitis to several species (*Saguinus fuscicollis, S. nigricollis,* and *S. oedipus*) of South American marmoset monkeys. The agent (designated GB) initially passaged in these animals was shown ultimately to be unrelated to HAV.[47,56] Subsequently, pedigreed MS-1 material (passaged in Joliet Prison volunteers) was successfully transmitted to these marmosets.[8] Moreover, other investigators found *S. mystax* marmosets even more susceptible, and this species has become the most frequently studied.[9,10,16,19,40,57-60] The CR326 strain of HAV was evaluated extensively in *S. mystax* marmosets by investigators at the Merck Institute,[9,10] and these studies led eventually to visualization of the virus in marmoset liver and serum, to development of CF and IAHA tests for HAV and anti-HAV, to careful characterization of virus properties, and to an overall acceleration of HAV research. The equal susceptibility of another marmoset, *S. labiatus,* a poorly categorized species also known as *Jacchus rufiventer,* has also been reported.[60] Of the other marmoset species evaluated, none has proved as susceptible or useful for preparation of liver-derived HAV antigen.[60] In susceptible marmosets, the incubation period for HAV is approximately 4 weeks, but, after serial passage, HAV adapts to this nonhuman primate host, as reflected by shortening of the incubation period, enhanced susceptibility, and increased HAV titers within the liver.[59,61]

Outbreaks of hepatitis in handlers of recently imported chimpanzees[62] fostered the suspicion that these nonhuman primates were also susceptible to HAV. Their susceptibility was not demonstrated until serologic tests became available, however. Unlike marmosets, which in their natural habitat and during capture remain free of exposure to HAV, serologic testing revealed that most jungle-caught chimpanzees harbored anti-HAV,[26] suggesting prior exposure and immunity to HAV challenge. Use of such immune animals probably accounted for earlier failures to infect chimpanzees experimentally.[63,64] By contrast, chimpanzees born and raised in protective captivity were found to be seronegative for anti-HAV and, when inoculated, were almost universally susceptible to HAV infection.[26,65,66] The illness in chimpanzees is subclinical and relatively mild but parallels that seen in man morphologically, biochemically, virologically, and serologically. Shedding of HAV in feces, biophysical properties of the virus, and the humoral immune response in chimpanzee infection follow the same pattern as that seen in human infection; however, mononuclear infiltration of portal tracts and liver parenchyma is quantitatively less severe.[67] The chimpanzee is the only nonhuman primate found to be susceptible to both HAV and HBV. Unlike marmosets, which occasionally succumb, chimpanzees experience neither mortality nor morbidity associated with HAV infection, and no chronic illness has been observed in either species. Unfortunately, both marmosets and chimpanzees for HAV research are of limited availability. Therefore, susceptibility to HAV of a large variety of Old and New World monkeys has been tested in several laboratories,[54] but no other nonhuman primate has proven as susceptible or as suitable an experimental model of human HAV as marmosets (*S. mystax* and *S. labiatus*) and chimpanzees.

VIRUS BIOLOGY AND HOST IMMUNE RESPONSE

From studies in marmosets, chimpanzees, and man, we have made great strides in delineating the natural sequence of virologic and serologic events during the course of viral hepatitis type A. Because the pattern is similar in all three groups, a synthesis of the information derived from studies of humans and nonhuman models is presented. Whether inoculation is by the oral or parenteral route, the incubation period is the same, approximately 2 to 4 weeks between inoculation or exposure and biochemical evidence of hepatitis.[41]

Liver

Within 1 to 2 weeks after inoculation or exposure, HAV can be detected in the liver by immunofluorescence[39] or by infectivity of homogenates. Peak levels of intrahepatocytic HAV have been detected approximately 20 to 25 days after inoculation. When monitored serially by immunofluorescence, HAV may appear in the liver as early as a week before fecal shedding, first in a finely granular pattern distributed diffusely throughout liver parenchyma, then increasing in intensity, and finally localizing to focal areas within hepatocytes and Kupffer cells.[39] Persistence of HAV in the liver has been demonstrated by immunofluorescence for as long as 8 weeks, long outlasting fecal excretion of the virus and elevation of serum aminotransferase activity (B.L. Murphy et al., unpublished observation). As noted, localization of HAV is restricted to the cytoplasm,[39] and in studies performed by electron microscopy, particles resembling HAV[16,20] and documented immunologically as such by immunoperoxidase staining[40] appear within cytoplasmic vesicles of hepatocytes and Kupffer cells.

Blood

Viremia has been demonstrated by infectivity as early as 12 days after inoculation,[68] is generally most pronounced during the late incubation period before symptoms or maximal elevations of aminotransferase activity occur, and in general, is brief and low in concentration. Once jaundice develops, or shortly after elevation of serum aminotransferase activity in anicteric persons, viremia probably lasts no more than a few days.[69] Detection of HAV late into convalescence by radioimmunoassay has been reported[28] but does not reflect infectivity as demonstrated in transmission studies and has not been confirmed. Chronic viremia has not been observed.

Feces

Shedding of HAV in stools occurs later than intrahepatic localization of the virus but is one of the earliest virologic events detectable with in vitro techniques in clinically available specimens. Fecal HAV excretion coincides with the onset of nonspecific symptoms, such as malaise, anorexia, and fatigue, and usually reaches a peak before biochemical and morphologic evidence of hepatitis can be detected (Fig. 2). Although the bulk of fecal excretion of HAV precedes peak serum aminotransferase elevation and the onset of jaun-

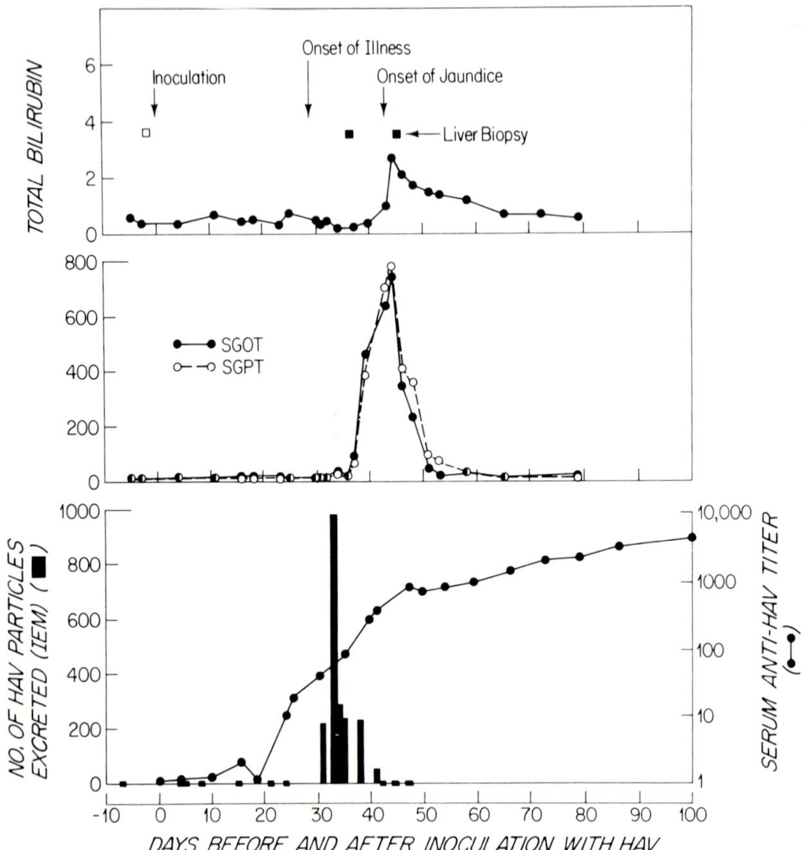

FIG. 2—Pattern of fecal excretion of hepatitis A virus (HAV) and development of antibody to HAV (anti-HAV) in relation to other indicators of acute viral hepatitis in a patient with experimental HAV infection.[12] HAV was detected by immune electron microscopy and quantitated by counting HAV particles in five squares of a 400-mesh electron microscope grid.[70] Fifty percent inhibition titer of anti-HAV was measured by competitive binding radioimmunoassay[52] (Reproduced here with permission of Overby LR, Abbott Laboratories, North Chicago, Illinois.) □ = no hepatic lesions, ■ = hepatic features compatible with acute viral hepatitis.

dice,[15,25,26,43,44,46,66,67,70-72] virus has been detected in infected persons, at lower levels, during the first 2 weeks and as late as 16 days after the onset of dark urine.[22,44,72,132] By the time a patient presents to a physician with hepatitis manifested by jaundice, levels of fecal HAV are usually inadequate for diagnostic purposes. Such predominantly early fecal HAV shedding coincides with early infectivity of feces from HAV patients, as described in human transmission studies performed during the 1940s and 1950s[7,69,73-75] and as deduced by epidemiologic observation.[71] Buoyant densities of HAV particles excreted at different times during illness are not constant.[76] Lower density ''empty'' particles appear earlier, while denser particles appear later. Suggestions have also been made that intensity of viral shedding in feces is proportional to severity of disease.[15,72]

As reiterated later, chronic fecal HAV shedding has not been documented and is unlikely to occur.

Other Body Fluids and Tissues

Hepatitis A virus has been visualized by IEM in *bile* during acute illness in infected chimpanzees,[20,21] but serial studies of HAV excretion in bile throughout illness have not been done. Although HAV has not been visualized in urine, infectivity of urine collected on the first day of jaundice has been demonstrated,[68] and one large hepatitis A outbreak has been attributed on circumstantial grounds to urinary contamination of food.[77] Conceivably, fecally contaminated urine accounted for these instances of transmission, for attempts to transmit type A hepatitis to susceptible chimpanzees with urine from hepatitisA patients have not been successful (J.L. Dienstag, R.H. Purcell, unpublished observations). Heptitis A virus was not detected by immunofluorescence in duodenum, jejunum, ileum, or transverse colon from any of 7 intravenously inoculated *S. mystax* marmosets sacrificed during acute illness.[60] Germinal centers of spleen and of abdominal lymph nodes, however, as well as glomeruli, were HAV-positive in at least some of the animals. Respiratory secretions, semen, and vaginal secretions have not been evaluated for the presence of HAV, but epidemiologic evidence does not favor infection by the respiratory route or through sexual contact.

Virus Replication

From the observations above, preliminary conclusions about HAV replication can be made. Hypothetically, the virus replicates in hepatocytes and is released into the circulation via sinusoids and into the biliary system via bile canaliculi. From the biliary tree, HAV gains access to the intestines and is excreted in feces. Although virus replication in the gut has been postulated,[75] no evidence for intestinal intraepithelial virus has been found in intravenously inoculated animals.[60] Conceivably, gut replication occurs in individuals infected by the oral route, but studies to test this possibility have not been performed. The presence of HAV in lymphoid tissue during acute illness[60] is consistent with the very early humoral immune response to HAV (see later) and probably does not represent extrahepatic virus replication. Similarly, glomerular deposits reflect deposition of HAV–anti-HAV complexes rather than renal replication of virus.[60]

Hepatic Morphologic and Biochemical Changes

Morphologic findings of portal and periportal mononuclear cell infiltration, focal necrosis of hepatocytes, and coagulative necrosis coincide with elevations of serum aminotransferase activities, both of which appear later than intrahepatic localization and fecal excretion of HAV. Such evidence of acute hepatitis first appears approximately 3 to 4 weeks after exposure, usually lasts no longer than 2 to 4 weeks, and in almost all cases resolves without distortion

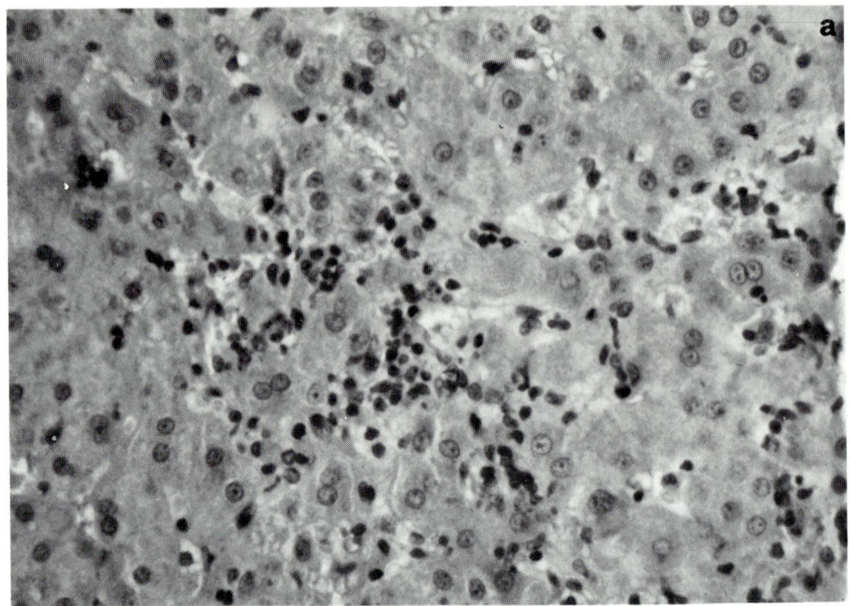

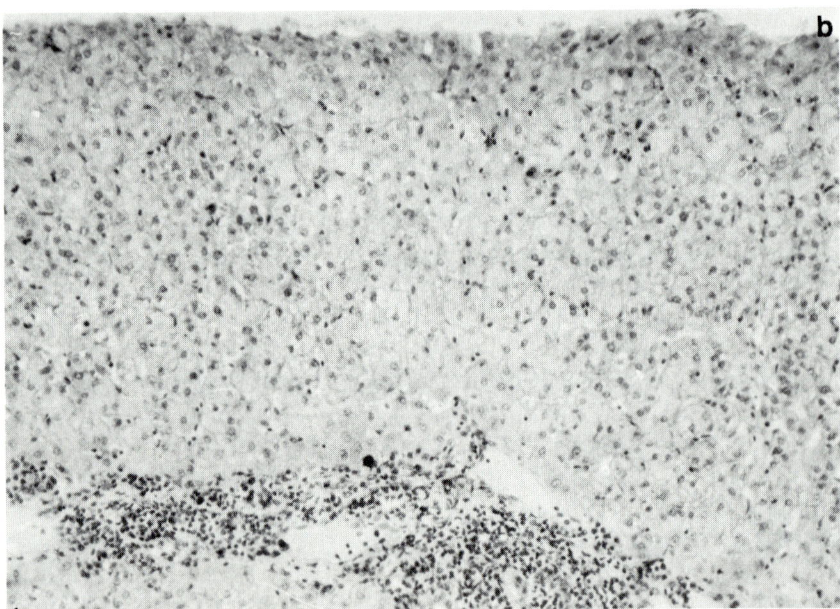

FIG. 3—Percutaneous liver biopsy sections of chimpanzees with hepatitis A virus infection (hematoxylin and eosin). (A) focal necrosis of hepatocytes in the periphery of the lobule with accumulation of lymphocytes and macrophages in the space of Disse and activation of sinusoidal lining cells (× 250). (b) Portal tract enlarged by a mononuclear infiltrate and minor periportal inflammation (× 100). (c) Extensive hepatitis with focal necrosis sparing the centrolobular zones (× 100). (Reproduced with permission from Dienstag JL, Popper H, Purcell RH: The pathology of viral hepatitis types A and B in chimpanzees: A comparison. Am J Pathol 83:131–148, 1976.)

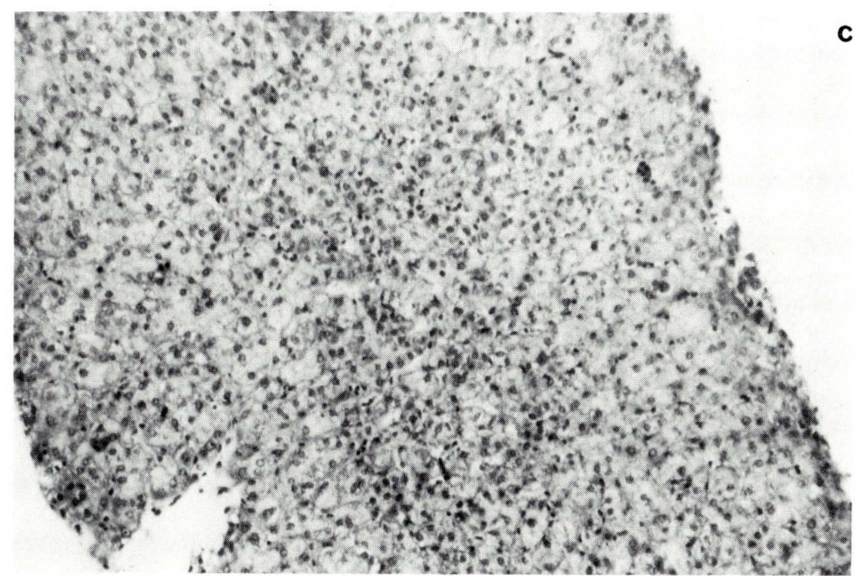

of architecture or evidence of chronic liver disease. Whereas focal necrosis is distributed diffusely, especially in centrizonal areas in marmosets infected with HAV and in chimpanzees infected with HBV, in HAV-infected chimpanzees, focal necrosis of hepatocytes occurs in the periphery of the lobule, sparing the central zone (Fig. 3).[67] In Joliet Prison volunteers also, necrosis of hepatocytes was localized to periportal areas (H. Popper, personal communication).

Humoral Immune Response

Antibody to HAV can be detected during acute illness by any of the assays described above except IAHA. For reasons that remain obscure, there is a delay of from 1 to 4 weeks after acute illness before anti-HAV is detectable by IAHA.[29-31,48,50,51,67,79,80] For the other assays, kinetics of anti-HAV development are more rapid, and detectable levels can often be seen before clinical symptoms (Fig. 2) and during a time when serum has been shown to be infectious.[11,22,26,28,30,31,48,49,51-54,67,72,78,79,81] Serum anti-HAV titers continue to rise during acute and convalescent periods and reach peak levels, sometimes on the order of 1×10^5, approximately 2 to 3 months after acute illness.[48-52,72,78-80] Although titers fall gradually, relatively high levels can be detected many years after infection[51,72] and probably persist indefinitely. As shown by several techniques, antibody appearing during early acute illness is predominantly IgM, while IgG antibody develops more slowly and reaches high levels during convalescence.[78,81] This early IgM rise may account partially or completely for the high IgM levels characteristic of acute type A hepatitis.[82] Individuals and experimental animals with anti-HAV are immune to reinfection with HAV but, if reinoculated, develop a transient boost in antibody titer (anamnestic response) with no evidence for viral replication or hepatitis.[83] In subclinical HAV infection identified by elevations of aminotransferase activity alone, anti-HAV seroconversions are observed regularly.[84] Moreover, immune responses typical of those seen in clinically apparent cases have also been detected in the absence of biochemical abnormalities in individuals previously felt to have escaped infection.[85]

As noted, both HAV and anti-HAV have been detected in the same acute phase serum samples.[28,60,81] In addition, anticomplementary activity,[49,86] depressed serum complement levels,[87] and deposition of HAV in glomeruli[60] have been observed during acute type A hepatitis. Despite such evidence for the appearance of circulating and tissue-depositing immune complexes, clinically apparent immune complex disease, such as that seen during acute and chronic type B hepatitis, is rarely noted during acute type A hepatitis. Skin rashes and arthralgias have been noted, however, in 8% and 10%, respectively, of 130 naval recruits in a large outbreak in San Diego (J.A. Routenberg, et al., unpublished observations).

Cellular Immune Response

Little attention has been devoted to studies of cellular immune mechanisms in viral hepatitis type A. First, assays to detect HAV infection have not been readily available, making selection of patients difficult; and second, the illness is usually brief and often does not come to medical attention. In addition, quantities of purified HAV sufficient for lymphocyte stimulation studies have not been generated. Mitogen responsiveness, cytotoxicity, and lymphokine elaboration of lymphocytes from patients with serologically proven hepatitis A have not been reported. In contrast, both an intrinsic defect in lymphocytes' ability to form rosettes with sheep red blood cells and an extrinsic defect mediated by the presence of a serum rosette inhibitory factor (RIF) in patients with serologically bona fide HAV infection have been found.[88] Moreover, RIF persisted in individuals whose acute type A hepatitis was slow to resolve. Whether cellular immune mechanisms, as postulated in the pathogensis of type B hepatitis, play a role in HAV infection remains to be determined. Conceivably, HAV, unlike HBV, behaves as a cytopathic agent and destroys hepatocytes without any contribution by host immunocytes. Several observations support this possibility. First, most enteroviruses are cytopathogenic, and HAV appears to be enteroviruslike; second, the incubation period of acute HAV infection in experimental animals may be as short as 7 days,[61] a brief period consistent with direct viral hepatocellular injury; third, although fecal excretion of HAV in stools has been observed in anicteric patients,[22,72] most anicteric individuals do not have detectable virus excretion,[15,72] suggesting a correlation between intensity of viral replication and severity of illness. Finally, there is no asymptomatic chronic HAV carrier state and thus no instance in which large quantities of virus appear in hepatocytes in the absence of cell necrosis.

Laboratory diagnosis

Until recently, a diagnosis of type A hepatitis was based on hepatitis B surface antigen (HBsAg) seronegativity and, perhaps, correlative epidemiologic information. More often than not, however, a diagnosis based on these criteria is incorrect. The only way to be certain of a diagnosis of type A hepatitis is to demonstrate virologic or serologic evidence of HAV infection. Because viremia is limited, its demonstration is difficult and impractical for diagnostic purposes. Although the virus is more readily found in feces, bile, and liver, none of these is a source for routine diagnostic specimens. Fecal shedding of HAV usually reaches its peak and declines in titer by the time a patient presents to a physician, bile is not a routinely accessible body fluid, and liver biopsies are rarely performed during acute viral hepatitis. Consequently, a diagnosis can be made most practically by demonstrating a specific antibody response.

If a rise in serum anti-HAV titer can be demonstrated between acute illness and convalescence, a diagnosis of acute HAV infection can be made. For IEM, CF, RIA, or ELISA, a very early acute phase serum sample should be compared to a sample drawn 1 to 2 months after acute illness. Detection of anti-HAV by IAHA is usually delayed, as previously noted, and during acute illness, a patient's serum may be anti-HAV-positive by one of the other techniques but negative by IAHA. Thus, when a late convalescent serum is unavailable, a combination of IAHA negativity with anti-HAV positivity by one of the other techniques may be presumptive evidence for a diagnosis of HAV infection.[79,89] If specificity of early anti-HAV positivity with IEM, RIA, or ELISA is demonstrable, this method for early diagnosis of type A hepatitis is quite reliable. Another approach to early diagnosis with a single serum sample involves demonstration of specific anti-HAV of the IgM class, which reaches a peak during early acute illness and ebbs gradually as acute illness subsides. Two to three months after acute illness, the contribution of IgM to anti-HAV is negligible, and IgM anti-HAV is rarely detected beyond 4 months. Therefore, distinction between IgM and IgG anti-HAV found in an acute phase serum discriminates acute phase from convalescent anti-HAV and can be used to make a diagnosis acutely. The presence of IgM anti-HAV can be determined morphologically by immune electron microscopy;[14,78] by testing 19 S (IgM) fractions for anti-HAV after sucrose gradient ultracentrifugation of serum[78] (B. Flehmig et al., personal communication); by absorption with goat antihuman IgM (heavy chain [μ] specific);[81] by failure of absorption with staphylococcal protein A, which binds avidly to IgG but not to IgM;[90] or by substituting radiolabeled anti-IgM for the second antibody in the "sandwich" solid phase radioimmunoassay for anti-HAV (Overby, personal communication). A commercial competitive binding radioimmunoassay, with HAV antigen purified from human stools, will be available (Abbott Laboratories, North Chicago, Illinois), and one of these simple modifications will make diagnosis during acute illness practical.

EPIDEMIOLOGY

Even before serologic tests were developed, studies in volunteers and natural outbreaks provided a wealth of epidemiologic information about HAV. Type A hepatitis has been recognized for many years as a disease transmitted primarily by the fecal-oral route, often in the context of large common-source outbreaks.[17,91] In temperate climates, epidemic waves of type A hepatitis tend to recur every 5 to 20 years, and there is seasonal variation in frequency of infection which peaks in late fall and early winter. These trends are no longer detectable in the United States, however, apparently because improved sanitation has led to an overall decrease in the incidence of HAV infections. Vehicles of exposure that have been implicated in the transmission of HAV include contaminated food, water, milk, shellfish, and subclinically infected nonhuman primates.[17,91] Outbreaks of type A hepatitis have been observed commonly among individuals housed together in institutions and within family units. Since the discovery of HAV and serologic tests to identify anti-HAV, seroepidemiologic studies have been done that have defined the extent of exposure to HAV and provided insight into its modes of spread.

Distribution of Exposure to HAV

Several difficulties confound estimates of the extent of exposure to HAV made without the benefit of serologic testing. First, testing for HBsAg revealed that many cases once considered type A ("infectious") hepatitis on clinical and epidemiologic grounds are actually caused by HBV. This error casts suspicion on surveillance records that differentiate without adequate substantiation between type A and type B hepatitis. Second, even when HBsAg testing is performed and is nonreactive, type A hepatitis is only one of several etiologic possibilities, including non-A, non-B hepatitis, and type B hepatitis with levels of HBsAg too low for detection. Third, underreporting of hepatitis cases invalidates statistical estimates, and fourth, the fact that much of HAV infection is inapparent makes accurate reporting impossible. Reliable estimates of HAV exposure based on serologic surveys are practical, however, and the distribution of exposure has been reported from diverse geographic locales (Table 1).[92-104] Regardless of geographic region, exposure to HAV, as determined by serologic testing, is considerably greater than expected on the basis of historical recollection of clinical hepatitis among the individuals tested. In one report no more than 3% to 5% of all persons studied, despite their considerable anti-HAV prevalences, recalled having experienced an episode of hepatitis.[98] This finding supports the belief that most infections with HAV are clinically inapparent.

Exposure to HAV increases with increasing age and with decreasing socioeconomic level in almost all populations studied. Figure 4 demonstrates prevalences of anti-HAV as a function of age in three sets of contrasting populations. In metropolitan New York residents, socioeconomic factors appear to determine the age at which primary infection occurs. The age-standardized prevalence of anti-HAV is 60% in persons of lower socioeconomic level, and 50% exposure in the population occurs by the third decade. In contrast, the prevalence in New York middle-class individuals is significantly lower, 41% ($p<0.01$), and 50% exposure does not occur until the fifth decade.[98] The pattern of anti-HAV acquisition observed in New York City contrasts with the pattern of exposure to poliomyelitis virus observed in the preimmunization era. Exposure to polio, another enterically spread agent, occurred very early in life and was virtually universal after adolescence.[105-107] The pattern of anti-HAV

TABLE 1.—*Prevalence of Antibody to HAV in Various Populations*

State/Country (Reference)	No. Tested	Anti-HAV Positive	State/Country (Reference)	No. Tested	Anti-HAV Positive
Pennsylvania[92]	197*	12%	France[97]	600	75%
Sweden[93]	591	13%	Senegal[95]	102	75%
Norway[94]	175	17%	Sri Lanka[103]	645	76%
Switzerland[95]	98	24%	Fanafuti[104]‡	574	80%
Tennessee[96]	245	37%	Mediterranean[94]**	70	81%
Switzerland[97]	700	39%	Upou[104]‡	49	82%
New York[98]	629	41%	Greece[97]	647	82%
Texas[99]	538	44%	Tahiti[101]‡	179	84%
Japan†	400	50%	Fiji[104]‡	293	84%
Australia[100]	1053	51%	Belgium[95]	133	87%
Ponape[101]‡	184	52%	Taiwan[95]	93	88%
Holland[97]	505	52%	Kenya††	138	88%
Germany[94]	661	55%	Bougainville[101]‡	164	88%
Poland§	128	60%	Israel[95]	112	94%
Australia[102]¶	959	62%	Rarotonga[104]‡	60	95%
Costa Rica[92]	300	72%	Nieu[104]‡	50	95%
			Yugoslavia[95]	100	97%

*High socioeconomic group.
†Y. Moritsugu, unpublished data.
‡South Pacific island.
§R. H. Purcell and A. Nowoslawski, unpublished data.
¶Serum collected 1954–1955.
**Assorted Mediterranean countries.
††D. P. Hansen, S. M. Feinstone, and R. H. Purcell, unpublished data.

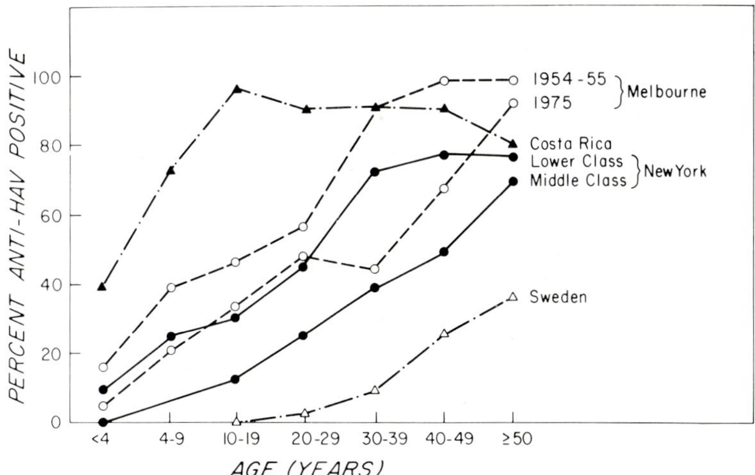

FIG. 4—Prevalence of exposure to hepatitis A virus (HAV) expressed as the percentage positive for antibody to HAV (anti-HAV) as a function of age. Note the contrasts between (A) lower- and middle-class populations in New York City;[98] (B) a developing country, Costa Rica,[92] and an advanced, modern urban society, Sweden;[93] and (C) populations in Melbourne sampled 20 years apart.[108]

acquisition in underdeveloped countries, however, is identical to the pattern of exposure to poliomyelitis before immunization was introduced. The differences in anti-HAV prevalences among countries of greatly different developmental status exaggerate the differences seen between lower- and middle-class New Yorkers. Exposure to HAV in underdeveloped countries where sanitary and hygienic conditions are relatively primitive is very high and is acquired in early childhood,[92,101-104] whereas exposure is low in highly urbanized, modern societies with excellent sanitation facilities in the population at large and almost absent in the younger generation born after the introduction of modern improvements in hygiene. Such a distinction is seen in the comparison between Sweden[93] and Costa Rica[92] shown in Fig. 4.

Figure 4 also depicts anti-HAV prevalences determined in age-stratified populations collected 20 years apart in Melbourne, Australia.[108] The lower prevalence of exposure in 1975 indicates that the disease is less common than it was in the mid-1950s. The prevalence of exposure in individuals older than 30 in 1975 is almost identical to that noted among individuals 20 years younger in 1954–1955, suggesting that few of the anti-HAV-positive individuals acquired infection after the second decade of life.

These observations indicate that for those whose living conditions or developmental status provide adequate hygiene, susceptibility to HAV appears to extend into early adulthood, consistent with the observation that children are more likely to be affected in common-source outbreaks among the poor and that adults are more likely to be affected in more well-to-do neighborhoods.[109-111] Moreover, the gradual increase in anti-HAV with age appears to be explained by a cohort effect; that is, the high anti-HAV prevalence of older individuals resulted from more universal exposure when these adults were children, before improvements in hygienic conditions had occurred, a change reflected in the brief period of 20 years in Melbourne.

From seroepidemiologic surveys of European countries, South Pacific islands, and Greenland comes additional information that supports the role of a cohort effect in age-related increases in anti-HAV. In non-Mediterranean European countries, HAV exposure was almost universal in individuals over the age of 40 but negligible in persons under 20 years of age, data consistent with a dramatic decline in the incidence of HAV infection during the last 20 to 40 years.[97] Evaluations of most South Pacific islands[101,104] reveal a very high prevalence of exposure and very early acquisition of infection (under 20 years of age), as described above for Costa Rica. In one of these islands, Ponape, however, exposure to HAV was limited to individuals above the age of 20, almost all of whom harbored anti-HAV.[101] It appears that HAV disappeared from the island after a period of peak activity 20 years before the serum samples tested were collected. The cohort of individuals exposed then remains anti-HAV-positive, while the younger generation, spared by the elimination of HAV infection from the island, remains susceptible. More than likely, a similar cohort effect is operative in urban populations and accounts for the high anti-HAV prevalence in older adults. As opposed to insular populations, however, in urban societies a low level of exposure persists in the young. Similar patterns of HAV inactivity have been reported in other isolated populations.[112,113] In these situations, large outbreaks of type A hepatitis were separated from earlier outbreaks by approximately 15 to 20 years, suggesting widespread immunity in adults as a result of the earlier outbreak. Serologic testing has confirmed this dichotomy between young and aged cohorts in Greenland. Anti-HAV was found in 93% of 41 persons born before the first epidemic in 1947–1948 but in only 3% of 29 persons born since then.[114] Thus, unlike type B hepatitis, which tends to remain *endemic* in populations, type A hepatitis endemicity appears to be limited to underdeveloped countries or to population groups with poor hygienic standards. In insular communities and modern societies with uniformly adequate hygiene, type A hepatitis tends to occur in *epidemics*.

Additional support for a cohort effect comes from the observed reduction in the number of children presenting with acute viral hepatitis to municipal hospitals over the last several decades (S. Krugman, personal communication) and the parallel decline in the number of reported and documented cases of type A hepatitis in children.[108,115] Moreover, in highly exposed populations, such as Senegal (Dakar)[95] and Upou (a Samoan island)[104] prevalence of anti-HAV actually declines after the age of 20, suggesting that exposure had occurred early in life and that anti-HAV may not remain detectable indefinitely in those infected at a very early age but not reexposed subsequently. Finally, if a cohort effect is operative, titers of anti-HAV in pooled gamma globulin should reflect this change. A preliminary evaluation did not show the appropriate trend.[116] However, titers of anti-HAV in globulin lots from the last 25 to 30 years prepared in Massachusetts, as measured by RIA in recently prepared lots, are approximately one-quarter to one-third lower than titers of globulin lots prepared more than 10 years ago (G. Grady, personal communication). This effect of cohort differences may explain why metropolitan areas of Belgium[95] and France,[97] which enjoy a high standard of living today, have such high prevalences of anti-HAV (Table 1).

Seroepidemiologic studies have shown that exposure to HAV is independent of sex and race. In New York City, exposure to HAV increased as a function of exposure to HBV[98] but in other places was independent of HBV exposure.[95,101,103,104] Why exposure to these viruses is parallel in some areas but not in others may be explained by individual, as yet undefined differences among geographic locales. In addition, because the two viruses share some modes of transmission but not others, international differences in parallelism between exposure to HAV and HBV conceivably may be related to local factors that promote common modes of exposure or that favor a mode of spread unique to one of the two viruses.

Modes of Transmission of HAV

The earliest seroepidemiologic studies confirmed the role of HAV in common-source outbreaks resulting from the classical modes of exposure listed above.[11,13,15,22,25,44,72,80,89,117,119] Subsequently, exposure to HAV was evaluated in populations representing enhanced enteric and nonpercutaneous interpersonal spread and in populations with enhanced parenteral and nonpercutaneous exposure to blood products.

In institutions for the mentally retarded, poor hygienic habits, especially unrestrained handling of secretions and excreta, predispose to transmission of infectious diseases spread by the fecal-oral route or by intimate contact. It is not surprising, then, that in this setting, exposure to hepatitis viruses is very high. At the Suffolk Developmental Center in New York, a high prevalence of exposure to both HAV (75%) and HBV (68%) was found.[120] Anti-HAV prevalences were similarly high for residents with Down's syndrome and with other forms of mental retardation, and prevalence correlated with length of institutionalization. These findings suggest that HAV is endemic at this institution, and a similarly high risk has been observed in institutions in Pennsylvania[92] and Melbourne[121] and at the Willowbrook State School.[122] At Willowbrook, *newly admitted* residents and staff had anti-HAV prevalences of 32% and 50%, respectively, not appreciably different from the frequency of exposure of a normal American urban population. In contrast, residents and staff who had been at the institution longer than 3 years had much higher prevalences of 95% and 75%, respectively.

Yet, although these institutions appear to harbor HAV endemically, other institutions for the mentally retarded differ. Only 42% and 23% of residents, respectively, of the Lynchburg Training School in Virginia[123] and the Western Carolina Center in North Carolina (W. T. Hall, personal communication) had detectable serum anti-HAV. In addition, none of 20 children under the age of 8 at two state schools in Pennsylvania were anti-HAV-positive.[92] High susceptibility among residents in some of the institutions with relatively low anti-HAV frequencies provides a ripe arena for large outbreaks, as have occurred at Lynchburg[124] and at the Wassaic State School in New York.[120] Thus in institutions for the mentally retarded, exposure to HAV, apparently fostered by improper handling of excreta, can be either endemic or epidemic.

Unlike institutionalization, which predisposes both to HAV and HBV infection, neither sexual promiscuity nor multiple exposure to blood products, which enhance HBV risk, play a role in transmitting type A hepatitis. Exposure to HBV is greater than fourfold higher in male homosexuals, who have frequent, intimate contact with many different sexual partners, than in the general population. Such sexual intimacy, which includes anal intercourse, does not enhance the spread of HAV, however. The 39% prevalence of anti-HAV in homosexuals in New York City was no greater than that in a comparable middle-class population.[98] Prospective serologic testing of patients receiving many units of blood for surgery failed to incriminate HAV in posttransfusion hepatitis.[125-128] Similarly, individuals exposed to blood products chronically and continually do not appear to be at enhanced risk of HAV exposure. Both patients and staff in hemodialysis units experience an inordinately high frequency of HBV exposure. The same is true for multiply transfused thalassemics and hemophiliacs and, to a lesser degree, for health care professionals. Exposure of these groups to HAV, however, is no greater than that seen in the general population and does not correlate with duration of exposure to blood.[129-133] Thus, although HAV can be transmitted by percutaneous injection, as demonstrated in experimental inoculation of volunteers[4,12,41] and experimental animals,[8-10,16,26,56,58-61,66,119] serologic studies fail to demonstrate a role in nature for percutaneous routes or high exposure to blood in the transmission of HAV.

Natural Perpetuation of HAV

Perpetuation of HBV in nature is facilitated by the existence of chronic carriers who serve as reservoirs of infection. The only evidence for the existence of a carrier state for HAV comes from a volunteer study conducted in the 1950s.[134] Fecal material obtained 14 months after the onset of illness from an infant with protracted hepatitis was inoculated into 4 prisoner volunteers, 1 of whom developed hepatitis 26 days later. Unfortunately, no material from this experiment has been saved for subsequent virologic validation of the observation. The suggestion that an outbreak of short-incubation postinoculation hepatitis was evidence for a chronic viremic HAV carrier state[135] cannot be upheld in light of recent serologic studies.[125-128] On the contrary, evidence is increasing that chronic intestinal or viremic carriage of HAV does not occur. Results of careful studies, such as those done at Willowbrook,[7] were compatible with a very brief viremia and fecal excretion of HAV, and more recent virologic studies during natural HAV outbreaks have failed to demonstrate prolonged fecal HAV shedding.[136]

Data cited to support the operation of a cohort effect to account for high anti-HAV prevalences in older populations also argue against the existence of chronic HAV carriers. Exposure to HAV in underdeveloped countries, follows a pattern of early acquisition characteristic for enteroviruses (in which, as a genus, chronic infection is not at all characteristic). In insular communities (Greenland, the Yukon, Ponape in the South Pacific), HAV can disappear entirely following a period of major virus activity,[101,104,112-114] making the argument that there is a chronic carrier state very tenuous. HAV rarely accounts for endemic infections in Greenland. Instead, it occurs in large outbreaks, is then entirely eliminated, and does not recur until many years later when a new susceptible generation has emerged and infection is reintroduced from outside the community.[113,114]

If there is no chronic carrier state for HAV, how does this virus maintain itself in nature between large outbreaks? One possibility suggested[104] is that there is an extrahuman reservoir, such as shellfish, which, although not infected, concentrates the hardy virus from large volumes of water. The perpetuation of infection in isolated populations may depend on chance reintroduction of the virus by visitors after a new susceptible generation emerges.[101,104] Nonepidemic, inapparent cases in urban centers, which heavily outweigh the number of apparent, reported cases, may serve as a reservoir of infection. This assumption is supported by the finding that 20% to 40% of sporadic hepatitis in urban adults is attributable to HAV.[22,137]

SELECTED CLINICAL FEATURES

Common clinical features of viral hepatitis type A are well known. Typically, the first signs and symptoms of illness are nonspecific and include fever (abrupt onset), epigastric and right upper quadrant pain, malaise, myalgias, arthralgias, fatigue, anorexia, nausea, vomiting, diarrhea, headache, and a blunting of olfactory-gustatory sense, followed shortly by darkening of urine, lightening of stool color, jaundice, and pruritus. Changes in hepatic enzyme activity in serum and in hepatic structure were described before. Although rashes have been reported during serologically bona fide HAV infection, the serum-sickness-like syndrome seen commonly during the prodrome of type B hepatitis is not observed during acute type A hepatitis. Considerable variability occurs in clinical expression of HAV infection; reports of the ratio of anicteric to icteric cases vary from 12:1 to 1:3.5.[15,138] Both the incidence of anicteric disease and the mildness of illness are more common in young children.

Prospective studies to evaluate the contribution of HAV to chronic liver disease have not been done, and suggestions that chronic liver disease may be caused by HAV have not been documented serologically. Inferences about the ability of HAV to cause chronic liver disease, however, may be derived from observations made during several studies of serologically documented type A hepatitis. Among children infected with the MS-1 strain of HAV at the Willowbrook State School, all clinical and biochemical indices of hepatitis returned to normal within 2 to 3 weeks of onset of acute illness.[7] Of 32 college-age young adults involved in the hepatitis outbreak at Holy Cross College, Worcester, Massachusettes,[139] 20% had minimal elevations of serum aminotransferase activity persisting for 143 days after exposure.[140] In an outbreak among adolescent and young adult naval recruits in October 1974,[15] 50% had normal serum aminotransferase activity after 3½ weeks of illness, but 11 (of 130) had abnormal enzyme activity persisting for more than 14 weeks and had morphologic lesions consistent with chronic hepatitis.[136] Subsequent evaluation of these patients, however, demonstrated resolution of clinical and biochemical abnormalities by the 24th week of illness. (J.A. Routenberg, J.L. Dienstag, unpublished data).

In patients with chronic active hepatitis, the prevalence of anti-HAV is no greater than in normal controls, nor is there a difference in anti-HAV prevalence between HBsAg-positive and negative cases.[132,141,142] In addition, fecal HAV shedding has not been observed in patients with chronic active hepatitis,[141] nor has intrahepatic HAV been observed by immunofluorescence in liver biopsies from these patients. No reports of serologically documented HAV infection accompanied by the development of ascites, hypoalbuminemia, chronic liver disease, or submassive hepatic necrosis have been published. Although HAV appears to be a relatively acute self-limited illness without sequelae, a few serologically documented cases of fulminant hepatitis A infection with encephalopathy have been reported.[137,141,143] The case fatality rate for HAV is very low, although high fatality rates have been reported among pregnant women.[144] No increase in severity of hepatitis in patients infected simultaneously with HAV and HBV has been seen.[145] Finally, serologic studies do not support a role for HAV in neonatal hepatitis and biliary atresia[146] or in Down's syndrome.[147]

PROPHYLAXIS

The seroepidemiologic surveys cited show that in many urbanized societies, susceptibility to HAV persists in adolescents. If infection is reintroduced through a common vehicle, this younger population is in danger of infection in epidemic proportions. For this reason, the prophylactic approach of choice is active immunization with a viral vaccine. Preparation of such a vaccine, however, must await the cultivation of HAV in tissue culture. In the absence of this alternative, prophylaxis against HAV infection depends on maintenance of high standards of environmental and personal hygiene and on timely administration of immune serum globulin (ISG). Long before serologic tests to identify HAV and anti-HAV were devised, the efficacy of intramuscular injection of ISG in preventing or ameliorating HAV infection and in conferring passive-active long-lasting immunity were shown.[4,75,138,148-150] Availability of serologic tests for anti-HAV has provided a means for determining susceptibility of exposed persons, measuring the titer of anti-HAV in ISG, and detecting serologic responses in individuals who develop no clinical or biochemical evidence of infection. A survey of 24 commercial globulin lots[50] revealed variability in anti-HAV titer (measured by IAHA) from 1:1,000 to 1:16,000. In 57 commercial globulin lots tested by RIA, 50% inhibition end-point titers, ranging from 1:200 to 1:3500, were found.[151] As expected from seroepidemiologic studies, globulin lots prepared from commercial donors (generally derived from lower socioeconomic persons) have higher anti-HAV titers than lots prepared from outdated blood obtained from volunteer blood donors (M.R. Hilleman, personal communication). We can also anticipate that older persons, whose prevalence of anti-HAV is high, would make better donors for pooled anti-HAV globulin than younger donors, with low anti-HAV prevalences, and that preselection of high anti-HAV donors would make feasible preparation of a high titer anti-HAV globulin ("HAIG").

Serologic reevaluations of earlier ISG administration studies provided the following observations:[85,152] (1) The ISG used by Krugman at Willowbrook had an anti-HAV titer of 1:3,200 and was mixed with HAV (MS-1 strain) prior to administration; the ISG evaluated by Hall had an anti-HAV titer of 1:10,000 and was administered to residents at an institution for the mentally retarded during an institutional outbreak. ISG was given in most cases prior to virus exposure. ISG was shown effective in preventing illness in both these studies. (2) Individuals with preexisting serum anti-HAV were immune to HAV infection during these studies. (3) All persons immunized prior to virus exposure in Hall's study, were protected from both *illness* and *infection*. In the study by Krugman, however, two immunized persons who had escaped illness— assessed clinically and biochemically—developed serologic evidence of infection. These studies provide serologic confirmation that ISG given early (prior to or simultaneously with virus exposure) prevents or ameliorates disease.

Public health recommendations for ISG administration to prevent type A hepatitis[153] may be subject to change if and when anti-HAV standardization of ISG is introduced. Presently, prophylaxis is recommended for travelers to endemic areas and for household contacts but not for casual contacts at work or school. Because of long delays between initial exposure and ultimate recognition of foodborne outbreaks, administration of ISG to exposed individuals rarely can be accomplished in time to provide protection. Therefore, widespread ISG prophylaxis in such situations is no longer recommended.[154]

NON-A, NON-B HEPATITIS

One of the most important derivatives of hepatitis A research has been its impact on direction of attention to non-A, non-B hepatitis agents. Originally defined in cases of non-B transfusion-associated hepatitis,[125-128] non-A, non-B agents appear to account for a sizable proportion of hepatitis in a variety of epidemiologic settings.[155] Although neither a virus particle nor an antigen has been detected, non-A, non-B hepatitis has recently been transmitted successfully in chimpanzees.[156-158]

ACKNOWLEDGMENTS

The author is grateful to Drs. Robert H. Purcell, Hans Popper, Wolf Szmuness, and John Gerin for their guidance in the author's studies referred to in this chapter; to Drs. Lacy R. Overby, Gert G. Frösner, and Ian D. Gust for providing preprints of unpublished manuscripts; and to Mrs. Hilda Gardner for preparation of the manuscript.

REFERENCES

1. Deinhardt F, Holmes AW: Epidemiology and etiology of viral hepatitis. Edited by H Popper and F Schaffner: Progress in Liver Diseases. Vol. II. New York, Grune & Stratton, 1965, pp 373–394

2. Mosley JW: Viral hepatitis: Recent studies of etiology. Edited by H Popper and F Schaffner: Progress in Liver Diseases. Vol. III. New York, Grune & Stratton, 1970, pp 252–268

3. Melnick JL, Hollinger FB: Hepatitis virology. Edited by H Popper and F Schaffner: Progress in Liver Diseases. Vol. IV. New York, Grune & Stratton, 1972, pp 345–365

4. Havens WP Jr, Paul JR: Infectious hepatitis and serum hepatitis. Edited by I Tamm and FL Horsfall: Viral and Rickettsial Infections of Man (ed 4). Philadelphia, JB Lippincott, 1965, pp 965–993

5. Purcell RH, Feinstone SM, Kapikian AZ: Recent advances in hepatitis A research. Edited by TJ Greenwalt and GA Jamieson: Transmissible Disease and Blood Transfusion. New York, Grune & Stratton, 1975, pp 11–26

6. Deinhardt F: Hepatitis in primates. Adv Virus Res 20:113–157, 1976

7. Krugman S, Ward R, Giles JP: The natural history of infectious hepatitis. Am J Med 32:717–728, 1962

8. Holmes AW, Wolfe L, Rosenblate H, Deinhardt F: Hepatitis in marmosets: Induction of disease with coded specimens from a human volunteer study. Science 165:816–817, 1969

9. Mascoli CC, Ittensohn OL, Villarejos VM, Arguedas JA, Provost PJ, Hilleman MR: Recovery of hepatitis agents in the marmoset from human cases occurring in Costa Rica. Proc Soc Exp Biol Med 142:276–282, 1973

10. Provost PJ, Ittensohn OL, Villarejos VM, Arguedas JA, Hilleman MR: Etiologic relationship of marmoset-propagated CR326 hepatitis A virus to hepatitis in man. Proc Soc Exp Biol Med 142:1257–1267, 1973

11. Feinstone SM, Kapikian AZ, Purcell RH: Hepatitis A: Detection by immune electron microscopy of a virus-like antigen associated with acute illness. Science 182:1026–1028, 1973

12. Boggs JD, Melnick JL, Conrad ME, Felsher BF: Viral hepatitis: Clinical and tissue culture studies. JAMA 214:1041–1046, 1970

13. Gravelle CR, Hornbeck CL, Maynard JE, Schable CA, Cook EH, Bradley DW: Hepatitis A: Report of a common-source outbreak with recovery of a possible etiologic agent. II. Laboratory studies. J Infect Dis 131:167–171, 1975

14. Locarnini SA, Ferris AA, Stott AC, Gust ID: The relationship between a 27-nm virus-like particle and hepatitis A as demonstrated by immune electron microscopy. Intervirology 4:110–118, 1974

15. Dienstag JL, Routenberg JA, Purcell RH,

Hooper RR, Harrison WO: Foodhandler-associated outbreak of hepatitis A: An immune electron microscopic study. Ann Intern Med 83:647–650, 1975

16. Provost PJ, Wolanski BS, Miller WJ, Ittensohn OL, McAleer WJ, Hilleman MR: Physical, chemical and morphologic dimensions of human hepatitis A virus strain CR326. Proc Soc Exp Biol Med 148: 532–539, 1975

17. Report of the WHO Expert Committee on Viral Hepatitis. Advances in viral hepatitis. World Health Organization Technical Report Series 602. Geneva, World Health Organization, 1977, pp 1–62

18. Cook EH, Bradley DW, Gravelle CR, Maynard JE: Ultrastructural studies of hepatitis A virus by electron microscopy. J Virol 20:687–689, 1976

19. Dienstag JL, Schulman AN, Gerety RJ, Hoofnagle JH, Lorenz DE, Purcell RH, Barker LF: Hepatitis A antigen isolated from liver and stool: Immunologic comparison of antisera prepared in guinea pigs. J Immunol 117:876–881, 1976

20. Schulman AN, Dienstag JL, Jackson DR, Hoofnagle JH, Gerety RJ, Purcell RH, Barker LF: Hepatitis A antigen particles in liver, bile, and stool of chimpanzees. J Infect Dis 134:80–84, 1976

21. Bradley DW, Hollinger FB, Hornbeck CL, Maynard JE: Isolation and characterization of hepatitis A virus. Am J Clin Pathol 65:876–889, 1976

22. Locarnini SA, Gust ID, Ferris AA, Stott AC, Wong ML: A prospective study of acute viral hepatitis with particular reference to hepatitis A. Bull WHO 54:199–206, 1976

23. Locarnini SA, Coulepis AG, Ferris AA, Lehmann NI, Gust ID: Purification of hepatitis A virus from human feces. Intervirology 10:300–308, 1978

24. Feinstone SM, Kapikian AZ, Gerin JL, Purcell RH: Buoyant density of the hepatitis A virus-like particle in cesium chloride. J Virol 13:1412–1414, 1974

25. Purcell RH, Dienstag JL, Feinstone SM, Kapikian AZ: Relationship of hepatitis A antigen to viral hepatitis. Am J Med Sci 270:61–71, 1975

26. Dienstag JL, Feinstone SM, Purcell RH, Hoofnagle JH, Barker LF, London WT, Popper H, Peterson JM, Kapikian AZ: Experimental infection of chimpanzees with hepatitis A virus. J Infect Dis 132:532–545, 1975

27. Bradley DW, Hornbeck CL, Gravelle CR, Cook EH, Maynard JE: News from the Center for Disease Control: CsCl banding of hepatitis A associated virus-like particles. J Infect Dis 131:304–306, 1975

28. Hollinger FB, Bradley DW, Maynard JE, Dreesman GR, Melnick JL: Detection of hepatitis A viral antigen by radioimmunoassay. J Immunol 115:1464–1466, 1975

29. Moritsugu Y, Dienstag JL, Valdesuso J, Wong DC, Wagner J, Routenberg JA, Purcell RH: Purification of hepatitis A antigen from feces and detection of antigen and antibody by immune adherence hemagglutination. Infect Immun 13:898–908, 1976

30. Purcell RH, Wong DC, Moritsugu Y, Dienstag JL, Routenberg JA, Boggs JD: A microtiter solid-phase radioimmunoassay for hepatitis A antigen and antibody. J Immunol 116:349–356, 1976

31. Hollinger FB, Bradley DW, Dreesman GR, Melnick JL: Detection of viral hepatitis type A. Am J Clin Pathol 65:854–865, 1976

32. Bradley DW, McCaustland KA, Schreeder MT, Cook EH, Gravelle CR, Maynard JE: Multiple buoyant densities of hepatitis A virus in cesium chloride gradients. J Med Virol 1:219–226, 1977

33. Bradley DW, Hornbeck CL, Cook EH, Maynard JE: Purification of hepatitis A virus from chimpanzee stools. J Virol 22: 228–231, 1977

34. Coulepis AG, Locarnini SA, Ferris AA, Lehmann NI, Gust ID: The polypeptides of hepatitis A virus. Intervirology 10:24–31, 1978

35. Siegl G, Frösner GG: Characterization and classification of virus particles associated with hepatitis A. I. Size, density, and sedimentation. J Virol 26:40–47, 1978

36. Rakela J, Fay OH, Stevenson D, Gordon I, Mosley JW: Similarities of two hepatitis A virus strains. Bull WHO 54:561–564, 1976

37. Rowlands DJ, Shirley MW, Sangar DV, Brown F: A high density component in several vertebrate enteroviruses. J Gen Virol 29:223–234, 1975

38. Siegl G, Frösner GG: Characterization and classification of virus particles associated with hepatitis A. II. Type and configuration of nucleic acid. J Virol 26:48–53, 1978

39. Mathiesen LR, Feinstone SM, Purcell RH, Wagner J: Detection of hepatitis A antigen by immunofluorescence. Infect Immun 18:524–530, 1977

40. Shimizu YK, Mathiesen LR, Lorenz D,

Drucker J, Feinstone SM, Wagner J, Purcell RH: Localization of hepatitis A antigen in liver tissue by peroxidase-conjugated antibody method. Light and electron microscopic studies. J Immunol 121:1671–1679, 1978

41. Krugman S, Giles JP, Hammond J: Infectious hepatitis: Evidence for two distinctive clinical, epidemiological, and immunological types of infection. JAMA 200:365–373, 1967

42. Crovari P, Cuneo-Crovari P, Mistretta AP, Tolentino P: Virus-like antigen associated with hepatitis A: Investigations in children's acute hepatitis. Bull 1st Sieroter Milanese 55:363–370, 1976

43. Coursaget P, Maupas P, Hibon P, Goudeau A, Sizaret P-Y, Despert F: Identification du virus de l'hépatite A dans les selles: Intérêt diagnostique et épidémiologique. Nouv Presse Méd 6:4109–4113, 1977

44. Hall WT, Bradley DW, Madden DL, Zimmerman DH, Brandt DEL: Comparison of sensitivity of radioimmunoassay and immune electron microscopy for detecting hepatitis A antigen in fecal extracts. Proc Soc Exp Biol Med 155:193–198, 1977

45. Skidmore SJ, Boxall EH: Small virus particles in faeces of patients with infectious hepatitis (hepatitis A). J Med Microbiol 10:43–48, 1977

46. Flehmig B, Frank H, Frösner GG, Gerth H-J: Hepatitis A-virus particles in stools of patients from a natural hepatitis outbreak in Germany. Med Microbiol Immunol 163:209–214, 1977

47. Holmes AW, Deinhardt F, Wolfe L, Froesner G, Peterson D, Casto B: Specific neutralization of human hepatitis type A in marmoset monkeys. Nature (London) 243:419–420, 1973

48. Dienstag JL, Alling DW, Purcell RH: Quantitation of antibody to hepatitis A antigen by immune electron microscopy. Infect Immun 13:1209–1213, 1976

49. Provost PJ, Ittensohn OL, Villarejos VM, Hilleman MR: A specific complement-fixation test for human hepatitis A employing CR326 virus antigen: Diagnosis and epidemiology. Proc Soc Exp Biol Med 148:962–969, 1975

50. Miller WJ, Provost PJ, McAleer WJ, Ittensohn OL, Villarejos VM, Hilleman MR: Specific immune adherence assay for human hepatitis A antibody. Application to diagnostic and epidemiologic investigation. Proc Soc Exp Biol Med 149:254–261, 1975

51. Krugman S, Friedman H, Lattimer C: Viral hepatitis, type A. Identification by specific complement fixation and immune adherence tests. N Engl J Med 292:1141–1143, 1975

52. Decker RH, Overby LR, Ling C-M, Frösner G, Deinhardt F, Boggs J: Serology of transmission of hepatitis A in humans. J Infect Dis (in press)

53. Mathiesen LR, Feinstone SM, Wong DC, Skinhoej P, Purcell RH: Enzyme linked immunosorbent assay for detection of hepatitis A antigen in stool and antibody to hepatitis A antigen in sera: Comparison with solid-phase radioimmunoassay, immune electron microscopy, and immune adherence hemmagglutination assay. J Clin Microbiol 7:184–193, 1978

54. Dienstag JL, Mathiesen LR, Purcell RH: Test methods and animal models for hepatitis A virus infection. Edited by GN Vyas, SN Cohen, and R Schmid: Viral Hepatitis. Philadelphia, Franklin Institute Press, 1978, pp 13–29

55. Deinhardt F, Holmes AW, Capps RB, Popper H: Studies on the transmission of human viral hepatitis to marmoset monkeys. I. Transmission of disease, serial passages and description of liver lesions. J Exp Med 125:673–689, 1967

56. Deinhardt F, Peterson D, Cross G, Wolfe L, Holmes AW: Hepatitis in marmosets. Am J Med Sci 270:73–80, 1975

57. Hillis WD: Viral hepatitis: An unconquered foe. Milit Med 133:343–354, 1968

58. Lorenz D, Barker L, Stevens D, Peterson M, Kirschstein R: Hepatitis in the marmoset, *Saguinus mystax*. Proc Soc Exp Biol Med 135:348–354, 1970

59. Maynard JE, Lorenz D, Bradley DW, Feinstone SM, Krushak DH, Barker LF, Purcell RH: Review of infectivity studies in nonhuman primates with virus-like particles associated with MS-1 hepatitis. Am J Med Sci 270:81–85, 1975

60. Mathiesen LR, Drucker J, Lorenz D, Wagner J, Gerety RJ, Purcell RH: Localization of hepatitis A antigen in marmoset organs during acute infection with hepatitis A virus. J Infect Dis 138:369–377, 1978

61. Provost PJ, Villarejos VM, Hilleman MR: Suitability of the Rufiventer marmoset as a host animal for human hepatitis A virus. Proc Soc Exp Biol Med 155:283–286, 1977

62. Hillis WD: An outbreak of infectious hepatitis among chimpanzee handlers at a United States Air Force Base. Am J Hygiene 73:316–328, 1961

63. Evans AS: Attempts to transmit the virus

of human hepatitis to primates other than man. Edited by JR Paul: Laboratory Propagation and Detection of the Agent of Hepatitis. Publ. No. 322. Washington, DC, National Academy of Sciences—National Research Council, 1954, pp 58–68

64. Deinhardt F, Courtois G, Dherte P, Osterrieth P, Ninane G, Henle G, Henle W: Studies of liver function tests in chimpanzees after inoculation with human infectious hepatitis virus. Am J Hygiene 75:311–321, 1962

65. Maynard JE, Bradley DW, Gravelle CR, Ebert JW, Krushak DH: News from Center for Disease Control: Preliminary studies of hepatitis A in chimpanzees. J Infect Dis 131:194–197, 1975

66. Thornton A, Tsiquaye KN, Zuckerman AJ: Studies on human hepatitis A virus in chimpanzees. Br J Exp Pathol 58:352–358, 1977

67. Dienstag JL, Popper H, Purcell RH: The pathology of viral hepatitis types A and B in chimpanzees: A comparison. Am J Pathol 83:131–148, 1976

68. Giles JP, Liebhaber H, Krugman S, Lattimer C: Early viremia and viruria in infectious hepatitis. Virology 24:107–108, 1964

69. Krugman S, Ward R, Giles JP, Bodansky O, Jacobs AM: Infectious hepatitis: Detection of virus during the incubation period and in clinically inapparent infection. N Engl J Med 261:729–734, 1959

70. Dienstag JL, Feinstone SM, Kapikian AZ, Purcell RH, Boggs JD, Conrad ME: Fecal shedding of hepatitis A antigen. Lancet 1:765–767, 1975

71. Rakela J, Mosley JW: Fecal excretion of hepatitis A virus in humans. J Infect Dis 135:933–938, 1977

72. Frösner GG, Overby LR, Flehmig B, Gerth H-J, Haas H, Decker RH, Ling C-M, Zuckerman AJ, Frösner H-R: Seroepidemiological investigation of patients and family contacts in an epidemic of hepatitis A. J Med Virol 1:163–173, 1977

73. Voegt HV: Zur aetiologie der hepatitis epidemica. Munch Med Wochenschr 89:76–79, 1942

74. Havens WP Jr: Period of infectivity of patients with experimentally induced infectious hepatitis. J Exp Med 83:251–258, 1946

75. Ward R, Krugman S, Giles JP, Jacobs AM, Bodansky O: Infectious hepatitis: Studies of its natural history and prevention. N Engl J Med 258:407–416, 1958

76. Bradley DW, Gravelle CR, Cook EH, Fields RM, Maynard JE: Cyclic excretion of hepatitis A virus in experimentally infected chimpanzees: Biophysical characterization of the associated HAV particles. J Med Virol 1:133–138, 1977

77. Joseph PR, Millar JD, Henderson DA: An outbreak of hepatitis traced to food contamination. N Engl J Med 273:188–194, 1965

78. Locarnini SA, Ferris AA, Lehmann NI, Gust ID: The antibody response following hepatitis A infection. Intervirology 8:309–318, 1977

79. Rakela J, Stevenson D, Edwards VM, Gordon I, Mosley JW: Antibodies to hepatitis A virus: Patterns by two procedures. J Clin Microbiol 5:110–111, 1977

80. Gust ID, Dienstag JL, Purcell RH, Lucas CR: Non-B hepatitis in Melbourne: A serological study of hepatitis A virus infection. Br Med J 1:193–195, 1977

81. Bradley DW, Maynard JE, Hindman SH, Hornbeck CL, Fields HA, McCaustland KA, Cook EH Jr: Serodiagnosis of viral hepatitis A: Detection of acute-phase immunoglobulin M anti-hepatitis A virus by radioimmunoassay. J Clin Microbiol 5:521–530, 1977

82. Giles JP, Krugman S: Viral hepatitis: Immunoglobulin response during the course of the disease. JAMA 208:497–503, 1969

83. Dienstag JL, Purcell RH: Viral hepatitis, type A: Etiology and epidemiology. Rush-Presbyterian-St Luke's Med Bull 15:104–114, 1976

84. Villarejos VM, Gutierrez-Diermissen A, Anderson-Visona, K, Rodriguez-Aragones A, Provost PJ, Hilleman MR: Development of immunity against hepatitis A virus by subclinical infection. Proc Soc Exp Biol Med 153:205–208, 1976

85. Krugman S: Effect of human immune serum globulin on infectivity of hepatitis A virus. J Infect Dis 134:70–74, 1976

86. Chang LW, O'Brien TF: Australia antigen serology in the Holy Cross football team hepatitis outbreak. Lancet 2:59–61, 1970

87. Baer GM, Walker JA, Yager PA: Studies of an outbreak of acute hepatitis A: I. Complement level fluctuation. J Med Virol 1:1–7, 1977

88. Chisari FV, Routenberg JA, Fiala M, Edgington TS: Extrinsic modulation of human T-lymphocyte E rosette function associated with prolonged hepatocellular injury after viral hepatitis. J Clin Invest 59:134–142, 1977

89. Rakela J, Nugent E, Mosley JW: Viral hepatitis: Enzyme assays and serologic pro-

cedures in the study of an epidemic. Am J Epidemiol 106:493–501, 1977

90. Bradley DW, Fields HA, McAustland KA, Maynard JE, Decker RH, Whittington R, Overby LR: Serodiagnosis of hepatitis A by a modified competitive binding radioimmunoassay for IgM anti-HAV. J Clin Microbiol (in press)

91. Mosley JW: The epidemiology of viral hepatitis: an overview. Am J Med Sci 270:253–270, 1975

92. Villarejos VM, Provost PJ, Ittensohn OL, McLean AA, Hilleman MR: Seroepidemiologic investigations of human hepatitis caused by A, B, and a possible third virus. Proc Soc Exp Biol Med 152:524–528, 1976

93. Frösner G, Iwarson S, Lindholm A, Norkrans G: Antikroppar mot hepatit A bland svenska blodgivare. Lakartidningen 75:544–545, 1978

94. Frösner GG, Frösner HR, Haas H, Dietz K, Sugg U, Schneider W: Haufigkeit von hepatitis-A-antikörpern in bevölkerungsgruppen verscheidener Europaischer lander. Schweiz Med Wochenschr 107:129–133, 1977

95. Szmuness W, Dienstag JL, Purcell RH, Stevens CE, Wong DC, Ikram H, Bar-Shany S, Beasley RP, Desmyter J, Gaon JA: The prevalence of antibody to hepatitis A antigen in various parts of the world. Am J Epidemiol 106:391–398, 1977

96. Hall WT, Mundon FK, Madden DL, DeSouza D, Kane JL: Distribution of antibody to hepatitis A antigen in a population of commercial plasma donors. J Clin Microbiol 6:132–135, 1977

97. Frösner GG, Deinhardt FW: The shifting epidemiology of hepatitis A in Europe. Edited by GN Vyas, SN Cohen, and R Schmid: Viral Hepatitis. Philadelphia, Franklin Institute Press, 1978, pp 732–733

98. Szmuness W, Dienstag JL, Purcell RH, Harley EJ, Stevens CE, Wong DC: Distribution of antibody to hepatitis A antigen in urban adult populations. N Engl J. Med 295:755–759, 1976

99. Maynard JE, Bradley DW, Hornbeck CL, Fields RM, Doto IL, Hollinger FB: Preliminary serologic studies of antibody to hepatitis A virus in populations in the United States. J Infect Dis 134:528–530, 1976

100. Lehmann NI, Gust ID: Prevalence of antibody to hepatitis A virus in two populations in Victoria, Australia. Med J Aust 2:731–732, 1977

101. Wong DC, Rosen L, Purcell RH: Sero- epidemiology of viral hepatitis in the South Pacific. Edited by GN Vyas, SN Cohen, and R. Schmid: Viral Hepatitis. Philadelphia, Franklin Institute Press, 1978, pp 733–734

102. Gust ID, Lewis FA, Lehmann NI: Prevalence of antibody to hepatitis A and polioviruses in an unimmunized urban population. Am J Epidemiol 107:54–56, 1978

103. Vitarana T, Kanapathipillai M, Gunasekera HDN, Lehmann NI, Dimitrikakis M, Gust ID: A seroepidemiological study of hepatitis A and hepatitis B infection in Sri Lanka. Asian J Infect Dis (in press)

104. Gust ID, Lehmann NI, Dimitrikakis M: A seroepidemiological study of infection with hepatitis A and B viruses in five Pacific islands. Am J Epidemiol (in press)

105. Paul JR: Epidemiology of poliomyelitis. WHO Monogr Ser 26:9–29, 1955

106. Walton M, Melnick JL: Poliomyelitis antibodies in two differing socioeconomic groups within the same city. Yale J Biol Med 27:350–370, 1955

107. Fox JP, Gelfand HM, LeBlanc DR, Conwell DP: Studies on the development of natural immunity to poliomyelitis in Louisiana. I. Over-all plan, methods and observations as to patterns of seroimmunity in the study group. Am J Hyg 65:344–363, 1957

108. Gust ID, Lehmann NI, Lucas CR: Relationship between prevalence of anti-HAV and age—a cohort effect? J Infect Dis 138:425–426, 1978

109. Szmuness W: Studies on intrafamilial spread of epidemic hepatitis. Epidemiol Rev 17:198–211, 1963

110. Lobel HO, McCollum RW: Some observations on the ecology of infectious hepatitis. Bull WHO 32:675–682, 1965

111. Goldstein GS, Wehrle PF: The influence of socioeconomic factors on the distribution of hepatitis in Syracuse NY. Am J Public Health 49:473–480, 1959

112. Maynard JE: Infectious hepatitis at Fort Yukon, Alaska—report of an outbreak, 1960–1961. Am J Public Health 53:31–39, 1963

113. Skinhøj P, McNair A, Andersen ST: Hepatitis and hepatitis B-antigen in Greenland. Am J Epidemiol 99:50–57, 1974

114. Skinhøj P, Mikkelsen F, Hollinger FB: Hepatitis A in Greenland: Importance of specific antibody testing in epidemiologic surveillance. Am J Epidemiol 105:140–147, 1977

115. Mosley JW: Epidemiologic implications of changing trends in type A and type B hepatitis. Edited by GN Vyas, HA Perkins, and R Schmid: Hepatitis and Blood Transfusion. New York, Grune & Stratton, 1972, pp 23–26

116. Dienstag JL, Szmuness W, Stevens CE, Purcell RH: Hepatitis A virus infection: New insights from seroepidemiologic studies. J Infect Dis 137:328–340, 1978

117. Dienstag JL, Gust ID, Lucas CR, Wong DC, Purcell RH: Mussel-associated viral hepatitis, type A: Serologic confirmation. Lancet 1:561–564, 1976

118. Dienstag JL, Davenport FM, McCollum RW, Hennessy AV, Klatskin G, Purcell RH: Nonhuman primate-associated viral hepatitis type A: Serologic evidence of hepatitis A virus infection. JAMA 236:462–464, 1976

119. Barker LF, Dienstag JL, Lorenz DE, Purcell RH, Wong DC, Feinstone SM, Peterson MR, Rosen MW: Serologic and animal inoculation studies of a communal outbreak of viral hepatitis, type A. Am J Med Sci 274:247–253, 1977

120. Szmuness W, Purcell RH, Dienstag JL, Stevens CE: Antibody to hepatitis A antigen in institutionalized mentally retarded patients. JAMA 237:1702–1705, 1977

121. Lehmann NI, Sharma DLS, Gust ID: The prevalence of antibody to the hepatitis A virus in a large institution for the mentally retarded. J Med Virol (in press)

122. Krugman S, Gocke DJ: Viral hepatitis. Edited by LJ Smith Jr: Major Problems in Internal Medicine. Vol XV. Philadelphia, WB Saunders, 1978, pp 23–25

123. Hall WT, Mundon FK, Madden DL: Antibody to hepatitis A in mentally retarded inpatients. Lancet 1:758–759, 1977

124. Matthew EB, Dietzman DE, Madden DL, Newman SJ, Sever JL, Nagler B, Bouton SM, Rostafinski M: A major epidemic of infectious hepatitis in an institution for the mentally retarded. Am J Epidemiol 98:199–215, 1973

125. Feinstone SM, Kapikian AZ, Purcell RH, Alter HJ, Holland PV: Transfusion-associated hepatitis not due to viral hepatitis type A or B. N Engl J Med 292:767–770, 1975

126. Knodell RG, Conrad ME, Dienstag JL, Bell CJ: Etiological spectrum of post-transfusion hepatitis. Gastroenterology 69:1278–1285, 1975

127. Alter HJ, Purcell RH, Holland PV, Feinstone SM, Morrow AG, Moritsugu Y: Clinical and serological analysis of transfusion-associated hepatitis. Lancet 2:838–841, 1975

128. Dienstag JL, Feinstone SM, Purcell RH, Wong DC, Alter HJ, Holland PV: Non-A, non-B post-transfusion hepatitis. Lancet 1:560–562, 1977.

129. Szmuness W, Dienstag JL, Purcell RH, Prince AM, Stevens CE, Levine RW: Hepatitis type A and hemodialysis: A seroepidemiologic study in 15 U.S. centers. Ann Intern Med 87:8–12, 1977

130. Stevens CE, Silbert JA, Miller DR, Dienstag JL, Purcell RH, Szmuness W: Serologic evidence of hepatitis A and B virus infections in thalassemia patients: A retrospective study. Transfusion 18:356–360, 1978

131. Papaevangelou G, Frösner G, Economidou J, Parcha S, Roumeliotou A: Prevalence of hepatitis A and B infections in multiply transfused thalassaemic patients. Br Med J 1:689–691, 1978

132. Gust ID, Lehmann NI, Lucas CR, Ferris AA, Locarnini SA: Studies on the epidemiology of hepatitis A in Melbourne. Edited by GN Vyas, SN Cohen, and R Schmid: Viral Hepatitis. Philadelphia, Franklin Institute Press, 1978, pp 105–112

133. Maynard JE: Viral hepatitus as an occupational hazard in the health care profession. Edited by GN Vyas, SN Cohen, and R Schmid: Viral Hepatitis. Philadelphia, Franklin Institute Press, 1978, pp 321–331

134. Stokes J Jr, Berk JE, Malamut LL, Drake ME, Barondess JA, Bashe WJ, Wolman IJ, Farquhar JD, Bevan B, Drummond RJ, Maycock Wd'A, Capps RB, Bennett AM: The carrier state in viral hepatitis. JAMA 154:1059–1065, 1954

135. Capps RB, Sborov V, Scheiffley CS: A syringe transmitted epidemic of infectious hepatitis. JAMA 136:819–824, 1948

136. Routenberg JA, Dienstag JL, Harrison WO, Kilpatrick MD, Hooper RR, Purcell RH, Fornes MF: A foodborne epidemic of hepatitis-A virus (HAV) infection among navy recruits (abstract). Gastroenterology 69:859, 1975

137. Dienstag JL, Alaama A, Mosley JW, Redeker AG, Purcell RH: Etiology of sporadic hepatitis B surface antigen-negative hepatitis. Ann Intern Med 87:1–6, 1977

138. Krugman S, Ward R, Giles JP, Jacobs AM: Infectious hepatitis: Studies on the effect of gamma globulin and on the incidence of inapparent infection. JAMA 174:823–830, 1960

139. Morse LJ, Bryan JA, Hurley JP, Murphy JF, O'Brien TF, Wacker WEC: The Holy Cross college football team hepatitis outbreak. JAMA 219:706–708, 1972

140. Wacker WEC, Riordan JF, Snodgrass PJ, Chang LW, Morse LJ, O'Brien TF, Reddy WJ: The Holy Cross hepatitis outbreak: Clinical and chemical abnormalities. Arch Intern Med 130:357–360, 1972

141. Rakela J, Redeker AG, Edwards VM, Decker R, Overby LR, Mosley JW: Hepatitis A virus infection in fulminant hepatitis and chronic active hepatitis. Gastroenterology 74:879–882, 1978

142. Lindberg J, Frösner G, Hansson BG, Hermodsson S, Iwarson S: Serologic markers of hepatitis A and B in chronic active hepatitis. Scand J Gastroenterol 13:525–527, 1978

144. Acute Hepatic Failure Study Group: Etiology of acute hepatic failure (abstract). Gastroenterology 73:1236, 1977

144. Viswanathan R: Certain epidemiological features of infectious hepatitis during the Delhi epidemic, 1955–56. Edited by FW Hartman, GA LoGrippo, JG Mateer, and J Barron: Hepatitis Frontiers. Boston, Little, Brown, 1957, pp 207–210

145. Hindman SH, Maynard JE, Bradley DW, Berquist KR, Denes AE: Simultaneous infection with type A and B hepatitis viruses. Am J Epidemiol 105:135–139, 1977

146. Balistreri W, Tabor E, Drucker J, Gerety R: Serologic markers of hepatitis A (HAV) and B (HBV) in biliary atresia (BA) and neonatal hepatitis (NH). Pediatr Res 12:429 (abstract), 1978

147. Sever JL, Kapikian AZ, Feinstone S, Purcell RH, Gilkeson MR: Hepatitis A and Down's syndrome: Lack of an association. J Infect Dis 134:198–200, 1976

148. Krugman S, Giles JP: Viral hepatitis: New light on an old disease. JAMA 212:1019–1029, 1970

149. Havens WP Jr, Paul JR: Prevention of infectious hepatitis with gamma globulin. JAMA 129:270–272, 1945

150. Stokes J Jr, Farquhar JA, Drake ME, Capps RB, Ward CS Jr, Kitts AW: Infectious hepatitis: Length of protection by immune serum globulin (gamma globulin) during epidemics. JAMA 147:714–719, 1951

151. Frösner GG, Haas H, Hotz G: Hepatitis-A antibody in commercial lots of immune serum globulin. Lancet 1:432–433, 1977

152. Hall WT, Madden DL, Mundon FK, Brandt DEL, Clarke NA: Protective effect of immune serum globulin (ISG) against hepatitis A infection in a natural epidemic. Am J Epidemiol 106:72–75, 1977

153. Public Health Service Advisory Committee on Immunization Practices: Immune globulins for protection against viral hepatitis. Morbid Mortal Weekly Report 26:425–428, 441–442, 1977

154. Denes AE, Smith JL, Hindman SH, Fleissner ML, Judelsohn R, Englender SJ, Tilson H, Maynard JE: Foodborne hepatitis A infection: A report of two urban restaurant-associated outbreaks. Am J Epidemiol 105:156–162, 1977

155. Alter HJ, Purcell RH, Feinstone SM, Holland PV, Morrow AG: Non-A, non-B hepatitis: A review and interim report of an ongoing prospective study. Edited by GN Vyas, SN Cohen, and R Schmid: Viral hepatitis. Philadelphia, Franklin Institute Press, 1978, pp 359–369

156. Alter JH, Purcell RH, Holland PV, Popper HJ: Transmissible agent in non-A non-B hepatitis. Lancet 1:459–463, 1978

157. Tabor E, Gerety RJ, Drucker JA, Seeff LB, Hoofnagle JH, Jackson DR, April M, Barker LF, Pineda-Tamondong G: Transmission of non-A, non-B hepatitis from man to chimpanzee. Lancet 1:463–466, 1978

158. Hollinger FB, Gitnick GL, Aach RD, Szmuness W, Mosley JA, Stevens CE, Peters RL, Weiner JM, Werch JB, Lander JL: Non-A, non-B hepatitis transmission in chimpanzees: A project of the transfusion-transmitted viruses study group. Intervirology 10:60–68, 1978

Chapter 20

Immunopathology of Hepatitis B

By LEONARDO BIANCHI, M.D., *and* FRED GUDAT, M.D.

THE IDENTIFICATION of specific hepatitis B (HB)-associated antigens and antibodies in liver tissue and blood, supplemented by in vitro measurements of cellular immunity, have greatly enhanced our knowledge about the natural history of HB. Thus, fairly characteristic virus expression patterns in tissue and correlated serologic reactions may be recognized.

The pathogenesis of the immunopathologic reactions, however, particularly the hepatocytic necrosis in the various forms of hepatitis B virus (HBV) infection, is far from understood. Whether viral antigens, host antigens, or both, expressed on the liver cell surface, are crucial in this respect is an unanswered question. On the effector side, the interaction of specific B- and T-lymphocyte-mediated immune reactions against such antigens have to be considered, and here, in vitro measurements of cellular immunity have yielded controversial results, probably because of critical differences in technical procedures. Moreover,the relevance of in vitro results for in vivo conditions is debatable.

This chapter focuses mainly on viral antigen expression in tissue and blood and the humoral immune responses. For the role of host antigens and cellular immunity, the reader is referred to Chapter 22. Our own results obtained on evaluation of 222 patients with chronic HBV infection are summarized in Tables 2 and 3. For methods and the histologic classification used, see references 1–4.

VIRAL ANTIGENS IN BLOOD

The 42-nm Dane particle as the complete infective virion of hepatitis B[5] is composed of at least two serologically and morphologically distinct antigens[6] (Fig 1A and B): A 27-nm core carrying the hepatitis B core antigen (HB$_c$Ag) is coated by an envelope carrying the hepatitis B surface antigen (HB$_s$Ag), including several subdeterminants.[7] The core contains DNA polymerase[8,9] and a circular double-stranded DNA.[10,11] HB$_s$Ag is produced in excess and appears in the blood as 20-nm spheres and tubular structures in addition to the Dane particle (Fig. 1A and B).

HB$_e$Ag/anti-HB$_e$ has been identified as an HB-associated antigen/antibody system unrelated to HB Ag precipitin lines,[12] although anti-HB$_e$-positive sera have been found capable of agglutinating Dane particles and tubules.[13] Speculations have considered HB$_e$Ag to be a virus-specific antigen,[14,15] the DNA polymerase itself,[16] a host-specific immunoglobulin[17] being anti-idiotypic, or an extra band of LDH$_5$ isoenzyme (complex of LDH$_5$+HB$_s$Ag+HB$_e$Ag).[18] HB$_e$Ag

From the Department of Pathology, University of Basel, Switzerland.

Original work was supported by the Swiss National Science Foundation (Grant No 6-1640-75).

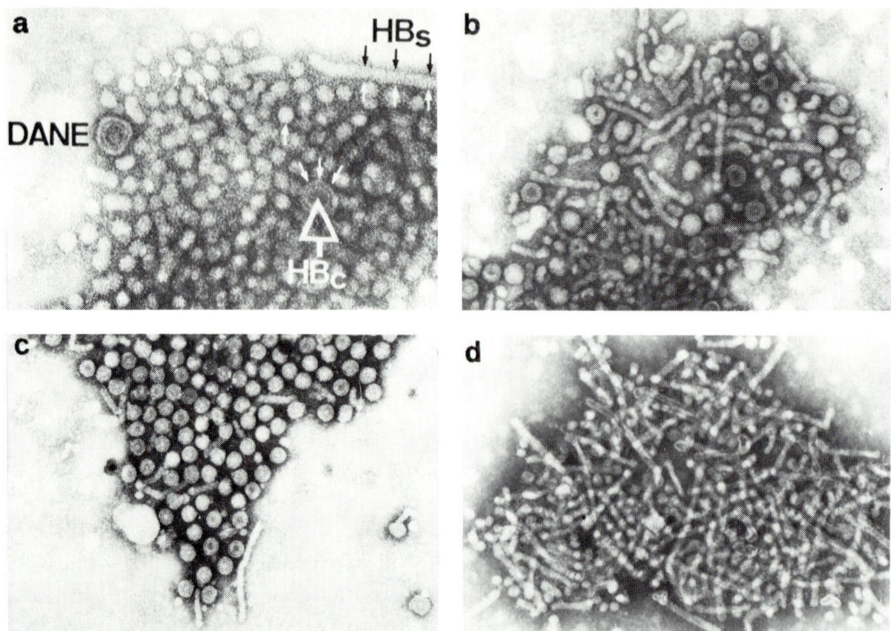

FIG. 1—HB Ag expression in blood. (A) HB Ag agglutinated by anti-HB$_s$ showing preponderance of 20-nm spherical particles and admixture of tubular HB$_s$Ag and Dane particles. Small arrows designate site of HB$_s$Ag determinants. Large arrow represents HB$_c$Ag. (B) Spontaneous HB Ag complex in a case of chronic active hepatitis B: predominance of Dane particles and tubular HB$_s$Ag. (C) Spontaneous HB Ag complex in a case of chronic nonaggressive hepatitis B with generalized HB$_c$Ag type, almost exclusively composed of Dane particles (Reproduced from Gudat F, Bianchi L: HB$_s$Ag: A target antigen on the liver cell? Edited by H Popper, L Bianchi, and W Reutter: Membrane Alterations as Basis of Liver Injury. Lancaster, MTP Press, 1977, pp 171–178 with permission of MTP.) (D) Spontaneous immune complex in a case of chronic nonaggressive HB of HB$_c$Ag-free HB$_s$Ag type. Note the almost exclusive involvement of tubular HB$_s$Ag and the absence of Dane particles.

activity in blood, and infectivity. It is, however, not a reliable marker either for aggressivity or for chronicity, since it may transiently appear in acute limited hepatitis B.[19]

HB Ag particles may also appear as circulating complexes in acute and chronic hepatitis.[20] These may show a predominance for Dane particles with or without admixture of tubules, mainly in cases of demonstrable HB$_c$Ag expression in tissue (Fig. 1C). Less frequently, pure tubular complexes may be found in carriers without detectable HB$_c$Ag or Dane particle formation (Fig. 1D). In some instances, mainly in acute HB, complexes predominantly of 20-nm HB$_s$Ag particles as seen following in vitro agglutination with anti-HB$_s$, may be found (Fig. 1A).

VIRAL ANTIGENS IN LIVER TISSUE

HB$_c$Ag is preferentially but not exclusively localized in liver cell nuclei (Fig. 2A)[3,21,22] and appears as noncoated spherical 24–27-nm structures (Fig.

2E).[3,23,24,24a] Excess formation of core particles can be recognized in rare instances even in conventional histologic hematoxylin- and eosin-stained slides by finely granular eosinophilic inclusions (Fig. 2F),[25] the so-called sanded nuclei.[26] For the formation of complete Dane particles, HB_cAg seems to be released from the nucleus through nuclear pores into the extracisternal perinuclear cytoplasm. In some instances of chronic HB, wavelike sequences occur in nuclear HB_cAg formation and cell-membrane-directed flow of core particles,[27] leading to different distribution patterns including a submembraneous HB_cAg accumulation (Fig. 2A–D). The dynamics and the definitive site of Dane particle formation, however, are not known.

HB_sAg is exclusively localized in the cytoplasm (Fig. 3A)[3,28-30] and appears as filamentous material within a proliferated and often distorted SER (Fig. 3F).[31] By light microscopy, HB_sAg-containing cells may readily be recognized as ground-glass hepatocytes (Fig. 3E).[29] They stain dark brown with orcein (Fig. 3B).[32]

Hb_sAg may also be demonstrated at the cell membrane in certain forms of hepatitis (Fig. 3C and D).[33,34] This membrane-associated HB_sAg is linked to nuclear and/or cytoplasmic (submembraneous) core expression in 72% to 100% of cases.[34]

HB_eAg is claimed to be localized in the cytoplasm by some[14] and in nuclei by others.[35] Our own preliminary studies were unable to confirm cytoplasmic localization but provided evidence for nuclear localization, although interference with the nuclear HB_cAg system is difficult to exclude.

PATHOGENESIS OF HEPATOCELLULAR INJURY AND OF CHRONIC FORMS OF HEPATITIS B

Evidence is accumulating that there is either no or only a low-grade cytopathogenicity of the HBV.[3,36-42] This is best exemplified by asymptomatic carriers or immunosuppressed patients who tolerate large amounts of viral antigens in liver tissue and blood without substantial liver cell damage. By contrast, spotty liver cell necrosis in acute hepatitis of apparently normergic persons illustrates that the hepatitic lesion results from host defense mechanisms eliminating hepatocytes altered by the noncytopathic virus.

Several facts indicate that notably immunologic interactions with viral antigens on liver cells cause the hepatocellular injury and provoke the various forms of HB. Whether humoral or cellular immunity is the main mediator of hepatocyte damage is not established, however.

Which antigens are the targets in acute and chronic HB is debated. Our discussion is centered on viral antigens as possible targets and on respective immune responses. This does not exclude the possibility that host antigens (e.g., liver-specific lipoprotein; see Chapter 22) may be involved simultaneously.

HB_sAg as a Target

The most likely candidate for a virus-derived target is HB_sAg. Its role in cell elimination is indicated by its association with the cell membrane (Fig. 3C and

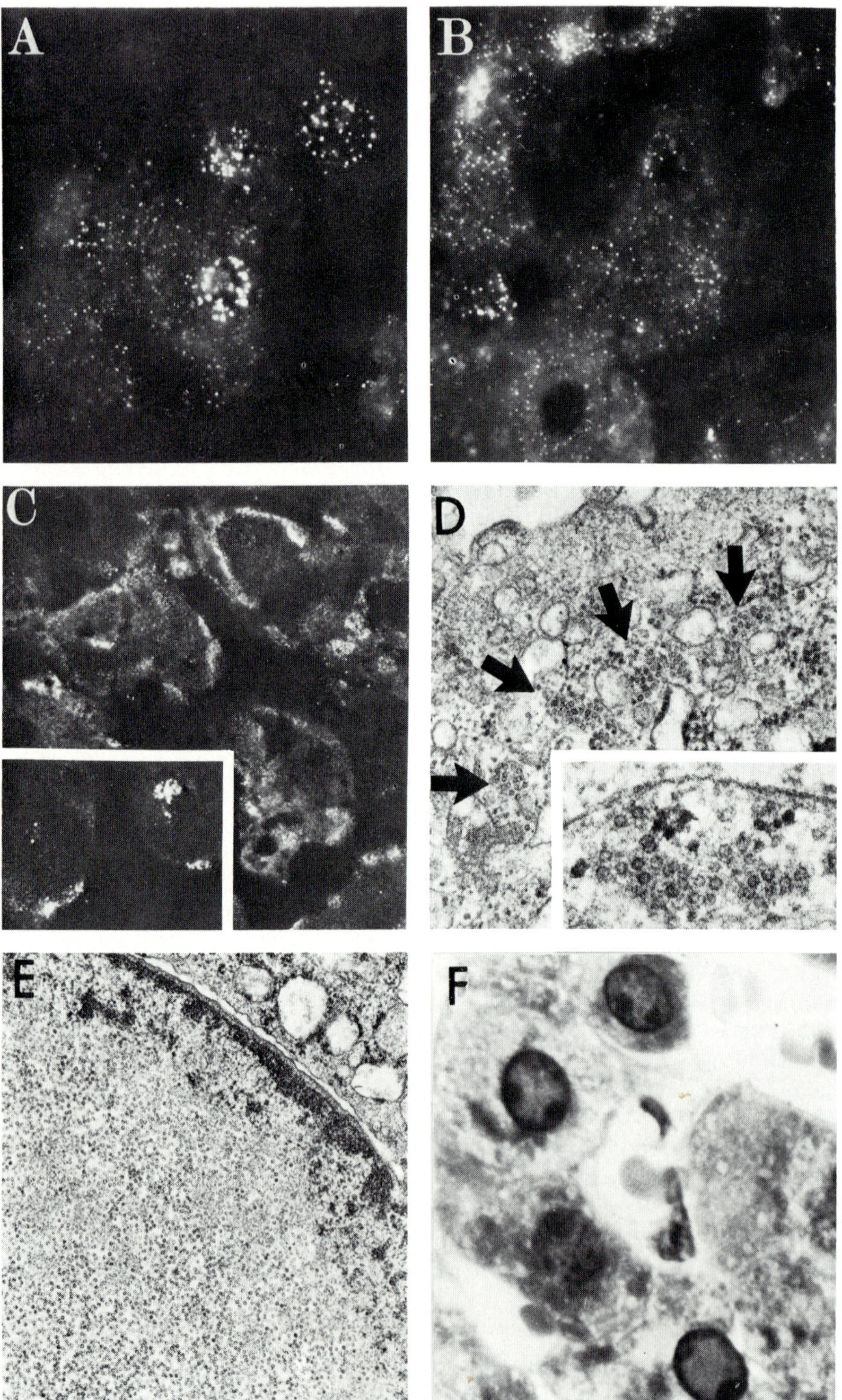

D) mainly in conditions with no or low-grade elimination, such as in effectively immunosuppressed patients.[22,34]

Several observations point to cellular immunity directed against HB_sAg as cause of cytopathogenicity: (1) the time relation between onset of acute illness and demonstration of cell-mediated immunity[36,37,43,44] including T-cell cytotoxicity against HB_sAg,[45] which is also demonstrable in chronic forms with liver cell damage; (2) the absence of cell damage and the tolerance of large amounts of viral antigens in effectively immunosuppressed renal transplant recipients,[3] in which cellular immunity is far more affected than humoral reactivity, and in carriers who tolerate viral antigens in the absence of demonstrable cell-mediated immunity to HB_sAg[46] and T-cell-mediated cytotoxicity in vitro.[45]

Anti-HBs-mediated cytotoxicity cannot be definitively excluded. The appearance of anti-HB_s usually indicates termination of HBV infection, although the antibody may appear long after the disappearance of HB_sAg from blood and liver. Radioimmunoassay does not detect anti-HB_s in all forms of active HBV infection. This, however, does not exclude trace amounts of antibody undetectable because of complexing to the target. Indeed, the observed immune complexes during acute viral hepatitis[20] indicate at least involvement of anti-HB_s in the elimination of intercellular and circulating HB_sAg. Antibody-mediated K-cell cytotoxicity has not been ruled out. Passively transferred anti-HB_s to HB Ag carriers does not appear to cause liver injury.[47,48]

Dane Particle/Tubule-related Antigens and HB_cAg as Targets

Of particular interest are Dane particle- and tubule-associated antigens that are different from HB_sAg and that seem to be involved in immune complex formation of the Dane particle/tubule type (Fig. 1C).[13,34] Elimination of Dane particles from blood and HB_cAg-producing cells from liver in chronic HB (HB_cAg-free HB_sAg type; see below) is followed by the appearance of antibodies that are capable of agglutinating Dane particles and tubules. Spherical HB_sAg particles in blood and hepatocytes are not affected by this elimination system.

The relation of HB_eAg and anti-HB_e to this Dane particle-associated antigen system has not been clarified, but it behaves identically in that HB_eAg is associated with Dane particles and with Dane particle/tubule complexes (L. Bian-

---

FIG. 2—HB_cAg expression in liver tissue. (A) Immunofluorescence demonstration of a nuclear and mixed nuclear-cytoplasmic HB_cAg distribution pattern. (B) HB_cAg in a mixed and pure cytoplasmic distribution. Note empty nucleus at bottom. (C) HB_cAg in pronounced submembraneous accumulation. Inset shows combination of nuclear and submembraneous HB_cAg. (D) Intracytoplasmic, extracisternal naked core particles (arrows) with submembraneous accumulation (inset). (E) Excess of intranuclear naked core particles. (F) Excess of intranuclear HB_cAg giving a sanded, pink appearance in light microscopy (H+E stain). (Figs. A-D reproduced from Gudat F, Bianchi L: Evidence for phasic sequences in nuclear HB_cAg formation and cell membrane-directed flow of core particles in chronic hepatitis B. Gastroenterology 73:1194–1197, 1977, copyright American Gastroenterological Society, with permission of *Gastroenterology*; Fig. E reproduced from Bianchi L, Gudat F: Sanded nuclei in hepatitis B. Lab Invest 35: 1–5, 1976, copyright US–Canadian Division of The International Academy of Pathology, with permission of Laboratory Investigations.)

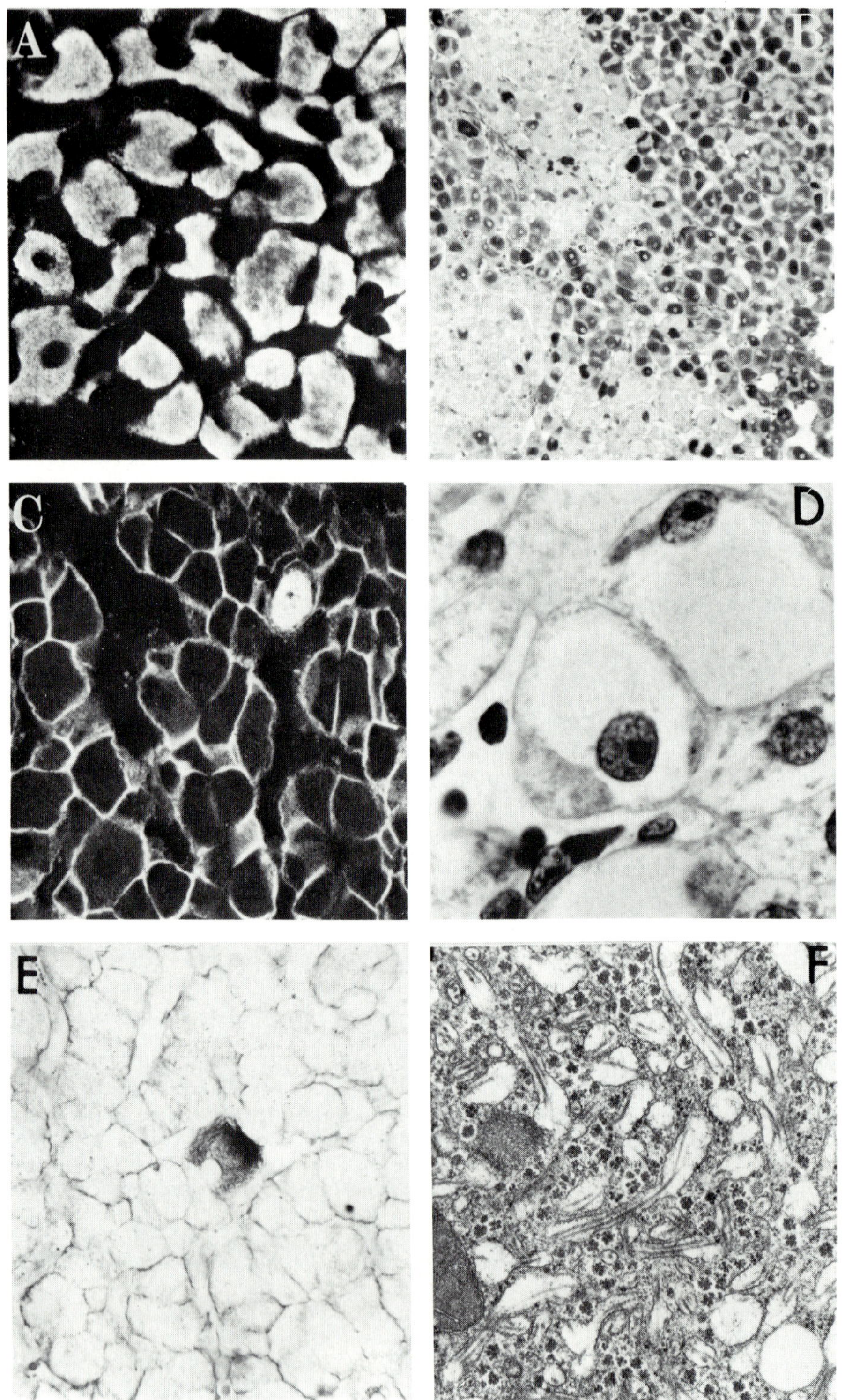

A
B
C
D
E
F

chi, F. Gudat, unpublished observations). By contrast, anti-HB$_e$-positive sera agglutinate Dane particles well, and anti-HB$_e$ is associated with absence of HB$_e$Ag and Dane particles. The hypothesis was advanced that LDH$_{5ex}$ might act as a target.[18] Cellular immunity against HB$_e$Ag and Dane particle-associated antigens in the various forms of HB has not been studied.

Besides the possibility that these antibodies may be involved in K-cell-mediated cytotoxicity for Dane particle-producing cells, such antigen/antibody complexes may have the opposite effect, namely of blocking or suppressing action on cellular immunity.[45]

HB$_c$Ag System as a Target

HB$_c$Ag has also been considered as a possible target antigen.[38] Indeed, HB$_c$Ag is found in close connection with the hepatocytic membrane by immunofluorescence.[22,27] Electron microscopy, however, demonstrated HB$_c$Ag particles only in the intracytoplasmic submembraneous region.[27] Also from a theoretical point of view the core of an enveloped virus is unlikely to be exposed on the cell surface. To our knowledge, HB$_c$Ag, unlike HB$_s$Ag, has never been demonstrated on the surface of hepatocytes in single cell studies.[49]

Cellular immunity to HB$_c$Ag has been reported in acute and chronic forms of HB,[40] indicating sensitization but not necessarily cytotoxic activity against hepatocytes.

Anti-HB$_c$ appears in virtually all forms of HBV infection, including those without cell damage.[50] This finding speaks against any role of anti-HB$_c$ in elimination and in cell damage. Particularly high titers of anti-HB$_c$ in chronic active hepatitis[50] might be a secondary phenomenon caused by prolonged immunization by core particles released from cells destroyed by other mechanisms.

In summary, elimination or persistence of infected cells may result from complex immune interactions of the T- and B-cell system. Under normergic conditions, mainly T lymphocytes mediate eradication of cells. Further evidence for this is the chronic active hepatitis with substantial liver cell damage in agammaglobulinemia, and these patients in fact run an even more severe course.[51-53] Moreover, the transiently increased severity of hepatitis after transfer of lymphocytes from convalescent patients, following administration of transfer factor[47,54] or of agents stimulating cellular immunity, such as levamisole,[55] supports T-cell-mediated hepatocytic damage. Antibodies seem to have mainly protective properties and are involved in inhibiting the spread of virus. Their blocking effect via immune complex formation[45] and their suggested

---

FIG. 3—HB$_s$Ag expression in liver tissue. (A) Immunofluorescence demonstration of intracytoplasmic HB$_s$Ag. Note negative nuclei. (B) Appearance of intracytoplasmic HB$_s$Ag with orcein staining. (C) Membrane-associated fluorescence for HB$_s$Ag in addition to intracytoplasmic HB$_s$Ag as seen in chronic HB with HB$_c$Ag expression. (D) Membrane-associated and intracytoplasmic HB$_s$Ag demonstrated by specific immune peroxidase method. (E) HB$_s$Ag-containing ground-glass cells in H+E stain. (F) Filamentous HB$_s$Ag within a proliferated and distorted SER of a ground-glass cell. (Reproduced from Gudat F et al: Pattern of core and surface expression in liver tissue reflects state of specific immune response in hepatitis B. Lab Invest 32:1–9, 1975, with permission of *Laboratory Investigations*.)

suppressive action on the viral genome in chronic hepatitis B[38] require confirmation by further investigations. In any event, the basic defect in chronic HB seems to be insufficient elimination owing to a specific immune disturbance. The role of T cell subpopulations and their relation to HL-A genes remain to be established.[37,39]

THE BASIC REACTION TYPES OF HEPATITIS B

The classification of hepatitis B proposed in this chapter was primarily derived from viral expression patterns related to complete or incomplete virus replication. As outlined in Table 1, HB_cAg and Dane particle synthesis and expression of associated antigens (e.g., HB_eAg) are taken as the basic discriminating features. These are supplemented by additional facultative, discriminating (e.g., membrane-associated HB_sAg), and nondiscriminating (e.g., intracellular HB_sAg) markers, allowing the recognition of four basic expression types with transitional forms (Fig. 4). This biologic classification correlates well with conventional histologic findings, indicating an intrinsic association between type and degree of inflammation and the state of virus infection. Whereas a limited infection lacks viral expression after the establishment of normergic inflammation, there is overt and persistent viral expression in chronic hepatitis of any histologic type, either with or without active core and Dane particle formation (Table 1, Fig. 4). Therefore, the identification of a histologic diagnosis with one of the basic expression types bears, in our view, on the evaluation of prognosis, therapy, and infectivity.

Elimination Type: Acute Self-limited Viral Hepatitis

Viral Antigens in Tissue and Tissue Reaction

At the height of classical acute spotty necrotic hepatitis no viral components are found in liver tissue despite HB Ag seropositivity, intense lobular inflammation, spotty hepatocytic necrosis and biochemical signs of liver cell damage

TABLE 1—*Characterization of Chronic Hepatitis B Infection*

		HBcAg-Free HBsAg Type	Focal HBcAg Type	Generalized HBcAg Type
Key Features	HBcAg in tissue	NO**	focal *	generalized
	Dane particles in blood (DP)	NO**	+	+
Additional Discriminating Features (facultative)	HBeAg	NO	+	+
	Anti-HBe	+	NO**	NO
	Membrane-associated HBsAg	NO	+	+
	Circulating immune complexes	(+)*** (tubules only)	+ (DP + tubules)	+ (DP + tubules)
Nondiscriminating Features	Intracytoplasmic HBsAg	+	+	+
	Anti-HBc	+	+	+/−
	Salient form of inflammation	none or nonaggressive	aggressive	nonaggressive or none

*Occasionally no HBcAg, but always Dane particles in blood
**Rare
***For exceptions see Table 2.

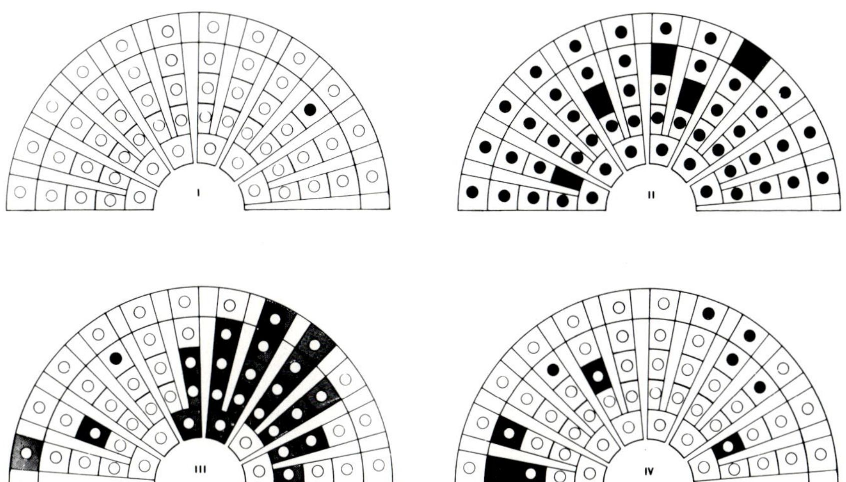

FIG. 4—Schematic representation of HB Ag expression patterns in liver tissue: (I) Elimination type: no viral components at the height of classical acute spotty necrotic hepatitis. Exceptionally, HB_cAg visible in early phases. (II) Generalized HB_cAg type, associated with chronic nonaggressive hepatitis. (III) Hb_cAg-free HB_sAg type, associated with chronic nonaggressive hepatitis. (IV) Focal HB_cAg type, associated with aggressive forms of hepatitis B. HB_cAg, full dots; HB_sAg, stippled blocks. (Reproduced from Gudat F et al: Pattern of core and surface expression in liver tissue reflects state of specific immune response in hepatitis B. Lab Invest 32:1–9, 1975, copyright US–Canadian Division of The International Academy of Pathology, with permission of *Laboratory Investigations*.)

(Figs. 4 and 8).[3] Consistent with experimental HBV infection in chimpanzees,[21] HB_cAg and HB_sAg may be demonstrated in the prenecrotic, preclinical (incubation) period.[38,56,57] The rare demonstration of some HB_cAg and of hepatocytic membrane-associated HB_sAg in the early phase of acute HB (Fig. 8) may therefore reflect ongoing elimination. At this stage, virus expression does not necessarily indicate elimination insufficiency and impending persistence. In late stages, however, this finding may be taken as a marker of possible persistence, even when histologic signs suggestive of chronicity[1,2] are not present in the biopsy.

Viral Antigens in Blood

The first evidence of HBV infection is the appearance of serum HB_sAg, followed by Dane particles, DNA polymerase, and HB_eAg.[58] HB Ag immune complexes may also be detected.[20]

Humoral Immunity

After the decline of DNA polymerase activity and coincident with the rise of the serum activities of aminotransferases, anti-HB_c is usually detected as the first marker of immunologic response (see Fig. 2 in Chapter 22),[58-61] followed by anti-HB_e. Anti-HB_s appears at variable times, sometimes as early as in the acute phase of infection, coincidently with rise in aminotransferase activities, or as late as several months after disappearance of serum HB_sAg;[58-61] during this interval, anti-HB_c and anti-HB_e may be the only marker of HBV infection.

The different biologic implications of the various humoral antibodies should be appreciated:

1. Seroconversion from HB_sAg to anti-HB_s reflects eradication of all virus-associated particles, termination of the HBV infection, and in most cases, cessation of hepatic inflammation. In some instances, however, inflammation may persist as chronic persistent hepatitis (CPH) or chronic active hepatitis (CAH) despite seroconversion (L. Bianchi, F. Gudat, unpublished observations). Anti-HB_s is assumed to have protective properties against reinfection.

2. The appearance of anti-HB_e seems to reflect specific immunologic elimination or suppression of active core replication in tissue and of Dane particles and HB_eAg in blood but not necessarily of 20-nm spherical and tubular HB_sAg particles. Anti-HB_e may therefore persist in the HB_cAg- and Dane particle-free HB_sAg carrier state (see p. 384).

3. By contrast, anti-HB_c is consistently detectable in nearly all forms of chronic HBV infection, regardless of Dane particle formation, including asymptomatic HB_cAg-free carriers, and therefore has no eliminating or protective effect. Furthermore, posthepatitic anti-HB_c may be short-lived, but anti-HB_c may also persist in HB Ag-negative persons without detectable liver disease. Anti-HB_c may provide a marker of continued HBV replication in the latter case.[38]

Cell-mediated Immunity

Cell-mediated immunity (CMI) against HB_sAg using in vitro lymphocyte transformation or macrophage inhibition tests[36,37,43,44,62] or T-cell cytotoxicity assays[45] has been demonstrated in early stages of the disease by some groups of investigators. Others, however, have found positive CMI only in late, convalescent stages.[63-66] High levels of serum HB_sAg might interfere with CMI in vitro. Furthermore, at least six serum factors interfering with in vitro lymphocyte reactivity have been described.[45,67-72] The interrelationships and the biologic significance of these factors remain to be clarified.[73] Transient CMI to a host liver-specific lipoprotein of the liver cell membrane (LSP) has also been detected in acute self-limited hepatitis (see Chapter 22).[44]

Interpretation of Findings in Acute Viral Hepatitis

Humoral and cellular immunity to HB_sAg in acute viral hepatitis may be found as early as the onset of illness and liver damage. The widespread presence of HB_cAg and HB_sAg in liver cells up to this point (i.e., during the prenecrotic, preclinical stage) may thus represent a phase of infection with viral expression and replication before the immune response is elicited (Fig. 8).[74] The absence of viral antigens from tissue at the height and in later stages of the disease may be the result of effective normergic humoral and cellular immune responses by which virus-infected cells with full viral antigen expression are eliminated by spotty necrosis, resulting in a self-limited disease. The eliminating acute hepatitis, as such, may thus be regarded as a beneficial event, and immunosuppression might prevent eradication of virus-producing cells and cause chronicity. Consequently, immunosuppressive therapy should be withheld.

Bridging hepatic necrosis in acute hepatitis may represent a special type of elimination leading to clearance of the virus and limited disease as in spotty necrotic hepatitis. If inefficient, however, persistent infection, usually with expression of the focal HB$_c$Ag type (see below) is observed. Likewise, an eliminating intralobular inflammatory bout during chronic HB may produce reduction of HB antigens from the tissue (but usually not disappearance from the blood).

Generalized HB$_c$Ag Type: Chronic Nonaggressive Hepatitis and Carrier State

Viral Antigens in Tissue and Tissue Reaction

The response to the infection in effectively immunosuppressed patients (e.g., kidney transplant recipients)[3] and in some patients without overt immune deficiency (spontaneous carriers) as well as in many children with neonatal hepatitis B[75] is not classical acute icteric hepatitis. Instead, a subclinical but chronic infection without biochemical abnormalities and hepatocytic damage, even at the electron-microscopic level (Fig. 5), consistent with a chronic carrier

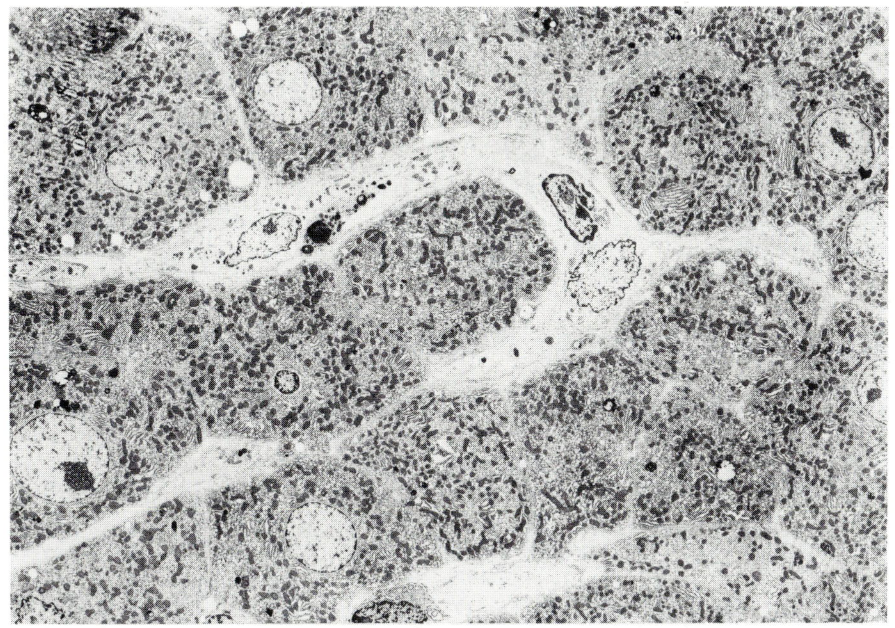

FIG. 5—Generalized HB$_c$Ag type, associated with chronic nonaggressive hepatitis in an effectively immunosuppressed kidney transplant recipient: Note lack of ultrastructural (and biochemical) hepatocellular damage despite demonstrable infection with core particles in 100% of liver cell nuclei.

state, may be found. This is accompanied by no inflammation at all or by a mild, chronic, nonaggressive inflammation, a term that in the present context includes CPH and nonspecific reactive hepatitis as well as one form of chronic lobular hepatitis[42] (Figs. 4 and 8). HB_cAg, however, is expressed in 60% to 100% of liver cell nuclei (Figs. 4 and 8, Tables 1 to 2). Cytoplasmic HB_sAg is expressed in up to 20% of liver cells. A striking honeycomblike pattern of membrane-associated HB_sAg is usually also noted (Fig. 3C and D).

This generalized HB_cAg type may develop in cancer patients and in others on long-term treatment with cytostatic and/or immunosuppressive agents.

Viral Antigens in Blood

The HB_cAg expression in tissue occurs parallel to the appearance of Dane particles in blood (Fig. 1B and C, Tables 1 to 2). The frequency of the HB_eAg in our material is 33% (Table 2) by the relatively insensitive Ouchterlony technique.

Humoral Immunity

Anti-HB_s and anti-HB_e are usually lacking, but immune complexes of the Dane particle/tubule type are found in half the cases (Table 2). In immunosuppressed patients, anti-HB_c may be lacking or present in very low titers (Table 3).

Cell-mediated Immunity

To our knowledge, CMI against HB_sAg or against liver-specific lipoprotein in effectively immunosuppressed patients exhibiting the generalized HB_cAg

TABLE 2—*Findings of HB-associated antigens and antibodies in 222 patients with chronic hepatitis B*

	HBcAg-Free HBsAg Type (n = 59)	Focal HBcAg Type (n = 142)	Generalized HBcAg Type (n = 21)*
Key Features and Additional Discriminating Features:			
HBcAg in tissue[1]	1.7%**	72.5%	100 %
Dane particles in blood (DP)[2]	10.4%**	75.9%	100 %
HBeAg[3]	0 %	21.3%	33.3%
Anti-HBe[3]	26.1%	3.8%**	0 %
Circulating immune complexes[2]	9.7%	73.5%	50 %
	(tubules only)	(DP + tubules)	(DP + tubules)
Non-discriminating Features:			
Anti-HBs[4]	0 %	10.2%	6.6%
Anti/HBc[1]	94.3%	96.8%	76.4%

*See also Table 3
[1]IF technic see ref. 3,4
[2]Immune electron microscopy see ref. 50
[3]Ouchterlony technic see ref. 27
[4]Aus-Ab (Abbott)
**Exceptional positive cases which otherwise show the typical serologic and histologic constellation of the respective type, probably representing transitional forms.

TABLE 3—*Findings of HB-associated antigens and antibodies in spontaneous and therapeutically induced generalized HBcAg type (same patients as in Table 2)*

	Generalized HBcAg Type		
	Spontaneous (n = 4)	Chemotherapy (n = 5)	Transplant Recipients (n = 12)
Key Features and Additional Discriminating Features:			
HBcAg in tissue	4/4	5/5	12/12
Dane particles in blood	4/4	2/2	12/12
HBeAg	1/4	1/3	3/8
Anti-HBe	0/4	0/3	0/8
Circulating immune complexes	3/3	1/2	5/11
Nondiscriminating Features:			
Anti-HBs	1/4	0/2	0/8
Anti-HBc	4/4	3/5	6/10*

*Low titers.
References for methods, see Table 2.

type has not been measured. It must be assumed, however, that effective therapeutic immunosuppression mainly affects cellular immunity as indicated by graft takes in transplant recipients.

The situation in spontaneous carriers of the generalized HB_cAg type is less clear. The carrier state in most studies is not defined with respect to HB_cAg- and Dane particle formation and patients of the generalized HB_cAg type are probably included in the heterogenous group of so-called asymptomatic carriers. They, like carriers without Dane particles (see later), are probably nonreactive against HB_sAg.

Interpretation of Findings in Chronic Nonaggressive Hepatitis Associated with the Generalized HB_cAg Type

In the absence of substantial humoral and cellular immunity, viral components are tolerated without detectable biochemical or electron-microscopic evidence of hepatocytic damage. This shows that HBV itself has little if any cytopathic properties. The visualization of membrane-associated HB_sAg is peculiar in such instances, since it reflects viral expression in the liver in fully developed, uninhibited form.

Generalized HB_cAg Type Without Therapeutical Immunosuppression

The generalized HB_cAg type associated with chronic nonaggressive hepatitis may occur spontaneously, mainly in two instances.

1. Neonatal hepatitis B infection, vertically transmitted from a Dane particle- and/or a DNA polymerase- and/or an HB_eAg-positive mother to her child[76] may show an identical (Fig. 6) or slightly different pattern.[75,77] The presentation of neonatal HB may be due to induction of absolute or partial immune tolerance to HBV which probably depends on the timing of trans-

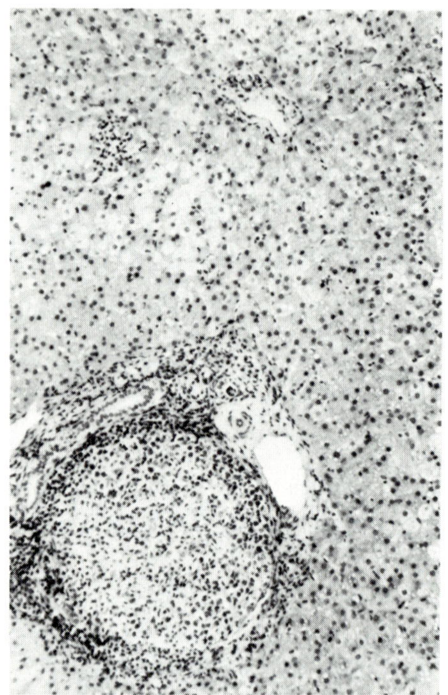

FIG. 6—Neonatal, vertically transmitted HB: generalized HB$_c$Ag type with chronic nonaggressive hepatitis. Note germinal center formation in portal tract and absence of substantial liver cell damage. (H+E stain.)

mission in the prenatal period. The inflammatory reaction and disease may vary, probably according to differences in immune responsiveness. Likewise, similar variations in the induction of immune tolerance may lead to differences in immune reactivity of the newborn.

2. Spontaneously occurring nonaggressive hepatitis of the generalized HB$_c$Ag type has been observed in the absence of any apparent immune disturbance. A specific unresponsiveness, perhaps linked to immune response and HL-A genes, may be postulated as an explanation for this and even for the other types of chronic HB. Similarities and differences between induced and spontaneous forms of the generalized HB$_c$Ag type are outlined in Figure 3.

HB$_c$Ag-free HB$_s$Ag Type: Chronic Nonaggressive Hepatitis and Carrier State

Viral Antigens in Tissue and Tissue Reaction

Abundant expression of HB$_s$Ag in up to 80% of liver cells in the absence of HB$_c$Ag from tissue (Figs. 3A and B, 4 and 8, Tables 1, 2, and 4) characterizes a second variant of chronic nonaggressive hepatitis not associated with therapy. Again, neither liver cell damage nor substantial biochemical abnormalities are noted. According to the degree of inflammation the condition may represent CPH[1,2] or, if only minor or no inflammation reaction is present, the HB$_c$Ag-free HB$_s$Ag carrier state.

TABLE 4—*Types of hepatitis and associated viral antigen expression patterns*

Acute Forms of Hepatitis	
1. Classical Acute Spotty Necrotic Hepatitis	— Elimination Type
2. Acute Hepatitis with Bridging Hepatic Necrosis	— Elimination Type
	— Focal HBcAg Type
3. Acute Hepatitis with Piecemeal Necrosis	— Focal HBcAg Type

Chronic Forms of Hepatitis	
1. Carrier	— Generalized HBcAg Type
	— HBcAg-free HBsAg Type
	— Generalized HBcAg Type
2. Chronic Persistent Hepatitis	— HBcAg-free HBsAg Type
	— Focal HBcAg Type
3. Chronic Active Hepatitis	— Focal HBcAg Type

Viral Antigens in Blood

In view of minimal HB_cAg formation, Dane particles and HB_eAg in serum are usually not detectable (Tables 1 and 2). This type of carrier is thus regarded as not very infective.

Humoral Immunity

Anti-HB_s is absent, but circulating spontaneous HB Ag complexes composed of tubular HB_sAg were detected in 9.7% of our cases (Fig. 1D; Table 2). Anti-HB_e is a marker for this carrier type. Anti-HB_c is found in virtually all cases (Tables 1 and 2).

Cell-mediated Immunity

So-called healthy carriers do not appear to have CMI to HB_sAg[36,43,46,64,66,78-82] including T-cell cytotoxicity.[45] CMI against HB_sAg was absent in the symptom-free "healthy" carrier, while in CPH of this expression type, slight inhibition of leukocyte migration by HB_sAg did occur.[46] CMI to HB_cAg and HB_eAg has not been tested.

Interpretation of Findings in the HB_cAg-free HB_sAg Carrier

A biologic explanation of this type of chronic HBV infection is not established. Lack of anti-HB_s, as well as lack of CMI against HB_sAg in vitro indicates complete immune unresponsiveness toward HB_sAg. Immune control, however, seems to be sufficiently effective to suppress or eliminate HB_cAg-expressing cells and Dane particle-associated antigens. An intact immune response toward HB_eAg and/or other Dane particle-associated antigens is an intriguing possibility for the pathogenesis of this type, since sera of these patients have anti-HB_e and Dane particle-agglutinating antibodies.

The viral genome may be assumed to be present in this HB_cAg-free HB_sAg carrier type. Evidence for this is the persistence of anti-HB_c and the unusual finding of single cores and/or Dane particles in patients of this group (Table 2). Future investigations have to pay more attention to mechanisms of viral genome expression on one side and specific immune or nonimmune repression on the other.[38]

A defective virus[83] or the influence of a helper virus[84] that might modulate the hepatitis B infection to an incomplete virus expression has also not been rigorously excluded.

Focal HB$_c$Ag Type: Aggressive Forms of Hepatitis B

Viral Antigens in Tissue and Tissue Reaction

Aggressive forms of hepatitis (e.g., CAH) are frequently associated with focal expression of HB$_c$Ag (up to 60% of liver cells), often together with membrane-associated HB$_s$Ag (Figs. 4 and 8; Tables 1, 2, and 4).[34] Cytoplasmic HB$_s$Ag is usually spotty and appears in up to 30% of hepatocytes.[3]

Inflammatory activity and the amount of HB$_c$Ag expression in liver tissue are inversely related. The more active the inflammation (i.e., with increasing efficiency of the immune response), the less the tissue expression of HB$_c$Ag and vice versa (shift to left side in Fig. 8).

Immunosuppressive therapy of CAH with piecemeal necrosis usually results in clinical improvement with decrease of the inflammatory reaction (e.g., shift from CAH to CPH). At the same time, HB$_c$Ag synthesis is better tolerated and the amount of HB$_c$Ag-expressing cells increases (shift toward the generalized HB$_c$Ag type; Fig. 8).

Focal HB$_c$Ag Type in Acute Hepatitis

This focal HB$_c$Ag type includes CAH with and without bridging hepatic necrosis (Table 4) and also certain acute forms characterized by piecemeal necrosis in the acute stage (Fig. 7),[1,2] referred to as "acute hepatitis with possible transition to chronicity." This is commonly associated with intravenous drug abuse but may occur independently, mainly in the elderly. Moreover, certain cases of acute hepatitis with bridging hepatic necrosis may be accompanied by this focal HB$_c$Ag type and these may more readily progress to CAH (Table 4).

Focal HB$_c$ Type in Chronic Nonaggressive Hepatitis

Some cases in our series of CPH are associated with the focal HB$_c$Ag type (Table 4). Progression to true CAH has been documented in half of these.

Viral Antigens in Blood

Concomitant with HB$_c$Ag expression in tissue, Dane particles (in 75.9%; Table 2), often associated with HB$_e$Ag, appear in the blood, implying high infectivity (Fig. 8).

Humoral Immunity

Anti-HB$_s$ may be detectable in up to 10% of the cases (Table 2). Furthermore, the aggressive focal HB$_c$Ag type carries the highest incidence of spontaneous immune complexes of the Dane particle/tubule type (73.5%; Fig. 1C). Anti-HB$_e$ appears rarely, but anti-HB$_c$ is regularly found, often in very high

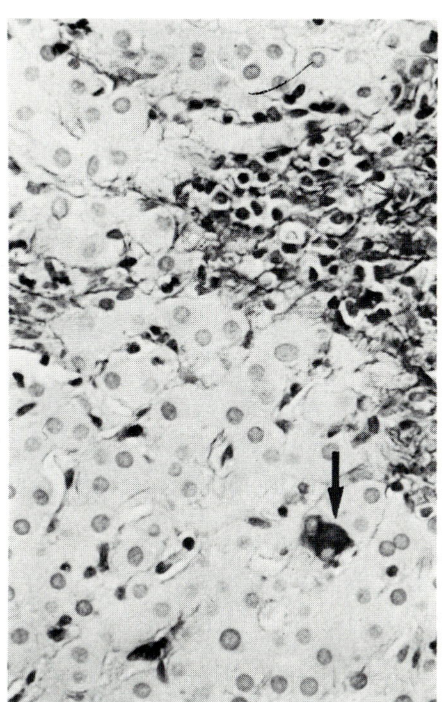

FIG. 7—Acute spotty necrotic hepatitis with piecemeal necrosis in an intravenous drug user (acute hepatitis with possible transition to chronicity). Note orcein-positive HB$_s$Ag-ion-containing hepatocyte (arrow) as part of a focal HB$_c$Ag type. (Orcein stain.)

titers.[85] Anti-HB$_c$ titers above $1:2^{12}$ by indirect immunofluorescence technique are highly indicative of chronic active hepatitis.[50]

Cell-mediated Immunity

Measurements of CMI to HB$_s$Ag in this type are controversial. Positive and negative CMI has been reported.[36,43,45,62,79,82,86,87] CMI against HB$_s$Ag was found in 80% of untreated CAH, whereas in treated cases, tests were positive only in 59%.[86] In vitro CMI to a liver-specific protein[88] was detected in 67% of HB$_s$Ag- or anti-HB$_s$-positive CAH and in 42% of cases without HB$_s$Ag or anti-HB$_s$.[86]

Interpretation of Findings in the Focal HB$_c$Ag Type

Persistence of HB$_c$Ag and membrane-associated HB$_s$Ag in tissue and findings of humoral and cellular immunity indicate that specific immunization to viral antigens is present but insufficient to eliminate the antigens. Therefore, there is continuous elimination of some but not all virus-containing cells, allowing the virus to propagate. This may explain chronicity and aggressive destruction of liver tissue.[74]

THE FOUR BASIC REACTION TYPES IN A DYNAMIC MODEL OF HEPATITIS B

If we envisage chronic hepatitis B to be the result of immune deficiency in which the expression of viral antigens is a function of insufficient elimination, a schematic diagram of HB integrating all four reaction types, as shown in Fig. 8, may be obtained. Taking the amount of detectable HB$_c$Ag in tissue as a

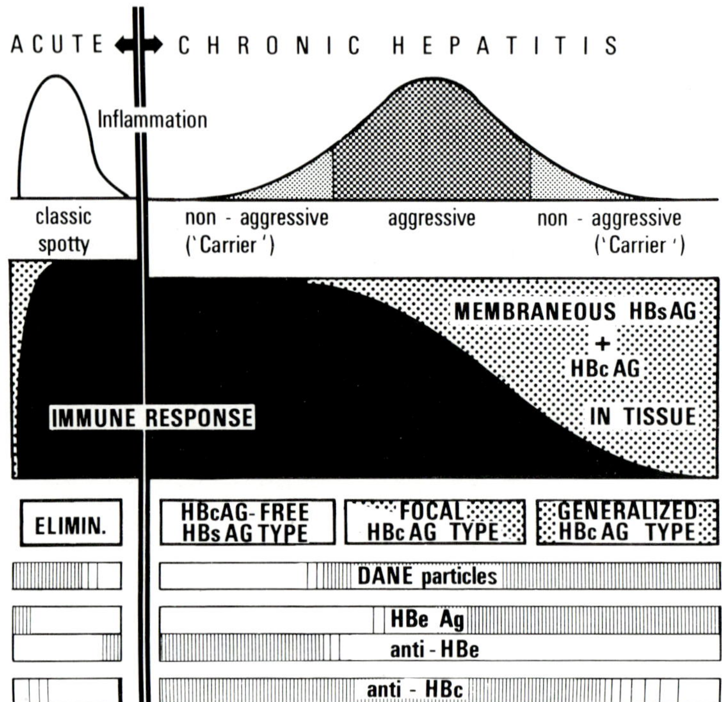

FIG. 8—Hypothetical scheme of the four basic reaction types in a dynamic model of HB. Section A: type and severity of inflammatory reaction. Section B: extent of nuclear HB$_c$Ag and membrane-associated HB$_s$Ag in relation to efficiency of the immune response. Section C: integration of the four basic viral expression types. Section D: HB-associated antigens and antibodies in blood. Type-associated findings are read vertically and may shift in either direction if immune response changes spontaneously or is therapeutically induced.

measure for the postulated immune insufficiency, the three types of chronic HB group into two extremes that have in common nonaggressive inflammation but differ fundamentally in Dane particle formation and associated markers. CAH lies in between with the greatest inflammatory reaction.

The four reaction patterns described, however, are not sharply delineated disease entities but rather characteristic types that imperceptibly merge into each other. Transitions may occur. Application and withdrawal of immunosuppressive agents result in simultaneous transition of both histologic findings and viral expression pattern. Occasional overlaps in a given biopsy specimen do not militate against such a dynamic system.

REFERENCES

1. Bianchi L, De Groote J, Desmet VJ, Gedigk P, Korb G, Popper H, Poulsen H, Scheuer PJ, Schmid M, Thaler H, Wepler W: Morphological criteria in viral hepatitis. Lancet 1:333–337, 1971.

2. Bianchi L, De Groote J, Desmet VJ, Gedigk P, Korb G, Popper H, Poulsen H, Scheuer PJ, Schmid M, Thaler H: Acute and chronic hepatitis revisited. Lancet 2:914–919, 1977

3. Gudat F, Bianchi L, Sonnabend W, Thiel G, Aenishaenslin W, Stalder GA: Pattern of core and surface expression in liver tissue reflects state of specific immune response in hepatitis B. Lab Invest 32:1–9, 1975

4. Gudat F, Bianchi L, Finch M, Krey G, Endo Y: Nuclear fluorescence of liver cells for IgG in viral hepatitis B: Significance and relation to hepatitis B-core and anti-hepatitis B-core formation. Klin Wochenschr 55:329–336, 1977

5. Almeida JD, Rubenstein D, Stott EJ: New antigen-antibody system in Australia-antigen-positive hepatitis. Lancet 2:1225–1227, 1971

6. Dane DS, Cameron CH, Briggs M: Virus-like particles in serum of patients with Australia-antigen associated hepatitis. Lancet 1:695–698, 1970

7. WHO Expert Committee on Viral Hepatitis: Advances in viral hepatitis. WHO Technical Report Series 602. Geneva, World Health Organization 1977

8. Kaplan PM, Gerin JL, Alter HJ: Hepatitis B-specific DNA polymerase activity during post-transfusion hepatitis. Nature 249: 762–764, 1974

9. Robinson WS, Greenman RL: DNA polymerase in the core of the human hepatitis B virus candidate. J Virol 13:1231–1236, 1974

10. Hirschman SZ, Gerber M, Garfinkel E: DNA purified from naked intranuclear particles of human liver infected with hepatitis B virus. Nature 251:540–542, 1974

11. Robinson WS, Clayton DA, Greenman RL: DNA of a human hepatitis B virus candidate. J Virol 14:384–391, 1974

12. Magnius LO, Espmark JA: New specificities in Australia antigen positive sera distinct from the Le Bouvier determinants. J Immunol 109:1017–1021, 1972

13. Neurath AR, Trepo C, Chen M, Prince AM: Identification of additional antigenic sites on Dane particles and the tubular forms of hepatitis B surface antigen. J Gen Virol 30:277–285, 1976

14. Trepo C, Vitvitski L, Neurath R, Hashimoto N, Schaefer R, Nemoz G, Prince AM: Detection of e antigen by immunofluorescence in cytoplasm of hepatocytes of HB$_s$Ag carriers. Lancet 1:486, 1976

15. Lam KC, Tong MJ, Rakela J: Release of e antigen from a Dane particle-rich preparation of hepatitis B virus. Infect Immun 16:403–404, 1977

16. Hirschman SZ: Integrator enzyme hypothesis for replication of hepatitis-B virus. Lancet 2:436–438, 1975

17. Neurath AR, Strick N: Host specificity of a serum marker for hepatitis B: Evidence that "e antigen" has the properties of an immunoglobulin. Proc Natl Acad Sci USA 74:1702–1706, 1977

18. Vyas GN, Peterson DL, Townsend RM: Hepatitis B "e" antigen: An apparent association with lactate dehydrogenase isozyme-5. Science 198:1068–1070, 1977

19. Norkrans G, Magnius L, Iwarson S: e Antigen in acute hepatitis B. Br Med J 1:740–742, 1976

20. Almeida JD, Waterson AP: Immune complexes in hepatitis. Lancet 2:983–986, 1969

21. Barker LF, Chisari FV, McGrath PP, Dalgard DW, Kirschstein RL, Almeida JD, Edgington TS, Sharp DG, Peterson MR: Transmission of type B viral hepatitis to chimpanzees. J Infect Dis 127:648–662, 1973

22. Ray MB, Desmet VJ, Bradburne AF, Desmyter J, Fevery J, De Groote J: Differential distribution of hepatitis B surface antigen and hepatitis B core antigen in the liver of hepatitis B patients. Gastroenterology 71:462–469, 1976

23. Nowoslawski A, Brzosko WJ, Madalinski K, Krawczynski K: Cellular localisation of Australia antigen in the liver of patients with lymphoproliferative disorders. Lancet 1:494–498, 1970

24. Huang S: Hepatitis-associated antigen hepatitis: An electron microscopic study of virus-like particles in liver cells. Am J Pathol 64:483–500, 1971

24a. Yamada G, Nakane PK: Hepatitis B core and surface antigens in liver tissue. Lab Invest 36:649–659, 1977

25. Huang SN, Millman I, O'Connell A, Aronoff A, Gault H, Blumberg BS: Virus-like

particles in Australia-antigen-associated hepatitis: An immunoelectron microscopic study of human liver. Am J Pathol 67:453–470, 1972

26. Bianchi L, Gudat F: Sanded nuclei in hepatitis B. Lab Invest 35:1–5, 1976

27. Gudat F, Bianchi L: Evidence for phasic sequences in nuclear HB$_c$Ag formation and cell membrane-directed flow of core particles in chronic hepatitis B. Gastroenterology 73:1194–1197, 1977

28. Hadziyannis S, Vissoulis C, Moussouros A, Afroudakis A: Cytoplasmic localisation of Australia antigen in the liver. Lancet 1:976–979, 1972

29. Hadziyannis S, Gerber MA, Vissoulis C, Popper H: Cytoplasmic hepatitis B antigen in ''ground-glass' hepatocytes of carriers. Arch Pathol 96:327–330, 1973

30. Huang SN: Immunohistochemical demonstration of hepatitis B core and surface antigens in paraffin sections. Lab Invest 33:88–95, 1975

31. Stein O, Fainaru M, Stein Y: Visualization of virus-like particles in endoplasmic reticulum of hepatocytes of Australia antigen carriers. Lab Invest 26:262–269, 1972

32. Shikata, T, Uzawa T, Yoshiwara N, Akatsuka T, Yamazaki S: Staining methods of Australia antigen in paraffin section. Detection of cytoplasmic inclusion bodies. Jpn J Exp Med 44:25–36, 1974

33. Ray MB, Desmet VJ, Fevery J, De Groote J, Bradburne, AF, Desmyter J: Distribution patterns of hepatitis B surface antigen (HB$_s$Ag) in the liver of hepatitis patients. J Clin Pathol 29:94–100, 1976

34. Gudat F, Bianchi L: HB$_s$Ag: A target antigen on the liver cell? Edited by H Popper, L Bianchi, and W Reutter: Membrane Alterations as Basis of Liver Injury. Lancaster, MTP Press, 1977, pp 171–178

35. Arnold W, Nielsen JO, Hardt F, Meyer zum Bueschenfelde KH: Localization of e-antigen in nuclei of hepatocytes in HB$_s$Ag-positive liver disease. Gut 19:994–996, 1977

36. Dudley FJ, Giustino V, Sherlock S: Cell-mediated immunity in patients positive for hepatitis-associated antigen. Br Med J 4:754–756, 1972

37. Eddleston ALWF: Aetiological factors in immune-mediated liver disease. Edited by A Ferguson and RNM MacSween: Immunological Aspects of the Liver and Gastrointestinal Tract. Lancaster, MTP Press, 1976, pp 291–317

38. Edgington TS, Chisari FV: Immunological aspects of hepatitis B virus infection. Am J Med Sci 270:213–227, 1975

39. Paronetto F: Immune mechanism in liver disease. Edited by A Ferguson and RNM MacSween: Immunological Aspects of the Liver and Gastrointestinal Tract. Lancaster, MTP Press, 1976, pp 319–343

40. Peterson JM, Dienstag JL, Purcell RH: Immune response to hepatitis viruses. Edited by AL Notkins: Viral immunology and immunopathology. New York, Academic Press, 1975, pp 213–235

41. Popper H: Clinical pathologic correlation in viral hepatitis: The effect of the virus on the liver. Am J Pathol 81:609–628, 1975

42. Popper H, Schaffner F: Chronic hepatitis. Taxonomic, etiologic and therapeutic problems. Edited by H Popper and F Schaffner: Progress in Liver Diseases. Vol. V. New York, Grune & Stratton, 1976, pp 531–558

43. Irwin GR Jr, Hierholzer WJ Jr, Cimis R, McCollum RW: Delayed hypersensitivity in hepatitis B: Clinical correlates of in vitro production of migration inhibition factor. J Infect Dis 130:580–587, 1974

44. Lee WM, Reed WD, Osman CG, Vahrman J, Zuckerman AJ, Eddleston ALWF, Williams R: Immune responses to the hepatitis B surface antigen and liver-specific liproprotein in acute type B hepatitis. Gut 18:250–257, 1977

45. El Sheikh N, Osman CG, Cullens H, Eddleston ALWF, Williams R: T lymphocyte-mediated cytotoxicity in HB$_s$Ag-positive liver disease. Clin Exp Immunol 31:150–157, 1978

46. Frei PC: Mécanismes immunitaires dans l'hépatite B. Aspects nouveaux et conséquences pratiques. Schweiz med Wochenschr 107:510–514, 1977

47. Kohler PF, Trembath J, Merrill DA: Immunotherapy with antibodh, lymphocytes and transfer factor in chronic hepatitis B. Clin Immunol Immunopathol 2:465–471, 1974

48. Reed WD, Eddleston ALWF, Cullens H, et al: Infusion of hepatitis-B antibody in antigen positive active chronic hepatitis. Lancet 2:1347–1351, 1973

49. Alberti A, Realdi G, Tremolada F, Spina GP: Liver cell surface localization of hepatitis B antigen and of immunoglobulins in acute and chronic hepatitis and in liver cirrhosis. Clin Exp Immunol 25:396–402, 1976

50. Endo Y, Gudat F, Bianchi L, Mihatsch M,

Gasser M, Stalder GA, Schmid M: Anti-HBc im Rahmen der Hepatitis-B-Virusinfektion: Korrelationen zu Entzündungsform und Virusexpression. Schweiz med Wochenschr 108:363–373, 1978

51. Good RA, Page AR: Fatal complications of virus hepatitis in two patients with agammaglobulinemia. Am J Med 29:804–810, 1960

52. Gelfand SG: Case report: Agammaglobulinemia associated with Australia-antigen-positive chronic active hepatitis. Postgrad Med 55:263–264, 1974

53. Tong MJ, Nies, KM, Redeker AG: Rapid progression of chronic active type B hepatitis in a patient with hypogammaglobulinemia. Gastroenterology 73:1418–1421, 1977

54. Jain S, Thomas HC, Sherlock S: Transfer factor in the attempted treatment of patients with HB$_s$Ag-positive chronic liver disease. Clin Exp Immunol 30:10–15, 1977

55. De Cree J, Verhaegen H, De Cock W, Brugmans J: The effect of levamisole on the immunologic response of HBAg positive patients. Digestion 10:306, 1974

56. Dienstag JL, Popper H, Purcell RH: The pathology of viral hepatitis types A and B in chimpanzees: A comparison. Am J Pathol 85:131–148, 1976

57. Arnold W, Meyer zum Bueschenfelde KH, Hess G, Knolle J: The diagnostic significance of intrahepatocellular hepatitis-B-surface-antigen (HB$_s$Ag), hepatitis-B-core-antigen (HB$_c$Ag) and IgG for the classification of inflammatory liver diseases. Klin Wochenschr 53:1069–1074, 1975

58. Krugman S, Hoofnagle JH, Gerety RJ, Kaplan PM, Gerin JL: Viral hepatitis, type B. DNA polymerase activity and antibody to hepatitis B core antigen. N Engl J Med 290:1331–1335, 1974

59. Bradley DW, Maynard JE, Bergquist KR, Krushak DH: Hepatitis B and serum DNA polymerase activities in chimpanzees. Nature 251:356–357, 1974

60. Hoofnagle JH, Gerety RJ, Barker LF: Antibody to hepatitis B core antigen. Am J Med Sci 270:179–187, 1975

61. Deinhardt F: Epidemiology and mode of transmission of viral hepatitis A and B. Am J Clin Path 65:890–897, 1976

62. Warnatz H: Immune reactions to hepatitis B antigen in acute and chronic hepatitis. Acta Hepatogastroent 21:237–244, 1974

63. Frei PC, Erard P, Zinkernagel R: Cell-mediated immunity to hepatitis-associated antigen (HAA) demonstrated by leukocyte migration test during and after acute B hepatitis. Biomedicine 19:379–383, 1973

64. Erard P: Technical study of the leukocyte migration inhibition test in agarose. Clin Exp Immunol 18:439–448, 1974

65. Reed WD, Mitchell CG, Eddleston ALWF, Lee WM, Williams R, Zuckerman AJ: Exposure and immunity to hepatitis-B virus in a liver unit. Lancet 1:581–583, 1974

66. Ibrahim AB, Vyas, GN, Perkins HA: Immune response to hepatitis B surface antigen. Infect Immun 11:137–141, 1975

67. Newberry UM, Shorey JW, Sanford JP, Combes B: Depression of lymphocyte reactivity to phythemagglutinin by serum from patients with liver disease. Cell Immunol 6:87–97, 1973

68. Schumacher K, Maerker-Alzer G, Wehmer U: A lymphocyte-inhibiting factor isolated from normal human liver. Nature 251:655–656, 1974

69. Chisari FV, Edgington TS: Lymphocyte E rosette inhibitory factor: a regulatory serum lipoprotein. J Exp Med 142:1092–1107, 1975

70. Wands JR, Perrotto JL, Alpert E, Isselbacher KJ: Cell-mediated immunity in acute and chronic hepatitis. J Clin Invest 55:921–929, 1975

71. Brattig N, Berg PA: Serum inhibitory factors (SIF) in patients with acute and chronic hepatitis and their clinical significance. Clin Exp Immunol 25:40–49, 1976

72. Curtiss LK, Edgington TS: Regulatory serum lipoproteins: Regulation of lymphocyte stimulation by a species of low density lipoprotein. J Immunol 116:1452–1458, 1976

73. Chisari FV, Routenberg JA, Edgington TS: Mechanisms responsible for defective human T-lymphocyte sheep erythrocyte rosette function associated with hepatitis B virus infections. J Clin Invest 57:1227–1238, 1976

74. Bianchi L, Zimmerli-Ning M, Gudat F: Viral hepatitis. Edited by RNM MacSween, PP Anthony, PJ Scheuer: Pathology of the Liver. Edinburgh, Churchill-Livingstone (in press)

75. Schweitzer IL, Dunn AEG, Peters RL, Spears RL: Viral hepatitis B in neonates and infants. Am J Med 55:762–771, 1973

76. Schweitzer IL, Edwards VM, Brezina M: e Antigen in HB$_s$Ag carrier mothers. N Engl J Med 283:940, 1975

77. Papaevangelou G, Hoofnagle J, Kremastinou J: Transplacental transmission of

hepatitis-B virus by symptom-free chronic carrier mothers. Lancet 2:746–748, 1974

78. Laiwah YAAC: Lymphocyte transformation by Australia antigen. Lancet 2:470–471, 1971

79. Ito K, Nakagawa J, Okimoto Y, Nakano H: Chronic hepatitis migration inhibition of leukocytes in the presence of Australia antigen. N Engl J Med 286:1005, 1972

80. Laiwah YAAC, Chaudhuri AKR, Anderson JR: Lymphocyte transformation and leucocyte migration-inhibition by Australia antigen. Clin Exp Immunol 15:27–34, 1973

81. Ibrahim AB, Vyas GN, Prince AM: Studies on delayed hypersensitivity to hepatitis B antigen in chimpanzees. Clin Exp Immunol 17:311–318, 1974

82. Lee WM, Reed WD, Mitchell CG, Woolf IL, Dymock IW, Eddleston ALWF, Williams R: Cell-mediated immunity to hepatitis B surface antigen in blood donors with persistent antigenaemia. Gut 16:416–420, 1975

83. Huang AS: Defective interfering viruses. Annu Rev Microbiol 27: 101–117, 1973

84. Mims CA: Factors in the mechanism of persistence of viral infections. Prog Med Virol 18:1–14, 1974

85. Bianchi L, Gudat F, Schmid M: Semiquantitative correlations between appearance of hepatitis B-antigen components in liver and blood in various forms of hepatitis B. Edited by R Preisig, J Bircher and G Paumgartner: The Liver. Quantitative Aspects of Structure and Function. Aulendorf, Editio Cantor, 1976, pp 99–105

86. Lee WM, Reed WD, Mitchell CG, Galbraith RM, Eddleston, ALWF, Zuckerman AJ, Williams R: Cellular and humoral immunity to hepatitis-B surface antigen in active chronic hepatitis. Br Med J 1:705–708, 1975

87. De Moura MC, Vernace SJ, Paronetto F: Cell-mediated immune reactivity to hepatitis B surface antigen in liver diseases. Gastroenterology 69:310–317, 1975

88. Meyer zum Bueschenfelde KH, Knolle J, Berger J: Celluläre Immunreaktionen gegenüber homologen leberspezifischen Antigenen (HLP) bei chronischen Leberentzündungen. Klin Wochenschr 52:246–248, 1974

Chapter 21

Hepatitis B Virus-Induced Immune Complex Disease

By ADAM NOWOSŁAWSKI, M.D.

THE TERM "immune complex disease" defines lesions that result from the deposition in tissues of circulating antigen-antibody complexes.[1,2] Most of our present knowledge of the pathogenetic events that characterize immune complex disease has been obtained in studies on acute and chronic serum sickness in experimental animals.[3-7]

SERUM SICKNESS AS IMMUNE COMPLEX DISEASE

Acute Serum Sickness

Acute serum sickness is produced by a single intravenous injection of a large amount of purified foreign protein. The injected protein is cleared from the circulation in three phases: (1) in the first few days its level drops as a result of the equilibration with the extravascular space; (2) it then declines slowly for several days, reflecting the catabolism of the antigen; and (3) the antigen rapidly disappears subsequent to its combination with antibody (the immune phase of antigen elimination). Increasing amounts of antigen-antibody complexes are formed in the circulation accompanied by a fall in the complement levels. It is in this last phase that lesions develop in the renal glomeruli, arteries, joints, and heart. Renal glomeruli swell and endothelial and mesangial cells proliferate with little or no plasma, cellular, and leukocytic exudation. Granular deposits of antigen, antibody, and the third component of complement (C3) are identified by immunofluorescence in a discontinuous linear pattern along the glomerular capillaries. This characteristic pattern has been accepted as a hallmark of immune complex disease. The glomerular lesions are completely reversible and undergo resolution coincident with the appearance of free antibody in the serum. Focal lesions that occur most frequently in medium-sized arteries of the heart, kidney, pancreas, and mesentery include segmental or diffuse fibrinoid necrosis of the media with fragmentation or loss of the internal elastic lamina, endothelial hyperplasia, and a diffuse infiltration by polymorphonuclear leukocytes. Globular and granular deposits of antigen, immunoglobulin, and complement can be detected in the subintimal areas for a short period of

From the Department of Immunopathology, National Institute of Hygiene, Warsaw, Poland.

The original work was supported by the MR-12 program of the Ministry of Health and Social Welfare and by a research grant from the Center for Disease Control, Atlanta, Georgia.

393

time only. Lesions occurring simultaneously in the heart and joints are characterized by mononuclear cell infiltrations of the endocardium and synovial membranes.

Chronic Serum Sickness

Chronic serum sickness is produced in experimental animals by daily intravenous injections of antigen in small amounts that are adjusted according to the antibody response, allowing for formation of circulating immune complexes in antigen excess.[4,6] Depending on the level of antibody response, various forms of chronic, often fatal, glomerulonephritis develop. These include transient acute, serum-sickness-like glomerulonephritis in animals with high-level antibody response and a wide spectrum of chronic diffuse glomerulonephritides, including membranous, membranous and proliferative, and mild mesangial proliferative in animals with intermediate or low-level antibody response. The animals that do not respond to the antigen by antibody production do not develop glomerulonephritis. Contrary to the acute serum sickness model, arterial lesions do not occur in these animals. However, a significant increase in the daily antigen dose aimed at increasing the levels of circulating immune complexes results in a simultaneous occurrence of necrotizing, acute, healing and healed lesions in arteries.[1,6,8] Large, coalescent, lumpy and granular deposits of antigen, immunoglobulins, and complement are identified by immunofluorescence along the glomerular capillaries. By electron microscopy, massive electron-dense deposits are visualized within the glomerular basement membrane and under the epithelium. In these, antigen was identified by immunoelectron microscopy.[9]

Serum Sickness in Viral Infections in Animals

The pathogenic role of viral antigen-antibody immune complexes has been recognized in several naturally occurring and experimental chronic viral infections in animals. The most extensively studied include infection with lactic dehydrogenase and lymphocytic choriomeningitis viruses in mice,[10-14] Aleutian disease in mink,[15-17] and equine infectious anemia.[18] All of these diseases are characterized by a limited pathogenicity of viral replication, low-level antibody response to viral antigens, persistence of virus antigen-antibody immune complexes in the circulation, and development of tissue lesions subsequent to the deposition of these complexes. Lesion-bound deposits of viral antigen, antibody, and complement were identified in renal glomeruli, medium-sized arteries, and the choroid plexus.[19-21]

HEPATITIS B IMMUNE COMPLEXES

The immune response in infection with hepatitis type B virus (HBV) is evoked by at least two distinct antigenic components of the spherical, double-shelled Dane particle[22-25] believed to be the complete HBV[26,27] (see Chapters 20 and 22). Hepatitis B surface antigen (HB$_s$Ag) constitutes the 7-nm thick coat of this particle, whereas the other antigenic specificity of this particle, hepatitis B core antigen (HB$_c$Ag), resides within its 27-nm core. By immunofluorescence and electron microscopy, HB_sAg was identified in the cytoplasm of hepatocytes and HB_cAg in their nuclei[28-31] (Figs. 1 and 2). Recent findings by immunoelectron microscopy suggest that both HB_sAg[32] and HB_cAg[33] are synthesized in the endoplasmic reticulum of hepatocytes. Two major morphologic forms of HB_sAg occur in the circulation: the spherical particle about 20 nm in diameter and the tubular form of approximately the same width and up to several hundred nanometers in length.[25,34] Free HB_cAg particles were not detected in the serum. In the course of clinically apparent and inapparent forms of the infection with HBV, large masses of surplus HB_sAg material are produced in hepatocytes and constantly released into the circulation.

HB_sAg appears in the sera of patients with acute hepatitis in most instances 2 to 8 weeks before the onset of jaundice or abnormal levels of serum transaminases (see Fig. 2 of Chapter 22). Antigenemia persists for 1 to 12 weeks and usually disappears during convalescence,[35-37] followed by the appearance of anti-HB_s. Anti-HB_c appears in the serum 2 to 10 weeks after HB_sAg, continues with antigenemia, and remains after its disappearance. HB_s antigenemia, mostly asymptomatic, may persist for longer periods of time in about 5% of patients convalescing from acute hepatitis.[37] Frequently, however, a persistent HB_sAg carrier state may follow mild and subclinical infection.[36,38] The majority of these chronic carriers show no clinical, biochemical, or histologic evidence of the disease, although their hepatocytes contain large amounts of HB_sAg and HB_cAg.[28,39] Some patients, however, display abnormal results of liver function tests, and histologic findings varying from chronic persistent hepatitis to chronic active hepatitis and cirrhosis.[40,41]

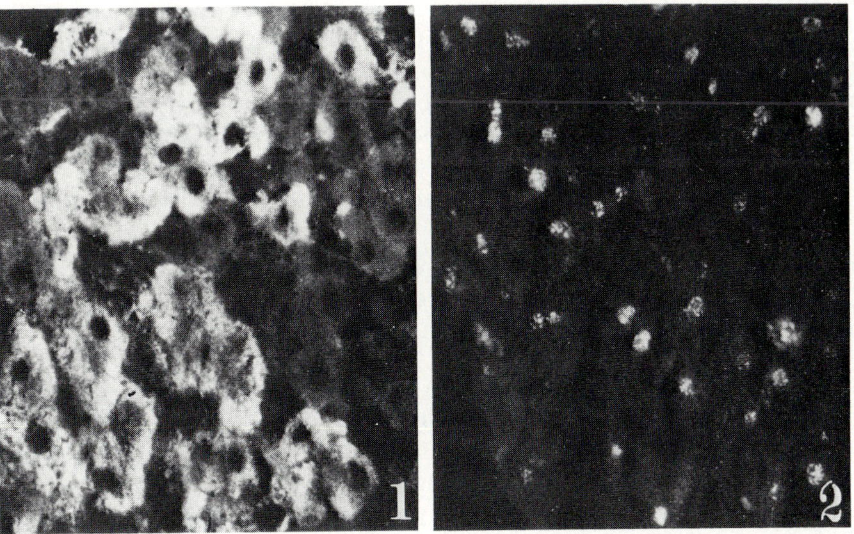

FIG. 1—Chronic active hepatitis. HB_sAg in the cytoplasm of hepatocytes ($\times$ 252). Anti-HB_s immunofluorescent reagent.

FIG. 2—Chronic active hepatitis. HB_cAg in the nuclei of hepatocytes ($\times$ 252). Anti-HB_c immunofluorescent reagent.

Types of Immune Complexes in Hepatitis B

Anticomplementary activity[42] and simultaneous occurrence of HB_sAg and anti-HB_s, apparently indicating HB_sAg immune complexes, were found in the sera of patients in the incubation period and the acute phase of hepatitis and in chronic hepatitis.[43-45] Differing features of serum HB_sAg immune complexes, revealed by immunoelectron microscopy in various forms of hepatitis, were interpreted to indicate different host responses: anti-HB_s excess in fulminant hepatitis, HB_sAg excess in chronic hepatitis, and no detectable antibody response in the chronic carrier state.[46] A distinct decrease in total complement activity and/or complement component levels was found early in acute hepatitis followed by a rise to very high levels and then a slow return to normal.[47,48]

The fall in the HB_sAg levels, in acute hepatitis coincident with the appearance of HB_sAg immune complexes and a decline in complement and complement component levels, followed by the appearance in the serum of anti-HB_s, indicates immune elimination of HB_sAg. During the prodromal stage of the disease in some patients, a serum-sickness-like syndrome is manifested by arthralgia and/or arthritis and skin rash.[47-50] Cryoproteins were detected in serum in the majority of patients with acute and chronic hepatitis type B and in chronic HB_sAg carriers. They contained both HB_sAg and anti-HB_s in most instances and occasionally contained complement (C3) and rheumatoid factor. Several of these patients had symptoms of acute and chronic serum sickness.[45] In all patients with distinct manifestations of the serum-sickness-like syndrome, that is, skin rash, severe polyarthritis, or angioedema, the isolated cryoproteins contained components of circulating immune complexes composed of IgG particularly complement-fixing subtypes IgG1 and IgG3, IgM, IgA, C3, C4, C5, HB_sAg, and anti-HB_s. The last two components were concentrated severalfold in the cryoprotein as compared to the whole serum. Moreover, anti-HB_s appeared in the complexes before it was detectable in the serum. These cryoprecipitable complexes also can activate both the classical and alternate complement pathway. These studies, showing a correlation between presence, composition, and concentration of the cryoproteins and development of the serum-sickness-like syndrome in acute hepatitis B, suggest the pathogenic potential of the circulating HB_sAg immune complexes.[51]

PATHOGENETIC ROLE OF HEPATITIS B IMMUNE COMPLEXES DEPOSITION IN LIVER

Several patterns of HB_sAg and HB_cAg localization have been described.[28,30,51,53] These suggest antigen synthesis, accumulation, and release relative to the host immune response aimed at the elimination of infected cells. The largest amounts of HB_sAg accumulating in the cytoplasm of hepatocytes in chronic asymptomatic carriers without an accompanying inflammation or hepatocytic damage indicate a low cytopathic potential of the process of HB_sAg synthesis. Most of the hepatocytes in the early phase of acute hepatitis show HB_sAg close to their surface.[29,54] At this stage, as well as in many cases of CAH, surface-bound IgG deposits were found in isolated hepatocytes that contained HB_sAg. In cases of chronic persistent hepatitis (CPH), however, the hepatocytic surface was devoid of these deposits.[55-57] Deposits of a mixture of IgG, IgM, and occasionally C3 were in the cytoplasm and nuclei of HB_sAg- and HB_cAg- containing hepatocytes, on their cell membranes, in the cytoplasm of Kupffer cells and, rarely, in the sinusoids in specimens of liver obtained by biopsy and at necropsy from patients with various forms of acute and chronic hepatitis.[29,58] IgG with anti-HB_s specificity was dissociated from these deposits by treatment with potassium thiocyanate.[58] The largest amounts of these intracellular complexes were found in fulminant hepatitis.[59] Serologic observation in fulminant hepatitis in which most patients showed unusually rapid clearance of HB_sAg, frequent coexistence of HB_sAg and anti-HB_s, and replacement by a high titer of anti-HB_s suggested that a vigorous immune elimination of HB_sAg may be involved in the pathogenesis of fulminant hepatitis.[60] Whether all these findings reflect the pathogenic mechanism of hepatocytic injury by circulating immune complexes,[61,62] an in situ immune complex formation, or an epiphenomenon[63] remains undetermined. The possibility of local in situ immune complex formation in various forms of hepatitis type B is also exemplified by the repeated finding of IgG and/or IgM and IgA in the HB_cAg-containing nuclei of hepatocytes. These IgG-HB_sAg complexes fix complement in vitro, and the IgG component could be eluted from the nuclei with buffers known to dissociate immune complexes.[64-67]

EXTRAHEPATIC HEPATITIS B IMMUNE COMPLEX DEPOSITION

Immunomorphologic studies of tissues obtained at necropsy of many patients who died from acute or chronic hepatitis or cirrhosis frequently revealed HB_sAg in several extrahepatic locations. These included, in order of decreasing frequency, germinal centers of lymph nodes and spleen (Figs. 3 and 4), blood vessel intima, and renal glomeruli.[58,59] At all these sites, deposits of HB_sAg were accompanied by a mixture of IgG, IgM, C3, and rarely IgA. All these deposits showed in vitro affinity for guinea pig complement. Germinal center activation, simple arteriolar hyalinosis or various stages of necrotizing arteritis, and diffuse glomerulonephritis of the mesangial proliferative or membranous and proliferative variety were found at the sites of these complexes.

All these data indicate that in spite of an overwhelming load of HB_sAg in the circulation, antibody response active in immune elimination of the antigen is maintained in acute and chronic hepatitis. This situation parallels that in most of the chronic viral infections in animals. The development of comparable lesions in renal glomeruli and blood vessel walls in these relatively noncytopathic infections has been attributed to the deposition of circulating immune complexes. Therefore, infection with HBV may be regarded as a potentially chronic disease with multiorgan involvement and a pronounced component of immunopathologic events. The overall pattern of these events conforms to that of experimental serum sickness of both the acute and chronic varieties and has its counterparts in several chronic viral infections in animals. HBV replication and/or production of its antigenic components in hepatocytes has apparently a limited cytopathic potential, and the course and outcome of this infection conceivably is largely determined by the variables of the host immune re-

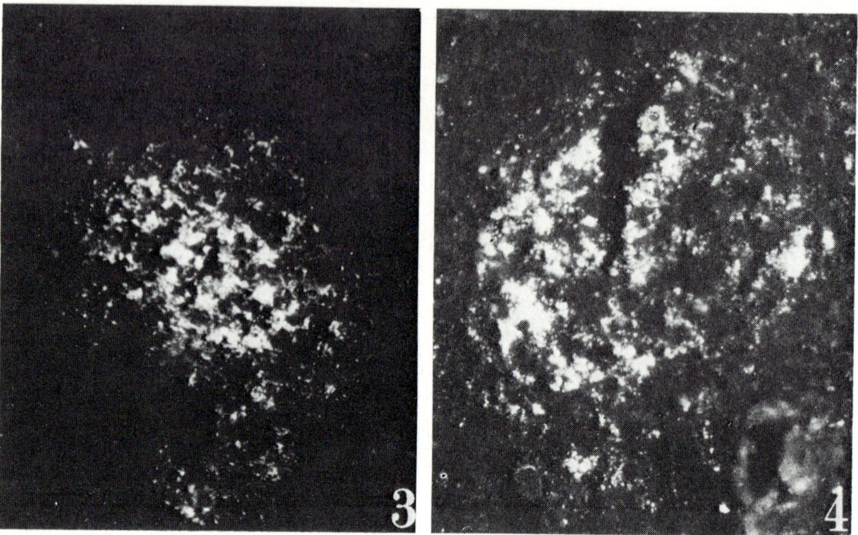

FIG. 3—Acute fulminant hepatitis. HB$_s$Ag deposit in an activated germinal center of a lymph node ($\times$ 100). Anti-HB$_s$ immunofluorescent reagent.

FIG. 4—Acute fulminant hepatitis. IgG deposits in an activated germinal center of a lymph node ($\times$ 100). Anti-IgG immunofluorescent reagent.

sponse. The spectrum of the possible forms of the host response toward the HBV antigens would be represented at one extreme by clinically inapparent infection with rapid immune elimination of the virus because of the preexisting immunity and/or low infecting dose of HBV[68,69] and on the other by an asymptomatic carrier state probably due to hyporeactivity to HBV antigens. Between the two extremes fall chronic hepatitis resulting from impaired immune response, acute self-limited hepatitis following a normal immune response, and rare acute fulminant and subacute hepatitis, both probably related to immune hyperreactivity to HBV antigens (see Chapter 22).

The formation of soluble HB$_s$Ag immune complexes in the circulation in most cases of acute hepatitis would thus be followed by their deposition at filtering sites: germinal centers of lymph nodes and spleen, blood vessel intima, the glomerular basement membrane, and most probably the synovial membrane and the choroid plexus. Subsequently, degenerative and inflammatory lesions ensue at these sites: hyaline and fibrinoid changes in blood vessel walls and membranous or proliferative lesions in renal glomeruli. In chronic hepatitis, continuous or intermittent formation of pathogenic HB$_s$AG immune complexes may be followed by a similar sequence. The trapping of these complexes at filtering sites is clinically inapparent or manifested by a transient serum-sickness-like syndrome only in most instances. Overload of HB$_s$Ag immune complexes deposited in renal glomeruli and/or blood vessel walls would ultimately lead to the lesion complex of glomerulonephritis or periarteritis in a few cases.

Glomerulonephritis

Since the first description of an HB$_s$Ag-immune-complex-mediated case of membranous glomerulonephritis in a patient with CAH,[70] several reports have appeared on the frequent association of HBV infection and glomerulonephritis. Most of these reports concerned adult patients with clinically diagnosed liver disease and superimposed signs of glomerulonephritis. In larger series of cases of glomerulonephritis in adults and children, the incidence of HB$_s$ antigenemia ranged from 6.8%[71] to 20%.[72] Immunofluorescent analysis of renal biopsy specimens, however, revealed glomerular deposits of HB$_s$Ag in 31%[73] and 34.5%[74] of similarly unselected cases that included various forms of glomerulonephritis and minimal glomerular lesions. These lumpy granular HB$_s$Ag deposits constituted an integral part of a homogenous mixture of IgG, IgM, C3, and occasionally IgA (Figs. 5 and 6) and showed a selective or predominant membranous or mesangial localization.[70,74-81] By electron microscopy, electron-dense deposits were identified in the epimembranous and/or intramembranous (Fig. 7) and mesangial localization.[70,74,77-79,81] Accumulations of spherical viruslike particles measuring 30–50 nm, particles measuring 50–100 nm, and tubular structures were detected within these deposits.[78,81] Immunoelectron microscopy confirmed the presence of amorphous masses of HB$_s$Ag within the electron-dense deposits in the glomerular basement membrane.[74] The accumulation of viruslike particles in both the glomerular basement membrane and the mesangium showed apparent concentration of HB$_s$Ag material.[78,81] The HB$_s$Ag immune complexes were not correlated with any particular form of glomerular disease. The most frequently encountered were the membranous form with usually mild to moderate glomerular cell proliferation,[70,71,74-76,78,79,81] membranoproliferative,[71,74,79,82] mesangioproliferative,[76] and apparently acute endocapillary proliferative glomerulonephritis.[74,80]

The coexisting hepatic alterations in some cases were clinically inapparent.[74]

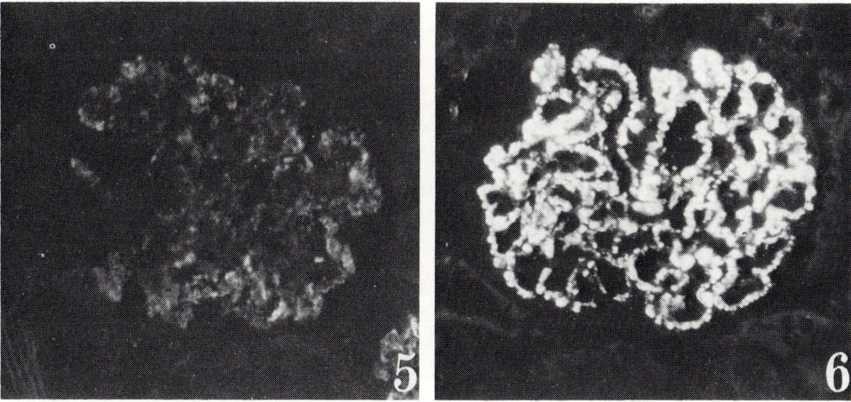

FIG. 5—Membranous glomerulonephritis. Discrete granular deposits of HB$_s$Ag along the glomerular capillaries (× 100). Anti-HB$_s$ immunofluorescent reagent.

FIG. 6—Membranous glomerulonephritis. Granular deposits of IgG along the glomerular capillaries (× 100). Immunofluorescent anti-IgG reagent.

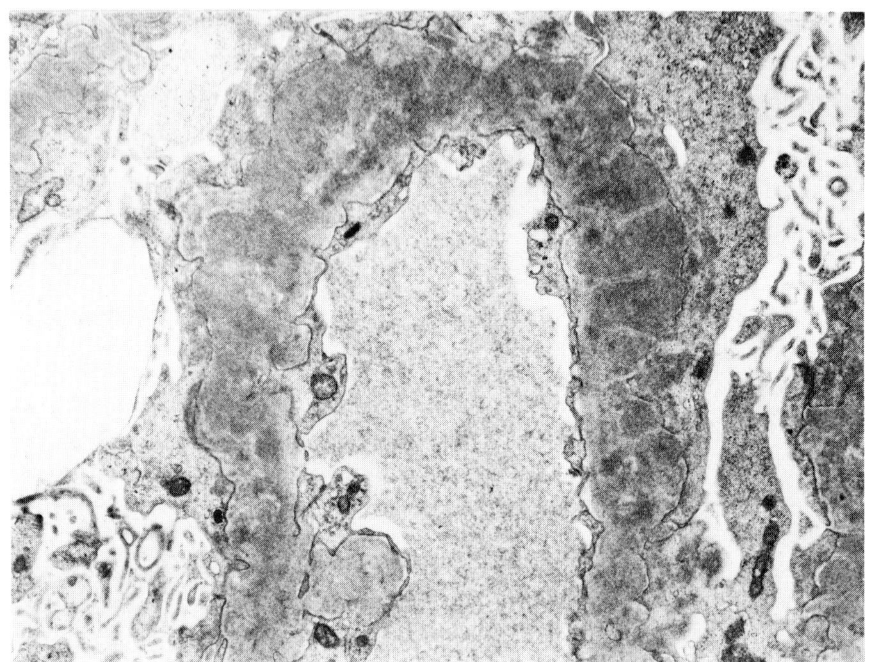

FIG. 7—Membranous glomerulonephritis. Coalescent electron-dense deposits in the glomerular basement membrane (× 12,000). Uranyl acetate and lead citrate.

In several instances, however, liver tissue obtained by biopsy or at necropsy revealed a broad spectrum of lesions, including massive hemorrhagic necrosis,[80] protracted acute hepatitis,[79] CAH,[77-79,82] CPH,[75] and cirrhosis.[76,81]

Continued production of HB_sAg was documented by protracted antigenemia in all cases and by identification of HB_sAg in the cytoplasm of hepatocytes in some.[79-81] Serum cryoprotein analysis, performed in a few instances, showed immunoglobulins, complement components, HB_sAg, and anti-HB_s, although the last could not be detected in the serum by the most sensitive methods.[78,80] Successful elution of high-titered anti-HB_s from affected glomeruli[80] provided additional evidence for the selective deposition of HB_sAg immune complexes in the glomeruli.

HB_cAg immune complexes may also participate in the pathogenesis of glomerulonephritis in children subclinically infected with HBV.[83] Deposits compatible in composition with HB_cAg immune complexes were detected by immunofluorescence and immunoelectron microscopy in about 15% of children with glomerulonephritis who were seropositive for HB_sAg and anti-HB_c. In most of these children, all with membranous glomerulonephritis, HB_cAg was the only HBV antigen detected in the glomerular deposits. Variable amounts of HB_sAg coexisted with HB_cAg in the remaining cases. By immunoelectron microscopy, HB_cAg specificity was identified within the amorphous electron-dense deposits in the glomerular basement membrane. High levels of anti-HB_c persisting in all these cases implies formation of nephritogenic HB_cAg immune complexes in an antibody-excess environment, a situation found also in Aleutian mink disease.[15-17] The source of this HB_c antigenic material remains unknown. The amorphous character of the electron-dense deposits suggests that it represents the nonparticulate HB_cAg material recently identified by immunoelectron microscopy in the nuclei and cytoplasm of hepatocytes[33] or derived from the cores of the Dane particles.

Periarteritis Nodosa

The pathogenetic role of HB_sAg immune complex deposition in blood vessel walls was suggested by the discovery of a frequent association of HB_s antigenemia with periarteritis nodosa.[84,85] In larger series of biopsy-proven cases of periarteritis nodosa, HB_sAg or anti-HB_s or both were detected with an incidence varying from 31%[86] to 69%.[87] The HB_sAg immune complex hypothesis was supported by frequent findings of circulating HB_sAg and anti-HB_s[87] and by the demonstration of HB_sAg immune complexes in the patients' sera by several methods including Clq precipitation, rate-zonal density-gradient centrifugation, and immunoelectron microscopy.[84,87,88] This hypothesis was further supported by immunofluorescent analysis of a muscle biopsy specimen that showed HB_sAg, IgM, and C3 deposits along the internal elastic lamina of the damaged arteries.[84] Similar localization of HB_sAg was encountered in a segment of a coronary artery from a patient who died in the course of lymphatic leukemia and periarteritis nodosa, although immunoglobulins were not detected.[64]

Long-term clinical studies on 9 patients with biopsy-proven periarteritis nodosa with HB_s antigenemia and on 11 additional patients without antigenemia did not provide a single clinical or laboratory criterion, except for overt signs of liver disease, if present, to differentiate these two groups of patients.[86] No correlation was found between periarteritis and liver disease. Symptoms of periarteritis occurred prior, during, and directly after acute hepatitis, but most frequently they were superimposed on CAH or CPH.[86,89]

HB_cAg in hepatocytic nuclei and HB_sAg in their cytoplasm, indicating ongoing infection with HBV, were found in all 11 unselected necropsy cases of periarteritis nodosa examined over 5 years.[90,91] The lesions in the liver varied from "minimal" to CAH. Chronic proliferative glomerulonephritis, either mesangial or endocapillary and extracapillary, with occasional focal fibrinoid necrosis of the glomerular tufts, was found in all but 1 case. Deposits of HB_sAg, IgG, IgM, and occasionally C3 were identified in the majority of these cases in the germinal centers of lymph nodes and spleen, suggesting circulating HB_sAg immune complexes. The largest amounts of these complexes were detected in the recent insudative and fibrinoid lesions in small arteries and arterioles (Figs. 8 and 9). Healing and healed lesions, both fibrotic and hyalinized (Figs. 10 and 11), contained lesser amounts or were devoid of these complexes. All these complexes showed strong in vitro affinity for guinea pig complement. Specificity of HB_sAg binding with immunoglobulins within these deposits was inferred from the results of the elution procedures that resulted in the dissociation of all HB_sAg from the lesion-bound immunoglobulins after treatment with solutions dissociating immune complexes. The presence of larger masses of HB_sAg immune complexes in recent vascular lesions, their lesser amounts

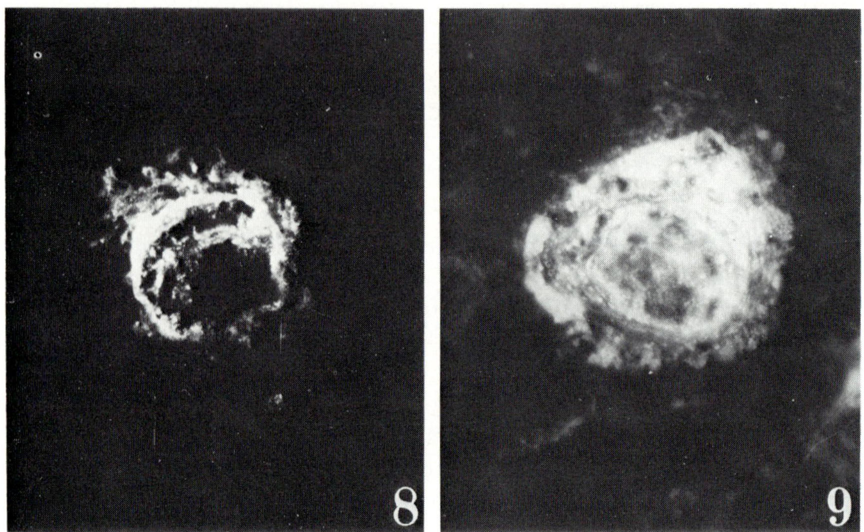

FIG. 8—Periarteritis nodosa. Large masses of HB$_s$Ag deposits in the necrotic intima and media of a small artery (× 100). Anti-HB$_s$ immunofluorescent reagent.

FIG. 9—Periarteritis nodosa. Diffuse incrustation by IgG deposits of the intima, media and adventitia of a small artery (× 100). Anti-IgG immunofluorescent reagent.

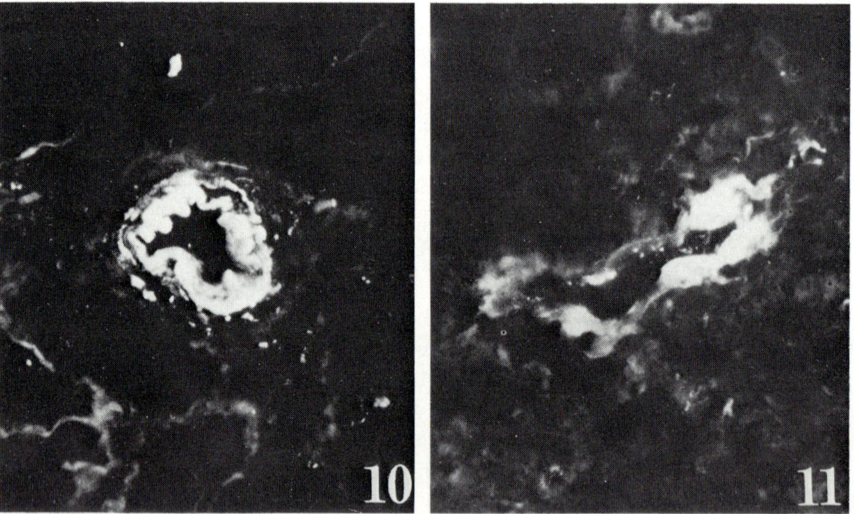

FIG. 10—Periarteritis nodosa. HB$_s$Ag in the hyaline lesions in the intima of a small artery (× 100). Anti-HB$_s$ immunofluorescent reagent.

FIG. 11—Periarteritis nodosa. IgM deposits in the hyaline lesions in the intima of a small artery (× 100). Anti-IgM fluorescent reagent.

in lesions undergoing involution, and their absence from healed lesions supported the hypothesis that the process of deposition is of primary pathogenetic significance. Furthermore, an extensive study of 55 biopsy-proven cases of periarteritis nodosa showed that the HB$_s$Ag titer might drop during exacerbation and that a dramatic clinical improvement followed by apparent recovery coincided with the clearance of serum HB_sAg and appearance of anti-HB_s.[87] Recently, circulating HB_sAg immune complexes and their changing levels were estimated by serial studies employing the Raji cell assay and antibody-dependent cell-mediated cytotoxicity (ADCC) in a patient with periarteritis nodosa. Both the serum concentration of HB_sAg immune complexes and the ADCC correlated with the disease activity.[92]

REFERENCES

1. Germuth FG Jr, Senterfit LB, Pollack AD: Immune complex disease. I. Experimental acute and chronic glomerulonephritis. Johns Hopkins Med J 120:225–234, 1967

2. McCluskey RT, Vassalli P: Serum sickness (immune complex disease). Edited by HZ Movat: Inflammation, Immunity and Hypersensitivity. New York, Harper and Row, 1971, pp 426–457

3. Germuth FG Jr: Comparative histologic and immunologic study in rabbits of induced hypersensitivity of serum sickness type. J Exp Med 97:257–269, 1953

4. Dixon FJ, Feldman JD, Vazquez JJ: Experimental glomerulonephritis: The pathogenesis of a laboratory model resembling the spectrum of human glomerulonephritis. J Exp Med 113:899–920, 1961

5. Dixon FJ: The role of antigen-antibody complexes in disease. Harvey Lect 58:21–52, 1963

6. Germuth FG Jr, Rodriguez E: Immunopathology of the Renal Glomerulus. Immune Complex Deposit and Antibasement Membrane Disease. Boston, Little, Brown and Company, 1973

7. Cochrane CG, Koffler D: Immune complex disease in experimental animals and man. Adv Immunol 16:185–264, 1973

8. Heptinstall RH, Germuth FG Jr: Experimental studies on the immunologic and histologic effects of prolonged exposure to antigen. Bull Johns Hopkins Hosp 100:71–79, 1957

9. Andres GA, Seegal BC, Hsu K, Rothenberg MS, Chapeau ML: Electron microscopic studies of experimental nephritis with ferritin-conjugated antibody: Localization of antigen-antibody complexes in rabbit glomeruli following repeated injections of bovine serum albumin. J Exp Med 117:691–704, 1963

10. Notkins A, Mahar S, Scheele C, Goffman J: Infectious virus-antibody complex in the blood of chronically infected mice. J Exp Med 124:81–97, 1966

11. Porter D, Porter H: Deposition of immune complexes in the kidneys of mice infected with lactic dehydrogenase virus. J Immunol 106:1264–1266, 1971

12. Oldstone MBA, Dixon FJ: Lactic dehydrogenase virus-induced immune complex type of glomerulonephritis. J Immunol 106:1260–1263, 1971

13. Oldstone MBA, Dixon FJ: Pathogenesis of chronic disease associated with persistent lymphocytic choriomeningitis viral infection. I. Relationship of antibody production to disease in neonatally infected mice. J Exp Med 129:483–505, 1969

14. Oldstone MBA, Dixon FJ: Immune complex disease in chronic viral infections. J Exp Med 134:32s–40s, 1971

15. Porter D, Larsen A: Aleutian disease of mink: Infectious virus-antibody complexes in the serum. Proc Soc Exp Biol Med 126:680–682, 1967

16. Porter D, Larsen A, Porter H: The pathogenesis of Aleutian disease of mink. III. Immune complex arteritis. Am J Pathol 71:331–341, 1973

17. Henson JB, Gorham JR, Padgett G, Davis W: Pathogenesis of the glomerular lesions in Aleutian disease of mink. Immunofluorescent studies. Arch Pathol 87:21–28, 1969

18. Banks K, Henson J, McGuire T: Immunologically mediated glomerulonephritis of horses. I. Pathogenesis in persistent infection by EIA virus. Lab Invest 26:701–707, 1972

19. Oldstone MBA, Lampert PW: Immune complex disease in chronic virus infection: involvement of the chorioid plexus. Adv Biosci 12:381–389, 1974

20. Oldstone MBA: Virus neutralization and virus-induced immune complex disease. PVROG Med Virol 19:84–119, 1975

21. Oldstone MBA, Dixon FJ: Immune complex disease associated with viral infections. Edited by AL Notkins: Viral Immunology and Immunopathology. New York, Academic Press, 1975, pp 341–356

22. Almeida JD, Rubenstein D, Stott EJ: New antigen-antibody system in Australia-antigen-positive hepatitis. Lancet 2:1225–1228, 1971

23. Brzosko WJ, Madaliński K, Krawczyński K, Nowosławski A: Duality of hepatitis B antigen and its antibody. I. Immunofluorescent studies. J Infect Dis 127:424–428, 1973

24. Hoofnagle JH, Gerety RJ, Barker LF: Antibody to hepatitis B virus core in man. Lancet 2:869–873, 1973

25. Dane DS, Cameron CH, Briggs M: Virus-like particles in serum of patients with Australia-antigen-associated hepatitis. Lancet 1:695–698, 1970

26. Peterson JM, Dienstag JL, Purcell RH: Immune response to hepatitis viruses. Edited by AL Notkins: Viral Immunology and Immunopathology. New York, Academic Press, 1975, pp 213–235

27. Zuckerman AJ: Hepatitis B: Nature of the virus and prospects for vaccine development. Edited by H Popper and F Schaffner: Progess in Liver Diseases. Vol. V. New York, Grune & Stratton, 1976, pp 326–336

28. Nowosławski A, Brzosko WJ, Madaliński K, Krawczyński K: Cellular localisation of Australia antigen in the liver of patients with lymphoproliferative disorders. Lancet 1:494–498, 1970

29. Edgington TS, Ritt DJ: Intrahepatic expression of serum hepatitis virus-associated antigens. J Exp Med 134:871–883, 1971

30. Huang SN: Hepatitis-associated antigen hepatitis. An electron microscopic study of virus-like particles in liver cells. Am J Pathol 64:483–500, 1971

31. Stein O, Fainaru M, Stein Y: Visualisation of virus-like particles in endoplasmic reticulum of hepatocytes of Australia antigen carriers. Lab Invest 26:262–269, 1972

32. Gerber MA, Hadziyannis S, Vissoulis C, Schaffner F, Paronetto F, Popper H: Electron microscopy and immunoelectron microscopy of cytoplasmic hepatitis B antigen in hepatocytes. Am J Pathol 75:489–502, 1974

33. Yamada G, Nakane PK: Hepatitis B core and surface antigens in liver tissue. Light and electron microscopic localization by the peroxidase-labeled antibody method. Lab Invest 36:649–659, 1977

34. Bayer ME, Blumberg BS, Werner B: Particles associated with Australia antigen in sera of patients with leukemia, Down's syndrome and hepatitis. Nature 218:1057, 1968

35. Prince AM: An antigen detected in the blood during the incubation period of serum hepatitis. Proc Natl Acad Sci USA 60:814–821, 1968

36. Giles JP, McCollum RW, Berndtson LW Jr, Krugman S: Viral hepatitis: Relationship of Australia/SH antigen to the Willowbrook MS-2 strain. N Engl J Med 281:119, 1969

37. Hoofnagle JH, Gerety RJ, Barker LF: Antibody to the hepatitis B core antigen. Am J Med Sci 270:179–187, 1975

38. Barker LF, Murray R: Acquisition of hepatitis-associated antigen. Clinical features in young adults. JAMA 216:1971–1976, 1971

39. Hanziyannis S, Moussouros A, Vissoulis CH: Cytoplasmic localization of Australia antigen in the liver. Lancet 1:976–979, 1972

40. Nielsen JP, Dietrichsen O, Elling P, Christoffersen P: Incidence and meaning of persistence of Australia antigen in patients with acute hepatitis: Development of chronic hepatitis. N Engl J Med 285:1157–1160, 1971

41. Reinicke V, Dybkjaer E, Poulsen H, Banke O, Lyllof K, Nordenfelt E: Transmission of hepatitis: Role of liver disease in Australia antigen-positive donors. N Engl J Med 286:867–870, 1972

42. Shulman NR, Barker LF: Virus-like antigen, antibody and antigen-antibody complexes in hepatitis measured by complement fixation. Science 165:304–306, 1969

43. Walsh RH, Yalow R, Berson SA: Detection of Australia antigen and antibody by means of radioimmunoassay techniques. J Infect Dis 121:550–554, 1970

44. Coller J, Millman I, Halbherr TC, Blumberg BS: Radioimmunoprecipitation assay for Au antigen, antibody and antigen-antibody complexes. Proc Soc Exp Biol Med 138:249–257, 1971

45. McIntosh RM, Koss MN, Gocke DJ: The nature and incidence of cryoproteins in hepatitis B antigen/HB$_s$Ag/positive patients. Q J Med 45:23–38, 1976

46. Almeida JD, Waterson AP: Immune complexes in hepatitis. Lancet 2:983–986, 1969

47. Alpert E, Isselbacher KJ, Schur PH: The

pathogenesis of arthritis associated with viral hepatitis: complement component studies. N Engl J Med 285:185–189, 1971

48. Kosmidis JC, Leader-Williams LK: Complement levels in acute infectious hepatitis and serum hepatitis. Clin Exp Immunol 11:31–35, 1972

49. Alacron GS, Townes AS: Arthritis in viral hepatitis. Report of two cases and review of the literature. Johns Hopkins Med J 132:1–15, 1973

50. Shumaker JB, Goldfinger SE, Alpert E, Isselbacher KJ: Arthritis and rash. Clues to anicteric viral hepatitis. Arch Intern Med 133:483–485, 1974

51. Wands IR, Mann E, Alpert E, Isselbacher KJ: The pathogenesis of arthritis associated with acute hepatitis B surface antigen-positive hepatitis. Complement activation and characterization of circulating immune complexes. J Clin Invest 55:930–936, 1975

52. Krawczyński K, Nazarewicz T, Brzosko WJ, Nowosławski A: Cellular localization of hepatitis-associated antigen in livers of patients with different forms of hepatitis. J Infect Dis 126:372–377, 1972

53. Gudat F, Bianchi L, Sonnabend W, Thiel G,. Aenishaenslin W, Stadler GA: Pattern of core and surface expression in liver tissue reflects state of specific immune response in hepatitis B. Lab Invest 32:1–9, 1975

54. Edgington TS, Chisari FV: Immunological aspects of hepatitis B virus infection. Am J Med Sci 270:213–227, 1975

55. Hopf U, Arnold W, Meyer zum Büschenfelde KH, Forster F, Bolte JP: Studies on the pathogenesis of chronic inflammatory liver diseases: Membrane-fixed IgG on isolated lymphocytes from patients. Clin Exp Immunol 22:1–8, 1975

56. Arnold W, Meyer zum Büschenfelde KK, Hess G, Knolle J: The diagnostic significance of intrahepacellular hepatitis-B-surface antigen (HB$_s$Ag), hepatitis-B-core-antigen (HB$_c$Ag) and IgG for the classification of inflammatory liver disease. Studies on the HB$_s$Ag-positive and negative patients. Klin Wochenschr 53:1069–1074, 1975

57. Alberti A, Realdi G, Tremolada F, Spina GP: Liver cell surface localization of hepatitis B antigen and of immunoglobulins in acute and chronic hepatitis and in liver cirrhosis. Clin Exp Immunol 25:396–402, 1976

58. Nowosławski A, Krawczyński K, Brzosko W, Madaliński K: Tissue localization of Australia antigen immune complexes in acute and chronic hepatitis and liver cirrhosis. Am J Pathol 68:31–55, 1972

59. Nowosławski A, Krawczyński K, Nazarewicz T, Ślusarczyk J: Immunopathological aspects of hepatitis type B. Am J Med Sci 270:229–239, 1975

60. Trepo CG, Robert D, Motin J, Trepo D, Sepetjian M, Prince AM: Hepatitis B antigen (HB$_s$Ag) and/or antibodies (anti-HB$_s$ and anti-HB$_c$) in fulminant hepatitis: Pathogenic and prognostic significance. Gut 17:10–13, 1976

61. Steiner JW: Investigations of allergic liver injury. I. Light fluorescent and electron microscopic study of the effects of soluble immune aggregates. Am J Pathol 38:411–436, 1961

62. Paronetto F, Popper H: Aggravation of hepatic lesions in mice by in vivo localization of immune complexes (Auer hepatitis). Am J Pathol 47:549–563, 1965

63. Popper H: Clinical pathologic correlation in viral hepatitis. The effect of virus on liver. Am J Pathol 81:609–628, 1975

64. Gerber MA, Brodin A, Steinberg D: Periarteritis nodosa, Australia antigen and lymphatic leukemia. N Engl J Med 286:14–17, 1972

65. Kater L, van Gorp LHK, Borat-Eilers E: Hepatitis: Intrahepatic expression of Au antigen and immune complexes in liver tissue. Vox Sang 24:27–32, 1973

66. Gerber MA, Sarno E, Vernace SJ: Immune complexes in hepatocytic nuclei of HB Ag-positive chronic hepatitis. N Engl J Med 294:922–925, 1976

67. Rizzeto K, Bonino F, Diana S, Verme G: Prognostic significance of in-vitro complement fixation in liver biopsy specimens from patients with acute viral hepatitis type B. Lancet 2:436–438, 1976

68. Barker L, Murray R: Relationship of virus dose to incubation time of clinical hepatitis and the time of appearance of hepatitis associated antigen. Am J Med Sci 263:27–33, 1972

69. Krugman S, Giles JP, Hammond J: Viral hepatitis type B/MS-2 strain/: Studies on active immunization. JAMA 217:41–45, 1971

70. Combes B, Stasny P, Shorey J, Eigenbrodt EH, Barrera A, Hull AR, Carter NW; Glomerulonephritis with deposits of Australia antigen-antibody complexes in glomerular membrane. Lancet 2:234–237, 1971

71. Lagrue G, Etievant MF, Sylvestre R, Hirbec G: Antigène Australie (Ag-HB) et glomérulonéphrites. Nouv Presse Méd 3:1870–1872, 1974

72. Vos GJH, Grobbelaar BG, Milner LV: A possible relationship between persistent hepatitis B antigenaemia and renal disease in southern african Bantu. S Afr Med J 47:911–913, 1973

73. Conté JJ, Fournié GJ: Antigène Australia et glomérulonéphrites. Nouv Press Méd 4:2741– 2742, 1975

74. Brzosko WJ, Krawczyński K, Nazarewicz T, Morzycka M, Nowosławski A: Glomerulonephritis associated with hepatitis B surface antigen immune complexes in children. Lancet 2:477–481, 1974

75. Bläker F, Hellwege HH, Kramer U, Thones W: Membranous nephropathy and hepatitis-B antigen. Lancet 2:955–956, 1974

76. Batai G, Ambrus M, Paál H, Nagy J, Deák Gy: Hepatitis-B antigenemia associated with progressive cirrhosis and membranous glomerulonephritis. Lancet 1:102–103, 1975

77. Strutta P, Camussi G, Ragui R, Vercellone A: Hepatitis-B antigenemia associated with active chronic hepatitis and mesangioproliferative glomerulonephritis. Lancet 2:179, 1975

78. Kohler PF, Crouin RE, Hammond WS, Olin D, Carr RI: Chronic membranous glomerulonephritis caused by hepatitis B antigen-antibody immune complexes. Ann Intern Med 81:448–453, 1974

79. Knieser MR, Jenis EH, Lowenthal DT, Bancroft WH, Burns W, Shalhoub R: Pathogenesis of renal disease associated with viral hepatitis. Arch Pathol 97:193–200, 1974

80. Ozawa T, Levisohn P, Orsini E, McIntosh RM: Acute immune complex disease associated with hepatitis. Etiopathogenic and immunopathologic studies of the renal lesion. Arch Pathol Lab Med 100:484–486, 1976

81. Moriyama M, Fukuda Y, Ishizaki M, Sugisaki Y, Masugi Y: Membranous glomerulonephritis associated with active liver cirrhosis both involved by HB_s antigen. Acta Pathol Jpn 26:237–250, 1976

82. Myers BD, Griffel B, Naveh D, Jankielowitz T, Klajman A: Membrano-proliferative glomerulonephritis associated with persistent viral hepatitis. Am J Clin Pathol 60:222–228, 1973

83. Ślusarczyk J, Michalak T, Nazarewicz T, Krawczyński K, Nowosławski A: Glomerulonephritis associated with HB_cAg immune complexes in children. (submitted for publication)

84. Gocke DJ, Hsu K, Morgan C, Bombardieri S, Lockshin M, Christian CL: Association between polyarteritis and Australia antigen. Lancet 2:1149–1153, 1970

85. Trepo C, Thivolet J: Antigène Australien, hépatite a virus et périartérite noueuse. Nouv Presse Med 78:1557, 1970

86. Sergent JS, Lockshin MD, Christian CL, Gocke DJ: Vasculitis with hepatitis B antigenemia: Long-term observations in nine patients. Medicine 55:1–18, 1976

87. Trepo CG, Zuckerman AJ, Bird RC, Prince AM: The role of circulating hepatitis B antigen/antibody immune complexes in the pathogenesis of vascular and hepatic manifestations in polyarteritis nodosa. J Clin Pathol 27:863–868, 1974

88. Prince AM, Trepo C: Role of immune complexes involving SH antigen in pathogenesis of chronic active hepatitis and polyarteritis nodosa. Lancet 1:1309–1312, 1971

89. Martini GA, Strohmeyer G, Sodomann CP: Die Panarteriitis nodosa bei chronischer Hepatitis mit Australia-Antigen Nachweis. Dtsch Med Wochenschr 97:642–645, 1972

90. Krawczyński K, Ślusarczyk J, Brzosko WJ, Nowosławski A: Viral antigen-antibody complexes and the pathogenesis of degenerative vascular lesions. Adv Biosci 12:435–443, 1974

91. Michalak T: Immune complexes of hepatitis B surface antigen in the pathogenesis of periarteritis nodosa. Am J Pathol 90:15–28, 1978

92. Fye KH, Becker MJ, Theofilopoulos AN, Moutsopoulos H, Feldman JL, Talal N: Immune complexes in hepatitis B antigen-associated periarteritis nodosa. Detection by antibody-dependent cell-mediated cytotoxicity and the Raji cell assay. Am J Med 62:783–791, 1977

Immunologic Liver Injury: The Role of Hepatitis B Viral Antigens and Liver Membrane Antigens as Targets

By K.-H. MEYER ZUM BÜSCHENFELDE,
T.H. HÜTTEROTH, W. ARNOLD, *and* U. HOPF.

INCREASING EVIDENCE suggests that hepatic injury in acute and chronic hepatitis is mediated by immunologic mechanisms (see Chapters 20 and 21). Evidence for humoral immunity has been obtained by the study of autoantibodies occurring in chronic active hepatitis and of antibodies against the hepatitis B viral antigens in acute and chronic hepatitis. The in vivo fixation of immunoglobulins to plasma membranes of isolated human hepatocytes in acute and chronic hepatitis suggests an antibody-mediated cytotoxicity. Cellular immune reactions have been shown against antigens of the hepatitis B virus and of plasma membranes of hepatocytes. Immune reactivity of lymphocytes from patients with chronic active hepatitis (CAH) against various target cells has been reported. Finally, evidence is accumulating that the induction of autoimmune reactions in response to liver injury may be related to genetic factors. Predominantly women with CAH reflect a genetic influence on the immune response to various insults. This demonstrates the complexity by which liver damage of diverse etiology may be caused. One of the main problems is that an immune attack cannot completely be accepted as the primary event. Studies with adequate controls for all variables that may play a role in different liver diseases are lacking. This chapter summarizes the knowledge about hepatitis B viral antigens and plasma membrane antigens of hepatocytes as target antigens in immunologic liver injury.

THE PROPERTIES AND LOCALIZATION OF TARGET ANTIGENS

Hepatitis B Viral Antigens

Three antigen-antibody systems have been differentiated in individuals infected with the hepatitis B virus (HBV): the hepatitis B surface antigen (HB_sAg) system, the hepatitis B core antigen (HB_cAg) system, and the hepatitis B e antigen (HB_eAg) system.

HB_sAg circulates in three different morphologic forms in sera of HB_sAg

---

From the Free University of Berlin, Charlottenburg Clinic, Department of Internal Medicine, Berlin, Federal Republic of Germany.

carriers: as a 22-nm spherical particle, as a filamentous form 22 nm in diameter but variable in length, and as the outer shell of the 42-nm Dane particle.

HB_cAg is morphologically distinguishable as a spherical 27-nm particle. It is found in the serum as the inner core of the Dane particle. A subpopulation of the Dane particles contains within the HB_cAg circular double-stranded DNA and DNA polymerase activity.[1,2] Therefore, the complete Dane particle is regarded as the complete hepatitis B virus. The nature of HB_eAg is still unknown.[3-8] Magnius et al. described HB_eAg as a soluble protein (11S gamma globulin) with a molecular weight of about 300,000.[3] Recent studies suggested that HB_eAg might be a part of the antigenic sites of the Dane particle surface,[4] might have properties of an immunoglobulin,[5] or might be associated with lactate dehydrogenase isoenzyme-5.[7] Besides the subtypes of HB_eAg (e_1, e_2, etc.), at least two different morphologic forms of HB_eAg are in the serum: a small free circulating one with a molecular weight of about 80,000 dalton and one closely associated with IgG (300,000 dalton). There is no evidence that HB_eAg itself is an immunoglobulin (Symposium "Viral Hepatitis," San Francisco, 1978, unpublished discussion remarks). Several studies confirmed the close correlation between the HB_eAg and Dane particles in the serum.[9-13] The high infectivity of the HB_eAg-positive sera has also been documented.[14,15]

The expression of the HB_sAg and HB_cAg in hepatocytes is well established. Using the direct immunofluorescent technique, HB_sAg is frequently detectable in the cytoplasm[16,17] and HB_cAg is in the nuclei of hepatocytes.[18-21] Recent studies have clearly demonstrated intranuclear localization of HB_eAg in close association with intranuclear HB_cAg.[22] By contrast with the observations of other investigators,[23] cytoplasmatic localization was not seen.

The statements concerning expression of hepatitis antigens in the hepatocellular membrane or fixation on the surface of the plasma membranes are controversial. HB_sAg has been demonstrated on isolated hepatocytes in the hepatocellular membrane during the very early phase of acute hepatitis B.[24] Using cryostat sections other authors claimed to have localized HB_sAg to the hepatocellular membrane in HB_sAg-positive CAH and chronic persistent hepatitis (CPH).[25-27] We were not able to demonstrate HB_sAg, HB_cAg and/or HB_eAg on the surface of isolated hepatocytes derived from patients with various HB_sAg positive liver diseases or from healthy HB_sAg carriers.[13] Immunoelectron-microscopic methods might clarify these discrepancies and identify one of the hepatitis B antigens or another neoantigen as the target antigen for liver injury on the surface of hepatocytes. The most likely candidate for such a target antigen in the hepatocellular membrane is still HB_sAg.

Liver Membrane Antigens

Liver-specific Protein

The liver-specific protein (LSP) is a macrolipoprotein present on the liver cell membrane. LSP shows complete organ specificity and incomplete species specificity. It was isolated from fresh human liver by homogenization, followed by ultracentrifugation, gel filtration on Sephadex G 100 and Sephadex G 200 or Sepharose 6B.[28] Isolated LSP is unstable in most buffer systems. This hampered the early studies, since it was necessary to use freshly prepared LSP.

Recently, LSP was found to be stable in a TRIS buffer system containing 1 mM EDTA.[29] Because of its lipoprotein nature, it is difficult to determine the molecular weight by gel filtration techniques. The appearance of LSP in the void volume of a Sepharose 4B column suggests a molecular weight greater than 20×10^6 dalton.[29] The apo-LSP was excluded from Sepharose 6B but included in Sepharose 4B. This suggests a molecular weight between 4×10^6 and 20×10^6. Whether LSP is composed of different subunits or whether it is an aggregate of identical subunits is unclear.

Lipid and apoprotein moieties were partially characterized after separation on LH-20 column chromatography. Thin layer chromatography of the three Sephadex LH-20 fractions shows that LSP contains large amounts of phosphatides and triglycerides. A further analysis of the phosphatides revealed cephalin, sphingomyelin, lecithin, and lysolecithin. LSP can be subdivided into several subcomponents, when polyacrylamide gel electrophoresis (PAGE) is performed in the presence of SDS (Sodium Dodecyl Sulfate). At least five major components and several minor components can be distinguished. The antigenicity of LSP depends on its lipid content. The delipidated apoprotein of LSP will not react with an antiserum against LSP by double immunodiffusion.[30]

LSP isolated from human, rat, rabbit, and guinea pig livers by PAGE demonstrated similar mobility of the corresponding macrolipoprotein from hepatocytes of different species.[30] Using heterologous antisera against purified LSP the membrane expression and membrane specificity was demonstrated on isolated human hepatocytes.[31] The lack of species specificity of LSP, shown by immunofluorescence in previous studies,[31a] was confirmed by immunodiffusion using an anti-LSP prepared in a sheep.

Preliminary studies suggest that LSP is not a component of the surface of the hepatitis B virus (Dane particles) or its gene products HB_sAg and HB_cAg. There was no identity between LSP and HB_eAg by immune diffusion analysis. Also LSP and a HB_sAg vaccine had no antigenic relationship.[33] These data do not support the possibility that hepatitis B virus immunization in men with HB_sAg from sera of chronic carriers may produce autoimmunity related to LSP.

Liver Membrane Antigen

An antibody was detected in serum of hypergammaglobulinemic patients with HB_sAg-negative CAH, that reacts with a membrane antigen of isolated rabbit hepatocytes.[34] This antibody was called liver membrane autoantibody (LMA). Further studies confirmed that LMA is closely correlated with the autoimmune type of CAH.[35] The corresponding antigen of the LMA, called liver membrane antigen (LM Ag) is like LSP in the 100,000-g supernatant of liver homogenates, although present in lower concentrations. Both are membrane antigens. LM Ag can be separated and purified by affinity chromatography using an insolubilized serum of patients with HB_sAg-negative, LMA-positive CAH. LM Ag has been further characterized by crossed immunoelectrophoresis. The LM Ag prepared from rabbit and human soluble liver proteins revealed a sharp precipitin pattern only with LMA but not when the agar contained anti-LSP; sera from HB_sAg-positive CAH; normal human or sheep serum; and antihuman plasma protein sera (Fig. 1A). The precipitin pattern of LSP purified by Sepharose 6B chromatography differed from that of LM Ag (Fig. 1B). In tandem-crossed immunoelectrophoresis the immunologic identity of LM Ag of different species could be shown.[108] While LSP seems to be involved in the immunopathogenesis of HB$_s$Ag-negative and -positive CAH, as shown by cell-mediated immunity against LSP[36-49] and by the detection of anti-LSP in radioimmunoassay,[50] LM Ag seems to be a target antigen mainly involved in the pathogenesis of autoimmune liver disease.

HUMORAL IMMUNE REACTIONS AGAINST TARGET ANTIGENS

Hepatitis B Antigens

Figure 2 shows the humoral immune reactions against HB$_s$Ag, HB$_c$Ag, and HB$_e$Ag during the normal course of acute hepatitis B. Some of these data are preliminary and need further confirmation.

Anti-HB$_s$ occurs characteristically 5 or 6 months after the onset of the disease (seroconversion). By contrast, high titers of anti-HB$_c$ are measurable during the clinical manifestations of acute hepatitis B, and the high anti-HB$_c$

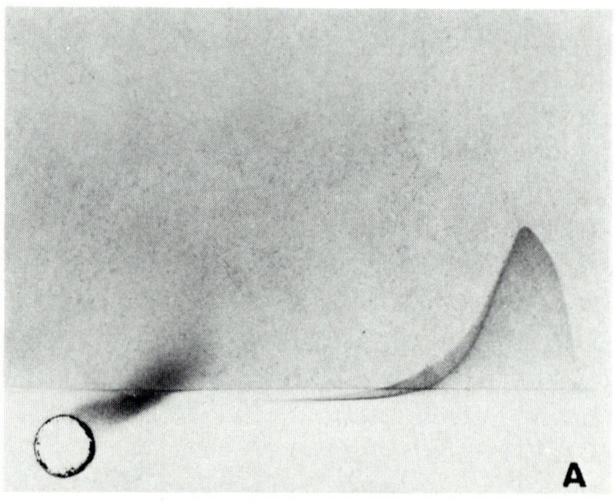

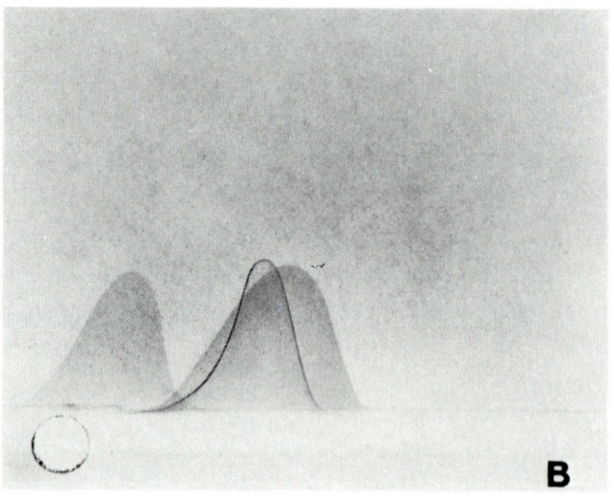

FIG. 1—(A) Lm Ag prepared by affinity chromatography of insolubilized serum of patients with LMA-positive, HB$_s$Ag-negative CAH tested against LMA serum gamma globulin in crossed immunoelectrophoresis. (B) LSP purified by Sepharose 6B chromatography tested against anti-LSP serum prepared in a sheep.

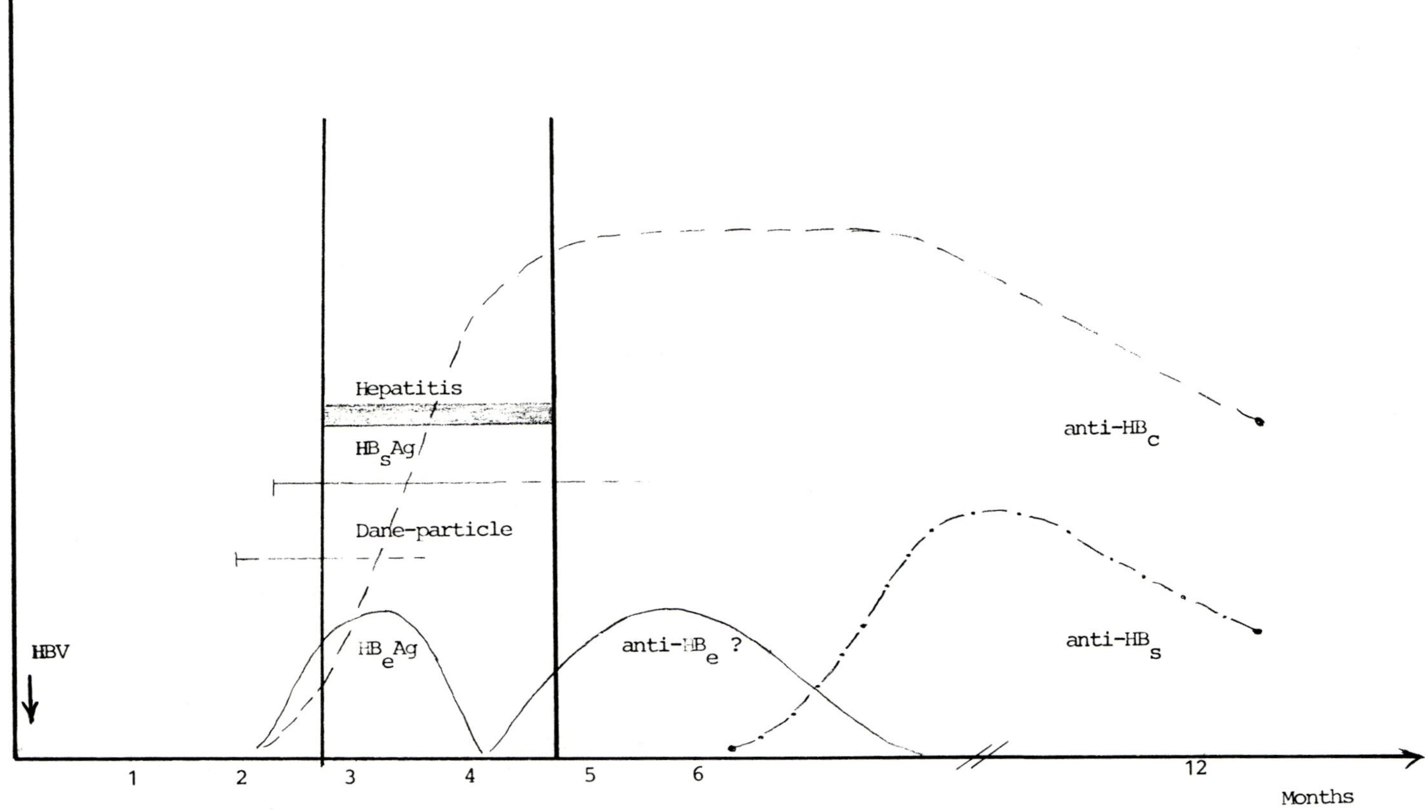

FIG. 2—Schematic representation of humoral immune reactions against hepatitis B antigen components.

411

titers might last for more than a year.[13,51] Only preliminary data are available concerning the occurrence of anti-HB$_e$ in acute hepatitis B. With a new radioimmunoassay, anti-HB$_e$ is found in low titers in the period between the clearance of HB$_s$Ag in the serum and the onset of seroconversion.[52] The characteristic findings in HB$_s$Ag-positive CAH and CPH are the extremely high titers of anti-HB$_c$ and the lack of humoral immune reactions against HB$_s$Ag and HB$_e$Ag. Longitudinal studies have shown no evidence for anti-HB$_s$ or anti-HB$_e$ production. "Healthy HB$_s$Ag carrier status"[9,12,13,53] is characterized by anti-HB$_c$ and the absence of HB$_e$Ag, DNA polymerase activity and Dane particles.[13] Table 1 summarizes the characteristic findings in this group of chronic HB$_s$Ag carriers.

Immunohistologic studies have shown, in addition, the in vivo fixation of immunoglobulins to the hepatocellular membrane in HB$_s$Ag-positive CAH and CPH.[34,58] This fixation of gamma globulin on hepatocytes is never detectable in healthy HB$_s$Ag carriers. The corresponding target antigen has not been identified. Furthermore, whether infectious antigen-antibody complexes might be fixed to the hepatocytes via C3 or Fc receptors is not settled.[55] Further discussion was raised by the detection of HB$_c$Ag/anti-HB$_c$ immune complexes in the nuclei of hepatocytes in such cases.[56,57] Whether this fixation of anti-HB$_c$ is an artifact or an in vivo fixation of this antibody is not clear.

Liver Membrane Antigens

While cell-mediated immunity against LSP has been demonstrated in various assay systems, disease-specific autoimmunity has been much more difficult to prove. Autoimmune phenomena have been well described, such as the occurrence of mitochondrial antibodies in primary biliary cirrhosis and of smooth muscle antibodies and antinuclear antibodies in most HB$_s$Ag-negative CAH.[31]

TABLE 1.—*Characteristic Findings in Chronic HB$_s$Ag Carriers*

		Healthy HB$_s$Ag Carriers	HB$_s$Ag-positive CAH or CPH
SERUM	HB$_s$Ag	+	+
	HB$_e$Ag	∅	+
	DNA polymerase	∅	+
	Dane particle	∅	+
Liver biopsy		Normal tissue	CAH/CPH
Immunohistology	HB$_s$Ag (cytoplasm)	+ +	(+)
	HB$_s$Ag (membrane)	?	+ ?
	HB$_c$Ag (nucleus)	∅	+ +
	HB$_e$Ag (nucleus)	∅	+ +
	IgG (nucleus/ membrane)	∅	+
Humoral immune	Anti-HB$_s$	∅	∅
Reactions	Anti-HB$_c$	∅ − + +	+ +
	Anti-HB$_e$	+ +	∅

None of these autoantibodies, however, is specific for a particular subgroup of liver disease or even restricted to liver disease only. To clarify these reactions, we investigated the in vitro and in vivo binding of IgG to isolated hepatocytes. The mechanical isolation of hepatocytes from rabbit liver and from human liver biopsy specimens without the use of enzymes has been described.[31a]

Isolated human hepatocytes from patients with CAH revealed two different patterns of in vivo fixed IgG, a linear one and a granular one.[34] The two patterns of IgG binding was assumed to be caused by different antibodies. In autoimmune type of CAH, the LMA is probably fixed in vivo on hepatocytes.

The search for LMA in various diseases indicates a specificity for inflammatory liver diseases.[35] LMA was found in 27 of 72 patients with HB_sAg-negative chronic active hepatitis and in 17 of 28 patients with HB_sAg-negative nonalcoholic cirrhosis.

LMA is not at all species-specific.[59] Isolated hepatocytes from mice, rats, rabbits, chicken, and sheep react with this antibody. A low percentage of binding was observed in isolated mouse and rat hepatocytes, a high percentage of binding cells was noted in man and rabbit. The membrane expression of the corresponding LM Ag appears to be restricted to the liver.

The interpretation of the granular IgG binding in HB_sAg-positive CAH is more difficult. Whether the IgG binding represents an antibody against a liver membrane component or whether IgG is bound in a different way is unclear. One explanation is binding via Fc or C3 receptors of IgG, which was demonstrated on human hepatocytes.[55] Circulating immune complexes are present in most patients with HB_sAg-positive CAH, as we could demonstrate with a modified Raji cell technique.[60] This raised the possibility that circulating immune complexes are bound to hepatocytes via Fc or C3 receptors of IgG.

A further demonstration of humoral immune reactions against liver membrane antigens is possible with Chang liver cells. Some Chang liver cell strains still express the liver-specific antigen on the cell surface but differ from human hepatocytes by the lack of Fc and C3 receptors of IgG.[61] We have employed one particular Chang liver cell line to study the IgG binding of patients with HB_sAg-positive and -negative CAH. Sera from 14 of 19 HB_sAg-positive CAH patients and from all of 7 patients with autoimmune-type CAH demonstrated fixation of IgG to Chang liver cells.[62] Normal controls showed no such binding. To further characterize the fixed antibodies, absorption studies were performed using human liver homogenate, purified LSP, and isolated rabbit hepatocytes. IgG binding to the membrane of Chang cells could be abolished completely by human liver homogenate.

Absorption studies with rabbit hepatocytes did not influence the IgG binding to Chang liver cells in either Hb_sAg-positive or autoimmune-type CAH, although the LMA activity had been absorbed completely. Absorption with purified LSP eliminated the IgG binding in HB_sAg-positive CAH, and partly did so from sera autoimmune-type CAH. The absorption studies suggest that at least two different autoantibodies are characteristic for CAH, the LMA typical for the autoimmune-type CAH and an anti-LSP autoantibody detectable in both HB_sAg-positive and -negative CAH. A radioimmunoassay has been described for the detection of circulating anti-LSP in human sera.[50] Circulating anti-LSP was found in 9 of 9 HB$_s$Ag-negative patients and in 8 of 9 HB$_s$Ag-positive patients with CAH. Patients with CPH had positive titers in 8 of 13 cases, usually at a lower titer than in CAH.

The Role of Immune Complexes and Receptors in Liver Injury

Antigenic substrates and immune complexes originating from the gastrointestinal tract are retained and altered by the normal liver[63-71] (see Chapter 17). The hepatic clearance function in patients with chronic liver disease may be reduced and antibodies formed against bacterial and dietary antigens.[72-74] The clearance activity of the liver has been attributed to the Kupffer cells as a part of the reticuloendothelial system (see Chapter 8). However the demonstrated receptors for IgG Fc and C3,[55] as well as for oligomeric IgA,[75] on isolated hepatocytes suggest involvement of the hepatocytes in the physiologic clearance of immune complexes.

The normal liver under physiologic conditions is largely resistant to damage by immune complexes. An unphysiologic challenge by immune aggregates can lead to hepatic injury, however. Earlier studies showed liver lesions induced by the administration of either preformed immune complexes or antigen in previously sensitized animals.[76-79] These areas of necrosis are considered to be a consequence of hepatic ischemia caused by the deposition of immune aggregates in sinusoids.[76] Preexisting hepatic lesions were amplified by immune complexes in an experimental model.[80] Mice pretreated with carbon tetrachloride developed extensive hepatocellular necrosis with inflammation after repeated administration of horse serum or bovine serum albumin. Diminished phagocytosis of Kupffer cells may be responsible for the increased deposition of immune complexes on hepatocytes and hepatic injury. This mechanism could also be operative in some cases of chronic active hepatitis.

Isolated hepatocytes from rabbits with experimental CAH,[32] as well as from patients with CAH,[34,58] had in vivo fixed IgG on their plasma membranes.

A granular pattern of the in vivo fixed IgG was observed in HB$_s$Ag-positive cases, possibly resembling membrane-attached immune complexes in the sera of these patients.[60] LMA in the autoimmune type of CAH seems to be fixed at the surface of hepatocytes. The in vivo fixed autoantibodies may block the hepatocellular receptors for IgG Fc or C3. Such a mechanism could play a role in the early development of hypergammaglobulinemia in the autoimmune type of CAH.

The importance of the in vivo fixed antibodies as well as immune complexes on the hepatocellular membrane for the induction and/or perpetuation of chronic liver disease needs further investigations.

CELL-MEDIATED IMMUNE REACTIONS IN ACUTE AND CHRONIC HEPATITIS

Cell-mediated Immunity (CMI) Against HB$_s$Ag

Cellular immune reactions against HB$_s$Ag have been demonstrated by three different techniques: the leukocyte migration inhibition test, lymphocyte stimulation, and cytotoxicity against HB$_s$Ag-coated target cells. The immune system is important for the elimination of the virus and its antigens.[81] An immune reaction against virus antigens and not the virus itself is postulated to be the pathogenetic principle for the liver cell damage. This hypothesis was supported by the demonstration of migration inhibition against HB_sAg in acute and chronic hepatitis B.[47,53,82-97]

Leukocyte migration inhibition was observed in patients with chronic liver diseases in 5 of 6 cases not persistently positive for HB_sAg, in none of 5 patients persistently HB_sAg-positive, and in 3 of 9 HB_sAg-negative patients.[82] The results suggest cellular hypoimmunity in HB_sAg-positive patients with chronic liver disease.

Patients were studied following acute hepatitis B with respect to immunity against HB_sAg by leukocyte migration inhibition and lymphocyte stimulation.[84] Significant migration inhibition and lymphocyte stimulation was observed in a group of patients following normal recovery from a hepatitis B infection. Correlation was good between the results of the two different test systems.

Cellular immunity was investigated in patients with various liver diseases using the one-step migration inhibition test.[92] Migration inhibition was shown in all of 9 patients with acute hepatitis B but only in 4 of 5 patients recovered from acute hepatitis B. Migration inhibition was not found in 8 patients each with HB_sAg-positive and -negative CAH. Using migration inhibition of leukocytes from patients with CAH, evidence was obtained for cellular immunity against HB_sAg in 8 of 12 positive patients and in 24 of 39 HB_sAg-negative patients. The percentage of migration-inhibition-positive patients was reduced by immunosuppressive therapy.

We used the two-stage migration inhibition test in our studies concerning cellular immunity against HB_sAg.[40,41] We investigated defined groups of acute hepatitis B, acute hepatitis non-B, HB_sAg-positive CAH and CPH, and healthy HB_sAg carriers.[91] During the first week of illness (clinical manifestations) most patients (8 of 11) with acute hepatitis B failed to show migration inhibition (CMI), whereas after 4 to 6 weeks, 12 of 13 patients had CMI against HB_sAg, when all patients no longer had HB_sAg in their sera. Six months after the onset of acute hepititis B, only 6 of 12 patients had CMI against HB_sAg.

Six patients with non-B hepatitis failed to have CMI against HB_sAg. We investigated 12 patients with HB_sAg-positive CAH over a period of 18 months: During the whole period, only 3 of 12 patients never had demonstrable migration inhibition; 9 of 12 patients showed inconsistent results of inhibition, stimulation, and/or migration against HB_sAg. The overall results were 29 of 64 showed migration, 18 of 64 showed stimulation, and 17 of 64 showed inhibition. Healthy HB_sAg carriers (17 of 22) failed to show CMI against HB_sAg.[91] Migration of leukocytes against HB_sAg was found in 4 of 13 patients with acute hepatitis B, in 7 of 12 patients after recovery, but only in 1 of 13 cases with HB_sAg-positive CAH.[98]

Cellular immunity appears to be a transient phenomenon at the time the antigen is cleared from the serum and liver tissue.

Lymphocyte Stimulation

The stimulation of lymphocytes by antigens and plant lectins to undergo blastic transformation is regarded as a test reflecting cellular immunity. Lymphocyte stimulation with HB$_s$Ag as antigen has been described by several authors.[83,84,90] Lymphocyte stimulation was observed with HB$_s$Ag-rich serum in patients following acute hepatitis B.[84] Significant stimulation was found in 6 patients studied up to 22 months following acute hepatitis.

Lympocyte transformation was studied using purified HB$_s$Ag in various disease groups.[90] While lymphocyte stimulation did not occur during the acute phase of hepatitis B, it did appear during early convalescence and was demonstrable up to 5 years after acute hepatitis. Patients with CAH and normal serum aminotransferase activity showed no transformation, and patients with increased aminotransferase activity showed a partial response to HB$_s$Ag. Healthy carriers of HB$_s$Ag and patients with CPH had no proliferative response to purified HB$_s$Ag. Thus, lymphocyte stimulation may be a more sensitive test for cellular immunity against HB$_s$Ag after hepatitis B infection.[83]

Cytotoxicity Against HB$_s$Ag-coated Target Cells

The cytotoxic effect of peripheral blood lymphocytes from patients with various inflammatory liver diseases against HB$_s$Ag-coated chicken red cells in a chromium release assay was studied.[99] Patients with acute hepatitis B (15 of 23) and 4 of 12 patients with CAH showed significant elevation of chromium release when compared to normal controls. None of 10 healthy carriers of HB$_s$Ag showed cytotoxicity. Studies with purified lymphocyte subpopulations demonstrated that the cytotoxic effect was associated with the T-lymphocyte fraction. The results suggested that liver damage in the early phase of hepatitis B is mediated by T lymphocytes reacting with hepatocytes bearing HB$_s$Ag on their membranes.

Cellular Immune Reactions Against LSP in Acute and Chronic Hepatitis

Our studies, as well as those by other investigators, were aimed at delineating the pathogenetic role of LSP as a target antigen in acute and chronic liver diseases. These investigations utilized three test systems to study cellular immune reactions against LSP, namely the leukocyte migration inhibition test,[37-41,47,91,101] lymphocyte stimulation,[36,45] and cytotoxicity assays.[44,49,100]

Leukocyte Migration Inhibition

Our group used the two-stage leukocyte migration inhibition test to study cellular immunity in patients with acute viral hepatitis. Migration inhibition was observed in approximately 30% of patients with acute hepatitis, irrespective of the loss of HB$_s$Ag in the serum during the acute phase of the disease. These studies suggested a loss of tolerance against LSP in acute hepatitis. This test was also applied to patients with CAH;[40] 29 of 34 (85%) untreated patients with hypergammaglobulinemic CAH and 8 of 19 patients with cryptogenic cirrhosis showed significant migration inhibition. Patients with CAH treated with immunosuppressive drugs, showed migration inhibition in only 4 of 23 cases. Only 1 of 9 patients with CPH showed migration inhibition.

This test was applied to characterize various subgroups of patients with CAH.[41] The presence of autoimmune markers and of HB$_s$Ag allowed subdivision into four groups. Migration inhibition was found in 85% of HB$_s$Ag-neg-

ative, autoimmune-marker-positive patients; in 46% of HB$_s$Ag-negative, au-
toimmune-marker-negative patients; in 29% of HB$_s$Ag-positive, autoimmune-
marker-negative patients; and in all 4 HB$_s$Ag-positive, autoimmune-marker-
positive patients. Migration inhibition was observed in 15 of 45 patients with
HB$_s$Ag-positive acute hepatitis after clearance of HB$_s$Ag, and in 7 of 17 patients
with protracted HB$_s$Ag-positive hepatitis. Twenty-six percent of patients with
various malignant diseases without overt liver disease demonstrated migration
inhibition with LSP as antigen. Another study from our group[91] was concerned
with the comparison of cellular immunity against HB$_s$Ag and LSP in acute and
chronic hepatitis. The results with HB$_s$Ag as antigen have been described
above. Cell-mediated immunity was observed in most patients with acute hepatitis B up to 6 weeks from the onset of the disease. After 4 to 6 months,
immunity against LSP could only rarely be detected. Patients with acute hepatitis non-B showed no cellular immunity against HB$_s$Ag and only in some
cases showed transient immunity against LSP. A longitudinal observation of
12 patients with HB$_s$Ag-positive CAH demonstrated cellular immunity against
LSP in a total of 40 of 61 tests. Similar results were obtained by other
groups.[37,38,47,101]

Lymphocyte Stimulation

Lymphocyte stimulation in patients with various inflammatory liver diseases
by autologous liver homogenate was found in 2 of 4 patients with primary
biliary cirrhosis and in 1 of 2 patients with chronic active hepatitis.[36] Lymphocytes from 34 patients with various liver diseases were stimulated in all lymphocyte transformation tests with liver-specific protein,[45] isolated according to
Meyer zum Büschenfelde at al.[28] Eight of 10 patients with CAH or CPH, 2 of
5 patients with nonalcoholic cirrhosis, and 6 of 19 patients with acute hepatitis
showed in vitro reactivity to LSP. One of 12 normal controls also had a positive
response. Stimulation with LSP did not correlate with the presence or absence
of HB$_s$Ag or with other biochemical parameters.

Cytotoxicity Against LSP-coated Target Cells

It is difficult to demonstrate cytotoxicity against LSP-coated target cells
because of the instability of purified LSP. Vogten et al.[49] described an assay
in which avian erythrocytes coated with LSP served as target cells for the
demonstration of the cytotoxic effect of lymphocytes from patients with
chronic liver diseases. Approximately 50% of patients with CAH showed cytotoxicity against LSP-coated cells without correlation with disease activity.
The activity could be blocked by addition of free LSP or aggregated IgG.

Cytotoxicity Against Various Target Cells

Test systems have been devised to demonstrate cytotoxic activity against
several target cells, such as human hepatocytes, rabbit hepatocytes, or cultured Chang liver cells. The limited availability and viability of autologous
human hepatocytes is the main obstacle in this system. The usefulness of
heterologous liver cells, such as rabbit hepatocytes is limited by the uncertain
antigenic identity, the short viability, and the very high effector-to-target-cell
ratio necessary to obtain cell lysis. Among cultured human cells, Chang cells
have been most extensively used. These cells, however, are dedifferentiated,

and the hepatic origin of these cells has been a matter of dispute.[102,103] Chang cell strains differ in the expression of the liver-specific lipoprotein.[61]

Cytotoxicity Against Human Hepatocytes

Increased cytotoxicity of lymphocytes from patients with CAH against autologous hepatocytes was noted when compared to normal lymphocytes.[43] Similar results were obtained with Chang cells as target cells. Since the cytotoxic effect was independent of the presence of human serum, T-cell-mediated cytotoxicity was postulated. The administration of prednisone in patients with CAH suppressed the cytotoxic effect. A similar methodologic approach was used with autologous human hepatocytes as target cells.[104] Increased cytotoxicity was found in 53% of CAH patients and decreased cytotoxicity was found in 32%, whereas the remaining patients with CAH had normal cytotoxicity. Patients exhibiting cytotoxicity against hepatocytes had a serum factor that was able to inhibit the phytohemaglutinin-induced lymphocyte transformation of normal lymphocytes. Patients with a short duration of disease tended to have greater cytotoxicity, and patients receiving steroid treatment tended to have a lesser cytotoxicity.

Cytotoxicity Against Rabbit Hepatocytes

Significant cytotoxicity was obtained in 20 of 22 patients with CAH using rabbit hepatocytes and in 2 of 6 patients with primary biliary cirrhosis.[44a] Serial studies showed decreasing cytotoxicity with steroid treatment. The cytotoxic effect could be blocked by addition of purified human LSP, suggesting that sensitization against this antigen plays a role in hepatic injury in CAH. These experiments were expanded to demonstrate by selective depletion of lymphocyte subpopulations that the cytotoxic effect resided in the B-cell-enriched fraction.[44] This suggested that K lymphocytes might be the effector cells. No difference was observed between HB_sAg-positive and -negative cases. In the early phase of acute hepatitis, significant cytotoxicity was found in 13 of 14 patients, but it occurred in only 5 of 9 patients 7 to 8 weeks after the onset of the disease.[100]

Cytotoxicity Against Cultured Cells

With cultured autologous liver 1 to 2 months after the establishment of cultures, significant cytotoxicity was found in 8 of 10 patients with CAH.[105] Also, 1 patient with primary biliary cirrhosis showed cytotoxicity against autologous cultured hepatocytes, while 4 of 5 patients with acute viral hepatitis were cytotoxic toward autologous liver cells. The organ specificity of the reaction could not be established. Cellular cytotoxicity against Chang cells was examined.[42] Increased cytotoxicity was observed in acute hepatitis (HB_sAg positive and HB_sAg negative) when compared to normal controls. Incubation with autologous or homologous HB_sAg-positive serum had an inhibitory effect, as had prednisone treatment in patients with CAH.

Spontaneous cell-mediated cytotoxicity (SCMC) and antibody-dependent cell-mediated cytotoxicity (ADCC) were reduced in primary biliary cirrhosis but not in CAH when tested against Chang cells and a mouse sarcoma cell line.[48] There was no difference in cytotoxicity when Chang cells were compared with mouse sarcoma cells, suggesting that this effect was not hepatocyte-specific. The lymphocytes mediating SCMC and ADCC were found in a surface-immunoglobulin-negative, Fc-receptor-positive cell fraction.

Binding of IgG from the sera of patients with CAH to Chang liver cells was observed.[46] Chang cells pretreated with CAH sera and tested with normal lymphocytes in a ^{51}Cr release assay showed increased cytotoxicity when compared to normal human serum. This suggested antibody-dependent cellular cytotoxicity.

OUTLOOK

The available evidence suggests that the HBV itself is not cytopathic. The host immune response is apparently responsible for tissue damage in HBV-induced acute and chronic hepatitis. One of the target antigens involved in the immune pathogenesis of acute hepatitis B seems to be HB_sAg. This antigen could be demonstrated on the membranes of hepatocytes in the very early phase of acute hepatitis B.[24] The second target antigen may be the membrane antigen LSP. Sensitization to this antigen can be found during the entire course of acute hepatitis B. The role of HB_eAg is unknown, but the early clearance of HB_eAg justifies further studies on the behavior of HB_eAg in acute hepatitis B, particularly studies of the HB_eAg titers and characterization of the known HB_eAg subtypes and/or HB_eAg/anti-HB_e immune complexes.

Immunologic mechanisms in chronic hepatitis are more complex. CAH is a disease of multiple etiologies. Three main types have been identified: HB_sAg-associated, autoimmune, and drug-induced CAH. In both HB_sAg-associated and autoimmune CAH, the membrane antigen LSP seems to be one of the most important target antigens. Whether T lymphocytes found in the liver of HB_sAg-positive CAH are LSP-activated is not established. Observations of lymphocyte populations in liver biopsy specimens from patients with CAH are compatible with a T-cell- and antibody-dependent cytotoxicity against hepatocytes.[106,107]

In addition to immune reactions against LSP, a further membrane antigen (LM Ag) seems to be involved in the immune pathogenesis of autoimmune CAH. The disease-specific autoantibody LMA can be demonstrated in vivo and in vitro on hepatocellular membranes.[34] One hypothesis explains the mechanisms of liver cell destruction in autoimmune CAH by a defect in suppressor T-cell function. Autoreactive B lymphocytes could, in the absence of suppressor T lymphocytes, produce continuously antimembrane-antibodies (anti-LSP?, LMA). The data from in vitro cytotoxicity assay systems supporting liver cell damage by immune mechanisms suffer from lack of adequate target cell systems. The use of autologous hepatocytes, cultured human hepatocytes, or of heterologous cells is open to methodologic criticism. A possible alternative may be the use of avian red cells coated with liver membrane antigens as cytotoxic assay systems.

The effector cell in cytotoxicity tests appears to be a surface-immunoglobulin-negative, Fc-receptor-positive cell, favoring an antibody-mediated cellular cytotoxicity. The possible role of macrophages has been largely ignored, and it is not known whether such data apply to the in vivo mechanisms.

REFERENCES

1. Kaplan PM, Grennman RL, Gevin JL, Purcell RH, Robinson WS: DNA polymerase associated with human hepatitis B antigen. J Virol 12:995–1005, 1973

2. Robinson WS, Clayton DA, Greenman RL: DNA of a human hepatitis B virus candidate. J Virol 14:384–391, 1974

3. Magnius LO, Lindholm A, Lundin P, Iwarson S: A new antigen-antibody system. Clinical significance in long-term carriers of hepatitis B surface antigen. JAMA 231:356–359, 1975

4. Neurath AR, Trepo C, Chen M, Prince AM: Identification of additional antigenic sites ou Dane particles and the tubular forms of hepatitis B surface antigen. J Gen Virol 30:277–285, 1976

5. Neurath AR, Strick N: Host specificity of a serum marker for hepatitis B: Evidence that "e-antigen" has the properties of an immunoglobulin. Proc Natl Acad Sci 74:1702–1706, 1977

6. Lam KG, Tong MJ, Rakela J: Release of e-antigen from a Dane particle-rich preparation of hepatitis B virus. Infect Immun 16:403–404, 1977

7. Vyas GN, Peterson DL, Towsend RM: Hepatitis B "e" antigen: An apparent association with lactate dehydrogenase isoenzyme. Science 198:1068–1070, 1977

8. Takahashi K, Yamashita S, Imai M, Miyakawa Y, Mayumi M: Failure of antibody to e to precipitate Dane particles containing DNA polymerase and hepatitis B core antigen activities. J Gen Virol (in press)

9. Nordenfeldt E, Kjellen L: Dane particles, DNA polymerase, and e-antigen in two different categories of hepatitis B antigen carriers. Intervirology 5:225–232, 1975

10. Eleftheriou N, Heathcote J, Thomas HC, Sherlock S: Incidence and clinical significance of e-antigen and antibody in acute and chronic liver disease. Lancet 2:1171–1173, 1975

11. Takahashi K, Imai M, Tsuda F, Takahashi T, Miyakawa Y, Mayumi M: Association of Dane particles with e antigen in the serum of asymptomatic carriers of hepatitis B surface antigen. J Immunol 117:102–105, 1976

12. Hess G, Nielsen JO, Arnold W, Meyer zum Büschenfelde KH: e-System and intrahepatocellular HB_cAg and HB_sAg in HB_sAg positive patients with liver diseases and healthy carriers. Scand J Gastroenterol 12:325–330, 1977

13. Arnold W, Hess G, Purcell RH, Kaplan PM, Gerin JL, Meyer zum Büschenfelde KH: Anti-HB_c, HB_eAg and DNA polymerase activity in healthy HB_sAg carriers and patients with inflammatory liver diseases. Klin Wochenschr 56:297–303, 1978

14. Alter HJ, Seef LB, Kaplan PM, McAucliffe VJ, Wright EC, Gerin JL, Purcell RH, Holland PV, Zimmermann HJ: Type B hepatitis: The infectivity of blood positive for e antigen and DNA polymerase after accidental needlestick exposure. N Engl J Med 295:909–913, 1976

15. Okada K, Kamiyama I, Inomata M, Imai M, Miyakawa Y, Mayumi M: e-Antigen and anti-e in the serum of asymptomatic carrier mothers as indicators of positive and negative transmission of hepatitis B virus to their infants. N Engl J Med 294:746–749, 1976

16. Almeida JD, Zuckerman AJ, Taylor PE: Immune electron microscopy of the Australia-SH (serum-hepatitis) antigen. Microbios 1:117–119, 1969

17. Brzosko WJ, Madalinski K, Krawczynski K, Nowoslawski A: Duality of hepatitis B antigen and its antibody. I. Immunofluorescence studies. J Infect Dis 127:424–428, 1973

18. Barker LF, Almeida JD, Hoofnagle JH, Gerety RJ, Jackson DR, McGrath PH P: Hepatitis B core antigen: Immunology and electron microscopy. J Virol 14:1552–1558, 1974

19. Huang SN: Structural and immunoreactive characteristics of hepatitis B core antigen. Am J Med Sci 270:131–139, 1975

20. Gudat F, Bianchi L, Sonnabend W, Thiel G, Aenishaenslin W, Stalder GA: Pattern of core and surface expression in liver tis-

sue reflects state of specific immune response in hepatitis B. Lab Invest 32:1–9, 1975

21. Arnold W, Meyer zum Büschenfelde KH, Hopf U, Kordebarlag C: Untersuchungen zur Hepatitis B-Antigen (HBA$_g$)-Fixation an peripheren Lymphozyten und isolierten Leberzellen bei Patienten mit entzündlichen Lebererkrankungen. Klin Wochenschr 53:231–235, 1975

22. Arnold W, Nielsen JO, Hardt F, Meyer zum Büschenfelde KH: Localization of *e*-antigen in nuclei of hepatocytes in HB$_s$Ag-positive liver diseases. Gut 19:994–996, 1977

23. Trepo C, Vitvitski L, Neurath R, Hashimoto N, Schaefer R, Nemoz G, Prince AM: Detection of *e*-antigen by immunofluorescence in cytoplasm of hepatocytes of HB$_s$Ag carriers. Lancet 1:486, 1976

24. Alberti A, Realdi G, Tremolada F, Spina GP: Liver cell surface localization of hepatitis B antigen and of immunoglobulins in acute and chronic hepatitis and in liver cirrhosis. Clin Exp Immunol 25:396–402, 1976

25. Ray MB, Desmet VJ, Fevery J, de Groote J, Bradburne AF, Desmyter J: Distribution patterns of hepatitis B surface antigen (HB$_s$Ag) in the liver of hepatitis patients: J Clin Pathol 29:94–100, 1976

26. Ray MB, Desmet VJ, Fevery J, de Groote J, Bradburne AF, Desmyter J: Hepatitis B surface antigen (HB$_s$Ag) in the liver of patients with hepatitis; a comparison with serological detection. J Clin Pathol 29:89–93, 1976

27. Bianchi L, Gudat F: Core- und Hüllenantigen des Dane-Partikels im Lebergewebe—Beziehungen zu den Verlaufsformen der Hepatitis B. Leber Magen Darm 5:180–187, 1977

28. Meyer zum Büschenfelde KH, Miescher PA: Liver-specific antigens. Purification and characterization. Clin Exp Immunol 10:89–102, 1972

29. McFarlane IG, Wojcicka BM, Zucker GM, Eddleston ALWF: Purification and characterization of human liver-specific membrane lipoprotein (LSP). Clin Exp Immunol 27:381–390, 1977

30. Meyer zum Büschenfelde KH: The nature of the target antigen LSP. Symposium: Immune Reactions in Liver Disease, London, 1977 (in press)

31. Meyer zum Büschenfelde KH, Hütteroth TH: Autoantibodies against liver membrane antigens in chronic active liver disease. Symposium: Immune Reactions in Liver Disease, London, 1977 (in press)

31a. Hopf U, Meyer zum Büschenfelde KH, Freudenberg J: Liver-specific antigens of different species. II. Localization of a membrane antigen at cell surface of isolated hepatocytes. Clin Exp Immunol 16:117–124, 1974

32. Hopf U, Meyer zum Büschenfelde KH: Studies on the pathogenesis of the experimental chronic active hepatitis in rabbits. II. Demonstration of immunoglobulin on isolated hepatocytes. Br J Exp Pathol 55:509–513, 1974

33. Hess G, Shih JW-K, Gerin JL, Purcell RH, Meyer zum Büschenfelde KH: Hepatitis B antigen: Lack of relationship to the liver-specific lipoprotein LSP. J Med Virol (in press)

34. Hopf U, Meyer zum Büschenfelde KH, Arnold W: Detection of a liver membrane autoantibody in HB$_s$Ag-negative chronic active hepatitis. N Engl J Med 294:578–582, 1976

35. Tage-Jensen U, Arnold W, Dietrichson O et al.: Liver-cell-membrane autoantibody specific for inflammatory liver diseases. Br Med J: 206–208, 1977

36. Tobias H, Safran AP, Schaffner F: Lymphocyte stimulation and chronic liver disease. Lancet 1:193–195, 1967

37. Bacon PA, Berry H, Pown R: Cell-mediated immune reactivity in liver disease. Gut 13:427–429, 1972

38. Miller J, Smith MGM, Mitchell CG et al: Cell mediated immunity to a human liver-specific antigen in patients with active chronic hepatitis and primary biliary cirrhosis. Lancet 2:296–297, 1972

39. Knolle J, Meyer zum Büschenfelde KH, Bolte JP et al: Zelluläre Immunreaktionen gegenüber dem Hepatitis-assoziierten Antigen (HAA) und homologem leberspezifischen Protein (HLP) bei akuten HAA-positiven Hepatitiden. Klin Wochenschr 51:1172–1173, 1973

40. Meyer zum Büschenfelde KH, Knolle J, Berger J: Celluläre Immunoreaktionen gegenüber homologen leberspezifischen Antigenen (HLP) bei chronischen Leberentzündungen. Klin Wochenschr 52:246–247, 1974

41. Meyer zum Büschenfelde KH, Alberti A, Arnold W, Freudenberg J: Organ-specificity and diagnostic value of cell-mediated

immunity against a liver-specific membrane protein: studies in hepatic and non-hepatic diseases. Klin Wochenschr 53:1061–1067, 1975

42. Wands JR, Perrotto L, Alpert E: Cell-mediated immunity in acute and chronic hepatitis. J Clin Invest 55:921–929, 1975

43. Wands JR, Isselbacher KJ: Lymphocyte cytotoxicity to autologous liver cells in chronic active hepatitis. Proc Natl Acad Sci USA 72:1301–1303, 1975

44. Cochrane AMG, Moussouros A, Thomson AD et al: Antibody-dependent cell-mediated (K cell) cytotoxicity against isolated hepatocytes in chronic active hepatitis. Lancet 1:441–444, 1976

44a.Thomson AD, Cochrane MAG, McFarlane IG et al: Lymphocyte cytotoxicity to isolated hepatocytes in chronic active hepatitis. Nature 252:721–722, 1974

45. Thestrup-Pedersen K, Ladefoged K, Andersen P: Lymphocyte transformation test with liver-specific protein and phytohaemagglutinin in patients with liver disease. Clin Exp Immunol 24:1–8, 1976

46. Kawanishi H: In vitro studies on IgG-mediated lymphocyte cytotoxicity in chronic active liver disease. Gastroenterology 73:549–555, 1977

47. Lee WM, Reed WD, Osman CG, et al: Immune responses to the hepatitis B surface antigen and liver specific lipoprotein in acute type B hepatitis. Gut 18:250–257, 1977

48. Vierling JM, Nelson DL, Strober W et al: In vitro cell-mediated cytotoxicity in primary biliary cirrhosis and chronic hepatitis. J Clin Invest 60:1116–1128, 1977

49. Vogten AJM, Hadzic N, Shorter RG et al: Cell-mediated cytotoxicity in chronic active liver disease: A new test system. Gastroenterology 74:883–889, 1978

50. Jensen DM, McFarlane IG, Portmann BS et al: Detection of antibodies directed against a liver-specific membrane lipoprotein in patients with acute and chronic active hepatitis. N Engl J Med 299:1–7, 1978

51. Hoofnagle JH, Gerety RJ, Ni LY, Barker LF: Antibody to hepatitis B core antigen. N Engl J Med 290:1336–1340, 1974

52. Aikawa T, Sairenji H, Furuta S, Kiyosawa K, Shikata T, Imai M, Miyakawa Y, Yanase Y, Mayumi M: Seroconversion from hepatitis B e antigen to anti-Hb$_e$ in acute hepatitis B virus infection. N Engl J Med 298:439–441, 1978

53. Knolle J, Born M, Hess G, Klinge O, Arnold W, Bitz H, Meyer zum Büschenfelde KH: Die Charakterisierung des klinisch gesunden Hepatitis-Antigen (HB$_s$Ag)-Trägers. Klinische, biochemische, histologische und immunologische Untersuchungen bei 129 Fällen einer prospektiven Studie. Klin Wochenschr 54:567–578, 1976

54. Arnold W, Meyer zum Büschenfelde KH, Hess G, Knolle J: The diagnostic significance of intrahepato-cellular hepatitis B-surface (HB$_s$Ag), hepatitis B-core-antigen (HB$_c$Ag) and IgG for the classification of inflammatory liver diseases (Studies in HB$_s$Ag-positive and -negative patients). Klin Wochenschr 53:1069–1074, 1975

55. Hopf U, Meyer zum Büschenfelde KH, Dierich MP: Demonstration of binding sites for IgG and the third component (C3) on isolated hepatocytes. J Immunol 117:639–645, 1976

56. Gerber MA, Sarno E, Vernace SJ: Immune complexes in hepatocytic nuclei HBAg-positive chronic hepatitis. N Engl J Med 294:922–925 1976

57. Arnold W, Meyer zum Büschenfelde KH: Immune complexes of HB$_c$Ag/anti-HB$_c$ in nuclei of HB$_s$Ag-positive chronic liver diseases. N Engl J Med 295:818, 1977

58. Hopf U, Arnold W, Meyer zum Büschenfelde KH, Förster E: Studies on the pathogenesis of chronic inflammatory liver disease. I. Membrane-fixed IgG on isolated hepatocytes from patients. Clin Exp Immunol 22:1–8, 1975

59. Hütteroth TH, Meyer zum Büschenfelde KH: Clinical relevance of the liver-specific lipoprotein (LSP). Acta Hepatogastroenterol 25:243–253, 1978

60. Hütteroth TH, Arnold W, Hopf U, Meyer zum Büschenfelde KH: Zirkulierende Immunkomplexe bei akuter Virushepatitis, chronisch-aktiver Hepatitis und Periarteriitis nodosa. Zschr Gastroenterol 6:395–402, 1978

61. Hütteroth TH, Meyer zum Büschenfelde KH: Antigenic relationship between Chang liver cells and human hepatocytes. Klin Wochenschr 56:525–527, 1978

62. Hütteroth TH, Meyer zum Büschenfelde KG: IgG binding to the plasma membrane of Chang liver cells in chronic active hepatitis. J Clin Lab Immunol (in press)

63. Chase MU: Inhibition of experimental drug allergy by prior feeding of the sensitizing agent. Proc Soc Exp Biol Med 61:257–259, 1946

64. Coons AH, Leduc EH, Kaplan MH: Localization of antigen in tissue cell. VI. The fate of injected foreign protein in mouse. J Exp Med 93:173–193, 1951

65. Cantor HM, Dumont AE: Hepatic suppression of sensitization to antigen absorbed into the portal system. Nature 215:744–745, 1967

66. Strauss W: Cytochemical observation on the relationship between lysosomes and phagosomes in kidney and liver by combined staining for acid phosphatase and intravenously injected horseradish peroxidase. J Cell Biol 20:497–507, 1964

67. Mannik W, Arend WP: Fate of preformed immune complexes in rabbits and rhesus monkeys. J Exp Med 134:19s–31s, 1971

68. Thomas CH, Vaez-Zadeh F: A homeostatic mechanism for the removal of antigen from the portal circulation. Immunology 26:375–382, 1974

69. Arnold W, Müller O, Mayersbach H v., Mitrenga D: The fate of injected human IgG in the mouse liver uptake, immunological inactivation and lysosomal reactions. Cell Tissue Res 156:359–376, 1975

70. Triger DR, Cynamon MH, Wright R: Studies on hepatic uptake of antigen. I. Comparison of inferior vena cava and portal vein routes of immunization. Immunology 25:941–950, 1973

71. Triger DR, Wright R: Studies on hepatic uptake of antigen. II. The effect of hepatotoxins in the immune response. Immunology 25:951–956, 1973

72. Protell RL, Solowary RD, Martin WJ, Schoenfield LJ, Summerskill WH: Anti-salmonella agglutinins in chronic active liver disease. Lancet 2:330–331, 1971

73. Bjørneboe M, Prytz H, Ørskov J: Antibodies to intestinal microbes in serum of patients with cirrhosis on the liver. Lancet 1:58–60, 1972

74. Triger DR, Alp MH, Wright R: Bacterial and dietary antibodies in liver disease. Lancet 1:60–63, 1972

75. Hopf U, Brandtzaeg P, Hütteroth TH, Meyer zum Büschenfelde KH: In vivo and in vitro fixation of IgA on the plasma membrane of hepatocytes. Scand J Immunol (in press)

76. Paronetto F, Woolf N, Koffler D, Popper H: Response of the liver to soluble antigen-antibody complexes. Gastroenterology 43:539–546, 1962

77. Paronetto F, Popper H: Aggravation of hepatic lesions in mice by an in vivo localization of immune complexes (Auer hepatitis) Am J Pathol 47:549–563, 1965

78. Blackwell JB: The effect on the liver of sensitized rats of intravenous injection of antigen. J Pathol Bacteriol 90:259–268, 1965

79. Fennel RH: Chronic liver disease induced in rats by repeated anaphylactic shock. Am J Pathol 47:173–182, 1965

80. Paronetto F, Popper H: Chronic liver injury induced by immunologic reactions: cirrhosis following immunization with heterologous sera. Am J Pathol 49:1087–1101, 1966

81. Dudley FJ, Giustino V, Sherlock S: Cell-mediated immunity in patients positive for hepatitis associated antigen. Br Med J 4:754–756, 1972

82. Ito K, Nakagawa J, Okimoto Y, Nakano H: Chronic hepatitis, migration inhibition of leucocytes in presence of Australia antigen. N Engl J Med 286:1005, 1972

83. De Gast GG, Houwen B, Nieweg HO: Specific lymphocyte stimulation by purified, heat-inactivated hepatitis B antigen. Br Med J 4:707–709, 1973

84. Yeung-Laiwah AAC, Chandhuri AKR, Anderson JR: Lymphocyte transformation and leucocyte migration inhibition by Australia antigen. Clin Exp Immunol 15:27–34, 1973

85. Erard Ph, Frei, PC, Peitreguin R, Hofstetter JR, Magnenat P: Etude de l'immunité cellulaire spécifique de l'antigene Australia. Rèsultants préliminaires dans different formes d'hepatite. Schweiz Med Wochenschr 104:1882–1185, 1974

86. Irwin GR, Hierholzer WJ, Cinis R, McCollum RW: Delayed hypersensitivity in hepatitis B: Clinical correlates of in vitro production of migration inhibition factor. J Infect Dis 130:580–587, 1974

87. Vyas GN, Ibrahim AB, Rao KR, Schmidt R: Tolerance to hepatitis B antigen: A hypothesis for its termination with "immune-RNA." Life Sci 15:261, 1974

88. De Horatius RJ, Henderson C, Strickland RG: T-cells and lymphocytotoxins in type B hepatitis and HB antigens carriers. Gastroenterology 29:683, 1974

89. Gerber MA, Phuangsab D, Sudin MS, Vittal SBW, Dourdourekas D, Steigmann F, Clowdus BF: Cell-mediated immune response to hepatitis B-antigen in patients with liver diseases. Am J Dig Dis 19:637–643, 1974

90. Tong MJ, Wallace AM, Robert D, Peters RL, Reynolds TB: Lymphocyte stimulation in hepatitis B infections. N Engl J Med 293:318–322, 1975

ber of electron-dense granules within the limiting membrane, giving a sandy appearance from which the generic name is derived (L. *arenosus*, "sandy"). Intracellular virus particles are found in either vesicles or extracellular invaginations, and the virion may be released from the cell by budding. The genus includes lymphocytic choriomeningitis virus, the Tacaribe complex viruses (hemorrhagic fever viruses of South America), and Lassa virus, all of which cross-react antigenically.

A further outbreak of Lassa fever, with a high mortality of 52% among 23 hospitalized patients, was reported in Jos, Nigeria, in 1970.[3] Dr. Jeannette M. Troup, who performed two autopsies while investigating Lassa fever and who was primarily responsible for drawing attention to the condition, contracted the infection and died of it. In March 1972, further cases of Lassa fever occurred among 4 patients and 7 members of the staff in a hospital in the Zorzor district of Liberia in West Africa; 4 died. The index case was a pregnant woman admitted to the obstetric ward, and all cases among the patients and members of the staff occurred in this ward. One of the fatal cases was an American missionary nurse who had direct contact with the blood of the index case.[4] A later report[5] records 64 more cases of Lassa fever admitted to hospital in Sierra Leone, Africa. Twenty-three (36%) died, and the case fatality ratio among pregnant women was 75% (6 out of 8). One of the 64 patients was a nurse who pricked her finger on a needle used for obtaining blood from a patient who subsequently died of clinical Lassa fever. This is the largest epidemic reported so far, and unlike the previous outbreaks in Nigeria and Liberia, it consisted primarily of community-acquired infection. Evidence was obtained of family outbreaks of the fever in which spread had occurred among those with the most intimate contact through infectious secretions or blood.

Since related arenaviruses have been isolated from wild rodents and bats, Lassa fever was also postulated to be a zoonosis. Monath et al.[6] trapped 641 small vertebrates during the epidemic of Lassa fever in Sierra Leone in 1972. Lassa virus was isolated from a single murine species, the multimammate rat *Mastomys natalensis*, which is a common commensal rodent in West Africa adapted to life both within houses and in the fields. Rodents of other species commonly found in the area of the epidemic (*Mus musculus* and *Rattus rattus*) were not infected. In 1976, a virus closely related serologically to Lassa virus was isolated from wild *Mastomys natalensis* captured in 1972 in Mozambique.[7] This finding more than doubles the potential area of Lassa-like virus distribution in Africa and stresses the need for great care in working with wild *Mastomys* rodents.

The mode of transmission of the virus from rodent to man or from man to man is not known yet. Similarly, the pathogenesis of Lassa virus infection in its natural host remains unknown. Perhaps, like other arenaviruses that induce a chronic virus carrier state in their natural hosts (e.g., lymphocytic choriomeningitis), Lassa virus causes a persistent infection with both horizontal and vertical transmission. Rodents may excrete the virus in urine and saliva and may thus contaminate food, water, or air. Monath et al.[6] suggest that a low level of sanitation, the storage of grain and food within houses, and the ease with which rodents infest mud and thatch houses enhance the contact between rodents and man. The means by which the virus is spread from person to person is not clear. Medical attendants or relatives providing direct personal care are most likely to contract the infection. Accidental inoculation with a sharp instrument or contact with affected blood has accounted for a few cases. Lassa virus has been isolated from the pharynx and urine of patients, so that indirect airborne spread of the virus, as well as mechanical transmission, is most likely.

The symptoms of Lassa fever, particularly early in the disease, are nonspecific. The differential diagnosis includes malaria, typhoid, yellow fever, influenza and measles. Prostration out of proportion to the degree of pyrexia has been described as the single most suggestive feature. Clinical findings may include conjunctivitis, pharyngitis, and tonsillitis with whitish exudative lesions and small vesicular lesions and ulcerations, lymphadenopathy, occasionally a faint maculopapular rash, and later hemorrhages. Jaundice has not been reported, although pathologically involvement of the liver is the most frequent finding.

The severity of the illness is stressed by a high case fatality ratio of 36% to 67% among patients admitted to hospital and a high risk of infection to medical personnel. Of 21 medical workers who contracted Lassa fever, 10 died. However, the relatively frequent finding of specific antibodies among persons without a history of illness suggests the existence of unrecognized or mild infections. In Africa, the virus was introduced into hospitals by African patients admitted with febrile illnesses that often mimic typhoid fever, malaria, or yellow fever. Secondary infections occurred among hospital staff and patients, but while the primary index cases were highly infectious, the secondary cases, for reasons that are not clear, were not. Only a few tertiary infections have been recorded. Intimate contact with the index case, e.g., relatives or medical attendants providing direct personal or nursing care, was associated with a high risk of infection. Cases have occurred among patients or hospital visitors who apparently had no direct contact with the index cases. The incubation period is 3 to 16 days. Diagnosis is by isolation of the virus and serologic tests.

Histologically, the liver is the principal target organ in human Lassa virus infection; there is a range of severity of the hepatitis produced by this virus.[8] The degree of inflammatory cell infiltration is small and unrelated to the extent of hepatocellular damage. Eosinophilic necrosis of individual hepatocytes is a constant finding, and larger foci of hepatocellular necrosis are frequently scattered through the lobules. Single hepatocytes in an otherwise intact liver cell plate undergo eosinophilic changes with eosinophilic cytoplasmic inclusions similar to those described in yellow fever. Other cells show homogeneous eosinophilic cytoplasmic staining with pyknosis or disappearance of the nucleus. Coalescence of necrotic foci, which bridge portal-to-portal and portal-to-central areas of the lobule, is a usual feature. Where the damage is more extensive, large portions of the individual lobules may be destroyed, but even in these areas the reticulin framework of the liver remains intact. The nonzonal distribution of necrosis distinguishes Lassa virus hepatitis from the classical lesion of yellow fever. At autopsy the extent of hepatic necrosis has been sufficient to implicate hepatic failure as a major cause of death.

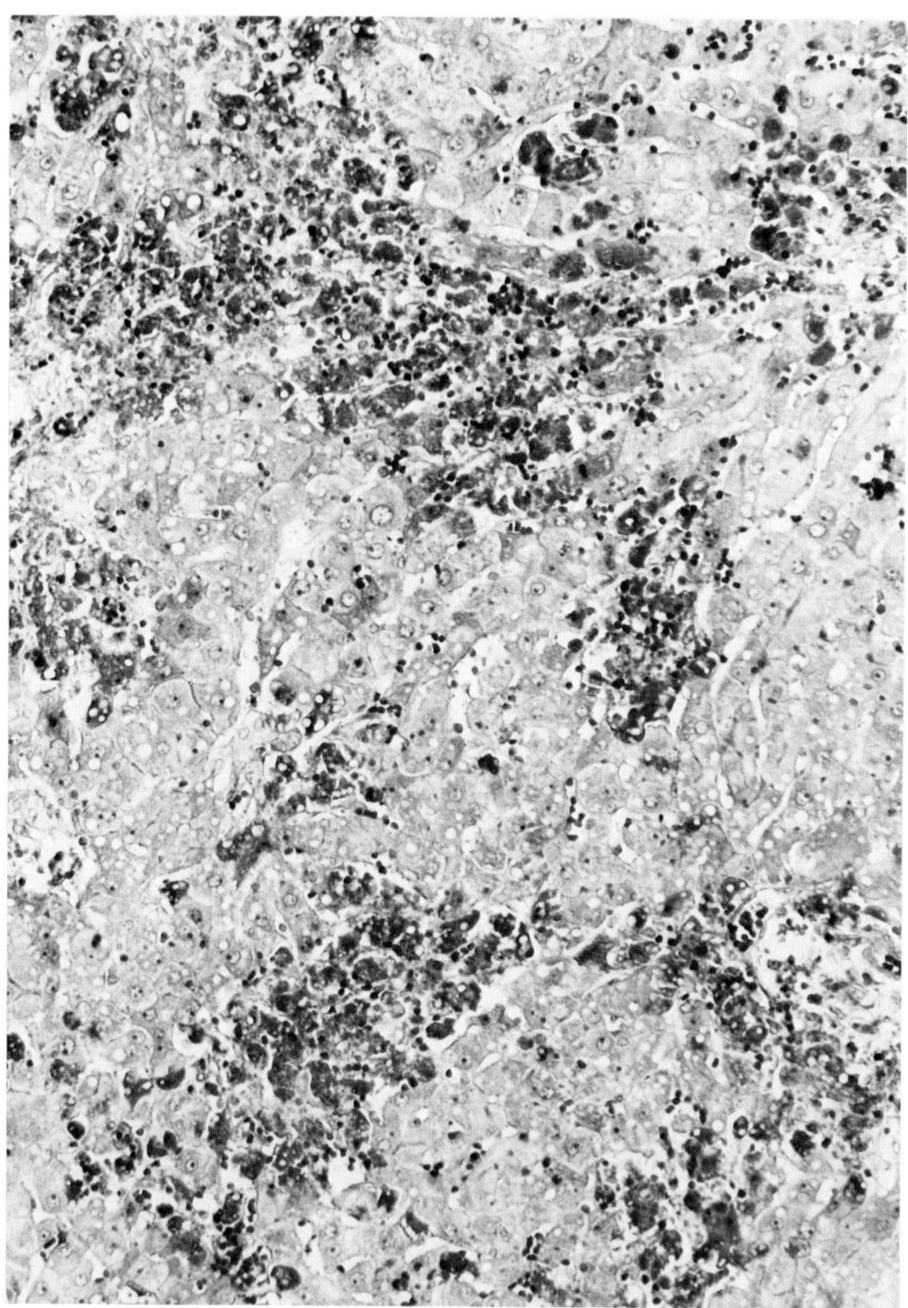

FIG. 1—Autopsy specimen of liver in Marburg virus disease. Necrosis of single and groups of hepatocytes (appearing dark) which are irregularly arranged. (Courtesy of Peter Gedigk For further details, see: Bechtelsheimer H, Korb G, Gedigk P: The morphology and pathogenesis of ''Marburg virus'' hepatitis. Hum Pathol 3:255–264, 1972.)

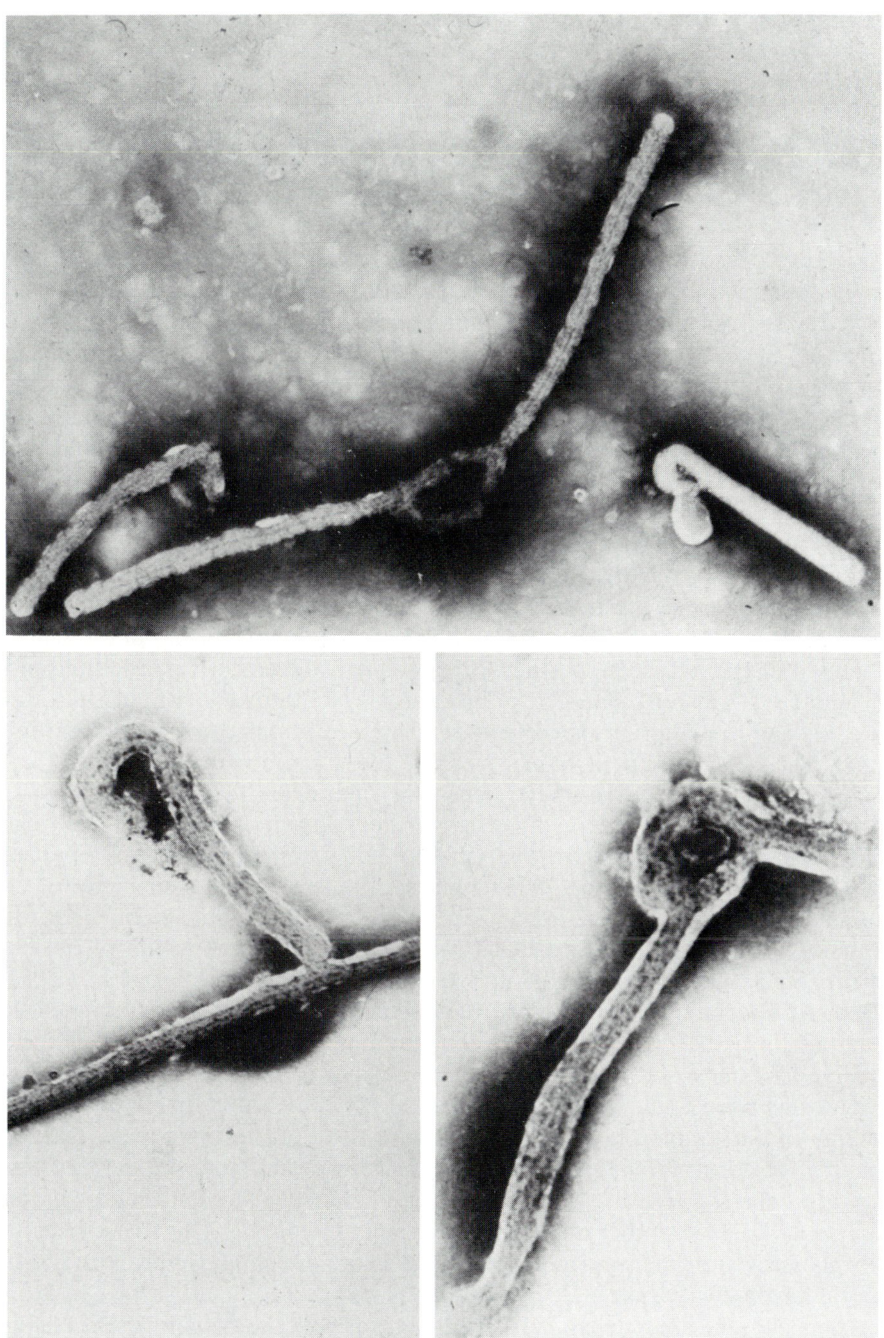

FIG. 2—Negatively stained preparation of Ebola virus (Zaire strain) showing filamentous forms of variable length, branching, enlarged heads, and coiled ends. Some of the particles contain an internal structure, others are empty (top micrograph, × 47,500; bottom micrograph, × 71,250). (Preparation by ETW Bowen and WJ Harris.)

At the ultrastructural level, many typical arenavirus particles are found in and near hepatocytes rather than in Kupffer cells. The virus matures by budding from cell membranes.

MARBURG VIRUS

Marburg virus disease,[9] commonly but incorrectly named "green monkey" disease, is a severe distinctive hemorrhagic febrile illness of man, first described in 1967 when 31 cases with 7 deaths in Germany and Yugoslavia were traced to direct contact with blood, organs, or tissue cell cultures from a batch of African green monkeys (*Cercopithicus aethiops*) that had been trapped in Uganda. Several secondary cases occurred in hospital personnel by contact with the blood of patients. One further case was apparently transmitted by sexual intercourse 83 days after the initial illness, and virus was isolated from the semen. The case fatality rate was 29% for the primary cases, but no deaths occurred in the 6 secondary cases. This previously unrecognized disease was caused by an infectious agent probably new to medical science.

The possible origin of the infection has been investigated since the 1967 outbreak. Complement-fixing antibodies to the Marburg virus were reported from a laboratory in the United States in many African monkeys, but conflicting results were obtained in other surveys, and the antigen used in the United States probably was not specific. Furthermore, before 1967, many thousands of monkeys had been handled in biomedical laboratories without such outbreaks, and in addition, experimental infection of monkeys proved uniformly fatal. The natural cycle of transmission of the virus in various species of animals and the origin of the infection remain unknown.

Marburg virus has been isolated experimentally in monkeys, guinea pigs, and a variety of cell cultures. The virus probably contains RNA and lipid and has an elongated cylindrical or filamentous shape. The outer diameter of the virus is about 70–110 nm, depending on the presence and thickness of the envelope and whether the particles are full or empty. The length of the filaments is variable, averaging about 600 nm, but much longer forms have been seen. All specimens had particles, often in large aggregates, that contained the sinuous forms but with a compact configuration. The most common morphologic appearance was that of a ring or doughnut form; both open and closed ring forms were found. An internal helix of about 20 nm in diameter could be seen. An outstanding feature of the mature form of the virus was a varying number of constrictions, and in particles with a visible internal helix, a constriction corresponded with a break in the helix so that each ring form contained a variable number of fragments of helix within it.[10] The basic structure of this virus is distinctive, and it does not share any antigenic properties with any other known virus.

Clinically, the illness characteristically begins with the sudden onset of fever, malaise, headache, and myalgia. Gastrointestinal symptoms soon follow and include nausea, vomiting, and often watery diarrhea. A maculopapular rash appears between the fifth and seventh day of illness, most marked on the buttocks, trunk, and outer aspects of the upper arms. Conjunctivitis is common. Most patients have functional evidence of liver damage during the second week of illness, but clinical jaundice has not been observed. Renal damage manifested by proteinuria, oliguria, and rising blood urea nitrogen levels has been observed. The patients develop a tendency to bleed, particularly from the gums and from needle punctures. Severe hemorrhages may occur, particularly into the gastrointestinal tract.

The first recognized outbreak of disease subsequent to the one initiated in the laboratories in Europe occurred in South Africa in February 1975. The primary case was a young Australian man who had hitchhiked through Rhodesia. He died in a Johannesburg hospital and shortly afterward his female travel companion and one of the nurses who had cared for him fell ill with the same disease. The women recovered. Virologic studies showed that this outbreak was caused by the Marburg virus. As in the original Marburg outbreak, virus was isolated from seminal fluid 83 days after the onset of illness, evidence that the virus can persist in the body for at least 2 to 3 months after the initial infection. In the Johannesburg episode, the virus was cultured from fluid aspirated from the anterior chamber of the eye 80 days after the onset of the illness.[11]

Gross morphologic changes found at autopsy were related to hemorrhages in the gastrointestinal tract and the lungs. The principal histologic lesions were limited to the liver, kidneys, and lungs, with the liver as the primary target organ.[12] Irregular foci of parenchymal necrosis become confluent so that hepatic lobular necrosis tends to be extensive without localization to any particular zone. Eosinophilic cytoplasmic degeneration, the formation of structures resembling Councilman bodies, and lysis of nuclei were characteristic. The basic architecture of the liver remained intact, and the inflammatory response was minimal. Kupffer cells were enlarged both in and around the necrotic areas and to a lesser extent in the rest of the liver; they frequently contained PAS-positive granules. The histologic appearance in autopsy specimens (Fig. 1) is sufficiently characteristic to raise the suspicion of an unusual viral infection.

The kinetics of viral maturation in the liver were investigated in vervet monkeys.[13] Early in the course of infection, many hepatocytes contained discrete cytoplasmic matrices which increased in number and complexity by the seventh day. Masses of uniformly packed filaments, arranged in parallel array, were found in these inclusions. These filaments or cylinders developed into the core structure of the virus particles as maturation occurred by budding through plasma or intracytoplasmic membranes.

EBOLA VIRUS INFECTION

Between August and November 1976, outbreaks of severe and frequently fatal viral hemorrhagic fever occurred in the equatorial provinces of Sudan and Zaire, causing widespread international concern. In Nzara, Sudan, 33 of 70 cases were fatal, and in Maridi, also in Sudan, the epidemic caused 229 cases, 117 of which were fatal. Of the 230 members of the staff in Maridi hospital, 76 were infected and 41 died. In Zaire, the number of cases was 237, including 211 death.[14] During laboratory investigations carried out to identify the virus, a member of the laboratory staff of the Microbiological Research Establishment, Porton Down in England, contracted the disease but recovered.[15]

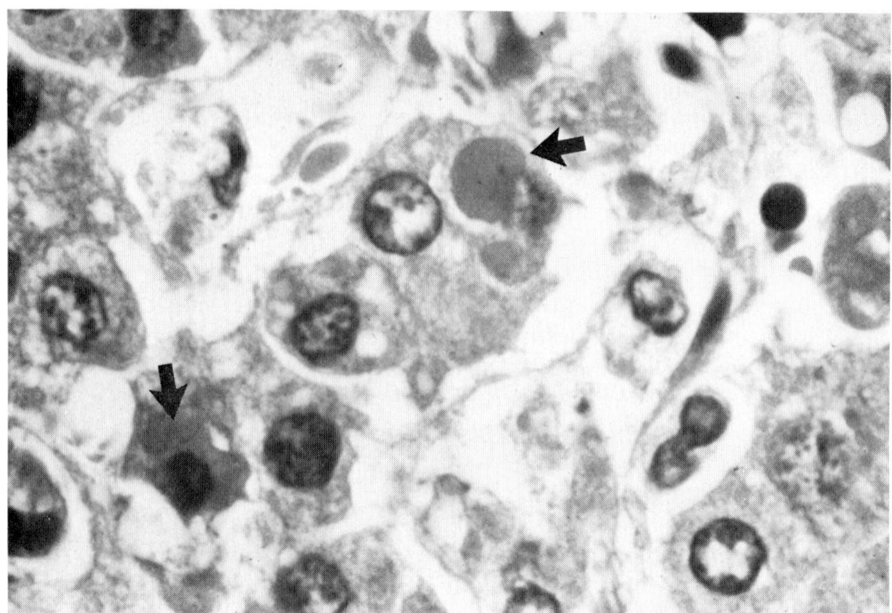

FIG. 3—Large eosinophilic intracytoplasmic inclusion bodies in human hepatocytes in Ebola infection (× 765). (Preparation by Dr F Murphy.)

The clinical picture was indistinguishable from Marburg virus disease. The incubation period ranged from 4 to 16 days, with an average of 7 days. The illness in Zaire was associated with fewer respiratory symptoms than in the Sudan and had a shorter clinical course and a higher fatality rate. Disseminated intravascular coagulopathy was a major feature of the disease, and bleeding occurred in the majority of cases, mainly from the gastrointestinal tract. Jaundice was present in about 5% of patients who died in Zaire.

The disease occurred in all age groups, with a predominance in adults. Transmission from person to person required close contact, particularly with blood or body fluids. The disease may be a zoonosis, but the natural host reservoir is unknown, although, as in Lassa fever, Ebola virus probably has an animal reservoir.

The prototype of the virus strains isolated has been named Ebola, after a small river in Zaire that flows north of Yambuku, the village of origin of the patient from whom the first isolate of the virus was obtained.

Ebola virus resembles Marburg virus in negatively stained preparations and consists of filamentous forms of variable length and cylindrical structures that are either U-shaped, shaped like the figure 6, or circular (Fig. 2). Branching of the filamentous form, as well as bizarre forms, is frequently observed. The diameter of the particles is about 80 nm, and length may reach 14,000 nm. A membrane envelope is present, as is a layer composed of short spikes about 10 nm in length. An internal helical structure is seen, but empty particles are also found, as well as particles containing segments of the internal nucleocapsid.

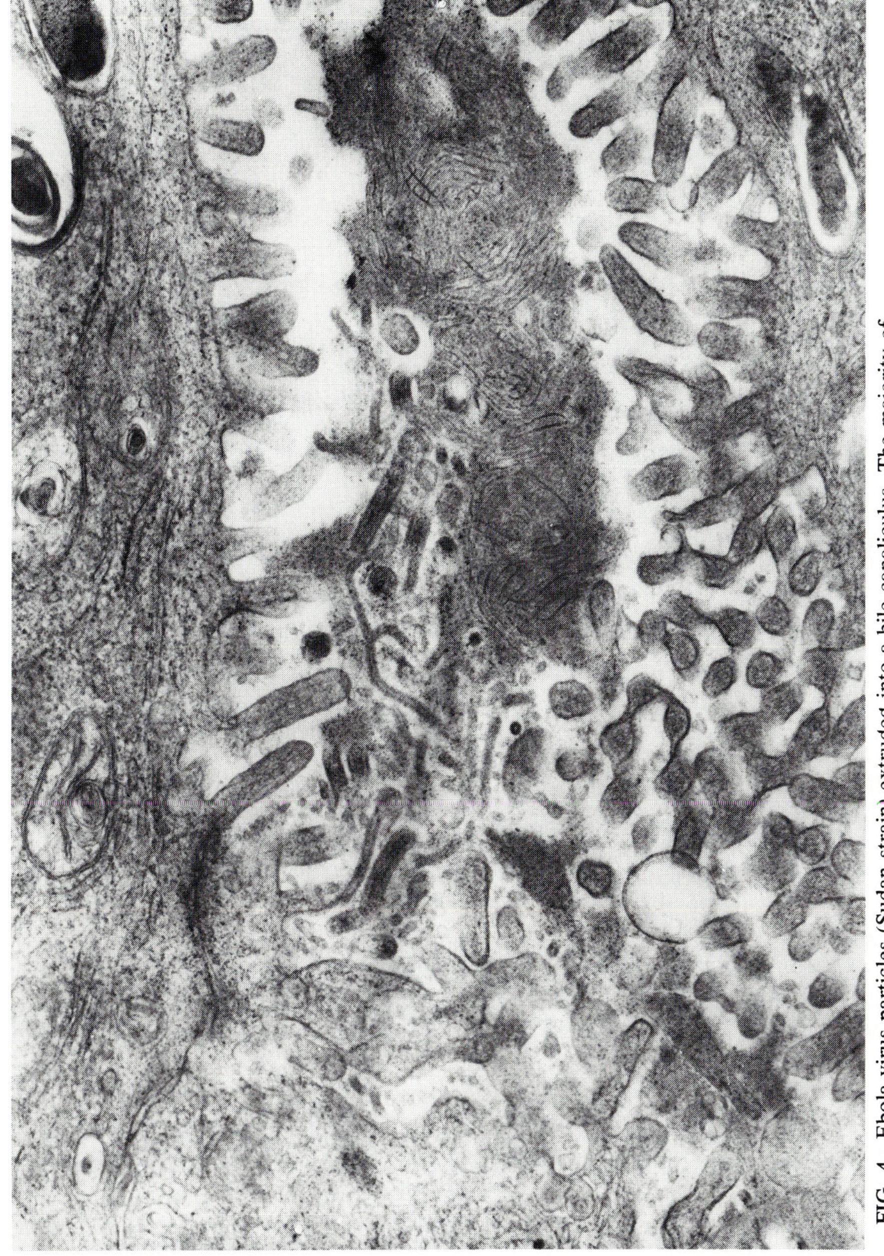

FIG. 4—Ebola virus particles (Sudan strain) extruded into a bile canaliculus. The majority of the particles are aberrant (× 44,100). (Preparation by Dr DS Ellis.)

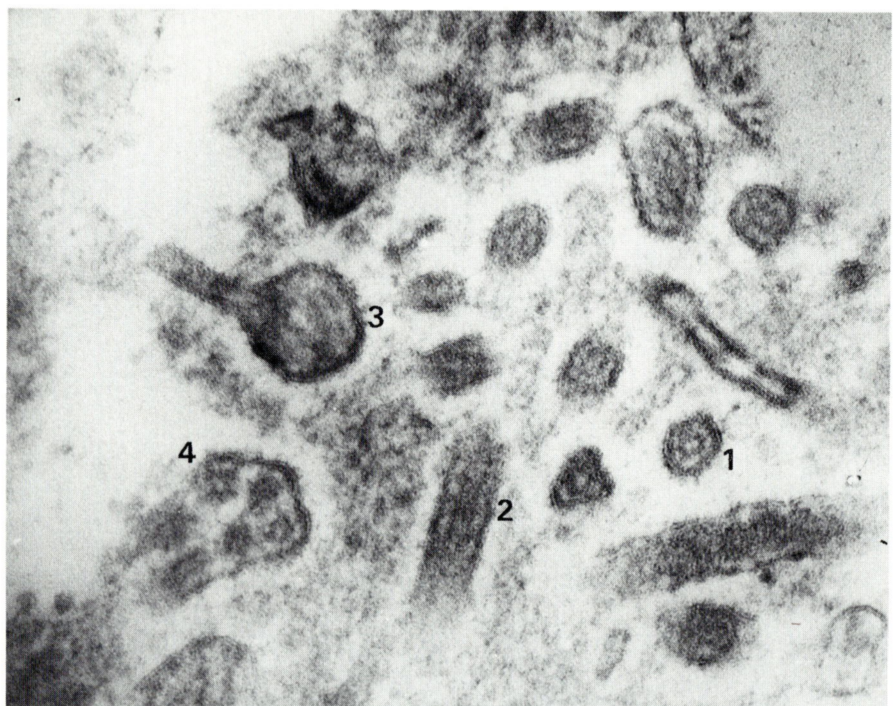

FIG. 5—A variety of forms of Ebola virus found in a thin section of a hepatocyte. (1) Cross section of a complete virus showing a core, above which there is an empty filamentous form. (2) Filamentous form with a core. (3) Enlarged head, possibly a pretorus form. (4) Viral membrane containing six cores. This is an aberrant form of the virus ($\times$ 107,100). (Preparation by Dr DS Ellis.)

Tissues from two autopsies carried out on patients with Ebola virus infection who died in the Sudan and three specimens from patients in Zaire revealed that the histologic lesions in the liver were identical with those of Marburg virus infection. The most prominent feature was focal necrosis of hepatocytes affecting principally the periportal and midzonal areas. Areas of coagulative necrosis of variable size were also common. Single or multiple intracytoplasmic eosinophilic inclusion bodies, ranging in size from 5 to 25 μm, were found in hepatocytes (Fig. 3). Small inclusions with indistinct margins and eosinophilic, nonvacuolated structures resembling Councilman bodies and early hyaline cytoplasmic changes were also seen. Thrombosis occurred in some of the central and portal veins. Portal tracts had little cellular infiltration.

Electron microscopy revealed the main concentrations of Ebola virus particles to be confined to the liver, where large aggregates were easily seen in dying hepatocytes and in the bile canaliculi. Precursors of the cores of this virus were found within intact hepatocytes, and these were aligned in membrane-bound aggregations. The complete virions, formed by incorporation from membranes from the surface through which the cores extruded, were mainly in the long tubular form. Many tubular forms had enlarged terminals or "heads" (Fig. 4–7), and some branched and torus forms were identified.[16]

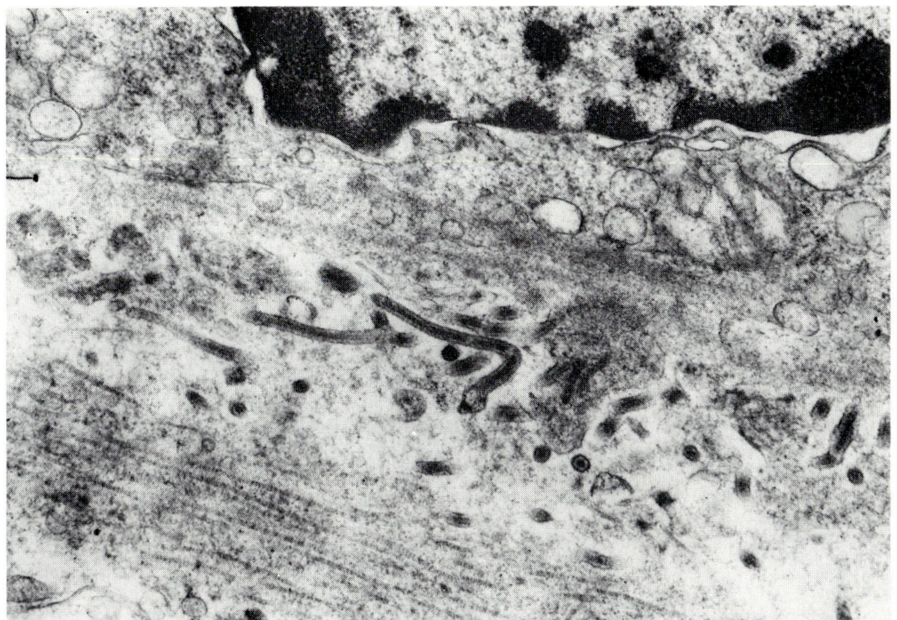

FIG. 6—Experimental transmission of the Zaire strain of Ebola virus to rhesus monkey. This liver section shows complete and occasional branching virus particles among still viable hepatocytes ($\times$ 31,500). (Preparation by Dr DS Ellis.)

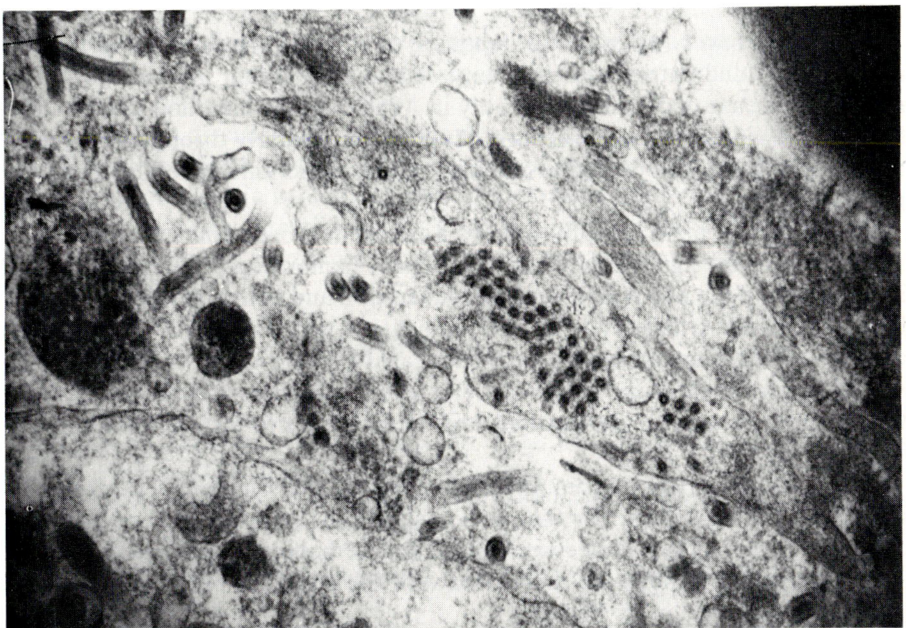

FIG. 7—Rhesus monkey liver showing an array of Ebola virus cores surrounded by complete and branching particles ($\times$ 37,500). (Preparation by Dr DS Ellis.)

of human Lassa fever. Bull WHO 52:535–545, 1975

9. Martini GA, Siegert R (eds): Marburg Virus Disease. Berlin, Springer Verlag, 1971, pp 1–230

10. Almeida JD, Waterson AP, Simpson DIH: Morphology and morphogenesis of the Marburg agent. Edited by GA Martini and R. Siegert: Marburg Virus Disease. Berlin, Springer Verlag, 1971, pp 84–97

11. Gear JSS, Cassel GA, Gear AJ, Trappler B, Clauser L, Meyers AM, Kew MC, Bothwell TH, Sher R, Miller GB, Schneider J, Koornhof HJ, Gomperts ED, Isaacson M, Gear JHS: Outbreak of Marburg virus disease in Johannesburg. Br Med J 4:489–493, 1975

12. Gedigk P, Bechtelsheimer H, Korb G: The morbid anatomy of Marburg virus disease. Ger Med Mon 14:68–77, 1969

13. Murphy FA, Simpson DIH, Whitfield SG, Zlotnik I, Carter GB: Marburg virus infection in monkeys. Ultrastructural studies. Lab Invest 24:279–291, 1971

14. Viral haemorrhagic fever. Wkly Epidem Rec 52:177–180, 1976

15. Emond RTD, Evans B, Bowen ETW, Lloyd G: A case of Ebola virus infection. Br Med J 2:541–544, 1977

16. Ellis DS, Simpson DIH, Francis DP, Knobloch J, Bowen ETW, Lolik P, Deng IM: The ultrastructure of Ebola virus particles in human liver. J Clin Pathol 31:201–208, 1978

17. Van Velder DJJ, Meyer JD, Olivier J, Gear JHS, McIntosh B: Rift Valley fever affecting humans in South Africa. S Afr Med J 51:867–871, 1977

18. Rift Valley fever. Wkly Epidem Rec 53:7–8, 1978

Chapter 24

The Pathogenesis of Hepatosplenic Schistosomiasis: From Man to Monkey to Mouse to Molecule

By KENNETH S. WARREN

SCHISTOSOMA MANSONI and *S. Japonicum* are inch-long flukes residing in the mesenteric venules of more than 100 million people. Each male and female worm pair produces hundreds to thousands of eggs daily, many of which are carried into the liver where they become impacted in the presinusoidal portal venules. Inflammation occurs around the eggs, and if they are present in large enough quantity, severe periportal fibrosis develops. This is accompanied by portal hypertension, congestive splenomegaly, and the development of portal-systemic collateral circulation, as exemplified by esophageal varices. Since there is no direct insult to the hepatocytes, liver function is relatively unimpaired.[1]

The eggs, which are responsible for the liver disease, are also the means of transmission of schistosomiasis. They secrete enzymes that enable them to pass out of the venules through the tissues of the gut and into the lumen, where they are passed in the feces. On entering fresh water the eggs hatch into free swimming miracidia. On penetration into certain species of snails, each miracidium multiplies into thousands of cercariae which destroy the hepatopancreas of the mollusks. Many of these fork-tailed cercariae pass out of the snail into the water. These organisms have the capacity to penetrate unbroken human skin. Within man, each larva develops into either a male or female schistosome during its migration from the skin to the mesenteric venules via the lungs and liver. The schistosomes themselves do not multiply within the human definitive host. Thus, infected individuals carry worm burdens varying from one to thousands. Epidemiologic studies reveal an overdispersed distribution of parasites in human populations, with most individuals bearing light and moderate infections. The intensity of infection in terms of the number of worm pairs and the number of eggs in the tissues and excreta correlates closely, both clinically and pathologically, with the occurrence of hepatosplenic disease, as has been shown in Brazil,[2,3] Uganda,[4] St. Lucia,[5] and Kenya.[6]

Our first knowledge of the pathogenesis of hepatosplenic schistosomiasis came from postmortem studies of man. Over the years, these were supplemented by clinical studies of the pathophysiology of the disease. Work in primates, notably chimpanzees, has added to our knowledge, but investigations in that most versatile of laboratory animals, the mouse, have particularly elu-

From the Rockefeller Foundation.

439

cidated the immunopathogenesis of schistosomiasis. Finally, we must turn to the molecular level to truly understand any biologic process. In the case of schistosomiasis, the isolation and purification of relevant antigens may even facilitate the development of a vaccine that will prevent disease in infected individuals.

MAN

The classical description of schistosomiasis of the liver was provided in 1904 by an English pathologist, William St. Clair Symmers, at Kasr El Ainy Hospital in Cairo, Egypt.[7] The severe periportal fibrosis that he observed, thick walls of white fibrous tissue surrounding the stoma of the large portal vessels, led him to the unusual name "clay-pipe stem cirrhosis" described "as if a number of white clay-pipe stems had been thrust at various angles through the surface." "Microscopically, there is a great increase of the periportal connective tissue, especially of the sublobular and larger portal canals rather than those of interlobular distribution. The fibers are wavy and parallel for the most part, but in certain places they are arranged concentrically. A small blood vessel may often be seen running up to such a mass of concentrically arranged young fibrous tissue, and lying in the center is an ovum, as if it had become impacted in the vessel and had by its presence produced the proliferation of tissue which resulted in cirrhosis. This cirrhosis is, I believe, due to the presence of the *Bilharzia* ovum . . . ." At about that time, schistosomiasis japonica was discovered in the Far East. While the liver disease of *S. japonicum* has not been studied as intensively as that of *S. mansoni*, they are generally considered to be similar entities, the major difference being the increased pathogenicity of the Far Eastern form owing to a tenfold greater egg output by the worms. A recent Japanese review of the subject begins by citing Symmers' pipe stem cirrhosis and then closely follows Andrade's descriptions of hepatosplenic schistosomiasis mansoni in Brazil.[8] The Japanese authors also agreed that the schistosome egg is the main pathogenic factor.[8] Sulit et al. in a description of 81 autopsy cases of hepatosplenic schistosomiasis in the Philippines, described the classical pathologic picture of this disease.[9] The possibility of significant differences in the etiologies of schistosomiasis mansoni and japonica is worthy of consideration, however, as *S. japonicum* and *S. mansoni* eggs differ in many ways other than the mere quantity of their output.[10]

Forty to fifty years after Symmers' description of "clay-pipe stem cirrhosis," Hashem in Egypt[11] and Bogliolo in Brazil[12] observed that the liver disease of schistosomiasis was not a form of cirrhosis but was essentially limited to periportal fibrosis, the patients having relatively little involvement of the hepatic parenchyma. The lobular arrangement of the hepatocytes was maintained, and there was essentially no nodular regeneration. Von Lichtenberg has observed that vascular lesions result from schistosome eggs, accompanied by diffuse portal inflammation and fibrous retraction.[13] These studies were extended by Andrade and Cheever using the plastic cast method to demonstrate extensive distortion and obstruction of small portal branches.[14] The network of small vessels surrounding the portal veins originally considered by

Bogliolo[12] to be venules has now been definitively shown by Andrade and Cheever in plastic cast studies of cadaver livers to be arterioles and to result in extensive arterialization of the liver.[14]

Another major contribution of pathologists is the demonstration of the relationship between the development of significant liver disease and the intensity of infection in terms of numbers of worm pairs and eggs in the tissues. Andrade studied patients with mild chronic schistosomiasis in which the liver did not show gross change at autopsy. Microscopically, occasional schistosome eggs with and without granulomas were seen, and there was mild portal inflammation with lymphocytes and histiocytes.[15] Cheever's classical studies in Brazil[16] and now in Egypt[17] have shown that the pathology in both regions is indistinguishable and that Symmers' fibrosis is clearly related to intensity of infection.

Although it has been claimed that *S. haematobium* may cause significant liver disease,[18] the extensive autopsy studies of Cheever and his colleagues in Egypt conclude that "Symmers' fibrosis was not seen in cases infected only with *S. haematobium* and was not related to the intensity of *S. haematobium* infection."[17]

Clinically, it took many years for the so-called Egyptian splenomegaly syndrome to be associated with Symmers' hepatic lesions, although the liver disease of schistosomiasis was recognized early elsewhere. Studies comparing hepatosplenic schistosomiasis and common cirrhosis revealed that these disease syndromes were very different. A retrospective investigation in Puerto Rico revealed that the patients with schistosomiasis were younger and had far less edema, ascites, and jaundice than those with cirrhosis.[19] Somewhat later, a prospective study in which Brazilian patients were rigorously divided into control groups, those with cirrhosis and those with compensated and decompensated hepatosplenic schistosomiasis, clearly revealed the remarkable clinical differences among these patients.[20] Although most of the compensated hepatosplenics had had hematemeses, none of them had ascites, and there was little edema or emaciation, no stigmata of chronic liver disease, and no jaundice. Mean results of liver function tests for the hepatosplenics were an albumin concentration of virtually 4g/dl, total bilirubin concentration of less than 1 mg/dl, and BSP retention of less than 6%. The blood ammonia levels (both venous and arterial) of these patients were virtually normal, and provocative ammonia-loading tests had little effect. A representative case is shown in Fig. 1. During hematemesis, blood ammonia levels were normal to mildly elevated, and none of the patients went into hepatic coma.[21] Following portacaval shunt, however, liver function deteriorated, often with the development of chronic portal-systemic encephalopathy.[20]

The mechanisms of the development of decompensated hepatosplenic schistosomiasis have essentially remained a mystery. Andrade has described a diffuse mononuclear infiltrate in the portal spaces and fibrous septa radiating from them.[22] Recently, however, Lyra et al. have reported that in comparison with controls and blood donors, patients with hepatosplenic schistosomiasis contain a significantly higher proportion of persistent carriers of hepatitis B surface antigen. The patients who were carriers of the antigen had more clinical signs

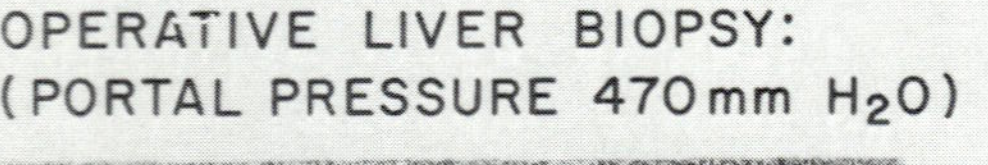

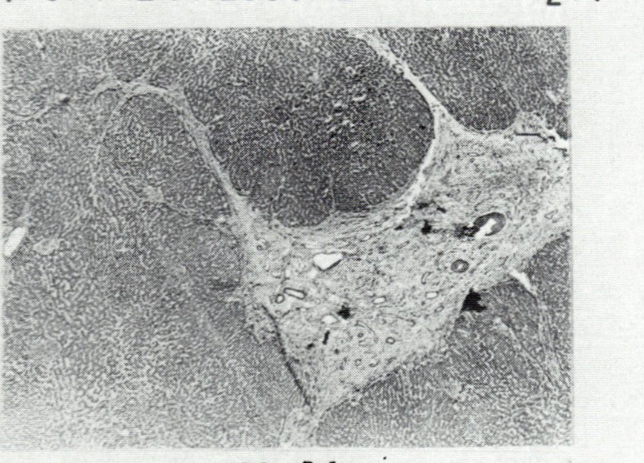

FIG 1—Representative Brazilian patient with hepatosplenic schistosomiasis mansoni.

of chronic liver disease and strikingly more chronic inflammation of the portal spaces on liver biopsy.[23]

Strangely enough, it was first suggested in a single case study of a Puerto Rican with hepatosplenic schistosomiasis in New York City that there was a presinusoidal block to liver blood flow with a high portal pressure and relatively normal wedged hepatic vein pressure,[24] and this has been extensively confirmed. Liver blood flow studies, notably those done in Brazil, have shown total liver blood flow within normal limits in most patients with hepatosplenic disease.[25]

Clinical immunologic studies in schistosomiasis are only beginning. Using parameters of cell- and humoral-mediated immunity, Cook et al. were not able to demonstrate any significant differences between patients with schistosomiasis with or without hepatosplenomegaly.[26] Rocklin's studies in Kenya did, however, reveal a reciprocal relationship between the size of granulomas in rectal biopsies and the quantity of a circulating antibody versus one of the major egg antigens.[27]

Recent studies in Egypt of collagen metabolism in hepatosplenic schistosomiasis using wedge liver biopsies with liver samples maintained in vitro have demonstrated greatly increased collagen content and striking collagen synthesis averaging seven times that of controls.[28]

With respect to schistosomiasis japonica the excellent studies of Sulit et al. in 16 cases revealed that clinically the problem was one of portal hypertension.[9] Standard liver function tests revealed insignificant impairment of parenchymal cell function. The wedged hepatic vein pressures were normal, while the splenic pulp pressures were greatly elevated. Splenoportography revealed evidence of portal hypertension with no obstruction of the extrahepatic venous system. Thus the clinical picture of hepatosplenic schistosomiasis japonica is remarkably similar to that of the mansoni variety described above.

MONKEY

Lower primates are essentially insusceptible to *Schistosoma mansoni* (tree shrew, slow loris, marmoset),[29] while higher primates are moderately susceptible (squirrel monkey, spider monkey, capuchin monkey stumptail monkey, irus monkey, rhesus monkey, baboon, chimpanzee).[30] The rhesus monkey, which has been the most extensively studied of the primates, has the particular characteristic of virtually eliminating its worm burden after several months of infection.[31] Extensive pathophysiologic studies in heavily infected rhesus monkeys over a period of 40 weeks, including surgical liver biopsies, splenoportograms, and blood and liver function tests, revealed the occurrence of only transient abnormalities.[32] There was no evidence of hepatic fibrosis or portal hypertension. Of the primates that develop chronic infections the grivet monkey was studied for as long as 31 months.[33] Although very heavy infections were present in some of these monkeys, only slight hepatic fibrosis was seen, and no portal hypertension or portal-systemic collateral circulation developed. Pathologic studies in 5 of 16 chimpanzees infected with *S. mansoni* did, however, reveal the occurrence of varying degrees of liver fibrosis.[34] One of them developed typical "clay-pipe stem" fibrosis and esophageal varices. Two chimpanzees showed some gross portal fibrosis seen as fine, spidery, greyish markings, one had even less, and the fifth animal's liver was normal in gross appearance. None of the animals had portal hypertension.

With respect to *S. japonicum* infection, studies have been performed in capuchin, grivet, and rhesus monkeys and baboons.[35] All of these animals were highly susceptible. A self-cure phenomenon was observed in the rhesus and grivet monkeys. Moderate portal fibrosis developed by the third month in capuchin monkeys but did not progress thereafter despite continued active infection; portal pressure remained normal, and collateral circulation did not develop. Only focal portal fibrosis was seen in the other host species. Extensive studies in chimpanzees infected with *S. japonicum* revealed chronic infections persisting as long as the animals were studied, up to 17 months.[36] Of 15 animals, 2 had no portal fibrosis, and 6 had fibrosis characterized as slender, 4 as variable, and 3 as broad. Some of the animals had portal-systemic collateral circulation, but none of the animals had portal hypertension. Nine of these animals were considered to have pipe stem fibrosis.

With respect to the pathogenesis of hepatosplenic schistosomiasis in the chimpanzee, it has been observed that fibrosis of the distal portal tracts and subcapsular septa in heavily infected animals appears to be related to the topography and the number of eggs deposited focally. Fibrosis of the large portal fields of the liver often occurred in areas where few or no eggs had been deposited; the etiology of this lesion has never been elucidated. Eggs and egg lesions were found mainly in the adjacent small portal triads.[34,36]

MOUSE

Since its earliest use in the study of schistosomiasis by Brumpt and Chevalier in 1931,[37] the mouse has become the laboratory animal of choice for studying schistosomiasis mansoni and japonica. All of the earlier work was essentially devoted to studies of the gross and microscopic pathologic findings in the livers of infected mice. Investigators using different systems of infecting animals and examining sections of liver under the microscope had variously concluded that the liver disease of schistosomiasis was due to toxins produced by the worms, eggs, and dead worms and to a combination of factors including toxins, eggs, and malnutrition.

The development of a disease syndrome in mice remarkably similar to hepatosplenic disease in man, including hepatomegaly, splenomegaly, portal hypertension, and esophageal varices with normal icterus index and serum albumin concentration, was then described.[38,39] The cause of this syndrome was then established by manipulating the infection in a manner similar to previous studies but using the development of the hepatosplenic disease syndrome as well as gross and microscopic abnormalities in order to determine the parasitic factor responsible for disease. The absence of significant hepatocellular toxins was demonstrated in the following ways: (1) the production of heavy unisexual infections, in the male or female, did not result in hepatosplenic disease or significant pathologic findings over long periods;[40] (2) the use of a drug, nicarbazin, which stopped egg production in bisexual infections, prevented the development of hepatosplenic disease;[41] (3) electron microscopy of hepatocytes in chronic bisexual infections showed no evidence of injury to the subcellular structures.[42] The failure of dead worms to produce hepatosplenic disease was demonstrated by treatment of mice with mature bisexual infections just prior to the onset of egg laying[40] and by repeated reinfection and treatment.[43] The essential role of eggs was revealed by experiments in which bisexual egg-producing infections invariably resulted in hepatomegaly, splenomegaly, portal hypertension, and esophageal varices.[40]

It was then demonstrated that worm burdens as low as one pair would result in hepatosplenic disease and that the mice would survive indefinitely.[44] Andrade, examining the sections of liver from mice infected for 25 weeks, stated that "the mild prolonged infection was accompanied by portal inflammation and later also by fibrosis which was similar to the early pipe-stem fibrosis as seen in human beings."[45] Stimulated by these observations, mice with low worm burdens were studied at various intervals over a period of 1 year.[46] The collagen content of the liver as determined by hydroxyproline measurements rose rapidly after 5 weeks of infection, reaching a steady state by 16 weeks. Egg count also reached a steady state at this time, as the rate of egg production was balanced by their destruction. At 8 weeks, large cellular granulomas around the eggs were distributed among the portal areas as discrete lesions (Fig. 2). At 16 weeks the granulomas were smaller, the collagen was condensed, and they were lined up one behind the other (Fig. 2). At 32 weeks, there was less inflammation, greater density of collagen, apparent resorption of eggs, and thickening owing to the addition of further lesions (Fig. 2). At 52 weeks, fibrosis was even more pronounced in some of the livers. In one of these animals the various stages in the evolution of the fibrosis were apparent, some areas containing fragments of egg shells with collagen in whorls around them and others in which the shells were apparently resorbed and the collagen was oriented in parallel strands.[46] Recent studies of collagen synthesis as measured by the formation of radiolabeled protein-bound hydroxyproline from ^{14}C-labeled proline in early infections in mice revealed a high rate of synthesis that was related to an increased pool of free proline.[47] Examination of the biochemical pathways and of the substrates involved revealed that arginine and not glutamate was the major precursor of the increased free proline pool in the livers of mice with schistosomiasis mansoni.[48]

Studies of liver blood flow in mice with hepatosplenic schistosomiasis and severe portal hypertension, as measured by hepatic uptake of radiocolloidal gold, revealed normal total liver blood flow.[49] Although it was suggested that this might be due to a great increase in the hepatic arterial flow in the presence of decreased portal venous flow, it was not until 1972 that such a phenomenon was proven.

Microcirculation studies in infected mice revealed neovascular formation in the older fibrotic granulomas and fibrotic tissues; ligation of the hepatic artery resulted in complete cessation of flow in these vessels, and, furthermore, in all the sinusoids and central venules under observation.[50] Thus, as the portal venous circulation was obstructed during the course of the schistosome infec-

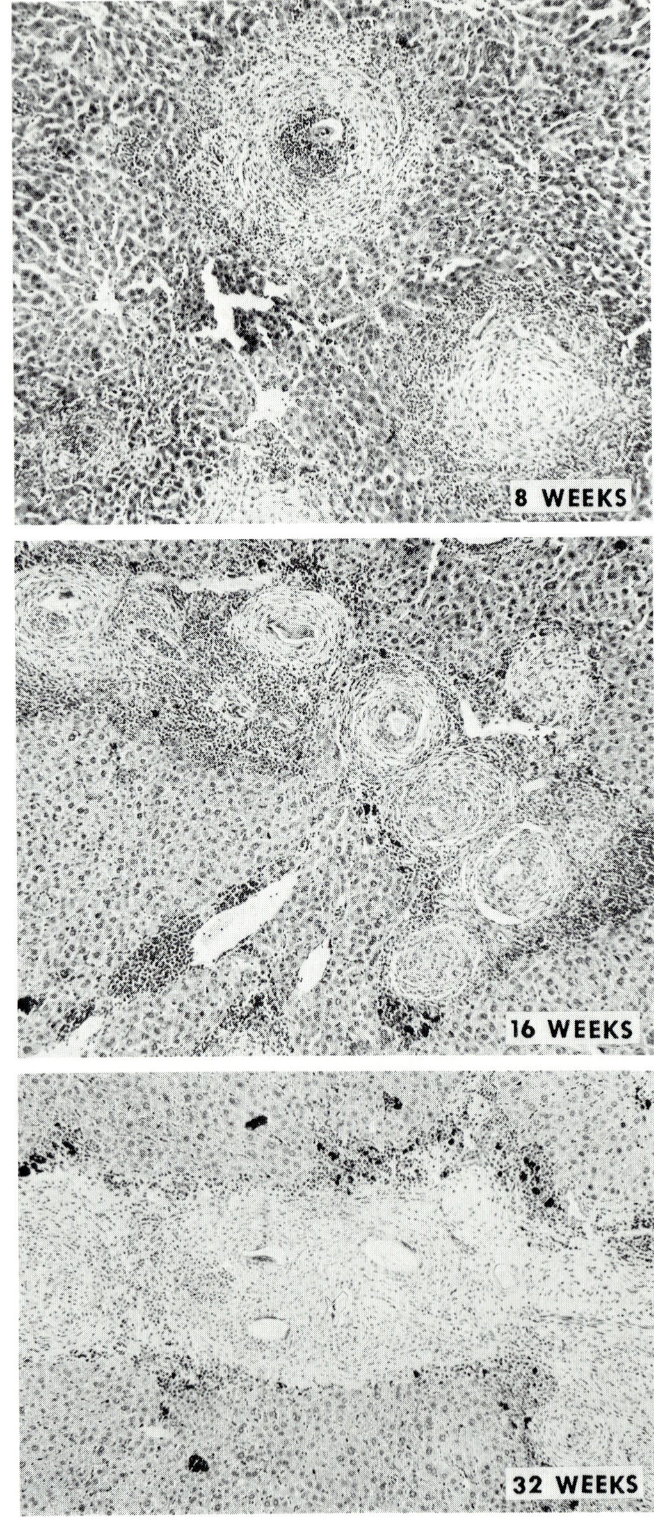

8 WEEKS
16 WEEKS
32 WEEKS

tion, total blood flow was maintained by a compensatory arterialization of the liver.

A major remaining question was the cause of the obstruction to portal blood flow: was it due to the eggs alone or to the inflammatory granulomatous reactions around them (often 100 times the volume of the eggs) and to the subsequent fibrotic scarring? Studies in animals with varying worm burdens suggested the importance of the granuloma in the pathogenesis of the disease: in early heavy infections when there were many eggs in the liver but little host response, there was little disease. Conversely, in long-term light infections, many eggs would often accumulate, but overall host response was also relatively slight, and again there was little disease. At 8 to 10 weeks, when host response was maximal, however, severe hepatosplenic disease was seen in the presence of relatively few eggs.[44] Subsequent studies in different species of inbred mice and other rodents revealed a direct relation between the size of the granulomas in the various species and the development of portal hypertension.[51] Suppression of granuloma formation in a variety of different experimental situations, including streptozotocin-induced diabetes,[52] cholera toxin,[53] toxoplasmosis,[54] and nude mice,[55] was associated with much milder disease. In one study of severely immunosuppressed mice, however, a higher mortality was observed than in control mice, and some necrosis was seen in cells surrounding the eggs; these experiments were confounded by secondary infection with gram-negative bacteria.[56] Nevertheless, some necrosis has been observed around eggs injected into nude mice in which granuloma formation is not only reduced but also appears to be defective.[57] This did not happen, however, around the small granulomas seen in mice with long-standing infections. It is not surprising that such a phenomenon would occur in a situation where there is either no host reaction whatsoever or defective reactivity, since the eggs secrete proteolytic enzymes. Even slight reactivity, if the cells are functioning properly, seems to prevent this reaction.

The most striking evidence for the essential role of the host granulomatous and fibrotic response to the eggs in the pathogenesis of hepatosplenic disease was the microcirculation studies of Bloch et al.[50] Direct observation in living animals showed that the eggs impacted in the presinusoidal portal venules often did not completely block blood flow and had no effect on the surrounding vessels. When the large granulomas formed, however, flow in the vessels ceased completely and was also compromised in the surrounding areas.

Under these circumstances, knowledge of the mechanism of granuloma formation was of great importance. A breakthrough in methodology was achieved by von Lichtenberg, who isolated living *S. mansoni* eggs from the livers of infected mice and injected them intravenously into the tail veins of groups of uninfected mice.[58] The eggs were trapped as individual emboli in the lungs, which were removed at different time intervals, sectioned, stained, and the size of the lesions around the eggs measured. While von Lichtenberg demonstrated the primary lesions, Warren and colleagues showed that secondary

---

FIG 2—Sections of mouse liver (hematoxylin and eosin stain) showing granulomas and fibrosis around *Schistosoma mansoni* eggs in mice infected for 8, 16, and 32 weeks. (From Warren KS: The pathogenesis of "clay pipe-stem cirrhosis" in mice with chronic schistosomiasis mansoni, with a note on the longevity of the schistosomes. Am J Pathol 49:477–489, 1966, with permission.)

exposure (the primary exposure being an intraperitoneal injection of eggs) resulted in anamnestic inflammatory reactivity, which was specific (there was no cross-reactivity with *Ascaris suum* eggs) and was transferable with lymph node or spleen cells but not with serum[59] (Fig. 3). These experiments strongly suggested that the *S. mansoni* egg granuloma was an immunologic reaction of the cell-mediated type.

Inhibition of granuloma formation by measures and conditions that strongly suppress cellular hypersensitivity, including antilymphocyte serum, neonatal thymectomy (in mice and chickens), Hodgkins'-like disease (SJL/J mice), cholera toxin, diabetes, niridazole and nude mice, was observed.[60] By contrast, inhibitors of humoral antibody-mediated responses, such as chronic x-irradiation, bursectomy (chickens), Friend virus leukemia, antineutrophil serum, cobra venom factor and anti mu serum, had no effect.[60]

Interrelationships between granuloma formation and in vivo forms and in vitro correlates of cellular hypersensitivity were then revealed. In mice, the onset of inflammation around the eggs closely approximated the development of delayed footpad swelling to soluble egg antigens.[61] In guinea pigs, there were close correlations between the beginning of granuloma formation and the soluble egg antigen-mediated delayed skin reactions, lymphocyte blastogenesis, and production of macrophage migration inhibitory factor.[62]

Using a technique in which intact granulomas could be isolated from the livers of infected mice,[63] mechanisms of granulomatous inflammation were then demonstrated in vitro. The production of the lymphokines macrophage migration inhibitory factor[64] and eosinophil stimulation promotor was revealed.[65] Using radiolabeled amino acids, protein synthesis was demonstrated, but only minute amounts, if any, of immunoglobulin production were shown.[66]

Investigations of granuloma formation around *S. japonicum* eggs, however, have suggested a different mechanism than that of *S. mansoni* granulomas.[67,68] Parasitologically, these lesions differ in that *S. japonicum* eggs are produced in large aggregates, while *S. mansoni* eggs enter the tissues singly. Pathologically, the lesions are different in schistosomiasis japonica in that eosinophilic abscesses occur early after egg-laying begins, there is much necrosis in the early lesions, and plasma cells are seen both in the granulomas and in areas of periportal inflammation.[67] Immunologically, precipitating antibodies appear soon after egg-laying begins, and footpad swelling from soluble *S. japonicum* egg antigens shows striking immediate and no delayed reactivity.[68]

Studies in mice exposed to different intensities of infection revealed, for the first time, that very low worm burdens (one to three pairs) would result in relatively uniform long-term chronic infections.[44] Sections from the livers of mice infected for 25 weeks revealed a considerable decrease in the size of the granulomatous lesions around living eggs in comparison with those around similar eggs at earlier stages.[45] Confirmation of these observations was later reported using the system of injection of living eggs into the pulmonary microvasculature of mice infected for periods from 2 to 32 weeks (the eggs produced by the worms are largely retained in the intestines and liver).[69] The mice infected for 2 weeks (prior to the onset of egg-laying) developed small granulomas similar to uninfected mice, while those infected for 8 weeks showed

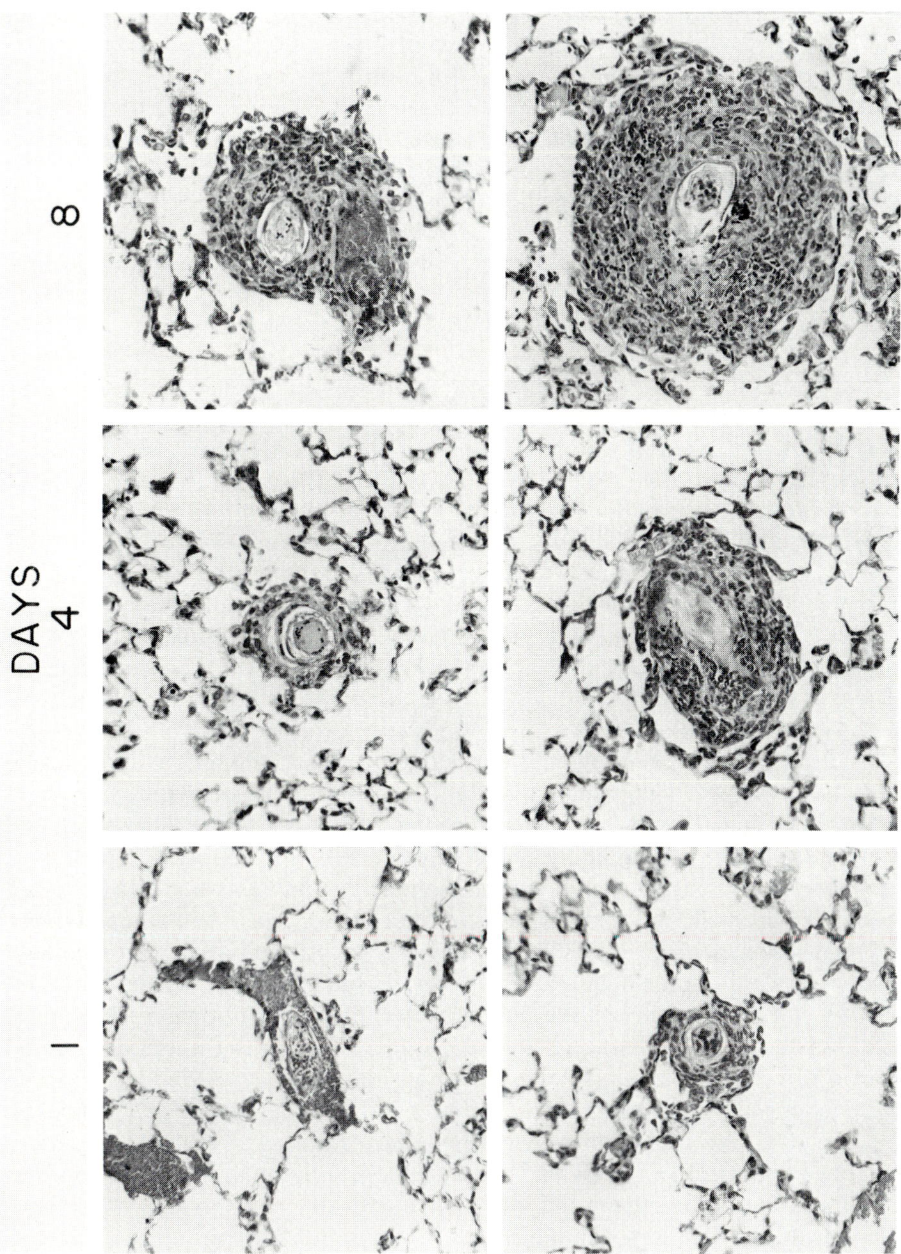

FIG 3—Granulomatous reaction 1, 4, and 8 days after intravenous injection of *Schistosoma mansoni* eggs into the lungs of mice injected intraperitoneally 3 days previously with lymph node cells from normal mice (top) and mice infected for 8 weeks with *S. mansoni* (bottom). Each lesion is representive of the means of 100 measured lesions. Hematoxylin and eosin stain (× 162). (Warren KS, Domingo EO, Cowan RBT: Granuloma formation around schistosome eggs as a manifestation of delayed hypersensitivity. Am J Pathol 51:735–756, 1967, with permission.)

accelerated, augmented granulomatous hypersensitivity. The mice infected for 16, 24, and 32 weeks, however, continued to have accelerated inflammation but also a constantly diminishing peak lesion size; by 24 and 32 weeks the peak lesions were much smaller than those seen in uninfected, unsensitized animals. The clinical effect of these changes was seen in mice with light infections studied for a period of 1 year.[46] The peak liver egg count was seen at 16 weeks, reaching a steady state thereafter as older eggs were being destroyed; the total liver collagen also peaked at 16 weeks and remained relatively constant thereafter. Mean peak granuloma size began to decrease from 8 weeks. Consistent with these results, liver and spleen weights and portal hypertension peaked at 16 weeks and declined by 52 weeks, respectively, by 15%, 46%, and 43%.[46]

A striking form of modulation of granulomatous reactivity was observed by Warren and Berry in 1972 in mice infected with different geographic strains of *S. japonicum*.[70] Each of the animals harbored only one worm pair, but since egg output of *S. japonicum* is ten times that of *S. mansoni*, it was assumed that all the mice would die between 10 and 20 weeks after infection. Surprisingly, mortality was exceedingly low, and groups of animals were studied for as long as 40 weeks. Although inflammation around the masses of *S. japonicum* eggs was massive at 8 weeks, there was virtually no reaction around the eggs at 40 weeks. Furthermore, in the most pathogenic of the strains, that from the Philippines, hepatosplenic disease peaked at 20 weeks but showed dramatic amelioration in all parameters (liver weight, spleen weight, portal hypertension, hematocrit) by 40 weeks.

Studies of the mechanism of this modulation of granulomatous hypersensitivity have shown a significant diminution in cell-mediated responses to soluble egg antigens coincident with the decrease in granuloma size.[71,72] These included delayed footpad swelling and failure of spleen cells to produce lymphokines. Lymphocyte blastogenesis not only to soluble egg antigens but also to T-cell mitogens was strikingly diminished, and heat-labile, passive cutaneous anaphylaxis antibody and peripheral eosinophilia decreased. While cell-mediated responses were diminishing, there was an exponential increase in hemagglutinating and heat-stable passive cutaneous anaphylaxis antibodies. The adoptive transfer of suppression of granuloma formation in the livers of infected mice (CBA/J) with either spleen or lymph node cells provided very strong evidence for a cellular mechanism for modulation.[73] Serum transfer studies in the sensitive lung granuloma system have also revealed a suppressive effect of large amounts of serum (R. P. Pelley, personal communication). It appears, therefore, that both cellular and humoral suppressive systems may be responsible for the modulation of granulomatous hypersensitivity around *S. mansoni* eggs in mice, although their relative importance has not been established.

MOLECULAR OBSERVATIONS

Soluble antigens were isolated from *S. mansoni* eggs in 1970 by homogenization and ultracentrifugation (100,000 g for 2 hr), which in minute quantities and without adjuvant induce sensitization to a delayed hypersensitivity type of granuloma around intact schistosome eggs.[74] This material is secreted by intact eggs and is found in high concentration in the fluid released during the hatching process. When adsorbed to bentonite particles, these soluble egg antigens (SEA) elicit hypersensitivity-type granuloma formation in specifically sensitized animals. SEA also both induces and elicits delayed footpad swelling in mice. These sensitizing amounts of SEA do not induce antibody formation detectable by a sensitive hemagglutination technique. In 1976 the identification and purification of three major antigens from SEA was described, and similar findings were soon reported using different experimental systems.[75-77] The original system involved identification of the antigens using serum from chronically infected animals (longer than 20 weeks) in which anti-SEA antibodies were high. Major serologic antigen$_1$ (MSA$_1$), the antigen present in greatest quantities, appeared most likely to play a major role in granuloma formation because it shared the same high stage and species specificity in terms of induction and elicitation of the lesions as the intact eggs, as determined by competitive inhibition studies using radioimmunoassay.[78] Both the method of isolation and further biochemical studies have suggested that MSA$_1$ is a glycoprotein of molecular weight 50,000, MSA$_2$ a glycoprotein of molecular weight greater than 200,000, and MSA$_3$ a protein of molecular weight 70,000.[79] The most recently published method of purification of MSA$_1$ involves isolation of eggs from the livers of infected mice, homogenization in a Ten Broeck grinder, ultracentrifugation at 100,000 g for 2 hr, desalting on Sephadex G 25, affinity chromatography on concanavallin A Sepharose with elution by methyl alpha mannose and ion exchange chromatography on DEAE cellulose.[80] With respect to granuloma formation, MSA$_1$-chronic infection serum complexes strongly sensitized to accelerated augmented lesions.[79] Experiments now in progress have shown that the concanavallin A Sepharose drop-through (containing mainly MSA$_2$ and MSA$_3$) is not sensitizing while the concanavallin A Sepharose eluate (mainly MSA$_1$) is more strongly sensitizing than crude SEA.

INTEGRATION AND OUTLOOK

In the past two decades there has been a virtual explosion of knowledge about schistosomiasis. Modern epidemiologic studies have uncovered the importance of intensity of infection in the development of human disease. Thus, hepatosplenic disease clusters in those with heavy worm burdens; fortunately, the distribution of intensity of infection is negative binomial with only a small proportion of the infected population carrying large numbers of worms.

Clinical studies have clearly shown that hepatosplenic schistosomiasis differs greatly from cirrhosis in that stigmata of liver parenchymal disease, ascites, edema, jaundice, and liver function test derangements are rare. Even under maximal stress, these patients do not develop portal-systemic encephalopathy. Circulation studies have tended to reveal normal total liver blood flow but a presinusoidal type of portal hypertension.

Pathologists have confirmed the original description in 1904 of hepatosplenic disease by Symmers. They have noted that this is a form of fibrosis of the liver and not cirrhosis, as the liver parenchymal cells are unharmed and regenerative nodules are uncommon. Quantitative studies again suggest that Symmers' fibrosis clusters in those with heavy infections. Plastic casts of the liver circulation have revealed a presinusoidal block to portal blood flow with compensatory arterialization of the liver.

Studies in primates have shown that some species are refractory to infection (usually those lower on the phylogenetic scale), that others are highly susceptible to infection but do not develop the classical pathologic features of hepatosplenic disease, and that some chimpanzees do attain a form of Symmers' fibrosis but without associated portal hypertension.

Mice develop a clinical syndrome remarkably similar to that seen in man, with hepatomegaly, splenomegaly, portal hypertension, and esophageal varices. Liver parenchymal cell function tends to be relatively unimpaired. Liver collagen content is greatly elevated in these animals, and synthesis is greatly increased. Total liver blood flow is normal, and microcirculation studies have revealed neovascular formation in the fibrous tissue, which is all arterial. The helminth factor that is responsible for the disease has been shown to be the egg, as previously suggested by Symmers in 1904, but the host granulomatous inflammatory and fibrotic response is essential for the development of hepatosplenic disease. The *S. mansoni* egg granuloma has clearly been shown to be an immunologic reaction of the delayed hypersensitivity type on the basis of the development of anamnestic reactivity that is specific and transferable with cells but not with serum, studies with immunosuppressive measures, coincidence with other forms of cell-mediated reactivity, and demonstration of lymphokine production in vitro. A spontaneous form of suppression of granulomatous reactivity has been demonstrated in chronically infected mice that appears to be due to suppressor cell mechanisms but may also have a component of humoral blockade.

The molecule responsible for the granulomatous reaction around the eggs and hence hepatosplenic disease appears to have been isolated in pure form. The specificity of this glycoprotein antigen for the *S. mansoni* egg is so high that it has enabled the development of a highly sensitive and specific radioimmunoassay for schistosomiasis mansoni. It is possible that repeated doses of antigen, chemically altered antigen, or antigen administered with certain adjuvants may induce the suppressor responses and thereby inhibit granuloma formation and hepatosplenic disease. Thus the final outcome of all of these investigations could well be the development of a vaccine which, while having no effect on infection, could prevent or ameliorate disease.

REFERENCES

1. Warren KS: The pathology of schistosome infections. Helm Abs 42:591–633, 1973
2. Kloetzel K: Splenomegaly in schistosomiasis mansoni. Am J Trop Med Hyg 11:472–476, 1962
3. Lehman JS Jr, Mott KE, Morrow RH Jr, Muniz TM, Boyer MH: The intensity and effects of infection with *Schistosoma mansoni* in a rural community in northeast Brazil. Am J Trop Med Hyg 25:285–294, 1976
4. Ongom VL, Bradley DJ: The epidemiology and consequences of *Schistosoma mansoni* infection in West Nile Uganda. I. Field studies of a community at Panyagoro. Trans R Soc Trop Med Hyg 66:835–851, 1972
5. Cook JA, Baker ST, Warren KS, Jordan P: A controlled study of morbidity of schistosomiasis mansoni in St. Lucian children, based on quantitative egg excretion. Am J Trop Med Hyg 23:625–633, 1974

6. Arap Siongok TK, Mahmoud AAF, Ouma JH, Warren KS, Muller AS, Handa AK, Houser HB: Morbidity in schistosomiasis mansoni in relation to intensity of infection: Study of a community in Machakos, Kenya. Am J Trop Med Hyg 25:273–284, 1976

7. Symmers WStC: Note on a new form of liver cirrhosis due to the presence of ova of *Bilharzia haematobia*. J Pathol Bacteriol 9:237–239, 1904

8. Tsutsumi H, Nakashima T: Pathology of liver cirrhosis due to *Schistosoma japonicum*. Edited by M. Yokogawa: Research in Filariasis and Schistosomiasis. Vol. 2. Baltimore, University Park Press, 1972, pp 113–131

9. Sulit YSM, Domingo EO, Dalmacio-Cruz AE, De Perolta DS, Imperial ES: Parasitic cirrhosis among Filipinos. J Philipp Med Assoc 40:1021–1038, 1964

10. Warren KS: Schistosomiasis japonica: Models for the pathogenesis of hepatosplenic, intestinal and cerebral disease. Jpn J Parasitol 20:40–44, 1971

11. Hashem M: The etiology and pathogenesis of the endemic form of hepatosplenomegaly "Egyptian splenomegaly." J Egypt Med Assoc 30:48–79, 1947

12. Bogliolo L: The anatomical picture of the liver in hepatosplenic schistosomiasis mansoni. Ann Trop Med Parasitol 51:1–14, 1957

13. von Lichtenberg F: Lesions of the intrahepatic portal radicles in Manson's schistosomiasis. Am J Pathol 31:757–771, 1955

14. Andrade ZA, Cheever AW: Alterations of the intrahepatic vasculature in hepatosplenic schistosomiasis mansoni. Am J Trop Med Hyg 20:425–432, 1971

15. Andrade ZA, Prata A: Asymptomatic schistosomiasis studied by needle biopsy of the liver. Am J Trop Med Hyg 12:854–858, 1963

16. Cheever AW: A quantitative post-mortem study of schistosomiasis mansoni in man. Am J Trop Med Hyg 17:38–64, 1968

17. Cheever AW, Kamel IA, Elwi AM, Mosimann JE, Donner R: *Schistosoma mansoni* and *Schistosoma haematobium* infections in Egypt. II. Quantitative parasitological findings at necropsy. Am J Trop Med Hyg 26:702–716, 1977

18. Carter RA, Shaldon S: The liver in schistosomiasis. Lancet 2:1003–1008, 1959

19. Rodriguez HF, Garcia-Palmieri MR, Rivera JV, Rodriguez-Molina R: A comparative study of portal and bilharzial cirrhosis. Gastroenterology 29:235–246, 1955

20. Warren KS, Rebouças G, Baptista AG: Ammonia metabolism and hepatic coma in hepatosplenic schistosomiasis. Patients studied before and after portacaval shunt. Ann Intern Med 62:1113–1133, 1965

21. Warren KS, Rebouças G: Blood ammonia during bleeding from esophageal varices in patients with hepatosplenic schistosomiasis. N Engl J Med 271:921–926, 1964

22. Andrade ZA: Hepatic schistosomiasis. Morphological aspects. Edited by H Popper and F Schaffner: Progress in Liver Disease. Vol. II. New York, Grune & Stratton, 1965

23. Lyra LG, Rebouças G, Andrade ZA: Hepatitis B surface antigen carrier state in hepatosplenic schistosomiasis. Gastroenterology 71:641–645, 1976

24. Aufses AH Jr, Schaffner F, Rosenthal WS, Herman BF: Portal venous pressure in pipestem fibrosis of the liver due to schistosomiasis. Am J Med 27:807–810, 1959

25. Coutinho A: Hemodynamic studies of portal hypertension in schistosomiasis. Am J Med 44:547–556, 1968

26. Cook JA, Woodstock L, Jordan J: Immunological studies in *Schistosoma mansoni* infection in St. Lucia. Ann Trop Med Parasitol 66:369–373, 1972

27. Rocklin RE, Brown A, Warren KS, Pelley RP, Houba V, Butterworth AF: Immunologic modulation in children with schistosomiasis. Clin Res 25:486A, 1977

28. Dunn MA, Kamel R, Kamel IA, Biempica L, El Kholy A, Hart PK, Rojkind M, Warren KS, Mahmoud AAF: Liver collagen synthesis in schistosomiasis. Gastroenterology (in press)

29. Warren KS, Jane JA: Comparative susceptibility to *Schistosoma mansoni* of the squirrel monkey, the slow loris and the tree shrew. Trans R Soc Trop Med Hyg 61:534–537, 1967

30. Sadun EH, von Lichtenberg F, Bruce JI: Susceptibility and comparative pathology of ten species of primates exposed to infection with *Schistosoma mansoni*. Am J Trop Med Hyg 15:705–718, 1966

31. Vogel H, Minning W: Uber die Erworbene Resistenz von Macacus Rhesus gegenuber *Schistosoma japonicum*. Z Tropenmed Parasitol 4:418–505, 1953

32. Bruce J, Warren KS, Sadun E: Observations on the pathophysiology of schistosomiasis mansoni in monkeys. Exp Parasitol 13:194–198, 1963

33. Cheever AW, Duvall RH: Single and re-

peated infections of grivet monkeys with *Schistosoma mansoni*: Parasitological and pathological observations over a 31 month period. Am J Trop Med Hyg 23:884–894, 1974

34. Sadun EH, von Lichtenberg F, Cheever AW, Erickson DG: Schistosomiasis mansoni in the chimpanzee. The natural history of chronic infections after single and multiple exposures. Am J Trop Med Hyg 19:258–277, 1970

35. Cheever AW, Erickson DG, Sadun EH, von Lichtenberg F: *Schistosoma japonicum* infections in monkeys and baboons: Parasitological and pathological findings. Am J Trop Med Hyg 23:51–64, 1974

36. von Lichtenberg F, Sadun EH, Cheever AW, Erickson DG, Johnson AJ, Boyce HW: Experimental infection with *Schistosoma japonicum* in chimpanzees. Parasitologic, clinical, serologic and pathological observations. Am J Trop Med Hyg 20:850–893, 1971

37. Brumpt E, Chevalier P: The spleen and spleno-hepatitis in experimental bilharziasis. Ann Parasitol 9:15–67, 1931

38. Warren KS, DeWitt WB: Production of portal hypertension and esophageal varices in the mouse. Proc Soc Exp Biol Med 98:99–101, 1958

39. DeWitt WB, Warren KS: Hepato-splenic schistosomiasis in mice. Am J Trop Med Hyg 8:440–446, 1959

40. Warren KS: The etiology of hepatosplenic schistosomiasis mansoni in mice. Am J Trop Med Hyg 10:870–876, 1961

41. Warren KS: Suppression of hepatosplenic schistosomiasis mansoni in mice by Nicarbazin, a drug that inhibits egg production by schistosomes. J Infec Dis 121:514–521, 1970

42. Stenger RJ, Warren KS, Johnson FA: An electron microscopic study of the liver parenchyma and schistosome pigment in murine hepatosplenic schistosomiasis. Am J Trop Med Hyg 16:473–482, 1967

43. Cheever AW, DeWitt WB, Warren KS: Repeated infection and treatment of mice with *Schistosoma mansoni*. Functional, anatomic and immunologic observations. Am J Trop Med Hyg 14:239–253, 1965

44. Warren KS: The contribution of worm burden and host response to the development of hepato-splenic schistosomiasis mansoni in mice. Am J Trop Med Hyg 12:34–39, 1963

45. Andrade ZA, Warren KS: Mild prolonged schistosomiasis in mice: alterations in host response with time and the development of portal fibrosis. Trans R Soc Trop Med Hyg 58:53–57, 1964

46. Warren KS: The pathogenesis of ''clay pipe-stem cirrhosis'' in mice with chronic schistosomiasis mansoni, with a note on the longevity of the schistosomes. Am J Pathol 49:477–489, 1966

47. Dunn MA, Rojkind M, Warren KS, Hait PK, Rifas L, Seifter S: Liver collagen synthesis in murine schistosomiasis. J Clin Invest 59:666–674, 1977

48. Dunn MA, Rojkind M, Hait PK, Warren KS: Conversion of arginine to proline in murine schistosomiasis. Gastroenterology 75:1010–1015, 1978

49. Cheever AW, Warren KS: Hepatic blood flow in mice with acute hepatosplenic schistosomiasis mansoni. Trans R Soc Trop Med Hyg 58:406–412, 1964

50. Bloch EH, Abdel Wahab MF, Warren KS: *In vivo* microscopic observations of the pathogenesis and pathophysiology of hepatosplenic schistosomiasis in the mouse liver. Am J Trop Med Hyg 21:546–557, 1972

51. Cheever AW: A comparative study of *Schistosoma mansoni* infections in mice, gerbils, multi-mammate rats and hamsters. I. The relation of portal hypertension to size of hepatic granulomas. Am J Trop Med Hyg 14:211–226, 1965

52. Mahmoud AAF, Cheever AW, Warren KS: Streptozotocin-induced diabetes mellitus and the host parasite relation in murine schistosomiasis mansoni. J Infect Dis 131:634–642, 1975

53. Warren KS, Mahmoud AAF, Boros DL, Rall TW, Mandel MA, Carpenter CCJ Jr: In vivo suppression by cholera toxin of cell-mediated and foreign body inflammatory responses. J Immunol 112:996–1007, 1974

54. Mahmoud AAF, Strickland GT, Warren KS: Toxoplasmosis and the host-parasite relationship in murine schistosomiasis mansoni. J Infect Dis 135:408–413, 1977

55. Phillips SM, DiConza JJ, Gold QA, Reid WA: Schistosomiasis in the congenitally athymic (nude) mouse. I. Thymic dependency of eosinophilia, granuloma formation and host morbidity. J Immunol 118:594–599, 1977

56. Buchanan RD, Fine DP, Colley DG: *Schistosoma mansoni* in mice depleted of thymus-dependent lymphocytes. II. Pathology; altered pathogenesis. Am J Pathol 71:207–218, 1973

57. Byram JE, von Lichtenberg F: Altered schistosome granuloma formation in nude mice. Am J Trop Med Hyg 26:944–956, 1977

58. von Lichtenberg F: Host response to eggs of *S. mansoni*. I. Granuloma formation in the unsensitized laboratory mouse. Am J Pathol 41:711–731, 1962

59. Warren KS, Domingo EO, Cowan RBT: Granuloma formation around schistosome eggs as a manifestation of delayed hypersensitivity. Am J Pathol 51:735–756, 1967

60. Warren KS: The pathology, pathbiology and pathogenesis of schistosomiasis. Nature 273:609–612, 1978

61. Hang LM, Warren KS, Boros DL: The *Schistosoma mansoni* egg granuloma: Antigenic secretions as the sole etiological factor. Exp Parasitol 35:288–298, 1974

62. Boros DL, Schwartz HJ, Powell A, Warren KS: Delayed hypersensitivity as manifested by granuloma formation, dermal reactivity, macrophage migration inhibition and lymphocyte transformation, induced and elicited in guinea pigs with soluble antigens of *Schistosoma mansoni* eggs. J Immunol 110:1118–1125, 1973

63. Pellegrino J, Brener Z: Method for isolating granulomas from mouse liver. J Parasitol 42:564, 1956

64. Boros DL, Warren KS, Pelley RP: The secretion of migration inhibitory factor by intact schistosome egg granulomas maintained in vitro. Nature 246:224–226, 1973

65. James SL, Colley DG: Eosinophils and immune mechanisms: Production of the lymphokine eosinophil stimulation promoter (ESP) in vitro by isolated intact granulomas. J Reticuloendothel Soc 18:283–293, 1975

66. Pelley RP, Boros DL, Warren KS: Lymphokine production and protein synthesis by isolated, cultured *Schistosoma mansoni* granulomas. J Immunol (in press)

67. Warren KS, Boros DL, Hang LM, Mahmoud AAF: The *Schistosoma japonicum* egg granuloma. Am J Pathol 80:279–294, 1975

68. Warren KS, Grove DI, Pelley RP: The *Schistosoma japonicum* egg granuloma. II. Cellular composition, granuloma size and immunologic concomitants. Am J Trop Med Hyg 27:271–275, 1978

69. Domingo EO, Warren KS: Endogenous desensitization: changing host granulomatous response to schistosome eggs at different stages of infection with *Schistosoma mansoni*. Am J Pathol 52:369–377, 1968

70. Warren KS, Berry EG: Induction of hepatosplenic disease by single pairs of the Philippine, Formosan, Japanese, and Chinese strains of *Schistosoma japonicum*. J Infect Dis 126:482–491, 1972

71. Boros DL, Pelley RP, Warren KS: Spontaneous modulation of granulomatous hypersensitivity in schistosomiasis mansoni. J Immunol 114:1437–1441, 1975

72. Colley DG: Immune responses to a soluble schistosomal egg antigen preparation during chronic primary infection with *Schistosoma mansoni*. J Immunol 115:150–156, 1975

73. Colley DG: Adoptive suppression of granuloma formation. J Exp Med 143:696–700, 1976

74. Boros DL, Warren KS: Delayed hypersensitivity-type granuloma formation and dermal reaction induced and elicited by a soluble factor isolated from *Schistosoma mansoni* eggs. J Exp Med 132:488–507, 1970

75. Pelley RP, Pelley RJ, Hamburger J, Peters PA, Warren KS: *Schistosoma mansoni* soluble egg antigens: I. Identification and purification of three major antigens, and the employment of radioimmunoassay for their further characterization. J Immunol 117:1553–1560, 1976

76. Boros DL, Tomford R, Warren KS: Induction of granulomatous and elicitation of cutaneous sensitivity by partially purified SEA of *Schistosoma mansoni*. J Immunol 118:373–376, 1977

77. Brown AP, Remold HG, Warren KS, David JR: Partial purification of antigens from eggs of *Schistosoma mansoni* which elicit delayed hypersensitivity. J Immunol 119:1257–1278, 1977

78. Hamburger J, Pelley RP, Warren KS: Purified *Schistosoma mansoni* egg antigens: Determinations of the stage and species specificity of their serological reactivity by radioimmunoassay. J Immunol 117:1561–1566, 1976

79. Pelley RP, Pelley RJ: *S. mansoni* soluble egg antigens. IV. Biochemistry of major serological antigens with particular emphasis on MSA_1. Edited by H. Van den Bossche: Biochemistry of Parasites and Host-Parasite Relationships. Amsterdam, Elsevier/North Holland Biomedical Press, 1976, pp 283–290

80. Pelley RP: Purification of *Schistosoma mansoni* egg antigens: Theory and practice. Am J Trop Med Hyg 26 (part 2): 104–112, 1977

Chapter 25

Mechanisms of Intrahepatic Cholestasis

By ELWYN ELIAS *and* JAMES L. BOYER

DEFINITION OF CHOLESTASIS

Physiologists, pathologists, and clinicians each view the problem of cholestasis from slightly different vantage points. To the experimental physiologist, any reduction in the rate of bile flow may represent cholestasis. The clinician thinks of cholestasis when a significant deficit in bile production produces symptoms and signs as a result of excessive accumulation of products normally excreted in bile (e.g., jaundice, pruritus, xanthelasma) and to the inadequate secretion of bile into the intestine (e.g., steatorrhea, fat-soluble vitamin deficiency). The pathologist who first used the term, however, recognized cholestasis by its effects on hepatic structure, particularly canalicular bile plugs and feathery degeneration of hepatocytes. Each, of course, is focusing on only an obvious consequence of what is now regarded as a primary disturbance in hepatic bile formation. The mechanisms by which bile secretion is impaired represent an area of intense investigational interest, and some newer concepts are reviewed in this chapter. Other reviews of this subject have also appeared.[1,2]

ANATOMIC AND BIOCHEMICAL EVIDENCE
FOR A LOBULAR GRADIENT

The characteristically centrolobular distribution of canalicular bile plugs in intrahepatic cholestasis probably reflects differences in function of the various zones within each lobule. Rappaport[3] introduced the concept of the microcirculatory unit in which an acinus of liver cells surrounds a central arteriole, portal venule, and bile radicle, and blood is drained by two peripheral tributaries of the hepatic vein. Blood traversing the sinusoid from portal area to hepatic vein radicle would bathe in sequence zone 1 hepatocytes (periportal), zone 2 hepatocytes, and zone 3 hepatocytes (pericentral). Substances removed from the bloodstream by the liver would diminish in concentration from portal to central veins, whereas substances secreted into the blood by the liver would increase along the same axis.

The concept of hepatic lobular gradients is not new; in 1923, Noel[4] referred to "zone de repos permanent," "zone de fonctionnement permanent," and "zone intermediaire variable," zones first exposed to portal blood being re-

Dr. Elias was supported by a grant from the Medical Research Council of Great Britain. Dr. Boyer is a recipient of an USPHS Academic Career Development Award—AM 70218.

From the Liver Study Unit, Department of Medicine, University of Chicago, Chicago, Illinois.

garded as most active. Heterogeneity among liver cells according to their intralobular distribution was demonstrated for diurnal glycogen content[5] and mitochondrial appearance.[4,6] Histochemical studies have also shown statistically significant differences in the activities of several enzymes between portal and central areas.[7,11] The oxygen tension of sinusoidal blood diminishes progressively between portal and central areas of the lobule, and hypoxia, when it occurs, would therefore tend to be most severe in the center of the lobule.

Centrolobular cells probably have the highest activities of inducible microsomes and drug-metabolizing enzymes.[12] The centrolobular necrosis associated with toxic intermediate products of drug metabolism (e.g., acetaminophen, bromobenzene, and halothane) possibly reflects this pattern of differences between hepatocytes and their metabolism according to their intralobular location. Localization by autoradiography following the intravenous injection of a tracer dose of labeled galactose showed a large concentration in the area surrounding the portal triads, with decreasing intensity in the direction of the central veins.[13] When the concentration of galactose in portal blood was low, hepatic extraction was almost complete, and this extraction of galactose from portal blood increased with rises in the administered dose until a plateau was reached, so that at higher concentrations, recovery from the hepatic vein of additional galactose was virtually complete. These data suggested successive recruitment and finally saturation of hepatocytes for uptake of galactose in each microcirculatory unit.

Evidence for a Lobular Gradient for Bile Secretion

Since bile acids are major secretagogues for bile and are efficiently extracted from blood by the normal liver, which in turn has a massive reserve capacity for their removal,[14,15] it is likely that they are normally cleared from portal blood predominantly by hepatocytes of zone 1 and that zone 3 is exposed to extremely low concentrations of circulating bile acids. Deane (1944)[5] and Forsgren (1935),[16] using histochemical methods, found that bile acids are totally[16] or predominantly[5] localized to portal zones of the lobule where the diameter of the bile canaliculus is also the largest.[17,18]

Additional morphologic evidence in support of the concept of a lobular gradient for bile acid uptake and secretion has been provided by transmission and scanning electron microscopy. The cross-sectional diameter of the hemi-bile canaliculus in control animals was significantly greater in periportal regions than in centrolobular regions.[18,19] Infusions of 40 μmole of either taurocholic acid or dehydrocholic acid significantly increased the diameter in central regions but not in periportal areas. Only during supraphysiologic infusion rates of dehydrocholic acid (DHC) (120 μmole/hr) did the diameter of canaliculi increase in periportal areas.[18] Comparable changes were observed by morphometric analysis in the compensating nonobstructed lobules of the liver following selective biliary obstruction (SBO).[19] No enlargement of biliary spaces occurred in portal regions but SBO produced an increase of canalicular size in centrolobular zones. In the same studies, hypertrophy of the centrolobular Golgi complex occurred in the compensatory nonobstructed lobe, so that the lobular gradient in the volume of Golgi-rich areas seen in control animals was abolished 2 days after SBO in nonobstructed lobules. Because of the polarization of the Golgi complex toward the biliary spaces, these morphometric findings were interpreted as evidence for involvement of the organelle in bile secretion. The striking Golgi hypertrophy and canalicular dilatation of centrolobular areas in response to SBO suggest compensatory recruitment of these cells for active bile secretion. Both these studies suggest that under basal conditions the portal zones of the liver lobule are most active, while "resting" centrolobular zones represent a latent reserve from which progressive recruitment occurs in response to increased bile acid loads. According to this hypothesis the proportions of hepatocytes involved in bile acid transport would vary according to fluctuations in magnitude of the bile acid enterohepatic circulation.[18]

Differential localization of bile acid uptake sites within the acinar zones of each microcirculatory liver unit was looked for,[20] but despite selective destruction of periportal (zone 1) hepatocytes by allyl alcohol, the remainder of the lobule retained the ability to transport bile acids into bile at rates faster than the basal bile salt secretory rate. Based on this evidence, sinusoidal uptake of bile acids can occur throughout the acinus, but since the maximum capacity of the cells to remove bile acids was not tested, a gradient in the concentration of bile acid uptake sites was not excluded. When zone 3 hepatocytes were selectively destroyed by bromobenzene, biliary bile acid concentration increased, suggesting that at physiologic bile acid loads, bile secretion from central zone hepatocytes is predominantly independent of bile acid (bile-acid-independent canalicular secretion—BAIF).[20]

HYPOTHESES AS TO WHY CANALICULAR CHOLESTASIS OCCURS PERICENTRALLY

On the basis of the factors discussed above and assuming a basal BAIF upon which a lobular gradient for bile-acid-dependent flow (BADF) is superimposed, two major hypotheses may be advanced to explain the characteristically centrolobular distribution of canalicular bile plugs in intrahepatic cholestasis. Since bile acid secretion into the canaliculus is a major determinant of bile flow, it can be seen that zone 1 is probably the chief contributor to bile-acid-dependent bile flow and that the cul-de-sac biliary canaliculi of zones 2 and 3 are perfused by much smaller amounts of biliary fluid, which is generated by mechanisms progressively independent of bile acids. Such zonal differences in bile acid transport and secretion would predispose to a primarily centrolobular distribution of intracanalicular precipitates during cholestasis. Concentrations of primary bile acids would most likely fall below their critical micellar concentration in centrolobular zones, and therefore their protective effect against injury by potentially toxic substances such as monohydroxy bile acids would be diminished. In addition, if the maximal activity of drug-metabolizing enzymes and the major site of BAIF production both coincide in centrolobular zones (zone 3), certain drugs, the toxicity of which is dependent on production of their metabolites, may have a major inhibitory effect on BAIF. This suggests a second hypothesis as to why canalicular cholestasis occurs pericentrally and might also explain why drug-induced liver injury commonly produces chole-stasis. Lobular gradients for O_2 and ATP would contribute further to these predilections for centrolobular zones of cholestatic liver injury.

MECHANISMS

The following mechanisms, though discussed separately, should not be thought of in isolation from one another, since they may be closely interrelated. While a final common pathway may possibly underlie many of the diverse abnormalities produced by cholestatic agents, it is more likely that for any one cholestatic agent, several mechanisms may be important in the induction of liver injury. The mechanisms proposed are derived from evidence accumulated in both human disease and experimental models based on these diseases; three major examples are cholestasis induced by (1) abnormalities in bile acid me-tabolism, including the secondary bile acid, lithocholic acid; (2) the commonly used tranquillizer chlorpromazine (CPZ); and (3) the estrogenic hormonal ste-roid, ethinyl estradiol (EE).

Abnormalities in Bile Acid Metabolism or Transport

Most interest in the possible hepatotoxic role of bile acids has centered upon the monohydroxy bile acids.[21,22] Lithocholic acid (3-hydroxycholanoic acid) is a secondary bile acid that undergoes an enterohepatic circulation and is con-tinuously produced in the intestine by bacterial 7α-dehydroxylation of chen-odeoxycholic acid. The possibility that this bile acid may accumulate in the liver under pathologic conditions in man with induction of hepatic injury and cholestasis led to interest in the model of lithocholate cholestasis that was greatly enhanced by the use of its precursor chenodeoxycholic acid in the medical treatment of gallstones. Elevated levels of lithocholic acid have been found in plasma and other fluids in some progressive cholestatic disorders of infancy, and although these observations have not been verified in many in-stances of neonatal cholestasis, there is a morphologic resemblance between the canalicular membrane abnormalities in experimental lithocholate chole-stasis and a progressive cholestatic disease of infancy (Byler's disease).[23-27] These similarities suggest that there may be a familial defect in bile acid me-tabolism that results in the accumulation of monohydroxy bile acids in the vicinity of the bile canaliculus in these patients. 3β-Hydroxy-5-cholenoate (3βHC) is another naturally occurring monohydroxy bile acid; it accounts for approximately 10% of the total bile acids in human meconium[28] and produces qualitatively similar, though less severe, ultrastructural changes as compared to those seen with lithocholic acid when infused into animals.[29] The tendency for the highest concentrations of 3βHC to occur in premature infants suggests that it accumulates as a result of its incomplete conversion to primary bile acids because of immaturity of the smooth endoplasmic reticulum (SER). Al-though there is no proof that the mechanism exists in adults, hypoactivity of the SER with impaired hydroxylation of bile acids had been proposed as a possible contributory mechanism underlying cholestasis.[30]

Not all putatively cholestatic bile acids are monohydroxylated. A defect in the conversion of 3α, 7α, 12α – trihydroxy-5β-cholestan-26-oic acid (THCA) to cholic acid has been observed in infants with intrahepatic cholestasis,[31] including two siblings,[32] which suggests an inherited metabolic defect. Possibly, excessive accumulation of this intermediary metabolite is of pathogenetic importance in certain cholestatic syndromes even though THCA does not produce cholestasis in animals.[33]

Bile flow diminishes progressively immediately following an infusion of sodium taurolithocholate and is also transiently inhibited following administration of a single bolus of lithocholic acid, indicating that lithocholate cholestasis is reversible.[34] Morphologic studies in the hamster and rat indicate that both lithocholic acid and taurolithocholic acid (TLC) have a primary effect on membrane structure.[34-37] The earliest morphologic changes are limited to the membrane of the bile canaliculus and occur simultaneously with the impairment of bile secretion. Later, bile ducts proliferate if lithocholic acid is fed chronically to rabbits or mice.[21,38] These observations suggest that the initial toxic effect of TLC is at the level of the bile canaliculus and the associated components within the surrounding pericanalicular ectoplasm. The ectoplasm increases substantially following TLC administration and is transformed in focal areas into unusual ectoplasmic lamellae that protrude into the lumen of the bile canaliculus. The limiting membrane of the canaliculus in some areas is disrupted, and intracellular organelles and membranous structures enter the lumen (Byler's bile). While irregular dilatations of the canalicular lumen are observed throughout the lobule, the most severe disruptions of the canalicular membrane are located in the blind-ended or terminal portions of canaliculi (found throughout the entire lobule).[37]

Complete prevention of TLC cholestasis occurs with simultaneous infusions of equimolar amounts of taurocholic acid that not only totally preempt the cholestatic effects of TLC but actually stimulate bile secretion.[39,40] The magnitude of this choleresis is equivalent to the effects on bile flow when taurocholic acid is infused alone. Dehydrocholate, which is a non-micelle-forming bile acid that normally stimulates bile secretion to a greater extent than taurocholic acid in the rat, only partially prevents the cholestatic effects of lithocholic acid.[40] Thus the protective effects of taurocholate are likely to be related to its detergent properties, in particular its ability to solubilize lecithin and lithocholic acid into mixed micelles during the process of biliary secretion. Since taurocholic acid may be taken up more efficiently than TLC by periportal cells, lesions might be expected to be localized to more central areas in the lobule where the ratio of lithocholate to taurocholate is greatest. However, although it is true that morphologic abnormalities of canaliculi occur primarily in hepatocytes that are located at the "headwaters" of the canalicular stream, they are seen in all zones of the lobule.

Whether these morphologic abnormalities in canalicular membranes are important in the pathogenesis of cholestasis remains unclear; they probably represent a toxic manifestation of lithocholic acid that is not essential to the initiation of cholestasis, since they can be prevented by infusing the sulfated form of lithocholic acid even though a mild degree of cholestasis persists.[37] Lithocholate infusions have also been shown to alter the lipid composition of liver plasma membranes enriched in bile canaliculi, and as discussed later, the mechanism of its cholestatic effect may be related to permeability changes induced in hepatocyte membranes.[41,42]

Although it is uncertain which fraction of bile is inhibited by TLC, work with the isolated perfused hamster liver suggests that lithocholic acid may block bile-acid-independent canalicular secretion,[43] which is thought to be largely dependent on sodium transport. TLC, however, has no effect on Na^+,K^+-ATPase activity in bile canalicular plasma membranes of the rat isolated immediately following cholestatic infusions of TLC,[22] thus making it less likely that TLC produces cholestasis by inhibiting the putative sodium-transport-dependent fraction of canalicular secretion.

Impairment of Bile Acid Synthesis

Impairment of bile acid synthesis occurs during cholestasis induced by EE[44] in rats and by CPZ in the rhesus monkey[45] and may contribute to diminished bile secretion in these models, since bile acids are major determinants of bile secretion.

Consequences of impaired bile acid transport include a diminished capacity to solubilize insoluble bile constituents such as cholesterol and monohydroxy bile acids in mixed micelles. Intrahepatic accumulation of nonsecreted bile acids may also produce hepatic necrosis or have detergent effects on cell membranes.[46]

Altered Canalicular Membrane Enzymes and BAIF

Both bile duct ligation and EE treatment result in increased specific activity of alkaline phosphatase but reduced 5'-nucleotidase and Mg^{2+}ATPase in rat liver plasma membranes, and reported kinetic studies demonstrated decreased amounts of the latter two enzymes rather than inhibition of their activity.[47] Although parallel findings in such widely differing experimental models favor their involvement in the pathogenesis of cholestasis, these findings have not yet been explained mechanistically.

Na^+,K^+-ATPase has received considerable attention as an enzyme possibly involved in the bile secretory process[48-52] and the pathogenesis of cholestasis. During diminished BAIF produced by cardiac glycosides,[52,53] thyroidectomy,[54] and lowered body temperature,[48-55] there is a coincident fall in the specific activity of Na^+,K^+-ATPase in liver plasma membrane fractions enriched in bile canaliculi. Conversely, enhanced BAIF produced by nonobstructed lobules following partial ligation of lobular bile ducts[56] or pretreatment with thyroid hormone was accompanied by increased specific activity of the enzyme.[54] During EE cholestasis in the rat, the diminution in total bile flow was attributable to inhibition of BAIF, which decreased from 40% in the normal rat to 27% in EE-treated animals.[57]

CPZ and its metabolites also inhibit membrane enzyme function, and in vitro data indicate that rat liver plasma membrane Na^+,K^+-ATPase is inhibited by 7,8 dihydroxy-CPZ at concentrations 100-fold lower than that required for CPZ.[58] The highly reactive CPZ free radical can be formed by liver microsomes[59] and then react with oxygen to form the stable CPZ sulfoxide metabolite.[60] Studies confirming the dose-dependent in vitro inhibitory effect of CPZ on rat liver plasma membrane Na^+,K^+-ATPase[58,61] showed that inhibition was enhanced by free radical formation but was less striking with sulfoxide metabolites of CPZ or when reduced glutathione was added.[61] Inhibition of bile flow in isolated perfused rat liver is enhanced by SKF-525A pretreatment, which might impair conversion of CPZ to the less toxic sulfoxide form of CPZ.[62]

The relevance of impaired Na^+,K^+-ATPase activity to CPZ-induced cholestasis must be questioned, however, since a similar effect on other membrane enzymes, including Mg^{2+}ATPase can be demonstrated, and a primary injury at the membrane of the bile ductule is likely to account for the findings of cholestasis in man.[63] Furthermore, despite evidence in favor of a close relationship between Na^+,K^+-ATPase and BAIF, direct evidence for its role in secretion of Na^+ into bile is lacking, and recent histochemical findings indicate that the enzyme is localized to the basal-lateral surface of the cell.[64] If Na^+,K^+-ATPase is not localized to the canalicular membrane, then new hypotheses need to be developed and tested to account for the production of BAIF. Bile acids themselves may modify their own choleretic response and taurocholate infusions in both rat and rhesus monkey augment BAIF.[56,65] Other ions may also be transported into bile, such as HCO^-_3 or Cl^-.[65a] Whatever the mechanisms, the lobular gradient theory for bile acid secretion predicts that a decrease in BAIF flow would be proportionately greater in centrolobular zones.[66]

Altered Permeability of the Canalicular Membranes or "Tight" Junction

The bile canalicular membrane of the hepatocyte and the interhepatocyte junctional complex are the major possible sites for permeability changes that occur during cholestasis. Theoretical curves have been described relating bile-plasma solute ratios for sucrose or inulin to their clearance in bile, two important determinants being diffusion permeability coefficients and the reflection factor which is a function of the sieving coefficient of the membrane.[67-69] Unfortunately, these values cannot be directly determined for the membrane of the bile canaliculus. When these mathematical models are applied in TLC[40] or estrone cholestasis,[70] however, a diffusion permeability coefficient several times higher than control value must be assumed in order for the curves to fit the experimentally determined bile/plasma solute ratios, an observation that implies that the permeability of the biliary system is increased. The increase in the bile/plasma concentration ratio for ^{14}C-sucrose and the increased back-diffusion of BSP from bile to plasma seen in estrone-treated rats may indicate increased permeability of the canalicular membrane.[70] Increased permeability of the biliary tree was also inferred from enhanced bile/plasma ratios of polyethylene glycol 8300 in EE-treated animals as compared to controls.[71] After retrograde intrabiliary injection (RII) of radioactive mannitol and sucrose, recovery of ^3H-sucrose from bile was decreased by EE but not by indocyanine green or hypothermia, although they also diminished bile flow.[72] ^3H-sucrose recovery from the biliary tree after RII in control animals was also decreased following taurocholate (TC) infusion, although, in this instance, bile flow was increased. When EE animals were treated with TC infusions, bile flow increased toward control levels, but recovery of inert solute after its RII was still further diminished. Therefore, EE and TC apparently had a synergistic effect in increasing biliary tree permeability but had an antagonistic effect on bile flow. By contrast with the EE model, morphologic damage to the bile canalicular membrane is readily detectable during TLC cholestasis,[35-37] a model that is also associated with an increase in biliary permeability to ^3H-inulin.[40] Protection from both membrane damage and an increase in biliary permeability occurred when simultaneous infusions of TC prevented cholestasis.[40,42] Such parallelism of morphologic and functional changes favors the canalicular membrane as a primary site for permeability changes in this model and could be due to incorporation of TLC into the membrane or to other alterations in membrane lipids or proteins. By disrupting the surrounding molecular packing of cholesterol and phospholipid acyl groups, intercalating molecules can increase the permeability of membranes to water and water-soluble substances. Concentrations of lithocholic acid (LCA) and cholesterol in rat liver plasma membranes were high after a 30-min LCA infusion.[42] The striking reduction in protein particles observed with freeze-fracture electron micrographs of bile canaliculi from LCA-treated animals may also be due to the incorporation of lithocholic acid and cholesterol within the bilayer which then becomes incapable of supporting protein within its lipid matrix.[36]

CPZ is an amphiphilic cationic detergent that also intercalates into lipid membranes, especially at a pH above its pK_a of 7.4, and causes an expansion of the cytoplasmic portion of erythrocyte ghost membranes, resulting in stomatocyte formation.[74]

Phospholipid/cholesterol ratios influence the permeability characteristics of lipid bilayers, and a relative molar increase in cholesterol increases membrane viscosity and inhibits transmembrane water movement.[75] EE treatment increases cholesterol (both free and ester forms) in rat liver surface membrane fractions without a change in phospholipid content.[76] Similarly, lithocholic acid and taurolithocholic acid have been shown to increase membrane cholesterol without affecting total phospholipid content.[42,77] Thus LCA, CPZ, and EE could all interfere with bile secretion through a common pathway by changing the lipid composition and microviscosity of the canalicular membrane. Changes in microviscosity also closely correlate with sodium pump activity, suggesting that the physical state of membrane lipids plays an important role in regulating ion transport. Na^+,K^+-ATPase activity is influenced by the lipid composition of the membrane, and cholesterol accumulation increases viscosity and produces an impairment of this enzyme's function.[78]

Changes in biliary permeability might also take place within the intercellular junctional complex that demarcates the canalicular space and provides a structural barrier between the lumen of the canaliculus and thesinusoidal-intercellular space.[79] In certain "leaky" epithelia, morphologic and electrophysiologic evidence indicates that the intercellular junctional complex is a major site of extracellular fluid movement, whereas resistance to transepithelial solute and water movement is high in functionally "tight" epithelia.[80] Although freeze-fracture studies of junctional anatomy are not always a reliable indicator of junctional permeability,[81,82] hepatocyte junctions seem to contain an intermediate number of junctional fibers when compared to classical "tight" and "leaky" epithelia.[83] In addition, experimental evidence suggests that bile-acid-induced osmotic gradients increase the permeability of the rat hepatocyte junctional complex to ionic lanthanum,[84] and permeability of these junctions to larger solutes has been demonstrated when colloidal lanthanum is injected via the bile duct or portal vein under conditions of increased pressure.[85,86] During cholestasis, an increase in junctional complex permeability might allow back-diffusion of solutes from the canaliculus. The finding that ^{14}C-sucrose concentration in bile is more than twice that of hepatocellular water[70] during estrogen cholestasis would be explained if sucrose diffusion is dependent on its plasma/bile concentration ratios (rather than cell water/bile), and occurs down its concentration gradient from plasma to bile via these paracellular routes.

Increases in either canalicular membrane or junctional complex permeability would allow reflux of luminal solute either into the cell, because of increased membrane permeability, or into the intercellular space, because of increased leakiness of the junctional complexes. Cholestasis would be the consequence of this loss of solute in either instance, since the osmotic gradient that normally favors water entry into bile would be dissipated. Conversely, an increase in resistance to permeation of either the canalicular membrane or the junctional complex could retard the primary movement of fluid and solute entry into the canalicular lumen and also result in cholestasis.

Microfilament Dysfunction

The liver, like all eukaryotic cells, contains polymerized actin in the form of microfilaments which are concentrated in the pericanalicular region of hepatocytes[87] (see Chapter 5). Microfilaments seem necessary for the normal process of bile formation, since both cytochalasin B, which detaches microfilaments from hepatocyte plasma membrane,[88,89] and phalloidin, which shifts the equilibrium of hepatocellular actin in favor of its readily visible filamentous polymerized form,[90] produce cholestasis in association with morphologic abnormalities of the bile canaliculus and its pericanalicular ectoplasm that are common to all forms of cholestasis in animals and man. Microfilaments also insert into the junctional complex and thus may also control the permeability of the paracellular route of ion and water movement into bile. Although direct evidence of a primary effect of cholestatic agents on microfilaments has not yet been unequivocally demonstrated, dysfunction of pericanalicular microfilaments could result in cholestasis by increasing the permeability of paracellular pathways and dissipation of the necessary bile acid and ion osmotic gradients, as has been suggested following administration of phalloidin.[90a] Pericanalicular actin filaments also may provide a contractile force that facilitates canalicular bile flow. Microfilaments and microtubules are also linked to integral membrane components and control their translational mobility within the membrane.[91] Loss of such control probably accounts for the reduced number of available insulin and human growth hormone receptor sites observed on the cell surface of cultured human lymphocytes following treatment with cytochalasin B[92] and altered microfilaments could conceivably result in a loss in canalicular membrane protein as well. Cytochalasin B inhibits Mg^{2+}-ATPase in bile canalicular membranes both in vivo and in vitro (I.M. Yousef, personal communication), and histochemical studies have localized Mg^{2+}-ATPase to bile canaliculi and to adjacent microfilaments.[93] If hepatocyte plasma membrane Mg^{2+}-ATPase represents a myosin ATPase that is activated by microfilament actin, then CPZ and EE, which decrease this enzyme in canalicular membrane preparations, may inhibit membrane motility and produce many of their diverse effects on hepatocyte membrane structure by inhibiting the cytoplasmic actomyosin mechanism. Similarly, integral membrane proteins, such as Na^+,K^+-ATPase, that have a vectorial transport function may be sensitive to alterations of their microenvironment within the membrane that result from microfilament dysfunction. Cytochalasin B has been shown both in vitro and in vivo to abolish ruthenium red staining of the glycoprotein-rich coat of the luminal aspect of bile canalicular membranes in parallel with detachment of microfilaments from the membranes[89] and also produces inhibition of Na^+,K^+-ATPase activity.[94] Thus, by virtue of their postulated roles in membrane flow, translocation of integral membrane proteins and regulation of intercellular junctional complexes, microfilament dysfunction might result in cholestasis via impairment of exocytotic transport processes, inhibition of membrane enzymatic functions, or enhancement of canalicular permeability.

Intracanalicular Precipitates

During taurolithocholate-induced cholestasis, clear crystalline deposits have been observed within and adjacent to canaliculi in rat liver,[29] and recent cytochemical studies combined with scanning electron microscopy have identified plugs of cholesterol-digitoxin complexes obliterating parts of biliary canaliculi within a few minutes of injection of a cholestatic dose of TLC.[95] Mixtures of CPZ and bile salts in concentrations above their critical micellar concentration in vitro form insoluble 1:1 CPZ/bile salt complexes, but precipitation is inhibited by the presence of phosphatidylcholine.[96] Despite their propensity to precipitate in bile, it is overly simplistic to postulate mechanical obstruction of canaliculi by these substances as a primary cause of cholestasis.

ROLE OF EXPERIMENTAL MODELS

Complete elucidation of the mechanisms producing intrahepatic cholestasis first awaits a better understanding of the mechanisms by which bile is normally formed. The experimental models reviewed here, while designed primarily to unravel pathophysiologic mechanisms, also serve to advance knowledge of the physiology of bile secretion.

REFERENCES

1. Plaa GL, Priestly BG: Intrahepatic cholestasis induced by drugs and chemicals. Pharmacol Rev 28:207–272, 1977
2. Javitt NB: Hepatic bile formation (second of two parts). N Engl J Med 295:1511–1516, 1976
3. Rappaport AM: The structural and functional unit in the human liver. (liver acinus). Anat Rec 130:673–689, 1958
4. Noël R: Recherches histo-physiologiques sur la cellule hepatique des mammifêres. Arch Anat Microsc Morphol Exp 19:1–158, 1923
5. Deane HW: A cytological study of the diurnal cycle of the liver of the mouse in relation to storage and secretion. Anat Rec 88:39–65, 1944
6. Novikoff AB: Mitochondria (chondriosomes). Edited by J Brachet and AE Mirsky: The Cell. Vol. 2. New York, Academic Press, 1961, pp 299–421
7. Shank RE, Morrison G, Cheng CH, Karl I, Schwartz R: Cell heterogeneity within the hepatic lobule (quantitative histochemistry). J Histochem Cytochem 7:237–239, 1959
8. Novikoff AB: Cell heterogeneity within the hepatic lobule of the rat (staining reactions). J Histochem Cytochem 7:240–244, 1959

9. Schumacher HH: Histochemical distribution pattern of respiratory enzymes in the liver lobule. Science 125:501–503, 1957

10. Wachstein M: Enzymatic histochemistry of the liver. Gastroenterology 37:525–537, 1959

11. Cohen PJ: Change in the distribution of succinic dehydrogenase within the rat hepatic lobule after ligation of the common bile duct. Anat Rec 153:429–444, 1965

12. Burger PC, Herdson PB: Phenobarbital-induced fine structural changes in rat liver. Am J Pathol 48:793–809, 1966

13. Goresky CA, Bach GG, Nadeau BE: On the uptake of materials by the intact liver. The transport and net removal of galactose. J Clin Invest 52:991-1009, 1973

14. Adler RD, Wannagat FJ, Ockner RK: Bile secretion in selective biliary obstruction. Adaptation of taurocholate transport maximum to increased secretory load in the rat. Gastroenterology 73:129–136, 1977

15. Paumgartner G, Santer K, Schwartz HP, Herz, R: Hepatic excretory transport maximum for free and conjugated cholate in the rat. Edited by G Paumgartner and R Preisig: The Liver: Quantitative Aspects of Structure and Function. Basel, Karger, 1973, pp 337–343

16. Forsgren E: Über die Rhythmic der Leberfunktion, des Stoffwechsels und des Schlafes. Sven Läk-sällsk Landl Bd 61:1–56, 1935

17. Novikoff AB, Hausman DH, Podber E: The localization of adenosine triphosphatase in liver: In situ staining and cell fractionation studies. J Histochem Cytochem 6:61–71, 1958

18. Layden TJ, Boyer JL: Influence of bile acids on bile canalicular membrane morphology and the lobular gradient in canalicular size. Lab Invest 39:110–119, 1978

19. Jones AL, Schumaker RD, Adler RD, Ockner RK, Mooney JS: A quantitative analysis of hepatic ultrastructure in rats after selective biliary obstruction. Edited by R Preisig, J Bircher, and G Paumgartner: The Liver: Quantitative Aspects of Function and Structure. Aulendorf, Editio Cantor, 1976, pp 36–51

20. Gumucio JJ, Balabaud C, Miller DL, DeMason LF, Appelman HD, Stoecker TJ, Franzblau DR: Bile secretion and liver cell heterogeneity in the rat. J Lab Clin Med 91:350–362, 1978

21. Palmer, RH: Toxic effects of lithocholate on the liver and biliary tree. Edited by W Taylor: The Hepatobiliary System—Fundamental and Pathological Mechanisms. New York, Plenum Press, 1976, pp 227–243

22. Boyer, JL, Layden TJ, Hruban Z: Mechanisms of cholestasis—taurolithocholate alters canalicular membrane composition, structure and permeability. Edited by H Popper, L Bianchi, and W Reutter: Membrane Alterations as Basis of Liver Injury. Lancaster, England, MTP Press, 1977, pp 353–369

23. Linarelli LG, Williams CN, Phillips MJ: Byler's disease: Fatal intrahepatic cholestasis. J Pediatr 81:484–492, 1972

24. Williams CN, Kaye R, Baker L, Hurwitz R, Senior JR: Progressive familial cholestatic cirrhosis and bile acid metabolism. J Pediatr 81:493–500, 1972

25. Banfield WJ, Thaler MM, Alagille D, Admirand WH: Bile acid concentrations in Byler's disease. Gastroenterology 67:A-2/779, 1974

26. DeVos R, De Wolf-Peeters C, Desmet V, Eggermont E, VanAcker K: Progressive intraheptic cholestasis (Byler's disease): Case report. Gut 16:943–950, 1975

27. Clayton RJ, Iber FL, Ruebner BH, McKusick VA: Byler's disease: Fatal familial intrahepatic cholestasis in an Amish kindred. Am J Dis Child 117:112–124, 1969

28. Back P, Ross K: Identification of 3β-hydroxy-5-cholenoic acid in human meconium. Hoppe Seylers Z Physiol Chem 354:83–89, 1973

29. Miyai K, Richardson AL, Mayr W, Javitt NB: Subcellular pathology of rat liver in cholestasis and choleresis induced by bile salts. 1. Effects of lithocholic, 3β-hydroxy-5-cholenoic, cholic and dehydrocholic acids. Lab Invest 36:249–258, 1977

30. Schaffner F, Popper H: Cholestasis is the result of hypoactive hypertrophic smooth endoplasmic reticulum in the hepatocyte. Lancet 2:355–359, 1969

31. Eyssen H, Parmentier G, Compernolle F, Boon J, Eggermont E: Trihydroxycoprostanic acid in the duedenal fluid of two children with intrahepatic bile duct anomalies. Biochim Biophys Acta 273:212–221, 1972

32. Hanson RF, Isenberg JN, Williams GC, Hachey D, Szczepanik P, Klein PD, Sharp HL: The metabolism of $3\alpha7\alpha12\alpha$-trihydroxy-5β-cholestan-26-oic acid in two siblings with cholestasis due to intrahepatic bile duct anomalies. An apparent inborn error of cholic acid synthesis. J Clin Invest 56:577–587, 1975

33. Hanson RF, Williams GC, Hachey D, Sharp

83. Friend DS, Gilula NB: Variations in tight and gap junctions in mammalian tissues. J Cell Biol 53:758–776, 1972

84. Layden TJ, Elias E, Boyer JL: Bile formation in the rat—the role of the paracellular ''shunt'' pathway. J Clin Invest 62:1375–1385, 1978

85. Schatzki PF: Bile canaliculus and space of Disse. Electron microscopic relationships as delineated by lanthanum. Lab Invest 20:87–93, 1969

86. Schatzki PF: The passage of radioactive lanthanum from the biliary to the vascular system. Z Zellforsch 119:451–459, 1971

87. Oda M, Price VM, Fisher MM, Phillips MJ: Ultrastructure of bile canaliculi with special reference to the surface coat and the pericanalicular web. Lab Invest 31:314–323, 1974

88. Phillips MJ, Oda M, Mak E, Fisher MM, Jeejeebhoy KN: Microfilament dysfunction as a possible cause of intrahepatic cholestasis. Gastroenterology 69:48–58, 1975

89. Oda M, Phillips MJ: Bile canalicular membrane pathology in cytochalasin B-induced cholestasis. Lab Invest 37:350–356, 1977

90. Gabbiani G, Montesano R, Tuchweber B, Salas M, Orci L: Phalloidin-induced hyperplasia of actin filaments in rat hepatocytes. Lab Invest 33:562–569, 1975

90a.Dubin M, Maurice M, Feldmnn G, Erlinger S: Phalloidin-induced cholestasis in the rat: Relation to changes in microfilaments. Gastroenterology 75:450–455, 1978

91. Nicolson GL: Transmembrane control of the receptors on normal and tumour cells. I. Cytoplasmic influence over cell surface components. Biochim Biophys Acta 457:57–108, 1976

92. VanObberghen E, De Meyts P, Roth J: Cell surface receptors for insulin and human growth hormone. Effect of microtubule and microfilament modifiers. J Biol Chem 251:6844–6851, 1976

93. Oda M, Phillips MJ: Electron microscopic cytochemical characterization of bile canaliculi and bile ducts in vitro. Virchows Arch [Zellpathol] 18:109–118, 1975

94. Barnett RE, Palazzotto J: Mechanism of the effects of lipid phase transitions on the Na^+K^+-ATPase, and the role of protein conformational changes. Ann NY Acad Sci 242:69–76, 1974

95. Bonvicini F, Gautier A, Gardiol D, Borel GA: Cholesterol in acute cholestasis induced by taurolithocholic acid. A cytochemical study in transmission and scanning electron microscopy. Lab Invest 38:487–495, 1978

96. Carey MC, Hirom PC, Small DM: A study of the physiochemical interactions between biliary lipids and chlorpromazine hydrochloride. Biochem J 153:519–531, 1976

Chapter 26

Cholestasis in the First Three Months of Life

By DANIEL ALAGILLE, M.D.

JAUNDICE is clinically always present in the neonatal period, as is hepato-megaly. Cholestasis, defined as impairment of excretion of conjugated bile acids and conjugated bilirubin is often responsible, but pruritus almost never appears before 3 months of age. Stools are completely or partially, permanently or variably acholic. The stool color is of major clinical importance and so must be carefully recorded during the first 10 days following admission to the pediatric ward. It is indicated by a colored rubber patch (white or light yellow), which is pasted on the infant's chart each day by the nurse.

In our experience, during the last 13 years, 288 cases in this neonatal age group showed intrahepatic cholestasis almost as frequently (49.3%) as extrahepatic biliary abnormalities (50.7%). One of the most challenging problems is the identification of cases of extrahepatic obstruction requiring surgery. The prognosis after hepatic portoenterostomy in extrahepatic biliary atresia has been claimed to be better if the operation is carried out before 3 months of age,[1-3] and therefore differentation between extrahepatic and intrahepatic cholestasis early could be crucial.

DIAGNOSIS OF EXTRAHEPATIC AND INTRAHEPATIC CHOLESTASIS

Clinical Data

From 1964 to 1975, we studied 288 infants (161 males and 127 females) who developed jaundice before the age of 3 months. Mean age was 18.7 days at the onset of jaundice, 2.9 months on admission, and 3.8 months at surgery.

Group I includes 142 cases of extrahepatic cholestasis, and group II includes 146 cases of intrahepatic cholestasis. The final diagnosis in each case was substantiated by the clinical outcome and/or the macroscopic and histologic findings.

Thirty-one clinical features (Table 1) were subjected to computer analysis. Thirteen of them differed significantly in groups I and II (Table 2).

From the Unité de Recherche d'Hépatologie Infantile INSERM U 56 & Clinique de Pédiatrie, Université Paris-Sud, Hôpital d'Enfants, 78 rue du Général-Leclerc, 94270 Bicêtre, France.

TABLE 1.—*Clinical Investigations*

General Characteristics	History	Physical Examination at Admission
Sex	Onset of jaundice	Age
Twin pregnancy	Course of jaundice	Weight
Birth weight	Onset of acholic stools	Height
Family history	Course of acholic stools	Head circumference
Consanguinity	Digestive disorders	Color of stools
Course of the pregnancy	Fever	Color of urine
Neonatal respiratory distress	Previous exploratory surgery	Clinical features of the liver
Neonatal hemolysis		Size of the spleen
Blood group		Edema
		Ascites
		Pruritus
		Rash
		Congenital anomalies
		Neurologic disorders
		Associated symptoms

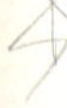

TABLE 2.—*Clinical Data That Differ Significantly in Groups I (Extrahepatic) and II (Intrahepatic) Cholestasis*

Variables	Group I*	Group II*	Significance
Males	45	66	≤ .001
Twin pregnancies	0.7	8	≤ .001
Congenital anomalies	17	32	≤ .01
Neurologic symptoms	8	21	≤ .01
Birth weight (grams)	3,226 ± 45†	2,678 ± 55†	≤ .001
Neonatal respiratory distress	5	22	≤ .001
Neonatal hemolysis	1.5	11	≤ .01
Onset of jaundice (days)	11 ± 1.5†	23 ± 2†	≤ .001
Course of jaundice:			
Progressive	80	66	≤ .01
Irregular	20	34	
Onset of acholic stools (days)	16 ± 1.5†	30 ± 2†	≤ .001
Prior course of acholic stools:			
Permanent	77	63	≤ .01
Intermittent	23	37	
Stool color 10 days after admission:			
White	79	26	≤ .001
Light Yellow	21	74	
Clinical features of the liver:			
Normal liver	1	12	
Hepatomegaly with normal consistency	12	35	≤ .001
Hepatomegaly with firm consistency	63	47	
Hepatomegaly with hard consistency	24	6	

*Values presented are expressed as percentage of patients in each group.

†Mean ± standard error.

Laboratory Data

Laboratory investigations, performed on admission, apart from the rose bengal test, were computerized (Table 3); only bilirubin, cholesterol, and protein blood levels were statistically different. Bile acids were always elevated, but because of insufficient data, this laboratory test was not subjected to statistical analysis.

TABLE 3.—*Biochemical Data That Differ Significantly in Groups I (Extrahepatic) and II (Intrahepatic) Cholestasis*

Variables		Group I (mean ± SE)*	Group II (mean ± SE)	Significance
Serum bilirubin level	(mg/dl)	10.0 ± 0.4	7.7 ± 0.5	≤ .001
Serum conjugated bilirubin	(mg/dl)	6.5 ± 0.3	4.4 ± 0.4	≤ .001
Serum cholesterol level	(g/dl)	0.29 ± 0.01	0.25 ± 0.01	≤ .01
Total serum protein	(g/dl)	6.7 ± 9.05	6.5 ± 0.1	≤ .05

*SE = Standard error

Histologic Data

Patients underwent a needle biopsy of the liver within 3 weeks following admission. The histologic data were analyzed by computer (Table 4). The absence of portal fibrosis appeared to be a strong argument against extrahepatic cholestasis. Bile thrombi in portal areas were seen only in group I, with the exception of 1 case in group II, presenting with alpha-1-antitrypsin deficiency.

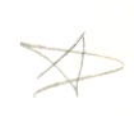

TABLE 4.—*Histopathologic Data that Differ Significantly in Groups I (Extrahepatic) and II (Intrahepatic) Cholestasis*

	Group I	Group II	Significance
No. of patients	36	106	
Bile ductular proliferation			
Absent	14*	70*	
Moderate	50	23	≤ .001
Prominent	36	7	
Portal fibrosis			
Absent	6	49	
Moderate	33	27	≤ .001
Prominent	56	20	
Annular	5	4	
Bile thrombi in portal area			
Absent	37	99	≤ .001
Present	63	1	
Focal necrosis			
Absent	82	84	≤ .05
Present	18	16	

*Values presented are expressed as percentage of patients in each group.

Discriminant Analysis

The 13 clinical, 4 biochemical, and 4 histologic findings that significantly differentiated groups I and II were used for a stepwise discriminant analysis to ascertain those that had the greatest diagnostic value. Of 17 clinical and biochemical features, the first 4 discriminant variables were as follows: (1) stool color within 10 days after admission, (2) birth weight, (3) age at onset of acholic stools, and (4) clinical features of liver involvement.

They permitted accurate distinction between extrahepatic and intrahepatic cholestasis in 83% of the patients tested. The addition of the fifth variable, (progressive or irregular course of jaundice) did not significantly improve this percentage.

The four significant histologic findings were then added to the preceding four discriminant variables; the resulting eight variables were programmed by the computer as follows: (1) bile ductular proliferation, (2) stool color within 10 days after admission, (3) birth weight, (4) age at onset of acholic stools, (5) focal liver cell necrosis, (6) intraportal bile thrombi, (7) clinical features of liver involvement, and (8) portal fibrosis. These eight observations permitted accurate identification of extrahepatic and intrahepatic cholestasis in 85% of the patients tested.

These results show that careful clinical investigation is of value in early differentiation between extrahepatic and intrahepatic obstruction; this point is of particular interest to pediatricians and surgeons working in centers where few such patients are encountered.[4] A still better differentiation, however, can be obtained through new biochemical tests claimed to be of discriminatory value. The most reliable tests are (1) I-rose bengal excretion,[5,6] (2) red blood cell peroxide hemolysis,[7] (3) vitamin E absorption,[8] (4) serum alpha-fetoprotein level,[9] and (5) determination of serum lipoprotein X before and after a short course of cholestyramine.[10] The accuracy of differentiation varied according to the technique and the investigators.[11]

EXTRAHEPATIC CHOLESTASIS

The most common cause of extrahepatic cholestasis in the first 3 months of life is biliary atresia, which was present in 133 of 142 cases of extrahepatic cholestasis in our series. Extrahepatic biliary atresia is a condition in which the common hepatic duct cannot be macroscopically identified. It is usually replaced by an apparently nonpatent cordlike structure. Extrahepatic biliary atresia may be associated with a cystic structure containing bile. The other causes are rare: paucity of interlobular ducts associated with extrahepatic biliary hypoplasia (4 cases), spontaneous perforation of bile ducts (3 cases), and choledochal cyst (2 cases). Extrahepatic biliary hypoplasia is a condition characterized by an extrahepatic bile duct of small size with patent lumen extending from the site of injection of contrast material to the porta hepatis. Extrahepatic biliary hypoplasia can be associated with extrahepatic biliary atresia or intrahepatic cholestasis of any cause.

In 1959, Kasai and Suzuki[12] proposed a new operation for "uncorrectable" biliary atresia, which was further modified in 1974.[13] Despite encouraging results obtained by Japanese[1] and French[3] surgeons, Kasai's approach was challenged for a long time by North American surgeons.[14,15] Only one group[16] achieved extensive experience with this procedure and obtained results similar to those of Japanese and French surgeons. At the international meeting held in Bethesda in March 1977,[17] general agreement was obtained concerning this procedure.

From September 1969 to December 1976, 91 infants in our group with "uncorrectable" extrahepatic biliary atresia were operated on using Kasai's procedure. We excluded infants with ascites or a prothrombin level below 50% after intramuscular vitamin K therapy. Three infants showing "correctable" extrahepatic biliary atresia were also excluded. Ten infants had already undergone surgery before referral to us, and postoperative success was more difficult to assess in these patients.

At laparotomy, extrahepatic bile ducts were either not visible to the naked eye or replaced by cordlike structures (fibrous remnants). Operative cholangiography was performed through the hypoplastic gallbladder in 18 infants and showed a threadlike communication with the duodenum but the absence of any duct connecting with the liver.

The gallbladder was absent or its lumen was so tiny that cholangiography was not possible in the other 73 infants. The excised fibrous remnants from the last 66 infants were serially cut and examined histologically, according to Kasai's technique;[13] complete obliteration of the hepatic duct and its replacement by dense fibrous tissue was always seen on several sections. The extrahepatic biliary atresia was associated with multiple abnormalities in 8 infants (Table 5) and with one isolated visceral malformation in 7 others. (Table 6).

TABLE 5.—*Associated Complex Malformations (8 Cases) in 142 Cases with Extrahepatic Biliary Atresia*

| | Accessory Spleens (5 Cases) | | Miscellaneous |
| | With _Situs Inversus_ | Without | |
	(3 cases)	(2 Cases)	(3 Cases)
Median liver	3	2	2
Preduodenal portal vein		2	2
Common mesentery		2	3
Annular pancreas			1
Complex heart disease	3		2
Dysplasia of acetabulum		1	

TABLE 6.—*Isolated Visceral Malformations (7 Cases) in 142 Cases with Extrahepatic Biliary Atresia*

Common mesentery	2 cases
Heart disease	3 cases
Cleft palate	2 cases
Microcephaly	1 case
Vertebral arch defect	1 case

These 91 patients were grouped according to the three types of surgical procedures performed:

Group I consisted of 53 infants who underwent hepatic portoenterostomy according to the original technique of Kasai.[12]

Group II consisted of 20 infants operated on since November 1975 who underwent classical hepatic portoenterostomy and jejunostomy of the jejunal loop used for the hepatic portoenterostomy.[13]

Group III consisted of 18 infants who were treated by hepatic portocholecystostomy as subsequently described by Kasai.[12]

Postoperative bile excretion was estimated from stool color, from daily bile flow at the jejunostomy, from liver function tests, and in the last 21 patients, from preoperative and postoperative rose bengal tests. Ampicillin and sulfonamides were administered orally for at least 1 year to patients of group I, intermittently to those of group II, and never in group III. Episodes of cholangitis were treated with intravenously administered antibiotics.

Results of Surgery

Five infants died during the first postoperative weeks. Bile flow was not restored in 36 out of 86 other infants (42%). Bile flow was restored in 50 patients (55%). There were 54 survivors (Table 7): 11 without bile flow restoration will die in the following 12 or 24 months. Thirty-three of the 91 operated patients survived with bile flow restored (36%): 20 of group I, 6 of group II, 7 of group III. Twenty-two were completely free of jaundice, and their long-term prognosis seems to be good (Table 7). The 11 other surviving patients remain partially icteric, and their long-term prognosis is dubious. Portal hypertension developed in 20 of the 33 survivors (Table 8). In 2 of them, surgical portacaval shunt was performed after severe gastrointestinal bleeding. Initially apparent esophageal varices in 5 of the 18 others disappeared later without surgical shunt.

TABLE 7.—*Survivors After Surgical Restoration of Bile Flow in 33 Cases of Extrahepatic Biliary Atresia*

Group	No. of Patients	Anicteric	Subicteric	?
I	20	12	7	1
II	6	3	2	1
III	7	7	0	0
Total	33	22	9	2

Histologic Study of Biliary Fibrous Remnants in Extrahepatic Biliary Atresia

The basis of Kasai's procedure is the persistence of patent biliary ducts or glandular epithelial cell clusters in the fibrous remnants at the porta hepatis. This led us to study the histologic changes in the extrahepatic biliary tree in the fibrous remnants removed from the porta hepatis in 66 infants during sur-

TABLE 8.—*Portal Hypertension in Survivors After Surgical Bile Flow Restoration in Extrahepatic Biliary Atresia*

Group	No. of Patients	No. of Patients with Portal Hypertension	Surgical Portacaval Shunt	Secondary Disappearance of Esophageal Varices
I	20	14	1	5
II	6	0	0	0
III	7	1	1	0
Total	33	15	2	5

gery for extrahepatic biliary atresia.[18] Serial sections confirmed the diagnosis of biliary atresia in each of the 66 cases by demonstrating complete ductal occlusion at some level of the extrahepatic biliary tree.

Three histologic patterns were identified at the porta hepatis:

Type I (17 cases): The specimens consisted of connective tissue, sometimes concentrically arranged. Neither lumen nor epithelium could be found. Nerves and dilated lymphatic vessels were present peripherally. The macroscopic reconstruction was difficult because no bile ducts or epithelial cell clusters were found.

Type II (28 cases): Connective tissue was abundant, without particular arrangement, in central and peripheral areas. One or several clusters of small lumens lined with cuboidal epithelium were seen peripherally, however. The lumens were empty, their sizes ranging from 50 to 80 μ. Many mononuclear and polymorphonuclear inflammatory cells were seen, essentially around the clusters. The macroscopic reconstruction showed epithelial cell clusters without a lumen. Their number was related to the size of the fibrous remnant.

Type III (21 cases): Bile ducts were easily found in the center of concentrically arranged connective tissue. They were lined with columnar epithelium, which was usually incomplete. Bile-containing macrophages and bundles of collagen were seen in and around the ducts. Epithelial cell clusters varied in number and were usually less numerous than in type II. Some of them were dilated, measuring as much as 350 μ, and contained bile plugs. Many inflammatory cells surrounded both biliary ducts and epithelial formations. The macroscopic reconstruction in this type always showed a patent biliary duct with more or less epithelial cell clusters. The three types correlated with the results of surgery (Table 9), with type III showing the highest success rate.

TABLE 9.—*Correlations Between Histologic Types of Fibrous Remnants and Postoperative Bile Flow Restoration in 66 Cases*

Type	No. of Patients	No. of Patients Operated On	Bile Flow Restoration +	−	Success Ratio
I	17	15	6	9	6/15
II	28	28	17	11	17/28
III	21	17	14	3	14/17

Statistical significance: χ^2: 6.0725
$p < 0.05$

INTRAHEPATIC CHOLESTASIS

For practical reasons, we propose to distinguish two main groups:

Group I (structural type) includes intrahepatic cholestasis with paucity of interlobular bile ducts (57 cases).

Group II (nonstructural type) includes intrahepatic cholestasis with present and normal interlobular bile ducts (91 cases).

Cholestasis in group I is related to a disturbance in the excretion of the bile (ductular cholestasis). Cholestasis in group II is related to a disturbance in the secretion of the bile (hepatocellular cholestasis).

Since we consider this distinction essential, we must be very precise about the presence or absence of ductules in the portal areas. Therefore, a laparotomy has to be performed in all patients, not only to confirm the patency of extrahepatic bile ducts but also to obtain large surgical biopsies from the left and right lobes of the liver. Only such biopsies permit the study of a sufficient number of portal areas. Special attention should be directed toward the size and number of portal areas, as well as the size and structural features of interlobular bile ducts.

The ratio of interlobular bile ducts to the number of portal areas was compared with normal livers from children of similar ages, and the differences were evaluated statistically by the Student's T-test: 0.0 to 0.4 in patients with the structural type of neonatal cholestatic liver disease, as compared with 0.9 to 1.8 in normal children ($p < 0.001$). This ratio cannot be easily assessed in the presence of extensive portal fibrosis, and pseudolobular proliferation widely developed. By contrast, in group I (structural type) the number of portal tracts is significantly reduced, as compared with controls.[19]

Some other histologic data are less important in this essential distinction between structural and nonstructural types of neonatal cholestatic liver disease including hepatocellular damage, such as clarification and ballooning and giant-cell transformation, which is commonly found in any liver disease at this early period of life.

Group I: Structural Type of Cholestasis (Table 10)

Infants with this structural type of intrahepatic cholestasis have a patent extrahepatic biliary tract and a decreased number of interlobular bile ducts. It is sometimes referred as "intrahepatic biliary atresia," "intrahepatic ductular hypoplasia," or "intrahepatic bile duct hypoplasia." Paucity of interlobular bile ducts is the term we have chosen. It is found associated with various extrahepatic congenital abnormalities in some patients, as part of a distinctive recognizable syndrome (syndromatic type). Further experience with new patients led us to reexamine the different conditions in which paucity of intrahepatic bile duct is observed.

Paucity of Interlobular Bile Ducts Associated with Other Developmental Abnormalities (Syndromatic Type)

Since our initial experience concerning 15 children,[20] 11 more patients with such a syndrome have been examined. Several reports of similar findings,[21-23]

TABLE 10.—*Group I: Structural Type of Intrahepatic Neonatal Cholestasis (Paucity of Interlobular Ducts)*

Syndromatic type (with associated malformations)		
Complete	26	
		39
Partial (without facies) abnormalities	13	
Nonsyndromatic type		18
Total cases		57

as well as some individual case reports communicated to us, have also confirmed the specificity of this syndrome. Both sexes are affected equally (13 girls and 13 boys). The four most frequent features include: chronic liver disease, characteristic facies, cardiovascular abnormalities, and vertebral arch defects. The earliest indication of the disease is persistent cholestasis, which appears during the first 3 months of life. An unusual feature of this cholestasis is the combination of intense pruritus which appears around the fourth to sixth month of life, with relatively moderate elevation in serum bilirubin concentration, and, in contrast, high concentrations of serum cholesterol. The stools are clay-colored or reveal the presence of bile. Hepatomegaly is a constant feature; the spleen can be enlarged, even in the absence of portal hypertension. As the disease progresses toward the second year of life, the serum bilirubin concentration becomes normal or moderately elevated (4–8 mg/dl); serum cholesterol rises to extremely high values ranging from 500 to 1,000 mg/dl; and xanthomas appear, suggesting the diagnosis when they were distributed over palms, extensor surfaces, and body creases. Alkaline phosphatase activity is increased three to five times normal. Protein synthesis by the liver is normal, as reflected by a normal serum albumin concentration and prothrombin time after vitamin K administration. Aminotransferase activities are moderately increased. HB_s Ag was absent in the 21 patients tested.

Many of these children improve spontaneously or with cholestyramine administration. Recurrent episodes of cholestasis occur, however, following intercurrent infections.

FACIES

The characteristic facies may permit the diagnosis at a glance in the first months of life; all patients resemble each other. The forehead is prominent, the eyes are set deeply and somewhat widely apart (mild hypertelorism) above a straight nose, and the chin is small and pointed.

CARDIOVASCULAR ABNORMALITIES

A harsh mid-systolic murmur is heard maximally in the third intercostal space at the left sternal border, and lung fields are normal on chest radiographs; electrocardiograms are normal or show a moderate and nonprogressing right ventricular hypertrophy. These findings are consistent with pulmonary artery hypoplasia or stenosis, confirmed in 13 children by angiography. One patient also had severe coarctation of the aorta that required surgery at the age of 6 years. Another patient had a tetralogy of Fallot and died at the age of 2 months.[24]

VERTEBRAL ARCH DEFECTS

Vertebral arch defects were observed in 15 patients. The anterior arches of one or several vertebrae are not fused, resulting in spina bifida defects without scoliosis. These abnormalities become more evident with age but can be seen during the first year of life. In our experience, they are different from other vertebral abnormalities commonly associated with congenital heart diseases.

OTHER FEATURES

Growth retardation was observed in 17 patients. Its presence did not seem to be related to the existence of vertebral defects or the degree of cholestasis. Stimulation with arginine results in the highest circulatory concentrations of growth hormone ever recorded in children with growth retardation.[25] Growth retardation spontaneously disappears with aging in some patients. Mental retardation was mild to moderately severe in 13 patients. A very weak tone of voice was present in some patients.

All 26 patients were admitted because of chronic liver disease; recognition of characteristic facies facilitated differential diagnosis between this syndrome and other causes of intrahepatic cholestasis in childhood. Thirteen additional patients (Table 10) can be included in this "syndrome" in spite of the absence of the characteristic face. They had paucity of interlobular bile ducts (13 patients), pulmonary artery hypoplasia or stenosis (10 patients), and/or vertebral arch defects (7 patients). Five of them were siblings of the patients described above and died before the age of 1 year. Thus the "syndrome" includes various developmental anomalies, paucity of the interlobular bile ducts being the most frequent. Recently, however, we examined a girl presenting all the features of the "syndrome," including the characteristic face, but without liver disease. Similar patients were also reported by others.[22]

This form of hypoplasia of interlobular bile ducts may carry a better prognosis than other types of intrahepatic cholestasis. Many patients have become relatively free of hepatic symptoms, and most have survived the first decade. By contrast, some patients may develop progressive periportal fibrosis with a severe course. Whether this fibrosis reflects progressive hypoplasia of the extrahepatic biliary tree secondary to a minimal bile flow and subsequent closure of the common duct remains to be demonstrated.

Parents are not affected by abnormalities, suggesting an autosomal recessive genetic basis for the disorder. Conversely, an autosomal dominant transmission has been proposed in the literature.[21,22]

Paucity of Interlobular Ducts Without Developmental Abnormalities (Nonsyndromatic Type)

During the past 20 years, 18 patients with the nonsyndromatic type of neonatal intrahepatic cholestasis have been investigated. All but 4 were full-term. Birth weights were less than 3 kg in 12 of them.

The patients developed jaundice, pale stools, dark urine, and hepatomegaly. Pruritus was a frequent finding but never appeared before the age of 5 months. Biochemical findings included high levels of serum bilirubin and alkaline phosphatase and aminotransferase activities. Total serum cholesterol level was abnormally high, ranging from 160 to 480 mg/dl. The biliary tree was explored surgically in the 18 patients after a few weeks or months with persistent cholestasis. Operative cholangiography demonstrated the patency of the extrahepatic biliary system in all patients. Subsequent gallbladder drainage relieved cholestasis in all patients, but removal of the tube led to recurrent jaundice in all. Wedge biopsy of the liver showed a reduced number or absence of bile ducts in portal areas, no or moderate periportal fibrosis, and mild inflammatory infiltration of portal tracts.

The course of illness was severe. Two patients died within a few months after birth, with intercurrent infections. The disease relentlessly progressed to biliary cirrhosis in 8 patients, and 6 of them died from progressive hepatic failure. The jaundice disappeared in 8 other patients, who have remained anicteric to the present, some more than 10 years later. Evidence of viral infection was found in only 1 patient, who developed congenital rubella, a finding formerly reported.[26] Six other infants have been tested for the presence of rubella, cytomegalovirus, and HB$_s$Ag infection, and none was found to be positive. By contrast, 4 of the 14 tested patients have been found to be deficient in alpha-1-antitrypsin with a phenotype Pi ZZ: these 4 patients developed neonatal cholestasis which persisted beyond the age of 6 months.[27]

The metabolism of bile acids was not investigated in the present series. Increased amounts of trihydroxycoprostanic acid, a cholic acid precursor, have been found in 2 families.[28,29] Chromosomal studies were not performed, but 1 patient has been described with Down's syndrome.[30]

Briefly, paucity of interlobular ducts can be observed in several situations. In one, it is part of multiple developmental abnormalities and has a relatively good prognosis. The others seem to result from a variety of insults and appear to have a rather bad prognosis.

Group II: Nonstructural Type of Cholestasis (Table 11)

The literature records disorders of this group under different synonyms, such as neonatal hepatitis and prolonged obstructive jaundice. The only essential difference between patients of groups I and II is that, in group II, interlobular bile ducts are always present and normal. In our 91 cases of this group, four main subgroups are recognized (Table 11).

Inspissated Bile Syndrome

The term "inspissated bile syndrome" was proposed by Hsia in 1952[31] in regard to cases of prolonged obstructive jaundice developing in 5% to 8% of babies with severe neonatal hemolysis (Rh or ABO problems). Significant manifestations of obstructive jaundice appear after initial hemolysis, during the first week of life, usually after many exchange transfusions. This cholestasis may last for 2 or 3 months in some infants. The proposed mechanism is either a defect in the excretory capacity of hepatocytes or subsequent secretion of excessive bilirubin into the bile canaliculi, resulting in inspissation of the bile. This condition is, in fact, rare; we observed only 3 infants with this disease during the last 13 years.

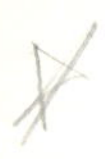

TABLE 11.—*Group II: Nonstructural Type of Intrahepatic Neonatal Cholestasis*

Inspissated bile syndrome	3	
Cytomegalovirus infection	8	
Rubella infection	2	17
Hepatitis B	7	
Alpha-1-antitrypsin deficiency	19	
Byler's disease	5	
Cystic fibrosis	2	31
Hereditary fructose intolerance	2	
Niemann-Pick disease	3	
"Giant-cell hepatitis"		
(Undetermined viruses)		40
(Undetermined inborn errors of metabolism)		
(Drugs)		
Total cases		91

Viruses

Cytomegalovirus, rubella, or HB virus infections are sometimes found in "neonatal hepatitis." In our experience, however, and in spite of systematic investigations, they were very rarely found as the cause of neonatal intrahepatic cholestasis. In these conditions, cholestasis, when present, can be total and permanent and may be confused with extrahepatic causes of cholestasis. By contrast, a high degree of suspicion arises when abnormal results of specific tests are found in patients hospitalized for a long time and susceptible to many superinfections.

Inborn Errors of Metabolism

The most frequent inborn error of metabolism associated with intrahepatic neonatal cholestasis is alpha-1-antitrypsin deficiency in infants with the Pi ZZ phenotype.[27] Jaundice and pruritus clear before 1 year of age, but hepatomegaly and laboratory evidence of partial cholestasis persist thereafter. We proposed that histopathologic study of the liver during the early cholestatic phase permits prediction of the course of the liver disease.[32]

The initial manifestations of familial benign recurrent cholestasis never begin before 1 year of age, so this condition does not occur in the neonatal period. Several reports have documented progressive intrahepatic cholestasis with autosomal recessive inheritance, frequently beginning in very early infancy. The first clinical symptoms of this condition, called Byler's disease or fatal (malignant) familial recurrent cholestasis, appear within the first 3 months of life (5 personal cases)[33] or somewhat later, before 1 year of age (6 personal cases) (Tables 12 and 13). In Byler's disease, the main biochemical anomalies are high blood levels of total bile acids and normal lipid and cholesterol concentrations in the blood. Histologically, portal fibrosis develops early and bile ductular proliferation is always present and normal. Death occurs in early childhood in some patients, while the others succumb to biliary cirrhosis by age 15 or 20. The suspected block in bile acid metabolism is not clearly identified. A relationship with lithocholic acid[34,35] or another abnormal bile acid[38] has not been established. The frequency of early intrahepatic cholestasis in cystic fibrosis is low (2 cases) despite a relatively high incidence of multinodular or focal biliary cirrhosis (20% to 25%). The clinical picture of hereditary fructose intolerance exceptionally is neonatal cholestasis (2 out of 52 patients). The same is true for Niemann-Pick disease (3 out of 23 patients) and galactosemia.

TABLE 12.—*Age of Clinical Onset in Cases of Byler's Disease Studied*

Case No.	Jaundice	Pruritus
1	5 days	
2	6 weeks	
3	6 weeks	
4	8 days	
5	4 days	
6		5 months
7	4 months	
8	10 months	10 months
9		4 months
10		8 months
11	5 months	5 months

TABLE 13.—*Age of Clinical Onset in Cases of Byler's Disease Reported in the Literature*

Case No.	Jaundice	Pruritus
Clayton et al.[40]		
1	3 months	
2	2½ months	
3	6 weeks	
4	9 months	
5	6 months	
6	8 months	
7	10 months	
Schubert[37]		
1		"Since early life"
Gray and Saunders[38]		
1	"Shortly after birth"	
2	6 weeks	
Hirooka and Ohno[39]		
1	6 months	
Linarelli et al.[34]		
1	3 months	
Williams et al.[35]		
1		3 months
2		5 months
3		6 months

"Giant-Cell Hepatitis"

Of 91 infants presenting with group II (nonstructural type) intrahepatic neonatal cholestasis, 40 had a histologic pattern in the liver of so-called giant-cell transformation. The cause of the liver disease in these patients remained unknown. This so-called neonatal hepatitis could be due to fetal infection by undetermined viruses, unidentified inborn errors of metabolism, or some drugs taken by the mother. Further studies are needed to explain this most common category of nonstructural type of neonatal intrahepatic cholestasis.

REFERENCES

1. Kasai M, Kimura S, Asakura Y, Suzuki H, Taira Y, Ohashi E. Surgical treatment of biliary atresia. J Pediatr Surg 3:665–675, 1968
2. Lilly JR: The Japanese operation for biliary atresia: Remedy or mischief? Pediatrics 55:12–19, 1975
3. Odièvre M, Valayer J, Razemon-Pinta M, Habib EC, Alagille D: Hepatic porto-enterostomy or cholecystostomy in the treatment of extrahepatic biliary atresia. J Pediatr 88:774–779, 1976
4. Chiba T, Kasai M: Differentiation of biliary atresia from neonatal hepatitis by routine clinical examinations. Tohoku J Exp Med 115:327–335, 1975
5. Ghadimi H, Sass-Kortsak A: Evaluation of the radioactive rose-bengal test for the differential diagnosis of obstructive jaundice in infants. N Engl J Med 265:351–358, 1961
6. Desbuquois B, Tron P, Alagille D: Etude de l'excretion fécale et urinaire du Rose Bengale marqué par l'iode radioactif au cours des ictères obstructifs du nouveau-né et du nourrisson. Arch Fr Pédiatr 25: 379–391, 1968
7. Lubin BH, Baehner RL, Schwartz E, Shohet SB, Nathan DG: The red cell peroxide hemolysis test in the differential diagnosis of obstructive jaundice in the newborn period. Pediatrics 48:562–565, 1971
8. Melhorn DK, Gross S, Izant RJ: The red cell hydrogen peroxide hemolysis test and vitamin E absorption in the differential diagnosis of jaundice in infancy. J Pediatr 81:1082–1087, 1972
9. Zaltzer PM, Fonkalsrud EW, Neerhout RC, Stiehm ER: Differentiation between neonatal hepatitis and biliary atresia by measuring serum alphafetoprotein. Lancet 1:373, 1974
10. Campbell DP, Poley JR, Alaupovic P, Smith EI: The differential diagnosis of neonatal hepatitis and biliary atresia. J Pediatr Surg 9:699–705, 1974
11. Mowat AP, Psacharopoulos HD, William R: Extrahepatic biliary atresia versus neonatal hepatitis. Review of 137 prospectively investigated infants. Arch Dis Child 51: 763–770, 1976
12. Kasai M and Suzuki S: A new operation for "non-correctable" biliary atresia: Hepatic porto-enterostomy. Shujutsu 13: 733–739, 1959
13. Kasai M: Treatment of biliary atresia with special reference to hepatic porto-enterostomy and its modifications. Prog Pediatr Surg 6:5–52, 1974
14. Campbell DP, Poley JR, Bhatia M, Idesmith E: Hepatic porto-enterostomy. Is it indicated in the treatment of biliary atresia? J Pediatr Surg 9:329–333, 1974
15. Koop CE: Biliary atresia and the Kasai operation. Pediatrics 55:9–11, 1975
16. Lilly JR, Altman RP: Hepatic porto-enterostomy (the Kasai operation) for biliary atresia. Surgery 89:76–86, 1975
17. International Workshop on Neonatal Hepatitis and Biliary Atresia. Bethesda, Fogarty International Center, March 1977, pp 21–23
18. Gautier M, Jehan P, Odièvre M: Histologic study of biliary fibrous remnants in 48 cases of extrahepatic biliary atresia. Correlation with postoperative bile flow restoration. J Pediatr 89:704–709, 1976
19. Hadchouel M, Hugon RN, Gautier M: Paucity of portal tracts associated with paucity of intrahepatic bile ducts. Arch Pathol (submitted)
20. Alagille D, Odièvre M, Gautier M, Dommergues JP: Hepatic ductular hypoplasia associated with characteristic facies, vertebral malformations, retarded physical, mental and sexual development and cardiac murmur. J Pediatr 86:63–71, 1975

21. Henriksen NT, Langmark F, Sorland SJ, Fausa O, Landaas S, Aagenaes O: Hereditary cholestasis combined with peripheral pulmonary stenosis and other anomalies. Acta Paediatr Scand 66:1–15, 1977

22. Watson GH, Miller B: Arteriohepatic dysplasia: Familial pulmonary arterial stenosis with neonatal liver disease. Arch Dis Child 48:459–466, 1973

23. Greenwood RD, Rosenthal A, Crocker AC, Nadas AS: Syndrome of intrahepatic biliary dysgenesis and cardiovascular malformations. Pediatrics 57:243–247, 1976

24. Case record of the Massachusetts General Hospital. N Engl J Med 293:1361–1368, 1975

25. Courtecuisse V, Dommergues JP, Girard F, Limal JM: Croissance staturale, anomalies osseuses et endocriniennes dans l'hypoplasie des voies biliaries intrahépatiques. Ann Pediatr 23:525–531, 1976

26. Heathcote J, Deodhar KP, Scheuer PJ, Sherlock S: Intrahepatic cholestasis in childhood. N Engl J Med 295: 801–805, 1976

27. Odièvre M, Martin JP, Hadchouel M, Alagille D: Alpha-1-antitrypsin deficiency and liver disease in children: Phenotypes, manifestations and prognosis. Pediatrics 47: 226–231, 1976

28. Eyssen H, Parmentier G, Compernolle F, Boon J, Eggermont E: Trihydroxycoprostanic acid in the duodenal fluid of two children with intrahepatic bile duct anomalies. Biochim Biophys Acta 273:212–221, 1972

29. Hanson RF, Isenberg JN, Williams GC, Hachey D, Szczepanik P, Klein PD, Sharp H: The metabolism of 3-alpha, 7-alpha, 12-alpha-trihydroxy 5-beta-cholestan-26-oic acid in two siblings with cholestasis due to intrahepatic bile duct anomalies. J Clin Invest 56:577–587, 1975

30. Puri P, Guiney EJ: Intrahepatic biliary atresia in Down's syndrome. J Pediatr Surg 10:423–424, 1975

31. Hsia DYY, Patterson P, Allen FH Jr, Diamond LK, Gellis SS: Prolonged obstructive jaundice in infancy. 1. General survey of 156 cases. Pediatrics 10:243–252, 1952

32. Hadchouel M, Gautier M: Histopathologic study of the liver disease in the early cholestatic phase of alpha-1-antitrypsin deficiency. J Pediatr 89:211–215, 1976

33. Odièvre M, Gautier M, Hadchouel M, Alagille D: Severe familial intrahepatic cholestasis. Arch Dis Child 48:806–812, 1973

34. Linarelli LG, Williams CN, Philipps MI: Byler's disease: Fatal intrahepatic cholestasis. J Pediatr 81:484–492, 1972

35. Williams CN, Kaye R, Baker L, Hurwitz R, Senior JR: Progressive familial cholestatic cirrhosis and bile acid metabolism. J Pediatr 81:493–500, 1972

36. Banfield WJ, Thaler MM, Alagille D, Admirand WH: Bile acid concentrations in Byler's disease (abstract). Gastroenterology 67:779, 1974

37. Schubert WK: Byler's disease: Fatal familial intrahepatic cholestasis in Amish kindred (discussion). J Pediatr 67:1027, 1965

38. Gray OP, Saunders RA: Familial intrahepatic cholestastic jaundice in infancy. Arch Dis Child 41:320–328, 1966

39. Hirooka M, Ono T: A case of familial intrahepatic cholestasis. Tohoku J Exp Med 94:293–306, 1968

40. Clayton RJ, Iber FL, Ruebner BH, McKusick VA: Byler's disease: Fatal familial intrahepatic cholestasis in Amish kindred. J Pediatr 567:1025–1028, 1965

Chapter 27

Primary Biliary Cirrhosis

By E. ROLLAND DICKSON, M.D.,
C. RICHARD FLEMING, M.D.,
and JURGEN LUDWIG, M.D.

PRIMARY BILIARY CIRRHOSIS is a chronic, progressive liver disease manifested by disturbance of bile secretion and by segmental inflammatory destruction of intrahepatic bile ducts. This process results in increasing loss of interlobular bile ducts, associated periportal hepatitis, and eventually cirrhosis with portal hypertension. The underlying histopathologic process is best described as chronic, nonsuppurative, destructive cholangitis[1]. The term "primary biliary cirrhosis," however, is shorter, universally recognized, and, by precedence, used most commonly (although it is also incorrect, confusing for the uninitiated, and not descriptive of any but the last stage of the disease). In this chapter, we use primary biliary cirrhosis (PBC) in its wider clinical sense, which does not always imply that cirrhosis is actually present.

ETIOLOGY

The cause and origin of PBC and the factors affecting its progression are unknown. Two possible clues to the pathogenesis are the female predominance and the frequent association with other autoimmune diseases. The female-to-male ratio approximates 9:1; furthermore, 10% of patients have their first symptoms during pregnancy.[1] Although speculation about hormonal imbalances related to the cause of PBC is intriguing, no evidence of such a relation exists.

IMMUNOLOGIC FEATURES

Many features of PBC suggest immunopathogenesis: granulomatous inflammation around intrahepatic bile ducts, hypergammaglobulinemia, presence of autoantibodies and complement fixation, circulating immune complexes, and association with other autoimmune diseases.

Hypergammaglobulinemia in PBC can be caused by any of the three major classes of immunoglobulins,[2-4] but the IgM fraction is the one most consistently elevated. The serum immunoglobulin changes are not diagnostic of PBC and are of limited value in differential diagnosis.

Several autoantibodies have been demonstrated in the immunoglobulin fraction of sera of PBC patients. The most significant clinically is the mitochondrial antibody (M antibody),[5] which has become the basis of a widely used diagnostic test for PBC. M antibody is complement-fixing and is directed against the inner membrane of mitochondria of all cells.[6,7] The antibody is present in high titer in 83% to 96% of patients and is located predominantly in the IgG fraction, although it may occur in the IgA and IgM fractions also. M antibody is not specific for PBC, since it may occur in lower frequency in other diseases, notably in about 20% of cases of chronic active hepatitis (CAH).[8] The M antibody does not disappear with steroid therapy or after hepatic transplantation. Other antibodies found in PBC are directed against nuclei (24% of cases), smooth muscle (49%), IgG (as rheumatoid factor, 60%), bile canaliculi (35%), and thyroid-specific antibodies (15%).[9]

Recent reports have indicated that immune complexes composed of antibodies and unknown antigens may circulate in PBC sera. Evidence for such complexes is the demonstration of cryoglobulins,[10,11] complement-binding IgG aggregates detected by Raji cell radioimmunoassay,[11-13] and split products of complement.[14,15] The Raji cell radioimmunoassay detects immune complexes that are bound by receptors for complement on the surface of a human cultured lymphocyte line (Raji cells). Such complexes, of 19s or greater in the majority of instances, were found in 65% of 88 PBC patients.[13] The incidence of elevated immune complexes was even higher (82%) in the subgroup of PBC cases with associated autoimmune disorders such as Sjögren's syndrome, rheumatoid-like arthritis, scleroderma, and Hashimoto's thyroiditis. In another study, cryoglobulins containing IgM and IgG were found in the sera of 18 of 20 patients with PBC. Efforts to demonstrate antibodies to mitochondria in these precipitates were unsuccessful.[11] Whether the immune-complex-like materials found in such patients contribute in any way to the evolution of PBC or whether they represent a secondary response to tissue injury is unknown.

Although the level of the fourth component of complement (C4) is decreased in many patients,[14,15] normal or increased levels of the third component (C3) have been reported;[3,4] both hypercatabolism and increased synthesis of C3 in PBC patients have been demonstrated,[14] suggesting activation of the complement system. An altered complement pathway is implied by the cleavage products of factor B found in plasma of 40% of patients with PBC in another study.[11]

Cell-mediated immune responses to skin testing in vivo and lymphocyte responses to mitogenic agents in vitro suggest diminished cellular immunity in PBC. Additionally, lymphocytes from approximately 50% of patients in one study were cytotoxic for hepatic cells, especially during the early histologic stages of PBC.[16] Cell-mediated cytotoxicity toward Chang liver cells has also been found in PBC.[17] The differences in target cells used and in patient selection hinder comparison of these two studies. Immunofluorescent examination of autopsy specimens or biopsy specimens of livers from PBC patients revealed scattered and focal collections of plasma cells containing IgG and particularly IgM, as well as immune deposits around bile ducts in early stages of the disease,[18] which suggest that immune complexes have an important part in its genesis.

No animal models with the exact entity of PBC have been discovered or produced, although the Bedlington terrier, which may develop a chronic, progressive liver disease associated with massive copper accumulation in the liver, may be useful to study.[19] Thus, much indirect evidence suggests that autoimmunity is among the possible causes of PBC, and yet other possible causes also deserve summary.

Infectious Agents

The discovery of hepatitis B surface antigen (HB_sAg) and subsequent recognition of its association with CAH led several investigators to determine the incidence of HB_sAg and anti-HB_sAg in PBC.[20-22] All available data suggest, however, that the rare presence of HB_sAg in PBC is coincidental. We found that 150 consecutive patients with PBC were HB_sAg-negative with the radioimmunoassay technique; most were tested on more than one occasion over a period of several years.

Genetic Factors

A report of a case in which alpha-1-antitrypsin (α_1-AT) deficiency coexisted with PBC led to the speculation that patients with PBC might be heterozygous for α_1-AT deficiency.[23] The concentration of α_1-AT in 28 patients with PBC was high-normal or elevated.[24] Furthermore, the common phenotypes were equally prevalent in patients with PBC and in healthy blood donors.[24]

Several examples of familial PBC have been documented. Examples of brothers,[25,26] sisters,[27,28] a brother and sister,[29] and a mother and daughter[30] have been described. We have examined three sets of sisters with PBC. A predisposition of family members to develop PBC is indicated by studies showing a high incidence of autoantibodies in asymptomatic relatives of patients with PBC.[26] Mitochondrial, smooth muscle, and antinuclear antibodies were detected in 7.4%, 11%, and 16%, respectively, of asymptomatic relatives, as compared with 0.4%, 1.9%, and 4.6% of the control populations. Among relatives of patients with PBC, 49% had one or more autoantibodies and 48% had elevated levels of one or more classes of immunoglobulins.[26] No relationship has been found between PBC and histocompatibility antigens, ABO blood groups, or rhesus blood groups.[31,32]

Drugs

Phenothiazines, methyltestosterone, and tolbutamide may cause intrahepatic cholestasis, which closely resembles PBC.[33-36] Among 36 patients with phenothiazine-induced liver injury, 6 (17%) had prolonged courses with manifestations that were difficult to distinguish from those of PBC.[34] Four of these 6 patients had clinical and biochemical features similar to those of PBC 14 to 36 months after diagnosis, and 2 patients developed xanthomas. Histologic features have been similar in the two conditions. Phenothiazine-induced jaundice is suggested by a history of drug exposure, acute onset (as opposed to the insidious onset of PBC), and eosinophilia in the peripheral blood or eosinophilic leukocytes in the portal tract and sinusoids. Mitochondrial antibodies have been detected in low titer in approximately 4% of patients with drug hepatitis, contrasting with 83% to 96% of patients with PBC.[9,37] Although liver injury caused by phenothiazines eventually resolved completely in most instances, it seems to have evolved into or unmasked PBC in some cases.

DESCRIPTIVE FEATURES

Clinical

PBC predominantly affects middle-aged women. Among 124 of our patients entering a treatment trial, 85% were females, and their mean age at presentation was 50 years, with a range of 28 to 77 years. Presenting complaints are not suggestive of the disease (except for generalized pruritus), and their onset tends to be gradual. The most common symptoms were fatigue (68%), pruritus (66%), and mild jaundice (50%). Pruritus may precede jaundice by as much as 10 years. Weight loss and anorexia were reported by about 25% of patients at initial presentation.

PBC can be recognized prior to the development of symptoms. This is largely the result of (1) widespread use of automated testing that may reveal an unexpected elevation of serum alkaline phosphatase activity, thus prompting more specific diagnostic studies; (2) greater availability of liver biopsy and enhanced expertise in recognition of histopathologic features; and (3) visualization of the biliary tract by nonsurgical techniques, such as percutaneous transhepatic cholangiography, endoscopic retrograde cholangiography, and ultrasonography. These latter procedures enabled us to exclude the various causes of extrahepatic biliary obstruction that may simulate PBC.

Approximately 20% of patients who entered our study were asymptomatic with respect to liver disease.[38] Of interest—and somewhat surprising—was that 43% of these asymptomatic patients had advanced histologic lesions (fibrosis or cirrhosis). Because its onset may be so gradual, the exact duration of PBC is difficult to determine. At a minimum, the duration can be considered as the period in which blood tests indicate cholestasis, and by this criterion, some of our asymptomatic patients with advanced histologic lesions have had their disease for 10 years or more. In contrast to an earlier opinion,[1] we believe that the course of PBC may extend for as long as 20 years or more.

Biochemical and Serologic Findings

The results of routine biochemical hepatic tests often show a pattern highly suggestive of the diagnosis. The most characteristic abnormality is striking elevation of the activity of serum alkaline phosphatase, present from the earliest point of recognition of PBC. Once elevated, the activity of serum alkaline phosphatase remains abnormal, although it may decrease slightly during the later stages of the disease. Hyperbilirubinemia is usually mild, with levels fluctuating over a period of years, but late in the disease it rises progressively. In contrast to the levels in chronic active liver disease, the serum aminotransferase activities are mildly to moderately elevated in PBC. Hypoalbuminemia and hypergammaglobulinemia tend to occur late, whereas IgM increases early (as demonstrated in more than 90% of our patients).

Mitochondrial antibody was found in 95% of our cases. There were no obvious differences between patients with M antibody and those without. When present, M antibody usually is detectable in high titers (median 1:160 or greater). The presence and titer of the M antibody do not correlate with the clinical or biochemical features, severity, or progression of the disease. Even so, the finding of M antibody is of diagnostic value. Experience in most centers suggests that M antibody occurs in less than 2% of patients with simple extra-hepatic obstruction, and then only in low titers.[39] About 20% of patients with CAH may be M-antibody-positive, but usually the titers are less than 1:40. The antibody is absent in cholestasis associated with inflammatory bowel disease and in viral hepatitis.

For diagnostic purposes, the most helpful combination of results from common biochemical and serologic tests includes (1) elevation of activity of serum alkaline phosphatase, (2) presence of M antibody (95% of cases), (3) elevation of IgM (90% of cases), (4) elevation of serum ceruloplasmin (90% of cases), and (5) elevated sedimentation rate (90% of cases).

In our patients, the serum cholesterol level ranged from 127 to 1,775 mg/dl (median 302) and was elevated in 52% of cases.

Clinical Signs

Generalized hyperpigmentation, a prominent feature in more than half of our patients, may antedate pruritus, develop simultaneously, or follow. Xanthelasma and excoriations were seen in 25% of cases at presentation. Hepatomegaly was present in 52% of cases and varied from mild to occasionally massive. Splenomegaly was present in 30% and cytopenia occurred in 38% of the 124 patients before they entered our treatment trial.

Roentgenologic Findings

Roentgenographic studies can be important in distinguishing PBC from extrahepatic biliary obstruction, a distinction that occasionally may be difficult. The clinical and laboratory differential diagnosis may be more problematic in males and in the 5% to 10% of PBC patients without M antibody. Furthermore, at least 30% to 40% of patients with PBC have radiologic evidence of gallstones.[40] In our experience, the great majority of PBC patients with cholelithiasis are asymptomatic.

Intravenous cholangiography may be unsuccessful because of hepatic dysfunction or jaundice. Percutaneous transhepatic cholangiography and endoscopic retrograde cholangiography have replaced surgical exploration in most instances. The extrahepatic biliary tree is normal on contrast visualization.[40,41] Intrahepatic biliary ducts may be normal but more commonly show evidence of diffuse and focal narrowing and shortening and diminished branching.[40,41] Usually the combination of normal extrahepatic bile ducts and characteristically abnormal intrahepatic bile ducts allows differentiation from other conditions, such as sclerosing cholangitis, carcinoma of the bile ducts, stones, and strictures.[41] In two postmortem cholangiograms, we found striking segmental dilatation of intrahepatic bile ducts.

HISTOPATHOLOGIC FINDINGS

Morphologic Diagnosis

Before patients are admitted to a prospective clinical trial, their liver biopsy specimens must be diagnostic for PBC or compatible with it. The florid duct lesion (which is the most important diagnostic feature of PBC) and other mor-

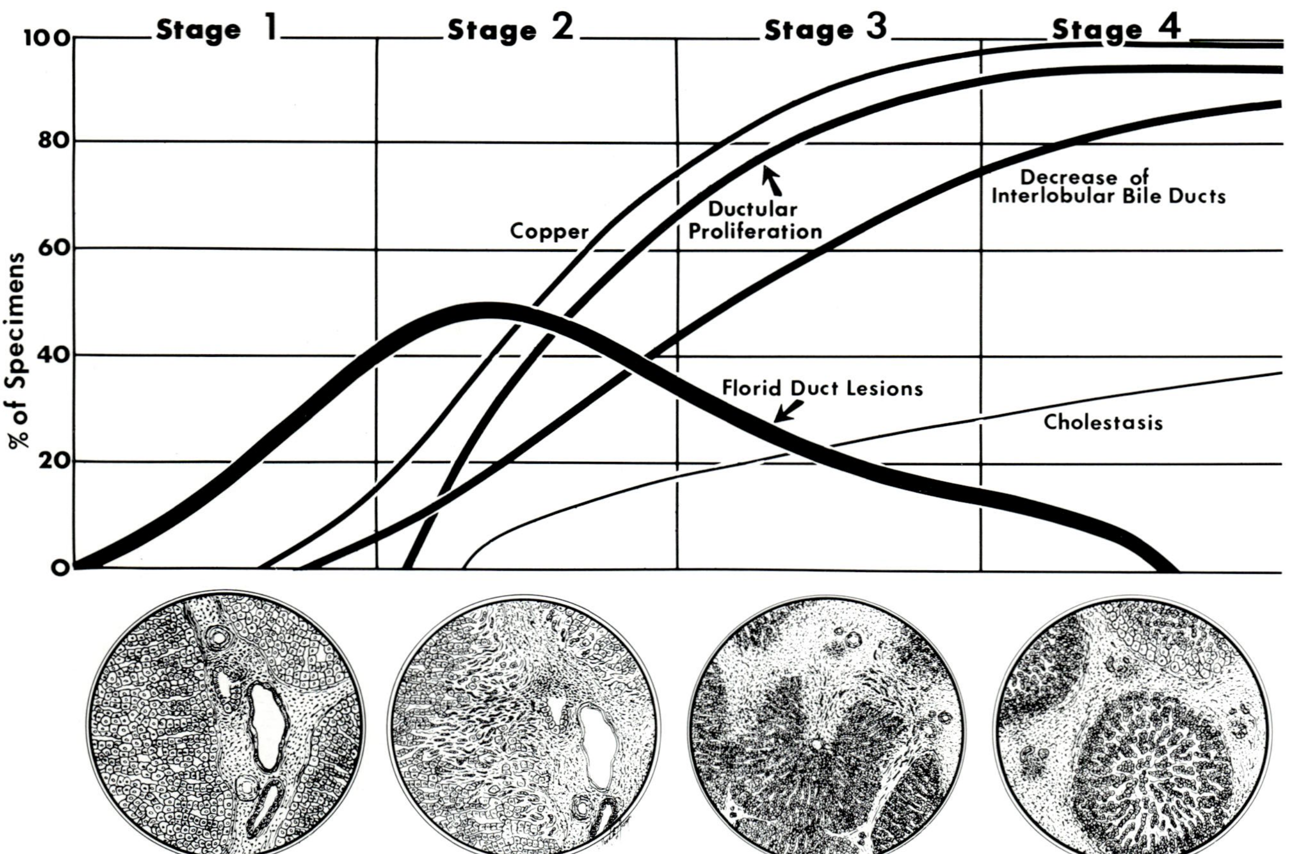

FIG. 1—Curves indicate approximate incidence of various histopathologic features in 219 single needle-biopsy specimens obtained during the four stages of PBC. Thus, florid duct lesions were found in 38% of all needle-biopsy specimens designated stage I and in 45% of those designated stage II, but in only 19% of stage III specimens and 15% of stage IV specimens. Bile stasis was rare in stage II and occurred in only 33% of specimens in stage IV. Shikata-stainable copper complexes were common in stages II and III, however, and occurred in all specimens in stage IV. Ductular proliferation had a similar pattern of incidence. The number of interlobular bile ducts decreased progressively as the disease advanced to cirrhosis. For definition of stages, see text.

phologic features have been well described,[1,42-44] and the descriptions will not be repeated here. Diagnostic difficulties arise often, primarily because the biopsy needle may fail to obtain a florid duct lesion. The incidence of florid duct lesions in single needle-biopsy specimens ranges from approximately 38% in stage I and 45% in stage II to 19% in stage III and 15% in stage IV (Fig. 1).

In the absence of fully developed florid duct lesions, components of these lesions are still of great diagnostic value in PBC of stage I or II. These include inflammatory cells within the walls of bile ducts, swelling of ductal epithelium, and scattered or clustered epithelioid cells in inflammatory portal infiltrates. Positive staining for copper also supports the diagnosis of PBC. The most useful diagnostic features in stage III or IV without florid duct lesions are decrease of interlobular bile ducts, intense copper staining in periportal hepatocytes or in those on the periphery of regenerative nodules,[45] and swelling of periportal hepatocytes (appearing as periportal pallor) or the swelling of hepatocytes in the periphery of regenerative nodules. This last-mentioned change may occur with or without bile stasis or Mallory bodies.

Stainable copper or stainable copper-protein complexes are a diagnostic feature of PBC[45,46] approaching in importance the decrease of interlobular bile ducts. Since, for unknown reasons, copper staining of liver biopsy specimens often is negative in other types of cholestatic disease despite increased chemical copper concentrations,[47] strongly positive staining for copper usually signifies PBC. In stages III and IV, copper was demonstrated in 82% and 90% of all specimens stained with rhodanine.[48] We found that the more sensitive Shikata stain demonstrated copper in 93% of 57 stage III specimens and in all of 32 stage IV specimens. Therefore, copper staining should be done in all instances where the diagnosis of PBC is considered.

Staging of PBC

Stages indicate how far the disease has progressed, and therefore staging is useful as a basis for a broad prognosis. The criteria used for staging PBC and other chronic liver diseases should reflect the morphologic progression of the disease, be applicable to routine specimens of ordinary size, and give results reproducible by many observers. In all instances, staging should be done by coded identification.

Currently, most pathologists who stage PBC use the method of Scheuer[42] or that of Popper and Schaffner.[43] There is little difference between the two. The stages are identified according to four pathologic features: stage I, inflammatory destruction of intrahepatic bile ducts; stage II, proliferation of ductules; stage III, fibrosis; and stage IV, cirrhosis. The disadvantages of these staging criteria are evident from the incidence curves for single needle-biopsy specimens (Fig. 1). Morphologic features that should indicate the early stages of PBC (namely inflammatory bile duct destruction in stage I and ductular proliferation in stage II) are not always present, particularly not in single needle-biopsy specimens. Furthermore, features of more than one stage may coexist, e.g., florid duct lesions, ductular proliferation, and fibrosis. Finally, in these staging systems, no provision is made for bridging necrosis. This lesion may occur in up to 30% of specimens, and in many cases its precirrhotic character has not been appreciated. Consequently, specimens with bridging necrosis have been assigned erroneously to stage I or II if florid duct lesions or ductular proliferation was present.

Proposed Staging System

We have named and defined the stages of PBC after features that are always present: stage I, portal stage (portal hepatitis); stage II, periportal stage (periportal hepatitis); stage III, septal stage (septal fibrosis or bridging necrosis or both); and stage IV, cirrhosis.[48] Figure 1 includes a schematic representation of the characteristics of our four stages. Neither our staging criteria nor those for stages II through IV of other classifications are based on diagnostic features of PBC; the diagnosis must be established before a specimen can be staged. Our classification is simple, uses a known terminology of chronic hepatitis,[49] and avoids common staging problems, for instance, portal hepatitis without cholangitis or periportal hepatitis without ductular proliferation. We believe that our staging system satisfies the above-mentioned requirements for morphologic staging.

Assessment of Response to Treatment

No set of morphologic features has been identified that would serve better than the above-mentioned staging methods for the evaluation of response to treatment. Copper stains may be suitable for monitoring of penicillamine trials. Although the rhodanine stain[50] is reliable and specific, we believe the Shikata stain is slightly more sensitive. We could not confirm the experience of other authors who found a satisfactory correlation between the results of histochemical and chemical copper studies.[44] We studied a larger number of specimens than they did, using essentially the same stains and methods.[50a]

The discrepancy between the results of copper staining and of chemical copper determinations became most apparent in instances where the histologic specimens stained strongly positive for copper. Uneven distribution of copper within biopsy specimens may account for this, and hence either method occasionally might yield unrepresentative results. Analysis of our data, however, indicates that other unknown factors may be involved. Methodologic limitations may hamper evaluation of individual cases, but copper staining appears to be helpful and valid when applied to large patient groups.

COPPER METABOLISM

Copper is a ubiquitous element, and under normal circumstances the healthy adult is in copper balance, the amount absorbed equaling the amount excreted. The major route of copper excretion is through the biliary tract, with negligible excretion in the urine. Studies using radioactive ^{64}Cu and ^{67}Cu indicate that the normal copper absorption by man is approximately 40% to 50%. After absorption from the proximal gastrointestinal tract, copper is transported in the plasma, mainly with the albumin fraction. Nearly all the absorbed copper is taken up by the liver. In the mammalian hepatocyte, copper is distributed into at least three major compartments[51]: some is excreted into the bile; some is held in a temporary storage pool; and a small fraction is incorporated into newly synthesized ceruloplasmin and thereafter released into the plasma. Impairment of biliary copper excretion results in accumulation of copper, particularly in the liver.

Primary Biliary Cirrhosis

In patients with PBC, the normal compensatory mechanisms (increased ceruloplasmin synthesis and increased cupruresis) fail to maintain the balance between the amount of copper absorbed and the amount excreted. Consequently, abnormalities of copper metabolism are one of the characteristic features of PBC. Hepatic copper concentrations in PBC may equal or exceed those in Wilson's disease or in prolonged extrahepatic biliary obstruction.[52] Furthermore, we have found elevated copper levels in other major organs, including the kidneys and spleen.[52] Multiorgan involvement suggests that PBC may be a generalized disorder of copper metabolism. In contrast to Wilson's disease, however, PBC is not accompanied by elevated copper levels in the brain.[52] As might be expected, pigmented corneal rings, similar to Kayser-Fleischer rings, have been observed by slit-lamp biomicroscopy in a few patients with PBC.[53,54]

Results of routine chemical tests reflecting copper metabolism (concentrations of copper in serum, urine, and liver and of ceruloplasmin) in patients with PBC are presented in Table 1.

TABLE 1.—*Pretreatment Copper and Ceruloplasmin Concentrations in 124 Mayo Clinic Patients With PBC*

	Copper			Ceruloplasmin, mg/dl
	Serum, μg/dl	Urine, μg/24 h	Liver, μg/g*	
(Normal)	(75–145)	(15–45)	(15–35)	(22.9–43.1)
Range	90–297	9–588	15–1600	22–100
Median	162	77	179	63
Patients abnormal	70%	75%	90%	90%

* Dry weight.

Other Diseases, with Implications for PBC

Various liver disorders may be accompanied by excessive copper accumulation within the liver. LaRusso et al.[55] reported some elevation of hepatic copper concentrations in the majority of 54 consecutive patients with severe chronic active liver disease. In only one instance, however, did the hepatic copper concentration exceed 250 μg/g dry weight, a level achieved in nearly all symptomatic cases of Wilson's disease. Hepatic copper concentrations exceeding 250 μg/g strongly suggest the presence of PBC, Wilson's disease, or extrahepatic obstruction of more than 12 months' duration. The effectiveness of D-penicillamine in Wilson's disease in decreasing hepatic copper concentrations and halting progression of liver injury has led to a trial of its efficacy in PBC (described in the section on management).

COMPLICATIONS

Hepatocellular failure is the usual cause of death in cases of PBC and, as in other types of cirrhosis, is often complicated by bleeding esophageal varices. Approximately 25% to 50% of patients with PBC bleed from varices at some time in the course of their disease. Variceal hemorrhage may be the first manifestation of PBC. Among 23 cases in one series,[56] 15 had bleeding varices as the first manifestation of the disease, an incidence much higher than the 2 of 24[57] and the 4 of 109[58] reported in other series. Generally, patients with PBC have less hepatocellular damage than do patients with posthepatitic or alcoholic cirrhosis, so they tolerate portal-systemic shunts reasonably well.[56,59] No operative deaths occurred among the 23 patients in the series mentioned above, and their mean survival was 3.4 years (range 1–8).[56] Although short-term survival is improved following a shunt, there is no change in the progression of the underlying disease.

Hyperlipidemia, a common complication, is characterized by elevated levels of phospholipid and free cholesterol, with normal or mildly elevated triglycerides. We found a mean serum cholesterol level of 377 mg/dl (SD = 206) in 83 symptomatic PBC patients and a mean of 285 mg/dl (SD = 110) in 21 who were asymptomatic.[38] The cholesterol level tends to rise concomitantly with direct bilirubin until the terminal stage of illness, when it usually declines. Ahrens and Kunkel[60] were able to predict that xanthelasma would occur in most patients whose total serum lipids exceeded 1,300 mg/dl, whereas xanthomas would not develop until total lipids exceeded 1,800 mg/dl for many months.

A low-density lipoprotein with alpha mobility (α_1-LDL), distinct from lipoprotein X, was detected in 40 of 77 patients with PBC.[61] Among lipoprotein profiles of 120,000 patients with other disease, α_1-LDL was found in only 5, of whom 4 had chronic hepatitis or sclerosing cholangitis associated with chronic ulcerative colitis. Particularly important diagnostically was the presence of α_1-LDL in 5 of 7 PBC patients who were seronegative for M antibody. Hence, α_1-LDL seems to be a reasonably specific but insensitive marker for PBC.

Malabsorption of fat, calcium, and vitamin D and impairment of hepatic protein synthesis contribute to the osteopenia observed in PBC. Calcium malabsorption is secondary to vitamin D deficiency and formation of insoluble calcium-fatty acid soaps. Vitamin D malabsorption is probably caused by decreased intraluminal concentration of bile acid micelles. Furthermore, excessive urinary loss of vitamin D_3 administered intravenously suggests that renal loss of endogenous or supplementary vitamin D may contribute to vitamin D deficiency.[62] Bone biopsies may show osteoporosis or osteomalacia or both.[63] Pathologic fractures usually are seen only in clinically and histologically advanced cases.

Among 40 randomly selected cases of PBC, serum vitamin A levels were below normal in 27 (68%),[64] with an inverse relation between these levels and the histologic severity. Clinical evidence of vitamin A deficiency in PBC is rare, although dark-field adaptation studies would probably detect abnormalities.

Hepatocellular carcinoma complicated PBC in 3 (6%) of the 52 cases in one series.[65] No cases were found among the 124 patients in our treatment trial; however, 2 patients not in the study have died as a result of hepatocellular carcinoma complicating PBC.

MANAGEMENT

No spontaneous, complete remissions of PBC have been reported, and no specific therapy has proven effective.

Relation to Chronic Active Hepatitis

PBC shares many morphologic and immunologic characteristics with CAH, a disease that has shown favorable response to corticosteroids either alone or in combination with azathioprine;[66] yet in PBC, each of these agents has been used without benefit. A 5-year controlled prospective trial in patients with symptomatic but precirrhotic PBC showed no difference between the drug and placebo groups in development of cirrhosis or in survival.[67] Indeed, corticosteroids are contraindicated because of the lack of long-term benefit and the acceleration of osteopenia.[68,69] A 3- to 6-month course of corticosteroids or steroids combined with azathioprine may be appropriate in cases with features of both PBC and CAH if a clear differential diagnosis is not possible.[70]

Supportive Therapy

Generalized pruritus is the earliest and most distressing symptom in the majority of cases. Cholestyramine has proved effective in relieving pruritus in most patients.[71] Phenobarbital (2–4 mg/kg/day) decreases pruritus in some patients and, taken before sleep, offers sedative and antipruritic effects that allow more adequate rest. Methyltestosterone gives prompt relief of pruritus but is associated with hirsutism and a striking increase of serum bilirubin. Therefore, it is reserved for those deeply jaundiced patients with intractable itching.[71] Fluorescent irradiation in total-body exposure cabinets for 9 to 12 min each week has relieved pruritus in PBC.[72]

Levels of serum 25-hydroxyvitamin D (25-OH-D) are below normal in most patients with PBC. Malabsorption of the fat-soluble vitamin D and impaired 25-hydroxylation in the liver may explain this, and double isotope techniques have shown that vitamin D malabsorption is the more important of these causes.[62] Intramuscular injection of vitamin D obviates the problem of its malabsorption, a complication that progresses with increasing cholestasis. Low serum 25-OH-D concentrations return to normal if sufficient intramuscular vitamin D substrate (100,000 U, once each month) is presented to the liver.[73] Vitamin D injections and the combination of low-fat diet with medium-chain triglycerides have resulted in significant increases in calcium retention, as determined by whole-body counting of calcium 47.[74,75] But despite normalizing of 25-OH-D with parenteral vitamin D, osteomalacia still may occur, and pathologic fractures may result. Bone pain ceased or diminished in one study, and histologic evidence of osteomalacia decreased after one to five monthly injections of 1,25-dihydroxycholecalciferol.[76] Hypoprothrombinemia and vitamin A deficiencies are treated with water-soluble vitamin K and A, respectively.

Experimental Therapy for PBC

Because of resemblances between PBC and Wilson's disease, wherein D-penicillamine (D-PCA) controls liver damage by lessening the hepatic concentration of copper, we initiated a therapeutic trial of D-PCA in PBC. We randomized 124 PBC patients to a D-PCA or a placebo group after stratification according to the presence or absence of complications (cirrhosis or varices) and the duration of disease (dividing at 3 years). In the 22 fatal cases, 21 pretreatment biopsy specimens were assigned to the cirrhotic stage and 1 to the septal stage. During 3½ years of treatment and follow-up, the mortality was 7 of 64 (11%) in the D-PCA group and 15 of 60 (25%) in the placebo group, a significant difference ($p<0.05$).

At 1 year, patients taking D-PCA had significantly lower values for serum bilirubin, IgM, and gamma globulins ($p<0.01$ for each) than did patients taking placebo. At 2 years the D-PCA patients had values lower than the placebo patients for IgM and gamma globulins ($p<0.01$ for each) and for alkaline phosphatase ($p<0.02$).

After 12 months, 7 of the 10 placebo patients with initial liver specimens staged I or II had progressed to stage III or IV, whereas 6 of the 7 D-PCA patients initially in stage I or II remained unchanged. Among patients whose initial liver biopsy specimens were of stage III or IV, no significant morphologic differences between the D-PCA and placebo groups were noted after 1 and 2 years of the study. The mean decrease of hepatic copper was much greater in the D-PCA group than in the placebo group: at 1 year, -146 versus -7 μg/g dry weight ($p<0.01$); and at 2 years, -180 versus -17 μg/g dry weight ($p<0.01$). Linear correlation is lacking between the reduction of hepatic copper and changes of other hepatic biochemical values in given cases, suggesting that the apparent therapeutic effects of D-PCA may be mediated through mechanisms other than decrease of hepatic copper. Two properties of D-PCA that may provide additional benefit are its ability to interfere with collagen maturation[77,78] and its ability to reduce the number of circulating T lymphocytes.[79,80]

The encouraging results obtained with D-PCA must be weighed against a 22% incidence of major toxicity (Table 2). Proteinuria (>1.2 g/24 hr) is the complication we have encountered most often, accounting for 8 of the 14 instances in which D-PCA therapy was discontinued. Nephrotic syndrome occurred in only 1 case, and the proteinuria disappeared in all within 6 months after discontinuance of D-PCA. Of particular interest was the development of proteinuria in 4 patients receiving placebo therapy. A glomerular lesion may be present in patients with PBC who are not taking D-PCA.

Severe cytopenia developed in 2 patients and resulted in the single drug-related death. Complications that did not require discontinuance of therapy included alterations in taste (6 patients) and nausea and vomiting (1 patient). Lupuslike reactions,[81] myasthenia gravis,[82] and polymyositis[83] have been observed by others.

The subtle onset and variable time course of PBC require that prospective

TABLE 2.—*Complications That Necessitated Discontinuance of* D-*Penicillamine Therapy*

	Patients, No.	
	D-PCA	Placebo
Proteinuria*	8	4
Cytopenia†	2‡	1
Miscellaneous§	4	0
Total	14/64 (22%)	5/60 (8%)

* >1.2 g/day.
† Leukocytes <3,000 or platelets <75,000/cu mm.
‡ 1 death, secondary to drug-induced marrow aplasia.
§ Anorexia, arthralgia, rash.

treatment trials extend over long periods and include large numbers of patients. Although fluctuation in the clinical and biochemical course of PBC is very common, liver lesions may remain static for many years. Therefore, survival is the most important criterion by which to judge therapeutic effectiveness. In the future, controlled trials should be continued to provide a data base that is indisputably firm.

REFERENCES

1. Foulk WT, BaggenstossAH, Butt HR: Primary biliary cirrhosis: Reevaluation by clinical and histologic study of 49 cases. Gastroenterology 47:354–374, 1964
2. Feizi T: Immunoglobulins in chronic liver disease. Gut 9:193–198, 1968
3. Hobbs JR: Serum proteins in liver disease. Proc R Soc Med 60:1250–1254, 1967
4. MacSween RNM, Horne CHW, Moffat AJ, Hughes HM: Serum protein levels in primary biliary cirrhosis. J Clin Pathol 25:789–792, 1972
5. Walker JG, Doniach D, Roitt IM, Sherlock S: Serological tests in diagnosis of primary biliary cirrhosis. Lancet 1:827–831, 1965
6. Berg PA, Muscatello U, Horne RW, Roitt IM, Doniach D: Mitochondrial antibodies in primary biliary cirrhosis. II. The complement fixing antigen as a component of mitochondrial inner membranes. Br J Exp Pathol 50:200–208, 1969
7. Ben-Yoseph Y, Shapira E, Doniach D: Further purification of the mitochondrial inner membrane autoantigen reacting with primary biliary cirrhosis sera. Immunology 26:311–321, 1974
8. Mackay IR: Lupoid hepatitis and primary biliary cirrhosis: autoimmune diseases of the liver? Bull Rheum Dis 18:487–494, 1968
9. Doniach D, Walker G: Immunopathology of liver disease. Prog Liver Dis 4:381–402, 1972
10. Roux MEB, Florin-Christensen A, Arana RM, Doniach D: Paraproteins with antibody activity in acute viral hepatitis and chronic autoimmune liver diseases. Gut 15:396–400, 1974
11. Wands JR, Dienstag JL, Bhan AK, Feller ER, Isselbacher KJ: Circulating immune complexes and complement activation in primary biliary cirrhosis. N Engl J Med 298:233–237, 1978
12. Gupta RC, Dickson ER, McDuffie FC, Baggenstoss AH: Circulating IgG complexes in primary biliary cirrhosis: A serial study in 40 patients followed for two years. Clin Exp Immunol (in press)
13. Gupta RC, Dickson ER, McDuffie FC: Circulating immune complexes and autoimmune features in primary biliary cirrhosis: implications for pathogenesis (abstract). Gastroenterology 73:1223, 1977
14. Potter BJ, Elias E, Jones EA: Hypercatabolism of the third component of complement in patients with primary biliary cirrhosis. J Lab Clin Med 88:427–439, 1976
15. Teisberg P, Gjone E: Circulating conversion products of C3 in liver disease: Evi-

dence for *in vivo* activation of the complement system. Clin Exp Immunol 14:509–514, 1973

16. Geubel AP, Keller RH, Summerskill WHJ, Dickson ER, Tomasi TB, Shorter RG: Lymphocyte cytotoxicity and inhibition studied with autologous liver cells: Observations in chronic active liver disease and the primary biliary cirrhosis syndrome. Gastroenterology 71:450–456, 1976

17. Vierling JM, Nelson DL, Strober W, Bundy BM, Jones EA: In vitro cell-mediated cytotoxicity in primary biliary cirrhosis and chronic hepatitis: Dysfunction of spontaneous cell-mediated cytotoxicity in primary biliary cirrhosis. J Clin Invest 60:1116–1128, 1977

18. Paronetto F, Schaffner F, Popper H: Immunocytochemical and serologic observations in primary biliary cirrhosis. N Engl J Med 271:1123–1128, 1964

19. Hardy RM, Stevens JB, Stowe CM: Chronic progressive hepatitis in Bedlington terriers associated with elevated liver copper concentrations. Minn Vet 15:13–24, 1975

20. Maddrey WC, Saito S, Shulman NR, Klatskin G: Coincidental Australia antigenemia in primary biliary cirrhosis. Ann Intern Med 76:705–709, 1972

21. MacSween RNM, Yeung Laiwah AAC, Busuttil AA, Thomas MA, Ross SK, Watkinson G, Millman I, Blumberg BS: Australia antigen and primary biliary cirrhosis. J Clin Pathol 26:335–339, 1973

22. Grady GF, Kaplan MM, Vyas GN: Antibody to hepatitis B core antigen in chronic hepatitis and primary biliary cirrhosis: Evaluation by a new autologous solid phase radioimmunoassay. Gastroenterology 72:590–593, 1977

23. Cars O, Stenram U, Strömberg A: Alpha-1-antitrypsin deficiency, mitochondrial antibodies and possible primary biliary cirrhosis: A case report and family study. Ups J Med Sci 80:93–98, 1975

24. Keuppers F, Dickson ER, Summerskill WHJ: Alpha$_1$-antitrypsin phenotypes in chronic active liver disease and primary biliary cirrhosis. Mayo Clin Proc 51:286–288, 1976

25. Bown R, Clark ML, Doniach D: Primary biliary cirrhosis in brothers. Postgrad Med J 51:110–115, 1975

26. Galbraith RM, Smith M, Mackenzie RM, Tee DE, Doniach D, Williams R: High prevalence of seroimmunologic abnormalities in relatives of patients with active chronic hepatitis or primary biliary cirrhosis. N Engl J Med 290:63–69, 1974

27. Chamuleau RAFM, Van Berge Henegouwen GP, Bronkhorst FB, Brandt KH: Primary biliary cirrhosis in sisters. Neth J Med 18:170–175, 1975

28. Chohan MR: Primary biliary cirrhosis in twin sisters. Gut 14:213–214. 1973

29. Schaffner F: Primary biliary cirrhosis. Clin Gastroenterol 4:351–366, 1975

30. Tong MJ, Nies KM, Reynolds TB, Quismorio FP: Immunological studies in familial primary biliary cirrhosis. Gastroenterology 71:305–307, 1976

31. Galbraith RM, Eddleston ALWF, Smith MGM, Williams R, McSween RNM, Watkinson G, Dick H, Kennedy LA, Batchelor JR: Histocompatability antigens in active chronic hepatitis and primary biliary cirrhosis. Br Med J 3:604–605, 1974

32. Hamlyn AN, Morris JS, Sherlock S: ABO blood groups, rhesus negativity, and primary biliary cirrhosis. Gut 15:480–481, 1974

33. Read AE, Harrison CV, Sherlock S: Chronic chlorpromazine jaundice: With particular reference to its relationship to primary biliary cirrhosis. Am J Med 31:249–258, 1961

34. Ishak KG, Irey NS: Hepatic injury associated with the phenothiazines: Clinicopathologic and follow-up study of 36 patients. Arch Pathol 93:283–304, 1972

35. Glober GA, Wilkerson JA: Biliary cirrhosis following the administration of methyltestosterone. JAMA 204:170–173, 1968

36. Gregory DH, Zaki GF, Sarcosi GA, Carey JB Jr: Chronic cholestasis following prolonged tolbutamide administration: associated with destructive cholangitis and cholangiolitis. Arch Pathol 84:194–201, 1967

37. Klatskin G, Kantor FS: Mitochondrial antibody in primary biliary cirrhosis and other diseases. Ann Intern Med 77:533–541, 1972

38. Fleming CR, Ludwig J, Dickson ER: Asymptomatic primary biliary cirrhosis: Presentation, histology, and results with D-penicillamine. Mayo Clin Proc 53:587–593, 1978

39. Sherlock S: Immunological disturbance in diseases of liver and thyroid. Proc R Soc Med 70:851–855, 1977

40. Summerfield JA, Elias E, Hungerford GD, Nikapota VLB, Dick R, Sherlock S: The biliary system in primary biliary cirrhosis:

A study by endoscopic retrograde cholangiopancreatography. Gastroenterology 70:240–243, 1976

41. Legge DA, Carlson HC, Dickson ER, Ludwig J: Cholangiographic findings in cholangiolitic hepatitis: Syndrome of primary biliary cirrhosis. Am J Roentgenol 113:16–20, 1971

42. Scheuer PJ: Liver Biopsy Interpretation (ed 2). Baltimore, Williams & Wilkins, 1973, pp 33–38

43. Popper H, Schaffner F: Nonsuppurative destructive chronic cholangitis and chronic hepatitis. Edited by H Popper and F Schaffner: Progress in Liver Diseases, Vol. III. New York, Grune & Stratton, 1970, pp 336–354

44. Irons RD, Schenk EA, Lee JCK: Cytochemical methods for copper: Semiquantitative screening procedure for identification of abnormal copper levels in liver. Arch Pathol Lab Med 101:298–301, 1977

45. Sipponen P, Salaspuro MP, Makkonen HM: Orcein positive hepatocellular material in histological diagnosis of primary biliary cirrhosis. Am Clin Res 7:273–277, 1975

46. Salaspuro M, Sipponen P: Demonstration of an intracellular copper-binding protein by orcein staining in long-standing cholestatic liver diseases. Gut 17:787–790, 1976

47. Jain S, Scheuer PJ, Archer B, Newman S, Sherlock S: Histochemical demonstration of liver copper and copper carrying protein in chronic liver disease (abstract). Gut 18:953–954, 1977

48. Ludwig J, Dickson ER, McDonald GSA: Staging of chronic nonsuppurative destructive cholangitis (syndrome of primary biliary cirrhosis). VirchowsArch [Pathol Anat] 379:103–112, 1978

49. Ludwig J: A review of lobular, portal, and periportal hepatitis: Interpretation of biopsy specimens without clinical data. Hum Pathol 8:269–276, 1977

50. Lindquist RR: Studies on the pathogenesis of hepatolenticular degeneration. II. Cytochemical methods for the localization of copper. Arch Pathol 87:370–379, 1969

50a. Ludwig J, McDonald GSA, Dickson ER, Elveback LR, McCall JT: Copper stains and the syndrome of primary biliary cirrhosis: An evaluation of staining methods and their usefulness for diagnosis and trials of D-penicillamine treatment. Arch Pathol Lab Med (in press)

51. Evans GW: Copper homeostasis in the mammalian system. Physiol Rev 53:535–570, 1973

52. Fleming CR, Dickson ER, Baggenstoss AH, McCall JT: Copper and primary biliary cirrhosis. Gastroenterology 67:1182–1187, 1974

53. Fleming CR, Dickson ER, Hollenhorst RW, Goldstein NP, McCall JT, Baggenstoss AH: Pigmented corneal rings in a patient with primary biliary cirrhosis. Gastroenterology 69:220–225, 1975

54. Fleming CR, Dickson ER, Wahner HW, Hollenhorst RW, McCall JT: Pigmented corneal rings in non-Wilsonian liver disease. Ann Intern Med 86:285–288, 1977

55. LaRusso NF, Summerskill WHJ, McCall JT: Abnormalities of chemical tests for copper metabolism in chronic active liver disease: Differentiation from Wilson's disease. Gastroenterology 70:653–655, 1976

56. Zeegen R, Dawson AM, Stansfeld AG, Hunt AH: Bleeding oesophageal varices as the presenting feature in primary biliary cirrhosis. Lancet 2:9–13, 1969

57. Lebrec D, Sicot C, Degott C, Benhamou J-P: Portal hypertension in primary biliary cirrhosis. Digestion 14:220–226, 1976

58. Kew MC, Varma RR, Dos Santos HA, Scheuer PJ, Sherlock S: Portal hypertension in primary biliary cirrhosis. Gut 12:830–834, 1971

59. Bauer JJ, Gelernt IM, Kreel I: Portosystemic shunting in patients with primary biliary cirrhosis: A good risk disease. Ann Surg 183:324–328, 1976

60. Ahrens EH Jr, Kunkel HG: The relationship between serum lipids and skin xanthomata in eighteen patients with primary biliary cirrhosis. J Clin Invest 28:1565–1574, 1949

61. Lauterburg BH, Ellefson RD, Dickson ER: $Alpha_1$ low density lipoprotein: A marker for primary biliary cirrhosis (abstract). Gastroenterology 74:1053, 1978

62. Krawitt EL, Grundman MJ, Mawer EB: Absorption, hydroxylation, and excretion of vitamin D_3 in primary biliary cirrhosis. Lancet 2:1246–1249, 1977

63. Atkinson M, Nordin BEC, Sherlock S: Malabsorption and bone disease in prolonged obstructive jaundice. Q J Med 25:299–312, 1956

64. Fleming CR, Ellefson RD, Dickson ER: unpublished data

65. MacSween RNM, Berg PA: Autoimmune diseases of the liver. Edited by A Ferguson and RNM MacSween: Immunological Aspects of the Liver and Gastrointestinal Tract. Baltimore, University Park Press, 1976, p 366

66. Summerskill WHJ, Korman MG, Ammon HV, Baggenstoss AH: Prednisone for chronic active liver disease: Dose, titration, standard dose, and combination with azathioprine compared. Gut 16:876–883, 1975

67. Heathcote J, Ross A, Sherlock S: A prospective controlled trial of azathioprine in primary biliary cirrhosis. Gastroenterology 70:656–660, 1976

68. Carman CT, Giansiracusa JE: Effect of steroid therapy on the clinical and laboratory features of primary biliary cirrhosis. Gastroenterology 28:193–207, 1955

69. Howat HT, Ralston AJ, Varley H, Wilson JAC: The late results of long-term treatment of primary biliary cirrhosis by corticosteroids. Rev Int Hepatol 16:227–238, 1966

70. Geubel AA, Baggenstoss AH, Summerskill WHJ: Responses to treatment can differentiate chronic active liver disease with cholangitic features from the primary biliary cirrhosis syndrome. Gastroenterology 71:444–449, 1976

71. Datta DV, Sherlock S: Cholestyramine for long term relief of the pruritus complicating intrahepatic cholestasis. Gastroenterology 50:323–332, 1966

72. Perlstein SM: Treatment of primary biliary cirrhosis (letter to the editor). Arch Dermatol 110:132, 1974

73. Skinner RK, Sherlock S, Long RG, Wills MR: 25-Hydroxylation of vitamin D in primary biliary cirrhosis. Lancet 1:720–721, 1977

74. Kehayoglou AK, Agnew JE, Holdsworth CD, Whelton MJ, Sherlock S: Bone disease and calcium absorption in primary biliary cirrhosis: With special reference to vitamin-D therapy. Lancet 1:715–718, 1968

75. Kehayoglou K, Hadziyannis S, Kostamis P, Malamos B: The effect of medium-chain triglyceride on ^{47}calcium absorption in patients with primary biliary cirrhosis. Gut 14:653–656, 1973

76. Long RG, Varghese Z, Meinhard EA, Skinner RK, Wills MR, Sherlock S: Parenteral 1,25-dihydroxycholecalciferol in hepatic osteomalacia. Br Med J 1:75–77, 1978

77. Deshmukh K, Nimni ME: A defect in the intramolecular and intermolecular cross-linking of collagen caused by penicillamine. II. Functional groups involved in the interaction process. J Biol Chem 244:1787–1795, 1969

78. Brunner G, Perings E, Creutzfeldt W: D-penicillamine in experimental cirrhosis. Edited by H Popper and K Becker: Collagen Metabolism in the Liver. New York, Stratton Intercontinental Medical Book Corporation, 1975, pp 191-195

79. Brandt L, Svensson B: Effect of penicillamine on peripheral-blood lymphocytes in rheumatoid arthritis (letter to the editor). Lancet 1:394–395, 1975

80. Roath S, Wills R: The effects of penicillamine on lymphocytes in culture. Postgrad Med J 50 (Suppl 2):56–57, 1974

81. Harpey JP, Caille B, Moulias R, Goust JM: Lupus-like syndrome induced by D-penicillamine in Wilson's disease (letter to the editor). Lancet 1:292, 1971

82. Gordon RA, Burnside JW: D-Penicillamine-induced myasthenia gravis in rheumatoid arthritis. Ann Intern Med 87:578–579, 1977

83. Cucher BG, Goldman AL: D-Penicillamine-induced polymyositis in rheumatoid arthritis. Ann Intern Med 85:615–616, 1976

Chapter 28

Visualization of the Bile Ducts

By DAVID S. ZIMMON, M.D., *and* ARTHUR R. CLEMETT, M.D.

FOR MANY YEARS the only method for visualization of the bile ducts was laparotomy with inspection, palpation, and biopsy of these remote and delicate structures. The initial diagnosis of biliary tract disease was characterized by an intense, lengthy, indirect evaluation that yielded a diagnosis by inference. Ultimately, exploratory laparotomy proved or disproved a clinical presumption and provided the only therapeutic approach. Frequently, no remedial lesion was found and the patient died shortly thereafter. The approach to biliary tract disease became polarized between an emphasis on a long, debilitating, low-yield work-up or abdominal exploration launched from a presumptive clinical diagnosis with the aim of correcting lesions, if possible.

Even today with the availability of remarkable modern diagnostic methods, prompt laparotomy may be advocated to evaluate patients suspected of biliary tract disease. This approach is limited by the radiologic facilities and techniques that can be applied in the operating room during laparotomy and the fact that errors in technique and judgment may occur early in the abdominal exploration even when "surgical jaundice" is present. Patients with parenchymal liver disease or other diseases not amenable to surgical management may be explored in error. The development of methods for managing biliary tract disease without abdominal operation has further limited the indications for laparotomy. Specific positive anatomic indications should be defined in advance of laparotomy. When laparotomy is indicated, operative time with its high risk and cost may be spared by superior preoperative procedures that define primary pathologic abnormalities or uncover occult primary or secondary lesions or anatomic variants of clinical importance.

CLINICAL DIAGNOSIS OF HEPATIC AND BILIARY TRACT DISEASE

For instance, a prospective analysis by Schenker et al. confirmed the accuracy of a meticulous history and physical examination in the differential diagnosis of jaundice.[1] History and physical examination alone yielded a diagnostic accuracy of 80% for cirrhosis, 77% for obstructive jaundice, and 70% for hepatitis in 61 patients. With the addition of simple laboratory tests, obstructive jaundice was diagnosed correctly in 90% of 20 patients. Why then the recent emphasis on sophisticated and expensive "tests" for the visualization

From the Department of Medicine, Gastroenterology Section, Veterans Administration Hospital, Departments of Radiology, Medicine and Surgery, St. Vincent's Hospital and Medical Center, and the New York University School of Medicine, New York, New York.

of the bile ducts? The goal of differential diagnosis in a jaundiced patient in the absence of methods for visualization of the bile ducts was to separate "medical" from "surgical" jaundice. But beyond the diagnostic problem lies the need for anatomic definition of the nature, origin, and extent of disease. Only with precise knowledge of pathologic anatomy can we take advantage of "nonsurgical" techniques that are alternatives to abdominal surgery or may be applied prior to abdominal surgery to reduce operative morbidity and mortality.

The following six clinical situations are presented to illustrate the value of biliary and pancreatic duct visualization and the therapeutic options opened by precise knowledge of the origin, nature, and extent of bile duct disease.

THE DIFFICULT CASE

In 10% of cases, even the experienced hepatologist is puzzled and requires liver biopsy[2] or direct cholangiography to establish a mechanical cause for cholestatsis. Because of widespread automated chemical profiles, the results of blood chemistry tests in patients with early cholestatic disease such as primary biliary cirrhosis or asymptomatic choledocholithiasis are only minimally abnormal. Eventually, with the definition of high-risk populations and the evolution of appropriate screening techniques, it will be possible to identify the early stages of carcinoma of the pancreas or bile ducts. By contrast with familiar presentations of gross jaundice, pain, or fever in these patients, bile duct dilatation is absent and cholestasis may fluctuate. Patients with known liver disease, cholelithiasis, or prior biliary surgery are difficult to evaluate without direct cholangiography to exclude bile duct disease (Fig. 1).

INTRAHEPATIC VERSUS EXTRAHEPATIC BILE DUCT OBSTRUCTION

Intrahepatic bile duct obstruction may occur without bile duct dilatation in infiltrative hepatic disease, such as lymphoma or infiltrating bile duct carcinoma. Metastatic carcinoma involving the porta hepatis or the liver may produce intrahepatic bile duct dilatation (Fig. 2).

DISTAL COMMON BILE DUCT OBSTRUCTION

Precise visualization of the anatomic features of both pancreatic and biliary ducts is essential to differentiate and manage distal bile duct obstruction. Cholelithiasis may be incidental. The proximal manifestations of neoplastic distal bile duct obstruction and choledocholithiasis may be identical. Even direct cholangiography with visualization of only the common bile duct may be inadequate to differentiate unresectable carcinoma of the pancreas from periampullary carcinomas that may be resected for cure[3] (Fig. 3A). This differential diagnosis is best established by visualizing both pancreatic and bile ducts with endoscopic retrograde cholangiopancreatography (ERCP)[4] (Fig. 3B). The differentiation of benign papillary stenosis from papillary neoplasia is particularly difficult and requires endoscopic visualization and biopsy of the papilla, some-

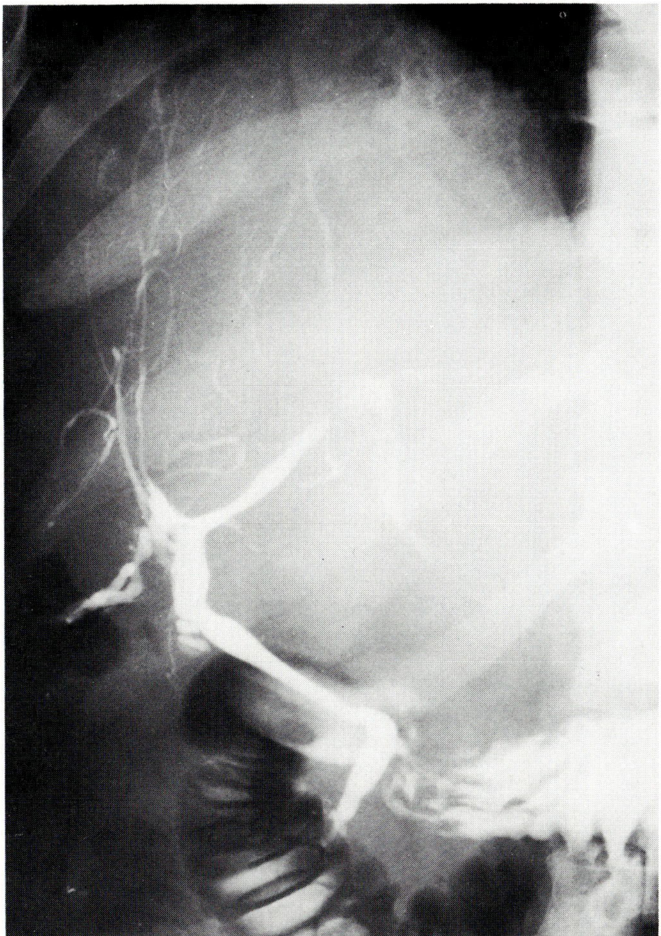

FIG. 1—ERCP in a jaundiced patient with chronic active hepatitis following cholecystectomy. Laboratory data suggested extrahepatic obstruction. The intrahepatic bile ducts are compressed and distorted by regeneration and fibrosis. Caudate lobe hypertrophy splays and displaces the right and left hepatic ducts inferiorly. Shrinkage of the right lobe with massive hypertrophy of the left lobe has shifted the porta hepatis to the right and angulated the common bile duct. A short cystic duct stump is visible. Extrahepatic bile duct obstruction was excluded by this examination. The compression with narrowing of the intrahepatic bile ducts and distorted anatomy, coupled with the presence of severe fibrosis and portal hypertension, would make a percutaneous transhepatic examination in this patient both liable to failure and hazardous.

times after endoscopic papillotomy to establish drainage and allow submucosal biopsy of the small neoplasm.

IDENTIFICATION OF ASSOCIATED PANCREATIC DISEASE AFFECTING THE DISTAL COMMON BILE DUCT

Pancreatitis is commonly associated with distal bile duct stenosis.[5] Pseudocysts in the head of the pancreas may compress the common bile duct, producing cholestasis.[6,7] Therapy in the cholestasis associated with pancreatitis

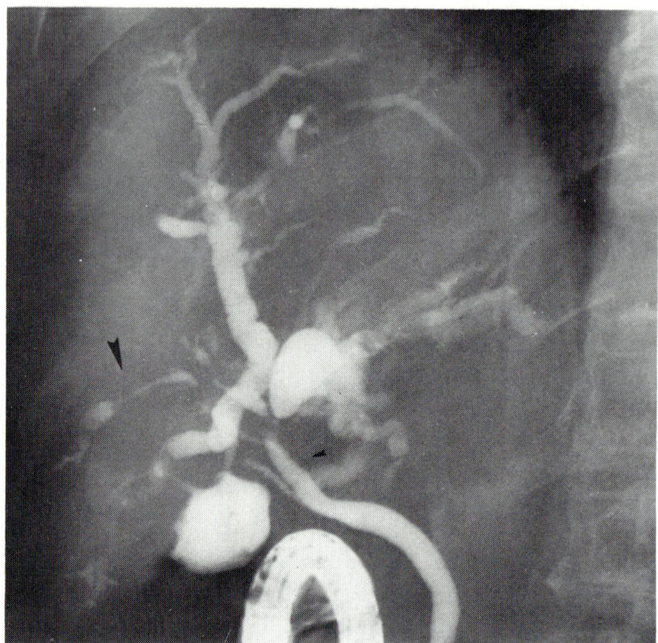

FIG. 2—ERCP in metastatic colon carcinoma of the liver and porta hepatis. There is extrinsic compression with stenosis and lateral displacement of the common hepatic duct (small arrowhead). The intrahepatic ducts are generally dilated, with multiple areas of duct distortion and displacement, tumor encasement, and duct occlusion (large arrowhead). In this case, bile duct obstruction at the porta hepatis and within the liver produced dilatation of intrahepatic ducts that could be misconstrued as indicative of extrahepatic bile duct obstruction.

should be directed primarily at the pancreatic disease and secondarily at achieving bile duct drainage. Commonly, drainage of a pseudocyst, if present, will decompress the biliary tree.[6] The differentiation of pancreatitis producing distal common bile duct obstruction from pancreatic carcinoma may be difficult at laparotomy. This differential diagnosis is best established by endoscopic retrograde pancreatography.[4,8-10]

THERAPEUTIC OPTIONS BASED ON THE ORIGIN, NATURE, AND EXTENT OF DISEASE

Many jaundiced patients may be managed without laparotomy or with preoperative procedures that reduce the morbidity and mortality of laparotomy. A frustrating diagnostic laparotomy in a seriously ill patient with carcinoma of the pancreas can be avoided by direct cholangiography coupled with endoscopic retrograde pancreatography or angiography that demonstrates unresectability[11,12] (Fig. 4). Jaundice may be relieved by a percutaneous biliary stent[13] without resorting to bypass operations. A tissue diagnosis may be obtained by percutaneous aspiration using the ductal lesion demonstrated by percutaneous transhepatic cholangiography (PTC) or ERCP or the vascular encasement demonstrated by angiography as a target.[14-16] If unresectable car-

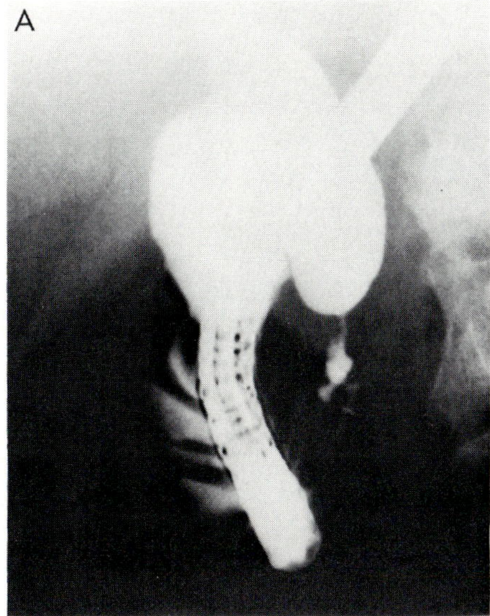

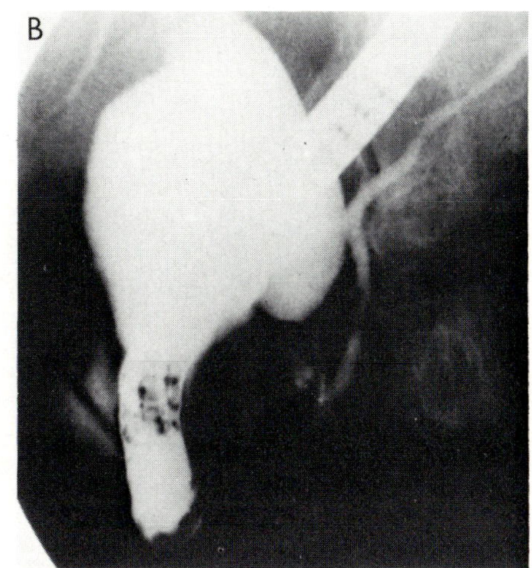

FIG. 3A—ERCP in periampullary cancer with obstruction of the distal common bile duct and striking proximal dilatation (arrow). A PTC might have given similar radiographic findings. Endoscopic examination of the papilla of Vater excluded papillary or duodenal malignancy.

FIG. 3B—ERCP shows the adjacent pancreatic duct displaced by this terminal bile duct tumor but essentially uninvolved, excluding carcinoma of the pancreas and indicating resectability and potential for cure.

cinoma of pancreas has been ruled out and periampullary cancer diagnosed, preoperative biliary drainage allows referral to a specialized center, where the patient may benefit from the reduced operative morbidity and mortality provided by a surgical team experienced in performing extensive pancreatic surgery.[3] The operative mortality is reduced by relieving biliary tract obstruction through endoscopic papillotomy of distal biliary tumors or percutaneous stents for external drainage.[13] Precise anatomic definition of the neoplastic lesions may be used to design ports for radiation therapy.[17-20]

Endoscopic management of choledocholithiasis or benign papillary stenosis is the procedure of choice in the postcholecystectomy patient.[21-25] Endoscopic papillotomy or sphincterotomy are valuable as temporizing procedures in patients with severe cholangitis or as a definitive procedure in patients who have not had cholecystectomy when removal of the common duct stones relieves cholestasis and the risk of cholecystectomy is great.

GALLBLADDER DISEASE

Direct cholangiography identifies cystic duct obstruction and determines the need for common duct exploration. When cystic duct obstruction coexists with acute cholecystitis, empyema of the gallbladder is present with the hazard of perforation. If the cystic duct is patent, resolution of cholecystitis is the rule, and the increased risk of emergency surgery can be avoided.[26]

The identification of variant anatomic features of the biliary tract is of great

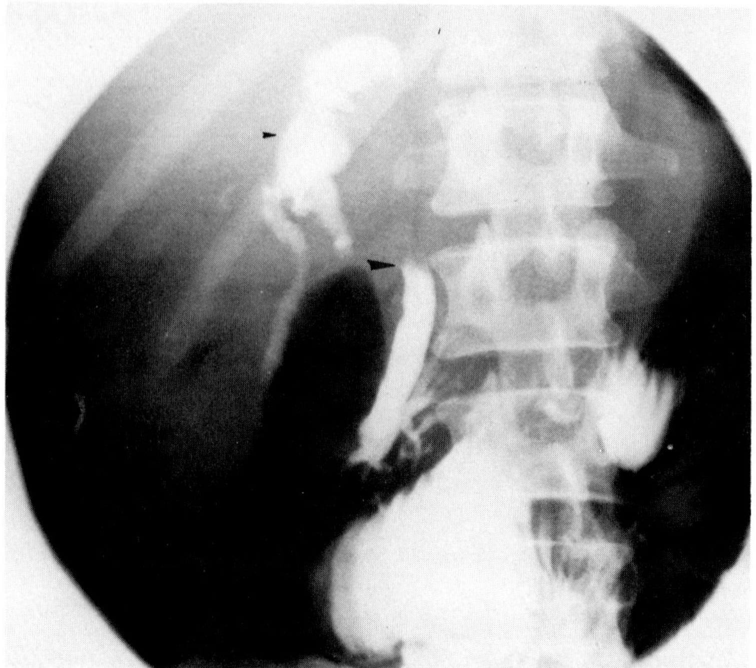

FIG. 4—ERCP in carcinoma of the pancreas. Obstruction of the pancreatic duct is visible to the right of the distal common bile duct. Extension of the tumor along the gastrohepatic ligament obstructs and displaces the common hepatic duct and cystic duct (large arrowhead) precluding cholecystoenterostomy. The intrahepatic bile ducts are markedly dilated (small arrowhead). The only option for palliation would be a percutaneous drain or stent and radiation or chemotherapy.

importance, since preoperatively it is difficult to estimate the magnitude of inflammation in the gastrohepatic ligament and the potential problems of defining lesions at the time of cholecystectomy. The unnecessary common duct exploration may be avoided and the occult common duct stone recognized.[27] Complicating papillary stenosis or occult periampullary neoplasia may be uncovered. Therapeutic options such as the use of endoscopic biliary surgery or temporary biliary drainage to control cholangitis or relieve high-grade biliary tract obstruction may be exercised.

Fortunately, the need for second operations to remove retained common duct stones or relieve papillary stenosis has been reduced by the techniques of endoscopic sphincterotomy and extraction of stones through T-tube tracts.[28-30] These options relieve the pressure on a surgeon to clear the bile duct at laparotomy. Nevertheless, many of these problems can be avoided by preoperative cholangiography.

DIAGNOSTIC TECHNIQUES

Screening Test

"Noninvasive" screening tests are rapidly evolving in terms of technique, instrumentation, and interpretation. They demand considerable skill and require confirmation (biopsy) or supplementation (direct cholangiography, pancreatography, or angiography).[31-34] Most reports are poorly documented as to technical accuracy or sensitivity. They constitute best case analyses of jaundiced patients, the majority of whom have pancreatic cancer where clinical evaluation yields upwards of 90% accuracy and little is gained by noninvasive confirmation. Screening tests are of value when performed by an individual or team of established skill. Since screening tests cannot provide the visualization of pathologic features in the bile or pancreatic ducts necessary for differential diagnosis and management, their role as preliminary studies is limited.

Both ultrasound and computerized tomography are not influenced by jaundice. They may replace oral cholecystography[35] or intravenous cholangiography in the jaundiced patient.[36] Ultrasound examination is valuable in identifying neoplasms or space-occupying lesions of the liver, cholelithiasis, or bile duct dilatation. Intra-abdominal gas, abdominal scars, abdominal tenderness, wounds and dressings, or intra-abdominal material (radiopaque contrast material, metal, calcification) impede the examination. Of importance is the problem of false-positive and false-negative observations and the difficulty encountered by the clinician in accepting and acting upon these, as yet unfamiliar diagnostic modalities.

The role of computerized tomography in the evaluation of the biliary tract and pancreas is inadequately defined (see Chapter 29). This technique is of value in imaging an intrahepatic cyst, tumor, or abscess.[34] Unfortunately, the currently expensive equipment is not available in many institutions, and it will take years to perfect interpretative skill and define clinical reliability. We have been disappointed by a high incidence of false-positive and false-negative computerized tomograms of the pancreas. Barium, intra-abdominal metal (vascular clips), residual contrast material after cholecystography, myelography, lymphangiography, and the absence of fat to define tissue planes limit the technique. Computerized tomography may not be considered noninvasive, since intravenous radiographic contrast agents are frequently required for the definition of intrahepatic mass lesions or dilated bile ducts, and the oral administration of contrast agents may be required to differentiate solid from hollow organs.

Unfortunately, there are as yet few studies on the number of examinations that are incomplete or useless as a result of technical defects, equipment failure, or the previously described impediments. The overall diagnostic accuracy of these techniques is probably no better than that of the experienced clinician utilizing history, physical examination, and basic laboratory data. Since these techniques rarely replace the specific anatomic diagnosis provided by direct cholangiography, pancreatography, angiography, or liver biopsy, their intermediate role between clinical judgment and definitive diagnostic procedures remains to be clarified (see Chapter 29).

In particular, it may be difficult to separate dilated bile ducts resulting from intrahepatic metastases from the dilated bile ducts caused by extrahepatic biliary tract obstruction.[34] The specific site of obstruction in the distal bile duct is difficult to determine.[37] The vital differential diagnosis of periampullary lesions including stone, benign stenosis, bile duct cancer, papillary cancer, and pancreatic cancer cannot be accomplished by ultrasound or computerized axial tomography. Dilatation of the pancreatic duct associated with periampullary cancer cannot be differentiated from that produced by carcinoma of the pancreas. Caution must be exercised to avoid the unwarranted assumption that the presence of cholelithiasis indicates stones in the bile duct as the cause of jaundice. The incidence of cholelithiasis in an aging population is sufficiently high to make an association between cholelithiasis and other types of disease producing jaundice common. The overall frequency of gallstone disease in a prospective necropsy study in Malmo was 44% (32% for males and 57% for females).[38] Of even greater interest is that 12% of these patients had stones in the common bile duct. The incidence of common bile duct stones in patients with prior cholecystectomy was 11%. This high incidence of cholelithiasis and choledocholithiasis indicates the level of "background noise" that must be filtered for the differential diagnosis of jaundice in an aging population.

Fiberoptic Esophagogastroduodenoscopy and Endoscopic Retrograde Cholangiopancreatography

Modern fiberoptic gastrointestinal endoscopy can be performed with remarkable ease and speed. No preparation is required, beyond assuring absence of food from the upper gastrointestinal tract. The procedure has a broad diagnostic spectrum, including not only the mass lesions and processes causing distortion of the gastrointestinal tract that are visible with barium contrast radiography but also the superficial inflammatory lesions including esophagitis, hiatus hernia, early esophageal stricture, gastritis, duodenitis, and peptic ulcer.[39] A diagnosis may be confirmed by biopsy, cytologic examination or bile sampling. Pancreatography yields precise definition of pancreatic ductal anatomic conditions and visualizes mass lesions. Mass lesions defined in the pancreatogram may be aspirated percutaneously.

Endoscopic cannulation of the bile duct allows the forceful injection of radiopaque contrast selectively into the cystic duct, gallbladder, and intrahepatic bile ducts. Visualization of the intrahepatic biliary tree allows the definition of infiltrative disease of the liver or cirrhosis and intrahepatic abscess or metastatic tumor.[40]

Endoscopy with ERCP as a Primary Diagnostic Procedure

In a selected series of 91 patients, aged 23 to 70, with a tentative diagnosis of rapidly evolving serious pancreatic or biliary tract disease that might have required prompt abdominal surgery, endoscopic visualization of the entire upper gastrointestinal tract and identification of the papilla of Vater was successful in all but one case.[41] This patient had an active duodenal ulcer with pyloric stenosis. Chronic pancreatitis was confirmed at laparotomy. A positive diagnosis was established in the remaining patients either by endoscopy or cholangiopancreatography in 77 of 91 (85%). Endoscopy yielded the diagnosis in 13 (17%), cholangiography in 39 (51%), and pancreatography in 25 (32%).

In 53 jaundiced patients, the cause was established by endoscopy in 11 and by retrograde radiographic studies in 33 for a success rate of 83% (44 of 53). Complete common duct obstruction demonstrated by subsequent PTC prevented collection of bile or retrograde cholangiography in 2 patients with choledocholithiasis. A normal extrahepatic biliary tree was shown by retrograde cholangiography in 25 of 29 patients (86%) with intrahepatic cholestasis.

The diagnosis of pancreatitis with a precipitating cause (gallstones) or complications (pseudocyst) was established in 27 patients. In 15 patients with acute pancreatitis, alcohol abuse was a factor in 11 and gallstones were present in 4. In 12 patients with chronic pancreatitis, pseudocyst was found in 2.

This integrated procedure narrows the diagnostic field and yet leaves little residua and may be followed immediately by laparotomy, liver biopsy, percutaneous cholangiography, angiography, intravenous pyelography, or evaluation of the colon. If a team is available to perform ERCP on an emergency basis for patients who may require immediate abdominal surgery, it seems reasonable to follow this advantageous route in the evaluation of less seriously ill individuals rather than following proposed algorithms that emphasize noninvasive procedures over invasion, that require numerous intervals for gut cleansing after barium or other radiopaque contrast agents, and that ultimately require a procedure that yields a definitive anatomic diagnosis.[42,43]

Indications for ERCP

After analysis of the procedure records of 1,089 attempts at ERCP, we defined groups of indications. Only one-third of the patient studies were investigated for cholestasis. ERCP immediately displaced intravenous cholangiography. Even with bilirubin levels below 3 mg/dl, intravenous cholangiography fails to visualize the bile duct adequately in 30% to 40% of patients and yields both false-positive and false-negative interpretive errors.[44]

ERCP is unique in visualizing the pancreatic duct in patients with pancretic disease for the diagnosis of neoplasm or inflammatory disease.[45-48]

Patients with gallbladder disease were either evaluated during an acute illness or presented as diagnostic problems where oral cholecystography and/or intravenous cholangiography had failed to visualize the gallbladder. ERCP may document the presence of gallstones, prove cystic duct obstruction, or demonstrate a rigid nondistensible gallbladder. High resolution cholangiography is essential in postcholecystectomy syndromes to rule out the presence of small stones retained in the common bile duct or cystic duct stump.

Overall Diagnostic Value

Diagnostic studies were achieved in 75.2% of 1,089 patients by endoscopic findings in 4.4%, cannulation with opacification of both pancreatic and biliary ducts in 45.4%, or single duct opacification demonstrating a diagnostic pattern in 25.4%.[44]

Diagnostic studies were achieved in 83.5% of 201 consecutive patients studied at St. Vincent's Hospital. Endoscopic findings were positive in 7.5%. Both pancreatic and bile ducts or a single diagnostic duct were visualized in 76%. A single nondiagnostic duct was cannulated in 9.5%. In only 7% of the patients was the papilla of Vater not cannulated.

With experience, the success rates increase and complications decrease.[44] Failure to cannulate a specific duct by an experienced operator indicates unusual anatomic conditions or disease within the duct system. During the 5 years from 1970 to 1975, the Erlangen group under the direction of L. Demling performed 2,507 examinations and increased their success rate from 88.3% to 94.5%. At the same time, the incidence of complications fell from 7.4% in 1970–1973 to 1.3% in 1975.[49]

Complications of ERCP

The anticholinergics originally used to achieve aperistalsis have been replaced by glucagon.[50] Therefore, the endoscopic complications of ERCP are similar in type and magnitude to those of upper gastrointestinal tract endoscopy and are rare.[51]

In the absence of duct obstruction, complications related to the injection of contrast agents were not observed in our series.[44] Limitation of injection of contrast material reduced the incidence of pancreatitis.[52] We have not observed serious complications of pancreatography in patients with pancreatitis or pseudocyst, although lethal complications have been reported.[53] In 235 patients studied for documented pancreatic disease, 8 patients (3.4%) experienced a brief self-limited exacerbation.[44] Early reports documented a 6% incidence of exacerbation or introduction of infection in the obstructed biliary tract after ERCP.[54] This has been reduced to less than 1% by disinfection of the endoscope,[55] prophylactic administration of systemic antibiotics when bile duct obstruction is recognized, and prompt endoscopic, percutaneous, or surgical drainage. Two deaths from sepsis after ERCP occurred when relief of biliary obstruction was not accomplished. The mortality rate for ERCP based on these 2 deaths is 2 out of 1,089 (0.18%).[44]

PERCUTANEOUS TRANSHEPATIC CHOLANGIOGRAPHY

Indications for PTC

PTC is only one of a number of useful percutaneous techniques that may be applied for the diagnosis and management of liver disease. Percutaneous liver biopsy,[2] portography,[56] portal pressure measurement, and bile drainage[13,57,58] should be considered and utilized when appropriate. PTC is used to visualize the biliary tree before abdominal operation or for percutaneous biliary drainage.

Diagnostic Value of PTC

Successful visualization of the bile duct is achieved in 90% of patients with "duct obstruction." The success rate in absence of duct dilatation is 70%.[59] Patients with bile duct obstruction from choledocholithiasis or infiltrating tumors of the porta hepatis may not have dilated intrahepatic bile ducts, and therefore PTC fails.

Technique for PTC

The early techniques utilized an anterior approach and a sheathed needle.[60,61] This has advantages over the currently popular Chiba University technique that uses a 23-gauge needle through a lateral approach.[59] The fine needle is designed to reduce the risk of hepatic puncture. The lateral approach is taken to "tamponade" the puncture with a mass of liver. These presumptions remain to be proven. Laceration of hepatic surface veins occurs with needle movement. The bare needle may dispose to surface lacerations.[62,63] The concept of puncture tamponade is dubious, since complications occur from laceration of structures in the porta hepatis or when the needle exists through the inferior surface of the liver as well as from puncture of ducts on or near the surface.[63,64]

Gram-negative sepsis with shock results from puncture of adjacent bile duct and vein. The pressure in the biliary tree in bile duct obstruction may exceed that of the venous system. The needle tract creates a direct bile-to-blood fistula.[65]

The bare needle technique requires that the needle be withdrawn at the completion of the procedure. Using a sheathed needle after the puncture, the procedure is completed with only the catheter in place. This may reduce the likelihood of capsule laceration. The catheter prevents passage of infected bile into the bloodstream and may remain in place until decompression is accomplished; or by utilizing the Seldinger technique, a larger catheter can be placed for drainage.[13,57,58] The gradual withdrawal of the catheter prevents bile leakage and bleeding when a large vessel has been punctured. The prevention of bile leakage of even a subclinical magnitude is important, as infected bile may contaminate the peritoneal cavity and prejudice the outcome of surgery.

Complication of PTC

Hines et al.[66] reported 102 examinations with a success rate of 78% using a 20- or 21-gauge bare needle. Pain suggesting bile leakage occurred in 7 patients. Six were operated upon, and bile in the peritoneal cavity was observed in 3 of them. Another patient developed frank bile peritonitis. A review of 1,629 procedures reported to that date revealed a success rate of 74% with 4 (0.25%) deaths and 82 (5%) complications. Okuda et al.,[59] using a 23-gauge bare needle (Chiba University), reported 314 cases with a success rate of 85%. In 234 patients with duct obstruction, cholangiography was successful in 91%, but complications such as fever (11 patients), fall in blood pressure (6), bile leakage (3), bile peritonitis (2), and bleeding (2) gave a complication rate of 10% in this group. Similar complications have been reported by Redeker[67] (10%) and Elias[68] (15%) in smaller groups of patients. These complications are not significantly different from those reported by Seldinger[69] in 1966 when he reviewed 1,218 cases with a 2.6% incidence of bile peritonitis. Improvement in diagnostic yield over the years results, at least in part, from improved image intensification fluoroscopy that allows the appreciation of contrast in fine bile ducts. Complications may be limited by following the contraindications proposed by Okuda et al.,[59] including bleeding tendency, sensitivity to iodine and other agents in the contrast medium, high or continuous fever around 38°C, poor general condition, extreme jaundice, ascites, moderate and severe anemia, and recent severe pain. They also advise prophylactic antibiotics for 24 hr before and 72 hr after the procedure.

The therapeutic potential of bare-needle PTC is limited to transient bile aspiration and the injection of antibiotics. Sheathed-needle techniques allow brief preoperative biliary drainage to reduce the incidence of hemorrhage, sepsis from bile-to-blood fistula, and intraperitoneal bile leakage. Nakayama et al. have shown that prolonged preoperative percutaneous bile drainage to reduce serum bilirubin below 5 mg/dl in resectable malignant lesions reduces operative mortality from 28.3% to 8.2% ($p<0.05$).[13] Presumably, similar benefits would accrue to patients with benign disease and cholangitis or jaundice who require abdominal operations.

Prolonged percutaneous drainage in patients with inoperable biliary tract obstruction, combined with radiation therapy or permanent percutaneous stents passed through the obstructing lesion, may be used instead of biliointestinal anastomosis to relieve pruritus and return bile to the digestive tract. The hazard or benefit of percutaneous techniques in patients with unresectable cancer has not been compared to the risks and benefits of bypass operations in these fragile patients. The potential for avoiding laparotomy with its inevitable disability and convalescence in patients with limited life expectancy is appealing.

Comparison of ERCP and PTC

When PTC is performed immediately prior to operation the preceding work-up must be extensive. Endoscopy combined with ERCP completes the diagnostic work-up of the upper gastrointestinal tract and may be performed on hospital admission.[41] The contraindications to PTC as proposed by Okuda[59] have been listed. ERCP has few, if any, contraindications.

The complication of ERCP are proportional to the disease uncovered and are rare in the absence of duct obstruction. Therefore, ERCP is the procedure of choice in patients suspected of having liver disease or who are poor operative risks when obstructive jaundice must be ruled out. Furthermore, the complications of ERCP are obvious, since they are limited to pancreatitis or cholangitis. The complications of PTC are random and may be subclinical in presentation although ultimately of vital importance.[63] Hemorrhage after PTC is unpredictable and requires meticulous follow-up after the procedure.

The anatomic constraints for PTC are few, and the technique is relatively simple. By contrast, ERCP is a complex endoscopic procedure that requires training and experience.

ERCP is therapeutic owing to its ability to force antibiotics into the biliary tree and perform endoscopic papillotomy or sphincterotomy as definitive therapy for choledocholithiasis.[22-24] Preoperative or palliative percutaneous biliary drainage or percutaneous biliary stents are important therapeutic extensions of PTC.[13,57,58]

A comparison of cost is difficult, since the major expense of both techniques is high-quality radiographic equipment and the radiologic team required to produce diagnostic films. Obviously, the needle for PTC is much less expensive than the $6,000 endoscope required for the performance of ERCP. By comparison with the initial expense and ongoing cost of a sophisticated image-intensification radiographic unit and the daily cost of hospitalization, however, these costs are trivial.

ERCP or PTC?

ERCP has a lesser incidence of serious complications and in expert hands a nearly equal incidence of successful biliary opacification, with an additional yield from endoscopy and pancreatography that makes it considerably superior to PTC.[4,44,70] The absence of risk for hemorrhage, bile-to-blood fistula, or intraperitoneal bile leak makes it easy to proceed with additional diagnostic procedures or operation. In addition, endoscopic biliary surgery is the therapeutic procedure of choice for some patients.

Integrated Approach to the Diagnosis of Pancreatic and Biliary Tract Disease

The diagnostic procedures of ERCP and PTC are not mutually exclusive. Before ERCP, it was our practice to perform endoscopy, followed by PTC and then liver biopsy. We now perform ERCP followed by PTC or liver biopsy.[70,71] Therapeutic procedures such as endoscopic sphincterotomy or percutaneous biliary drainage can be undertaken without delay. With this approach the diagnostic and therapeutic advantages of all these procedures are combined.

The techniques described here for visualization of the biliary and pancreatic ducts, either by themselves or when coupled with percutaneous biopsy or cytology, establish the nature, origin, and extent of cholestatic liver disease. Knowledge of the pathologic features in patients with bile duct obstruction permits the clinician to exercise therapeutic options not previously available. Endoscopic techniques for removal of common duct stones or relief of distal biliary stenosis and percutaneous methods for biliary drainage or the placing of stents through obstructions are important alternatives to abdominal operations and, when used preoperatively, reduce the hazard of surgery. An accurate preoperative diagnosis is essential if diagnostic and technical errors during surgery are to be avoided. Progress in the diagnosis and management of cholestasis is predicated on visualization of the biliary and pancreatic ducts.

REFERENCES

1. Schenker S, Balint J, Schiff L: Differential diagnosis of jaundice. Am J Dig Dis 7:449–463, 1962
2. Morris JS, Gallo GA, Scheuer PJ, Path MRC, Sherlock S: Percutaneous liver biopsy in patients with large bile duct obstruction. Gastroenterology 68:750–754, 1975
3. Warren KW, Choe DS, Plaza J, Relihan M: Results of radical resection for periampullary cancer. Ann Surg 181:534–540, 1975
4. Clemett AR: Endoscopic retrograde cholangiography. Edited by RN Berk and AR Clemett: Radiology of the Gallbladder and Bile Ducts. Philadelphia, WB Saunders Co, 1977, pp 255–271
5. Sarles H, Sarles JC, Camatte R, Muratore R, Gaini M, Guien C, Pastor J, LeRoy F: Observations in 205 confirmed cases of acute pancreatitis, recurring pancreatitis and chronic pancreatitis. Gut 6:545–559, 1965
6. Hsu KD, Trehan N, Falkenstein DB, Zimmon DS: Jaundice from pancreatic pseudocyst: Diagnosis by endoscopic retrograde cholangiography. NY State J Med 76:2030–2032, 1976
7. Warshaw AL, Schapiro RH, Ferrucci JT, Galdabini JJ: Persistent obstructive jaundice, cholangitis and biliary cirrhosis due to common duct stenosis in chronic pancreatitis. Gastroenterology 70:562–567, 1976

8. Rohrmann CA, Silvis SE, Vennes JA: Evaluation of the endoscopic pancreatogram. Radiology 113:297–304, 1974

9. Garabedian M, Shamszad M: Pancreatography in the diagnosis of carcinoma of the pancreas. Med Clin North Am 59:239–246, 1975

10. Kasugai T: Recent advances in endoscopic retrograde cholangiopancreatography. Digestion 13:76–99, 1975

11. Beall MS, Dyer GA, Stephenson HE, Jr: Disappointments in the management of patients with malignancy of pancreas, duodenum, and common bile duct. Arch Surg 101:461–465, 1970

12. Crile G, Jr: The advantages of bypass operations over radical pancreatoduodenectomy in the treatment of pancreatic carcinoma. Surg Gynecol Obstet 130:1049–1053, 1970

13. Nakayama T, Ikeda A, Okuda K: Percutaneous transhepatic drainage of the biliary tract. Gastroenterology 74:554–559, 1978

14. Oscarson J, Stormby N, Sundgren R: Selective angiography in fine-needle aspiration cytodiagnosis of gastric and pancreatic tumors. Acta Radiol 12:737–749, 1972

15. Shorey BA: Aspiration biopsy of carcinoma of the pancreas. Gut 16:645–647, 1975

16. Smith EH, Bartrum RJ, Chang YC, D'Orsi CJ, Lokich J, Abbruzzese A, Dantono J: Percutaneous aspiration biopsy of the pancreas under ultrasonic guidance. N Engl J Med 292:825–828, 1975

17. Green N, Mikkelsen WP, Kernen JA: Cancer of the common hepatic bile ducts: Palliative radiotherapy. Radiology 109:687–689, 1973

18. Smoron GL: Radiation therapy of carcinoma of gallbladder and biliary tract. Cancer 40:1422–1424, 1977

19. Hudgins PT, Meoz RT: Radiation therapy for obstructive jaundice secondary to tumor malignancy. Int J Radiat Biol 1:1195–1198, 1976

20. Kopelson G, Harisiadis L, Tretter P: The role of radiation therapy in cancer of the extra-hepatic biliary system: An analysis of thirteen patients and a review of the literature of the effectiveness of surgery, chemotherapy, and radiotherapy. Int J Radiat Biol 2:883–894, 1977

21. Zimmon DS, Falkenstein DB, Kessler RE: Endoscopic papillotomy for choledocholithiasis. N Engl J Med 293:1181–1182, 1975

22. Zimmon DS, Falkenstein DB, Kessler RE: Management of biliary calculi by retrograde endoscopic instrumentation (lithocenosis). Gastrointest Endosc 23:82–86, 1976

23. Koch H, Röch W, Schaffner O, Demling L: Endoscopic papillotomy. Gastroenterology 73:1393–1396, 1977

24. Sàfràny L: Duodenoscopic sphincterotomy and gallstones removal. Gastroenterology 72:338–343, 1977

25. Koch H: Operative endoscopy. Gastrointest Endosc 24:65–68, 1977

26. McSherry CK, Glenn F: Surgical aspects of biliary tract disease. Am J Med 51:651–658, 1971

27. Waye LW, Admirand WH, Dunphy JE: Management of choledocholithiasis. Ann Surg 176:347–359, 1972

28. Mazzariello R: Review of 220 cases of residual biliary tract calculi treated without reoperation: an eight-year study. Surgery 73:299–306, 1973

29. Burhenne HJ: Nonoperative retained biliary tract stone extraction: A new roentgenologic technique. Am J Roentgenol Radium Ther Nucl Med 117:388–399, 1973

30. Bean WJ, Smith SL, Calonje MA: Percutaneous removal of residual biliary tract stones. Radiology 113:1–9, 1974

31. Morin ME, Baker DA, Marsan RE: Demonstration of dilated biliary ducts by total-body opacification. Radiology 121:307–309, 1976

32. Goldstein LI, Sample WF, Kadell BM, Weiner M: Gray-scale ultrasonography and thin-needle cholangiography. JAMA 238:1041–1044, 1977

33. Taylor KJW, Rosenfield AT: Grey-scale ultrasonography in the differential diagnosis of jaundice. Arch Surg 112:820–825, 1977

34. Havrill TR, Haaga JR, Alfidi RJ, Reich NE: Computed tomography and obstructive biliary disease. Am J Roentgenol 128:765–768, 1977

35. Bartrum RJ, Jr, Crow HC, Foote SR: Ultrasonic and radiographic cholecystography. N Engl J Med 296:538–541, 1977

36. Vicary FR, Cusick G, Shirley IM, Blackwell RJ: Ultrasound and jaundice. Gut 18:161–164, 1977

37. Taylor KJW, Rosenfield AT, Dembner AG: Ultrasonography in cholestatic jaundice (letter). N Engl J Med 298:1364–1365, 1978

38. Lindström CG: Frequency of gallstone dis-

ease in a well-defined Swedish population. Scand J Gastro 12:341–347, 1977

39. Schuman BM: The gastroscopic yield from the negative upper gastrointestinal series. Gastrointest Endosc 19:79–80, 1972

40. Falkenstein DB, Riccobono C, Sidhu G, Abrams RM, Seliger G, Zimmon DS: The endoscopic intrahepatic cholangiogram: Clinico-pathological correlation with post-mortem cholangiograms. Invest Radiol 10:358–365, 1975

41. Zimmon DS, Breslaw J, Kessler RE: Endoscopy with endoscopic cholangiopancreatography: The combination as a primary diagnostic procedure. JAMA 233:447–449, 1975

42. Margulis AR: Cholestasis in ulcerative colitis: radiologic evaluation. Gastroenterology 73:362–363, 1977

43. Case records of the Massachusetts General Hospital. N Engl J Med 297:1054–1059, 1977

44. Kessler RE, Falkenstein DB, Clemett AR, Zimmon DS: Indications, clinical value and complications of endoscopic retrograde cholangiopancreatography. Surg Gynecol Obstet 142:865–870, 1976

45. Stadelmann O, Sàfraàny L, Löffler A: Endoscopic retrograde cholangiopancreatography in the diagnosis of pancreatic cancer. Endoscopy 6:84–88, 1974

46. Fukumoto K, Kakajima M, Murakami K, Kawai K: Diagnosis of pancreatic cancer by endoscopic pancreatocholangiography. Am J Gastroenterol 62:210–213, 1974

47. Rohrmann CA, Silvis SE, Vennes JA: The significance of pancreatic ductal obstruction in differential diagnosis of the abnormal endoscopic retrograde pancreatogram. Radiology 121:311–314, 1976

48. Zimmon DS, Falkenstein DB, Abrams RM, Seliger G, Kessler RE: Endoscopic retrograde cholangiopancreatography (ERCP) in the diagnosis of pancreatic inflammatory disease. Radiology 3:287–292, 1974

49. Belohlavek D, Koch H, Rösch W, Schaffner O, Maeder HU, Flory J, Classen M, Demling L: 5 Years experience in endoscopic retrograde cholangiopancreaticography (ERCP). Endoscopy 8:115–118, 1976

50. Zimmon DS, Falkenstein DB, Riccobono C, Aaron B: Complications of endoscopic retrograde cholangiopancreatography: Analysis of 300 consecutive cases. Gastroenterology 69:303–309, 1975

51. Mandelstam P, Sugawa C, Silvis SE, Nebel OT, Rogers BHG: Complications associated with esophagogastroduodenoscopy and with esophageal dilation. Gastrointest Endosc 23:16–19, 1976

52. Ruppin H, Amon R, Ettl W, Classen M, Demling L: Acute pancreatitis after endoscopic/radiological pancreatography. Endoscopy 6:94–98, 1974

53. Ammann RW, Deyhle P, Butikofer E: Fatal necrotizing pancreatitis after peroral cholangiopancreatography. Gastroenterology 64:320–323, 1973

54. Vennes JA, Jacobson JR, Silvis SE: Endoscopic cholangiography for biliary system diagnosis. Ann Intern Med 80:61–64, 1974

55. Elson CO, Hattori K, Blackstone MO: Polymicrobial sepsis following endoscopic retrograde cholangiopancreatography. Gastroenterology 69:507–510, 1975

56. Viamonte JRM, LePage JR, Lunderquist A, Pereiras R, Russel E, Viamonte M, Camacho M: Selective catheterization of the portal vein and its tributaries. Radiology 114:457–460, 1975

57. Tylén U, Hoevels J, Vang J: Percutaneous transhepatic cholangiography with external drainage of obstructive biliary lesions. Surg Gynecol Obstet 144:13–18, 1977

58. Mori K, Misumi A, Sugiyama M, Okabe M, Matsuoka T, Ishii J, Akagi M: Percutaneous transhepatic bile drainage. Ann Surg 185:111–115, 1977

59. Okuda K, Tanikawa K, Emura T, Kuratomi S, Jinnouchi S, Urabe K, Sumikoshi T, Kanda Y, Fukuyama Y, Musha H, Mori H, Shimokawa Y, Yakushiji F, Matsuura Y: Nonsurgical, percutaneous transhepatic cholangiography—diagnostic significance in medical problems of the liver. Am J Dig Dis 19:21–36, 1974

60. Shaldon S, Barber KM, Young WB: Percutaneous transhepatic cholangiography: a modified technic. Gastroenterology 42:371–379, 1962

61. Clemett AR: Percutaneous transhepatic cholangiography. Edited by RN Berk and AR Clemett: Radiology of the Gallbladder and Bile Ducts. Philadelphia, WB Saunders Co, 1977, pp 241–254

62. Juler GL, Conroy RM, Fuelleman RW: Bile leakage following percutaneous transhepatic cholangiography with the Chiba needle. Arch Surg 112:954–958, 1977

63. Mori W, Mukawa K: Wound healing and complications of the liver after percuta-

neous transhepatic cholangiography. Acta Hepatogastroenterol 24:86–92, 1977

64. Gothlin J, Tranberg KG: Complications of percutaneous transhepatic cholangiography (PTC). Am J Roentgenol Radium Ther Nucl Med 117:426–431, 1973

65. Koch RL, Gorder JL: Bile-blood fistula: a complication of percutaneous transhepatic cholangiography. Radiology 93:67–68, 1969

66. Hines C Jr, Ferrante WA, Davis WD Jr, Tutton RA: Percutaneous transhepatic cholangiography experience with 102 procedures. Am J Dig Dis 17:868–874, 1972

67. Redeker AG, Karvountzis GG, Richman RH, Harisawa M: Percutaneous transhepatic cholangiography. JAMA 231:386–387, 1975

68. Elias E, Hamlyn AN, Jain S, Long RG, Summerfield JA, Dick R, Sherlock S: A randomized trial of percutaneous transhepatic cholangiography versus endoscopic retrograde cholangiography for bile visualization in cholestasis. Gastroenterology 71:439–443, 1976

69. Seldinger SI: Percutaneous transhepatic cholangiography. Acta Radiol (Suppl) 253:1–134, 1966

70. Conn HO, Redeker AG, Zimmon DS: PTC versus ERC—an editor's dream. Gastroenterology 71:520–521, 1976

71. Huchzermeyer H, Luska G, Otto P: The value of the combination of antegrade and retrograde cholangiography in the diagnosis of bile duct obstruction. Endoscopy 7:126–133, 1975

Chapter 29

Ultrasonography and Computed Tomography of the Liver

By HSU-CHONG YEH, M.D.

ULTRASONOGRAPHY (gray scale B-scan) and computed tomography (CT) are rapidly growing medical imaging systems that have proven to be very useful for the evaluation of lesions in the liver. They are both noninvasive techniques and are capable of demonstrating true cross-sectional anatomy of the body. Although the physical basis of scanning is quite different, the details of the images they produce are very similar. Many differences exist in the techniques and elements of informations, however, and hence, there are advantages and disadvantages in either modality. The basic differences are as follows:

1. A nonionizing sound wave is used in ultrasonography. No harmful effect has been shown from diagnostic ultrasound imaging; x-ray is used in CT.
2. The ultrasonograph demonstrates the echoes of sound from the tissues. The echoes arise at the interfaces between tissues of different densities and elasticities. The ultrasound beam is sensitive to much smaller density differences than the x-ray beam. From both echo pattern (or sonographic texture) and the attenuation of sound, normal or abnormal tissue may be differentiated. Tissues of the same density may have different types of sonographic textures and may be highly echogenic or poorly echogenic, depending on the homogeneity of the cellular structure of the tissue. CT demonstrates the attenuation value (or density) of the tissue. The attenuation value is an average for the tissue sampled, and values of the normal and pathologic tissues overlap.[1]
3. Ultrasonography is limited by bones (e.g., ribs) and gas-filled bowel loops or stomach because of poor penetration of the sound beam through these structures. CT is not limited by these structures. The bowel gas and respiratory motion may cause multiple streak artifacts, however, obscuring lesions in the liver and decreasing the accuracy in density reading. With newer equipment, scanning can be finished in a much shorter time (6 sec or less) and with suspended breathing, the streak artifacts are decreased.[2]
4. Ultrasonography is more versatile. Different planes of scanning, either longitudinal or oblique, can be easily obtained. However, the diagnostic accuracy of ultrasonography is greatly affected by the quality of the equipment, the skill of operator, and the experience of hhe interpretator. The diagnostic accuracy of CT is also affected by the quality of equipment and

---

From the Department of Radiology, Mount Sinai School of Medicine and the Mount Sinai Hospital, New York, New York.

519

portal vein first appears in the left lobe as a horizontal tubular structure. In the lower section, the left main branch joins the right main branch at the porta hepatis. The right main branch takes an oblique course posterolaterally from the porta hepatis (Fig. 1B and C). The portal vein is located anterior to the caudate lobe. It runs along the right free edge of the lesser omentum with the common bile duct and the hepatic artery.

The hepatic vein can also be seen in both the sonograph and the CT. In the sonograph, the "wall" of the hepatic vein is less echogenic than the "wall" of the portal vein because of lack of surrounding connecting tissue. Their courses are toward the inferior vena cava, i.e., posteriorly and superiorly. Since only transverse scans are done with CT, usually transverse sections of the veins, i.e., a round or oval shape, are seen.

With presently available equipment, intrahepatic bile ducts cannot be seen by sonography. The common bile duct and common hepatic duct may be seen on right paramedial longitudinal B-scans as a small tubular structure anterior to and intersecting the portal vein (Fig. 1A). After intersecting the portal vein, the common bile duct usually dips posteriorly[7] and then passes behind the first part of the duodenum. The bile ducts are usually not seen on CT unless Cholografin is injected intravenously. After the injection of Cholografin, only the main branches of the intrahepatic bile ducts and the extrahepatic bile duct are visualized,[8] and there is only a slight increase in the density of liver parenchyma.[9]

By sonography, the internal echoes of the normal hepatic parenchyma are weak and homogeneously distributed (Fig. 2). By CT, the attenuation value of the liver parenchyma varies, ranging from 40 to 70 Hounsfield units.[10] The density is the same throughout the same liver, however, and the hepatic parenchyma therefore appears homogeneous except for areas of low density in the portal canals and hepatic veins. The density of the liver is usually higher than the densities of spleen, pancreas, and kidneys. After the intravenous injection of contrast material, (e.g., Renografin), the density of hepatic parenchyma increases to 80–90 Hounsfield units.[11]

The size and the thickness of the left lobe is quite variable. When it is wide

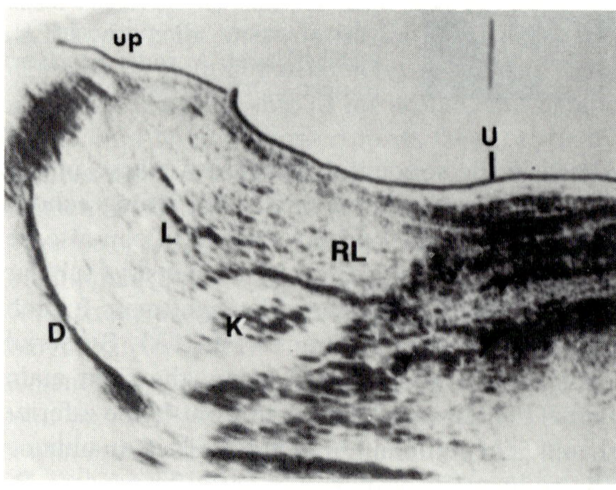

FIG. 2—Normal liver. Right longitudinal B-scan. Note the diffuse homogeneous weak echoes in the liver. RL, Riedel's lobe.

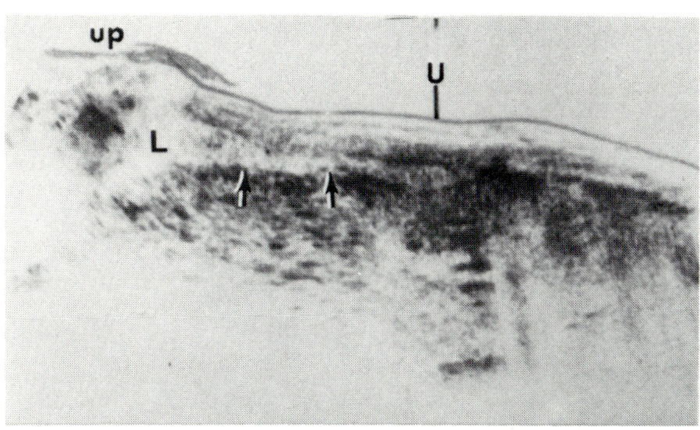

FIG. 3—Normal liver. Left longitudinal B-scan. The wide and thin left lobe (arrows) in this case simulates a large tumor in the radionuclide scan.

and thin (Fig. 3), an area of low uptake or "large filling defect" may be seen on a radionuclide scan simulating a space-occupying lesion. The sonograph and CT, however, will clearly demonstrate the anatomic features. The right lobe is less variable, but an inferior extension of its right lower aspect may be located over and beyond the right kidney (i.e., Riedel's lobe) (Fig. 2). A thin Riedel's lobe may also simulate a space-occupying lesion on a radionuclide scan.[4] Again, the sonograph and CT will clearly demonstrate the anatomic base for the "low uptake" in radionuclide scan.

CHOLESTATIC JAUNDICE

Ultrasonography and CT are useful for the evaluation of patients with the clinical features of cholestatic jaundice. In experienced hands, both modalities have obtained a high degree of diagnostic accuracy (both close to 97%) in differentiating obstructive (or surgical) jaundice from hepatocellular (or medical) jaundice.[8,12] The accuracy is almost 100% by sonography in patients with moderate to severe jaundice.[13] Since variable scanning planes, such as longitudinal and oblique scans, are easy to obtain by sonography, and since the bile ducts stand out as an echo-free tubular structure, the common hepatic and common bile ducts are easier to identify in the sonograph than in the CT. Even normal ducts can often be seen. Therefore, in general, the sonograph is superior to the CT in the evaluation of patients with cholestatic jaundice.

Greatly dilated intrahepatic bile ducts may be seen as stellate tubular structures converging toward the porta hepatis (Fig. 4). Sonographically, they are echo-free structures, similar to branches of portal veins but more numerous and tortuous. The right and left hepatic ducts are usually anterior to the right and left branches of the portal veins but are much smaller. When they are dilated, double parallel channels[14] ("shotgun" sign[15]) may become apparent (Fig. 4B). This may also be observed between the common bile duct and the portal vein. Since they intersect at various angles, however, when a longitudinal section of common bile duct is seen, a transverse or oblique section (i.e., round or oval shape) of the portal vein may be seen behind it. Posterior enhanced echoes are more likely to be seen behind a greatly dilated common bile than behind the portal vein. A pulsed Doppler device may detect blood flow in the portal vein system but not in bile ducts.

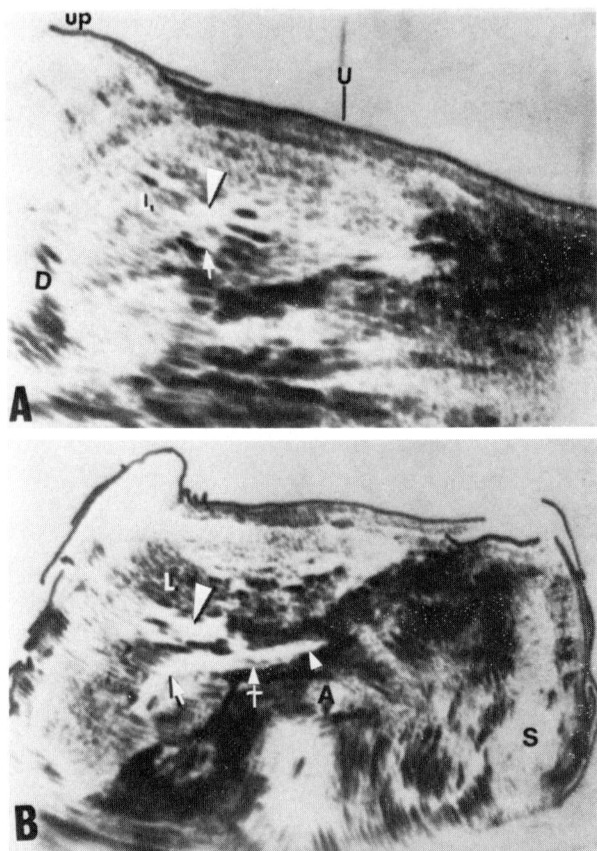

FIG. 4—Obstructive jaundice caused by carcinoma of the pancreas (not shown). (A) Right longitudinal B-scan. Stellate dilated bile ducts (large arrowhead) are seen anterior to the right branch of the portal vein (small arrowhead). (B) Transverse B-scan. The dilated bile ducts are again seen anterior to the portal system. Arrow = right branch of the portal vein; broken arrow = portal vein at the porta hepatis; small arrowhead = splenic vein.

Diffuse coarse flecks of strong echoes are seen in the liver in ascending cholangitis.[4]

By CT, striking dilatation of intrahepatic bile ducts also appears as stellate tubular structures converging toward the porta hepatis (Fig. 5). They are low-density structures similar to portal veins. The density of the bile ducts is that of water, however, and the density of the portal vein branches is that of blood. Because of the relatively small size of these structures, the partial volume effect, and the respiratory motion, the density reading may not be accurate. The density of the portal vein branches may be very low in patients with severe anemia, simulating bile ducts.[8] When in doubt, contrast medium should be injected intravenously. After the injection, the density of the portal vein branches will increase more than that of the hepatic parenchyma. Therefore, the portal vein branches will become less obvious because of a decrease in the density difference between them and the adjacent hepatic parenchyma. The

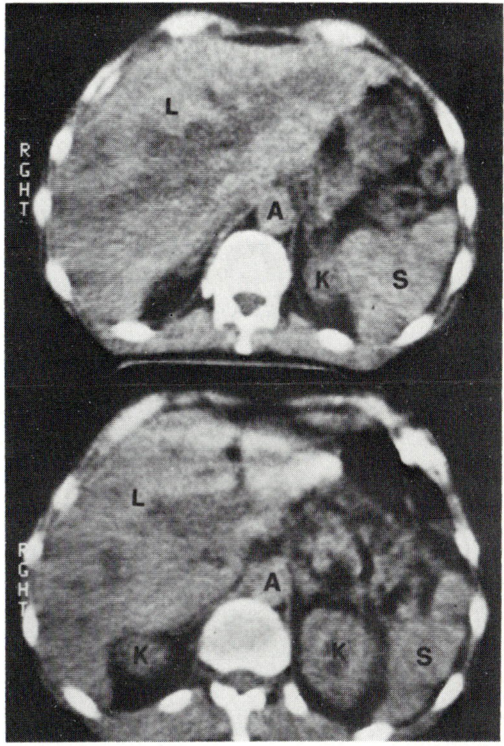

FIG. 5—Obstructive jaundice resulting from carcinoma of the pancreas (not shown). (A) CT shows greatly dilated and tortuous bile ducts (low-density structures) that converge toward the porta hepatis. (B) Slightly lower scan. Some of the dilated bile ducts are round or oval in shape on transverse section. K, kidney.

density of dilated bile ducts will not change, however. Therefore, they appear more lucent with respect to the contrast-medium-enhanced density of the hepatic parenchyma. The cross section of a dilated bile duct or a portal vein branch is round (Figs. 1C, 5B) and of lower density than that of hepatic parenchyma, similar to a small tumor. After the injection of contrast medium, a tumor may increase its density only slightly, and appear more lucent in contrast to the adjacent hepatic parenchyma, similar to a dilated bile duct. If the structure can be followed to the porta hepatis on serial sections, identity of the duct or vein can be better established.

Sclerosing cholangitis may simulate dilated bile ducts on CT. This is probably caused by periductal inflammation and edema. The density is greater than that of water, however.[10]

Finding a dilated gallbladder in a patient with jaundice is supportive evidence of obstructive jaundice, usually resulting from carcinoma. A dilated gallbladder, however, may be caused by obstruction in the gallbladder neck, cystic duct, or common bile duct. Therefore, this is not as specific a sign for the diagnosis of obstructive jaundice as dilated bile ducts. Since the size of the normal gallbladder may be quite variable, when in doubt, a fatty meal should be given. Lack of contraction after a fatty meal adds more evidence for obstruction.

The site of obstruction can be located in 85% of the cases by sonography.[13] The causes of obstruction, such as tumor, stone, or pancreatitis, are also detected by sonography and CT. Simultaneous dilatation of the common bile and pancreatic ducts may be seen in carcinoma of the head of the pancreas or of the ampulla of Vater.[16]

Generally, dilated bile ducts indicate extrahepatic obstruction. When dilated bile ducts are not seen or when a normal common bile duct is visualized in the sonograph, the diagnosis of intrahepatic (or medical) jaundice can be made in a majority of cases. This does not completely exclude a common bile duct stone, however. In patients with intrahepatic tumors, only some of the intrahepatic bile ducts may be dilated.[12]

After an obstruction is relieved, dilatation of the bile ducts may persist for many months. Therefore, the serum bilirubin level is a more sensitive indication of release of obstruction than the sonograph[12] or the CT.

CYSTIC LESIONS

A cyst is best seen in the sonograph because it stands out as an echo-free lesion with a smooth sharp border (Fig. 6). Because of good penetration of the sound through the cyst, there are strong posterior echoes that further enhance the detectability of the lesion. By CT, a cyst is also clearly seen because its low density is that of water. Polycystic disease is thus easily detected with

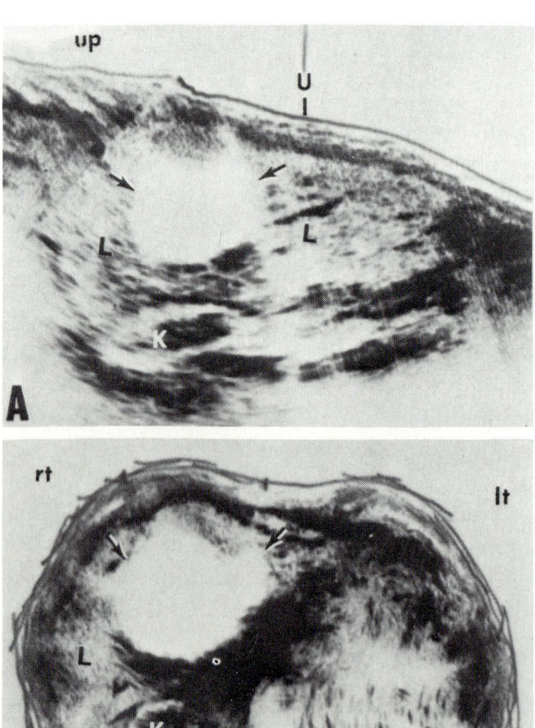

FIG. 6—A cyst in the liver. (A) Right longitudinal B-scan. The cyst (arrows) is completely free of echoes. (B) Transverse B-scan.

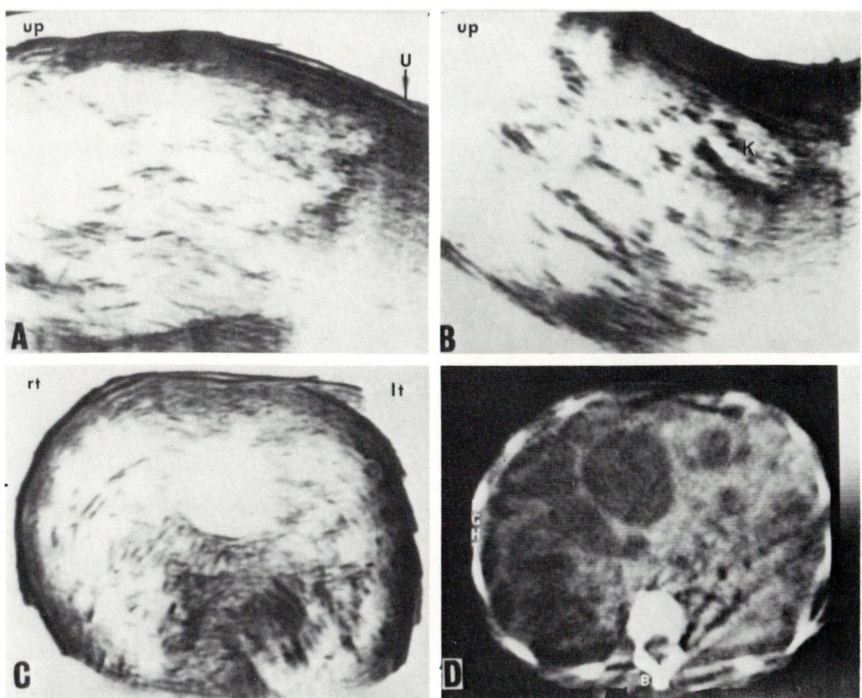

FIG. 7—Polycystic liver without involvement of kidneys. (A) Right longitudinal B-scan. The liver is greatly enlarged and full of cysts. (B) Right posterior longitudinal B-scan. The kidney (K) is normal. Multiple cysts in the liver are seen. (C) Transverse B-scan. (D) CT corresponding to (C). The cysts are of water density.

both modalities (Fig. 7). Since about one-third of patients with polycystic livers also have polycystic kidneys, both liver and kidneys should be included in the examination of such patients. Cysts may also be found in the pancreas in some cases.

When the cysts are very small and numerous, the individual cyst may not be clearly delineated in the sonograph; only the strongly echogenic cyst walls are seen. Therefore, sonography will show a diffuse, strong echo pattern. With CT, the "septa" between the small cyst may not be seen, and the involved area appears homogeneous with low density.

An intrahepatic gallbladder may simulate a cyst,[6] in which case a fatty meal may cause the gallbladder to contract. The diagnosis can be made with both sonography and CT.

Three sonographic features have been observed with echinococcal cysts[17]: (1) similarity to simple cysts; (2) cysts with complex internal structures owing to the organization of the cyst; and (3) cysts within a cystic structure as a result of daughter cysts within the cysts. With CT, two distinct patterns have been observed[18]: (1) *Echinococcus granularis* causes a cystic lesion that contains daughter cysts, and peripheral calcifications may be seen, which is a pathognomonic feature; and (2) *Echinococcus alveolaris* usually grows invasively to become an ill-defined mass that may be indiscernible from a malignant tumor; spotty calcifications may be seen in the lesion.

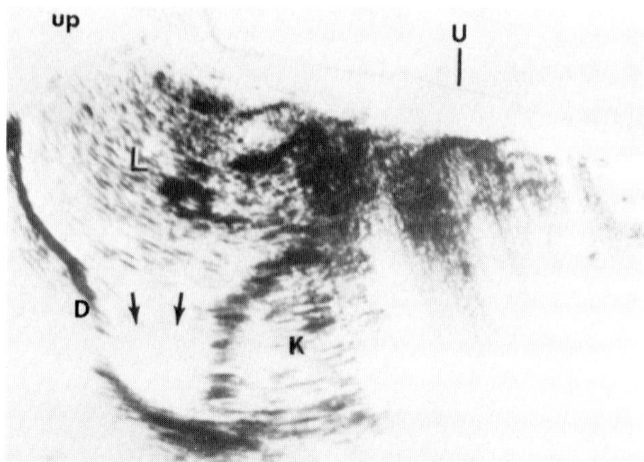

FIG. 8—Liver abscess. Right longitudinal B-scan. The border (arrows) of the abscess is ill defined. The diaphragm is well seen.

Multiple cystic lesions are recognized in Caroli's disease by sonography[4] and CT.[16] These are caused by segmental dilatation of bile ducts.

ABSCESSES

An abscess is similar to a cyst because of its poor echogenecity (in the sonograph) and low density (in CT). Its wall may be more ill defined (Fig. 8) and more irregular than a cyst, however. Some internal echoes may be present because of necrotic tissue debris, in which case, the lesion may simulate a solid mass or a necrotic tumor in the sonograph. The density of an abscess is usually higher than that of water but lower than that of soft tissue and about the same as a necrotic tumor.[8] The differential diagnosis may require clinical correlation. A higher density abscess may simulate a lower density tumor in CT.[8] Although a chronic abscess may have a thickened wall,[4] a greatly thickened "wall" is more likely to be a necrotic tumor than an abscess (Fig. 9). When the abscess is healing, the decrease in size may appear more pronounced by sonography than by radionuclide scanning. This may be due to the persistence of a devitalized area surrounding the abscess; after collapse of an abscess, the devitalized area is revealed on a radionuclide scan as a defect.[6]

A liver abscess located beneath the diaphragm may simulate a subdiaphragmatic abscess, since the capsule of liver is difficult to identify. Empyema indenting on the dome of liver may simulate a liver abscess on CT.[10] In the sonograph, however, a longitudinal scan will clearly show the diaphragm as an intensely echogenic band, and differentiation between empyema and a subphrenic or hepatic abscess can be made.[19] A subhepatic abscess appears as an echo-free lesion between the liver and the right kidney (i.e., Morison's pouch) or beneath the liver anteriorly on right paramedial longitudinal B-scanning.

HEMATOMA

A hematoma may be subcapsular or central. The subcapsular hematoma is usually lenticular in shape or lies mantlelike over the liver substance (Fig. 10).

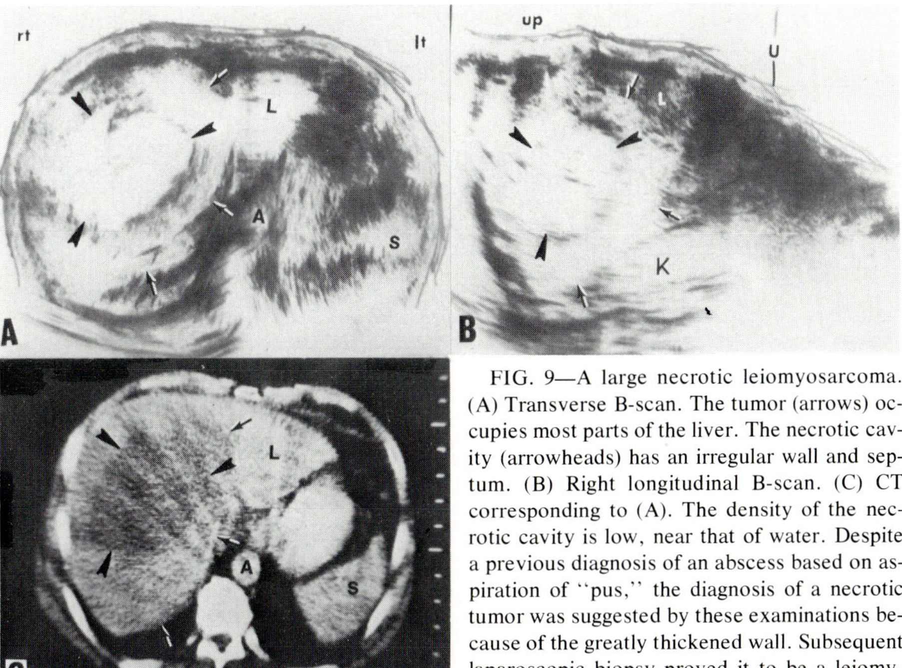

FIG. 9—A large necrotic leiomyosarcoma. (A) Transverse B-scan. The tumor (arrows) occupies most parts of the liver. The necrotic cavity (arrowheads) has an irregular wall and septum. (B) Right longitudinal B-scan. (C) CT corresponding to (A). The density of the necrotic cavity is low, near that of water. Despite a previous diagnosis of an abscess based on aspiration of "pus," the diagnosis of a necrotic tumor was suggested by these examinations because of the greatly thickened wall. Subsequent laparoscopic biopsy proved it to be a leiomyosarcoma.

It may simulate a subphrenic abscess. Both subcapsular hematoma and subphrenic abscess may extend along the superior and lateral surfaces of the liver. The subcapsular hematoma, however, may extend down to the free edge of the liver. A central hematoma is variable in shape. On sonograph, hematomas are usually free of echoes. When the blood is clotted, however, internal echoes may be seen. On CT, a recent hematoma is almost equally as dense as the hepatic parenchyma; therefore, it may not be obvious (Fig. 10C). After the injection of contrast medium, the density of the hematoma does not change. Therefore, it becomes more apparent against the contrast-medium-enhanced hepatic parenchyma as a lucent lesion. When a hematoma is older than 3 to 6 weeks, the density decreases to become only slightly greater than that of water (seroma).[8] Therefore, it is readily detectable on CT without injection of contrast medium. An organized subcapsular hematoma may have a thick wall.[8]

TUMORS

Both ultrasonography and CT are highly accurate for detecting masses in the liver, 90% accuracy being achieved with ultrasonography.[4] The accuracy of the radionuclide scan ranges from 72% to 90%,[20] and the accuracy of CT is similar.[9] The findings of sonography and CT are more specific than those of radionuclide scanning, however. The sonograph and CT are capable of differentiating a solid mass from a cyst. By contrast, a filling "defect" in radionuclide scan may represent a solid mass, a cyst, or not uncommonly, simply a normal anatomic variation such as the porta hepatis, the gallbladder fossa, a

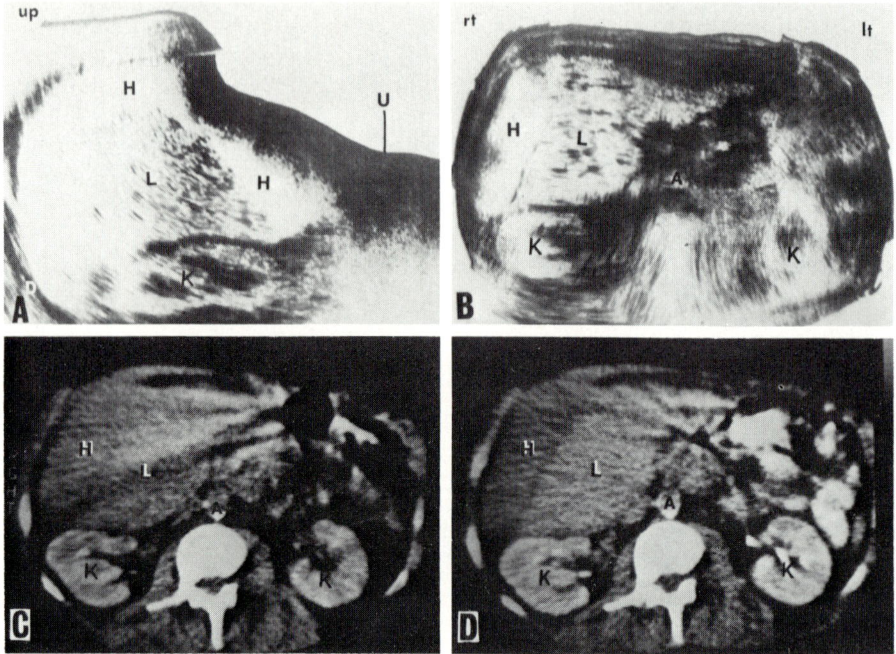

FIG. 10—Subcapsular hematoma after needle biopsy. (A) Right longitudinal B-scan. The hematoma (H) is anterior to the hepatic parenchyma. (B) Transverse B-scan. The hematoma extends laterally. (C) CT corresponding to (B). This recent hematoma is not well seen without injection of contrast medium. (D) After injection, the hematoma appears lucent compared to the contrast enhanced parenchyma. (10A and 10B from Yeh H-C, Wolf BS: Ultrasonograph in ascites. Radiology 124:783–790, 1977 with permission from Radiology.)

wide but thin left lobe of the liver (Fig. 3), or a thin Riedel's lobe. Therefore, although the radionuclide scan is highly sensitive for space-occupying lesions of the liver, it is not very specific and has a high false-positive rate (17% as compared to 8% with sonography[20]). The radionuclide scan is a good screening test, but when a filling detect is found, sonography or CT should be done for confirmation as well as for further characterization of the lesion.

There are several sonographic patterns of tumors of the liver[21,22]: (1) a relatively echogenic mass (Fig. 11A); (2) a relatively echo-free mass (Fig. 11B); (3) a bull's eye or targetlike lesion in which the central echoes are increased while the peripheral ones are diminished; (4) a mass with an echo-free center that may be caused by a necrotic cavity (Fig. 9); (5) a large mass difficult to characterize (Fig. 12); (6) a mixture or combination of the above patterns (Fig. 12); (7) a completely echo-free mass, which is a rare occurrence but may be seen in the metastatic lesions of a solid tumor, such as a leiomyosarcoma or lymphoma, or a cystic tumor, such as a cystadenocarcinoma of the ovary or pancreas; (8) diffuse alteration or inhomogeneity of the internal echo pattern of the liver as a result of diffuse involvement by small or irregular masses.

During his initial experience with gray scale sonography, Taylor reported that tumors of the liver show a diminished echo pattern and that highly echogenic masses occur only after treatment.[23] Although Taylor still assumes that a highly echogenic tumor in an untreated patient is rare,[4] others have found

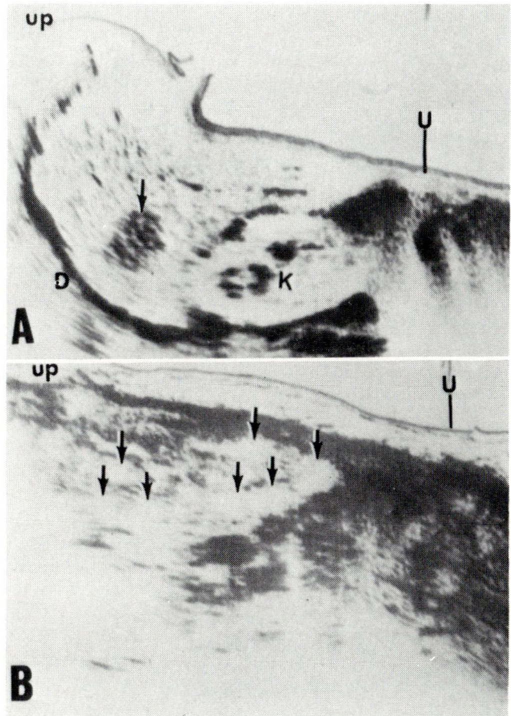

FIG. 11—Metastatic prostate cancer, (A) Right longitudinal B-scan. The tumor (arrow) is highly echogenic. The patient had no treatment before the examination. (B) Right paramedial longitudinal B-scan in another patient. Multiple, poorly echogenic masses (arrows) are seen. The patient had chemotherapy, but the poor echogenecity is not necessarily caused by it.

that more than half of their patients with highly echogenic tumors had no treatment.[21,22] In the author's experience, in fact, not only were many of the highly echogenic tumors seen in untreated patients, but some highly echogenic tumors disappeared or became poorly echogenic lesions shortly after chemotherapy (Fig. 12). Diminished echoes in a tumor may be caused by a relatively homogenous cellular structure, edema, hemorrhage, or necrosis. The possible factors causing increased echoes in a tumor are (1) hypervascularity, since the hypervascular tumors have higher incidence (75%) of high echogenecity; (2) a glandular structure, especially a mucinous adenocarcinoma of colon;[4,21] (3) collagenous or fibrous tissue; and (4) breakdown or fragmentation of necrotic tissue. When necrotic tissue becomes almost or completely liquified, however, an echo-free lesion appears.

A definite association between the sonographic patterns and the histologic types of the tumors has not been found. Any of the sonographic patterns may occur in many different kinds of tumors. On the other hand, one kind of tumor may show different types of sonographic patterns in different patients (Fig. 11) or even in the same patient (Fig. 12). No convincing association between the vascularity of a tumor seen on angiogram and the sonographic pattern has been described. Although many (more than 75% of the cases in one series[22]) of the hypervascular tumors are highly echogenic, poorly echogenic patterns also occur. Even hemangiomas are highly variable, in the author's experience, ranging from highly echogenic to very poorly echogenic, as well as combinations of these. In one series,[21] the majority (20 of 24 cases) of the metastatic lesions from colon carcinoma were large highly echogenic masses. Lymphomas tend

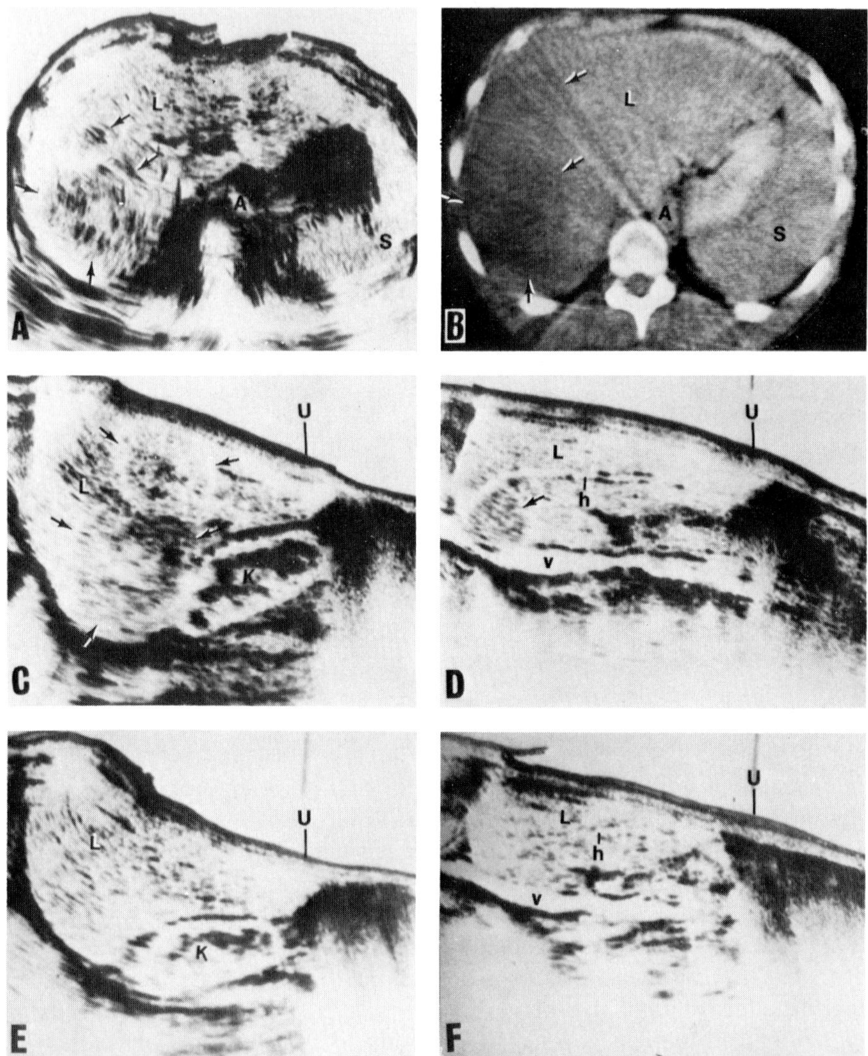

FIG. 12—Metastases from an embryonal cell carcinoma of testis. (A) Transverse B-scan. The tumors (arrows) are seen in the right lobe of the liver. (B) CT scan corresponding to (A). The tumors are of low density. (C) Right longitudinal B-scan. The echo pattern of the tumors (arrows) is difficult to characterize but appears to be surrounded by a thin "halo." (D) Right paramedial longitudinal B-scan. A well-defined highly echogenic mass (arrow) is in the superior aspect of the caudate lobe, indenting the inferior vena cava. (E) Four and one-half months after chemotherapy, the liver is much smaller, and only small, poorly echogenic lesions are vaguely seen. (F) On right paramedial longitudinal B-scan, the tumor is no longer seen.

to be poorly echogenic[4,21] or almost echo-free because of a homogeneous cellular structure. When a homogeneous tumor is totally free of echoes, it may simulate a cyst;[6] in this case, CT scan shows the lesion to be of tumor density, and the diagnosis of a homogeneous tumor rather than a cyst can be made.[3] Primary hepatic carcinoma is more commonly a solitary, well-defined, poorly echogenic mass (Fig. 13), but it may also be multiple masses or show a diffuse

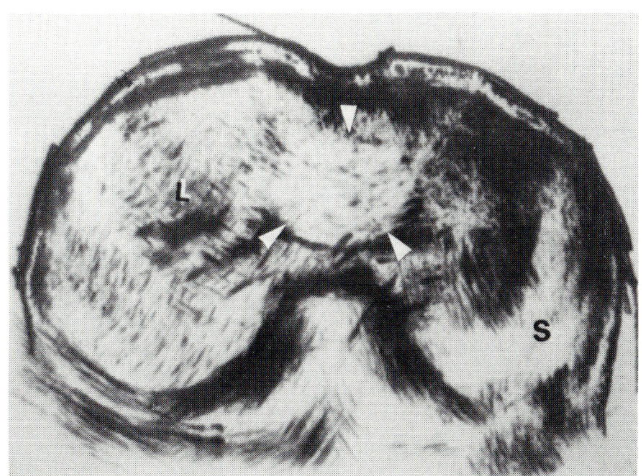

FIG. 13—Primary hepatic carcinoma. Transverse B-scan. A poorly echogenic solitary mass (arrowhead) is seen.

alteration of the echo pattern in the liver. The benign adenoma is rare and may occur after use of oral contraceptives; in one reported case,[4] it was highly echogenic.

The relative incidence of these echo patterns varies from series to series. The more common ones are a poorly echogenic type,[4] a highly echogenic type,[20] and diffuse alteration of the echopattern.[21]

With CT, most tumors of the liver are relatively lucent, usually 10–20 Hounsfield units less than the adjacent hepatic parenchyma.[24] Only occasionally is the tumor denser than the parenchyma. The difference in densities between the tumor and the parenchyma is frequently so small that the tumor may be easily overlooked. A narrow window setting may bring out more contrast to make it more easily recognizable. Intravenous injection of contrast medium usually further increases the visibility of the tumor, since after injection, the density of the hepatic parenchyma is increased more than that of the tumor, so that the latter appears lucent. Sometimes, the tumor can be seen only after contrast injection. Therefore, scanning without contrast injection may not exclude a tumor in the liver.

Injection of contrast medium considerably increases the density of some vascular tumor so that it becomes as dense as the hepatic parenchyma and, hence, becomes less visible than before injection. This is similar to the effect on the portal vein after contrast injection. Therefore, a small tumor of this kind may be difficult to differentiate from a branch of the portal vein.[8] Some of the highly vascular parts of a cavernous hemangioma become denser than hepatic parenchyma after contrast infusion.[16] Other hemangiomas may not be visible (isodense) before contrast injection, they become visible as a large relatively lucent lesion after injection.[25] Calcifications may be seen in metastasis to the liver, most commonly from cancer of the colon.[26] Other tumors that may also show calcifications are carcinoids, pseudomucinous cystadenomas of the ovary, adenocarcinomas of the stomach, and islet cell tumors of the pancreas. The calcification is best seen with CT, which clearly visualizes calcifications not visible in a conventional radiograph.[8] By sonography, calcifications may cause acoustic shadows.[26]

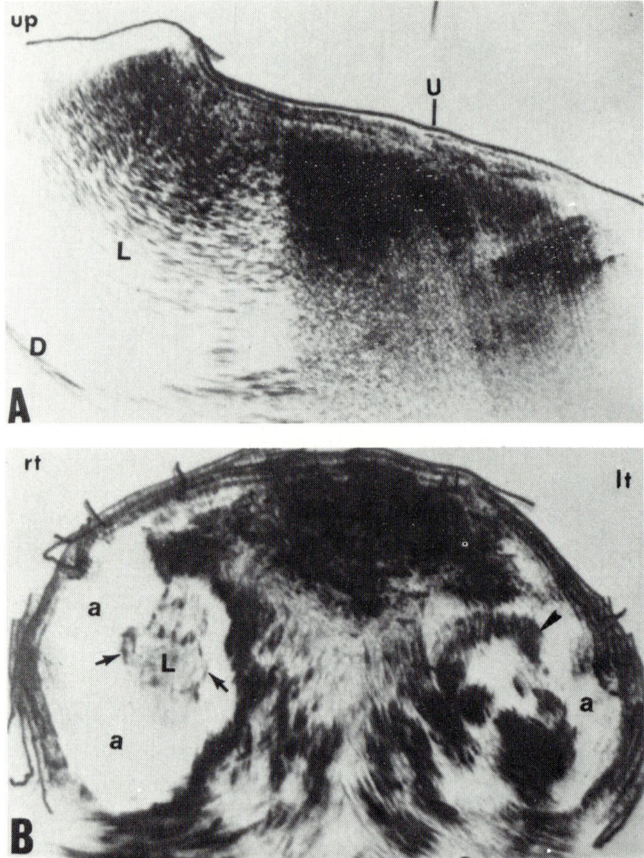

FIG. 14—Cirrhosis of liver. (A) Right longitudinal B-scan. Echoes in the liver are diffusely increased, and sound penetration is poor. (B) Transverse B-scan in another patient; the liver is small and nodular (arrows). Much ascites (a) surrounds the liver and bowel loops (arrowhead).

A tumor or cyst of 1 cm in size may be seen with CT, but it may be difficult to differentiate from a large portal triad.[16] Diffusely infiltrative metastases may not be detected on CT. The histologic type or origin of the tumor cannot be determined on CT.[16]

NEEDLE ASPIRATION OR BIOPSY OF FOCAL LESIONS

Since both sonography and CT are capable of demonstrating the true cross-sectional anatomic features of the abdomen, a lesion can be localized accurately in three dimensions. It is therefore, possible with sonography or CT to guide the needle so that it enters at an optimal spot on the skin to reach the lesion. An aspiration-biopsy transducer may be used with sonography. Both aspiration of abscesses and biopsy of tumors have been done with sonography and CT, and CT-guided percutaneous transhepatic cholangiography has also been successful,[9] although it is quite cumbersome and time-consuming.

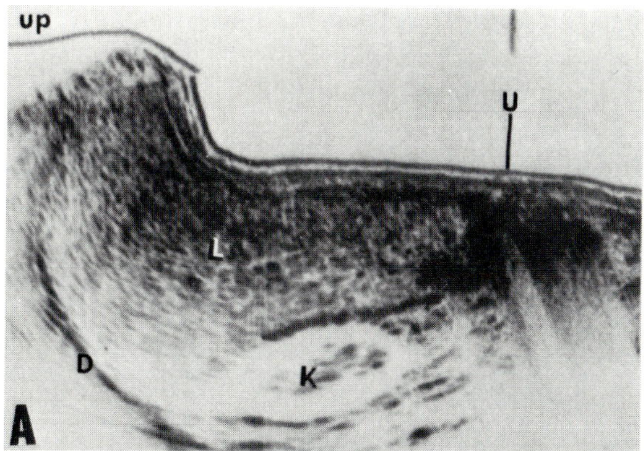

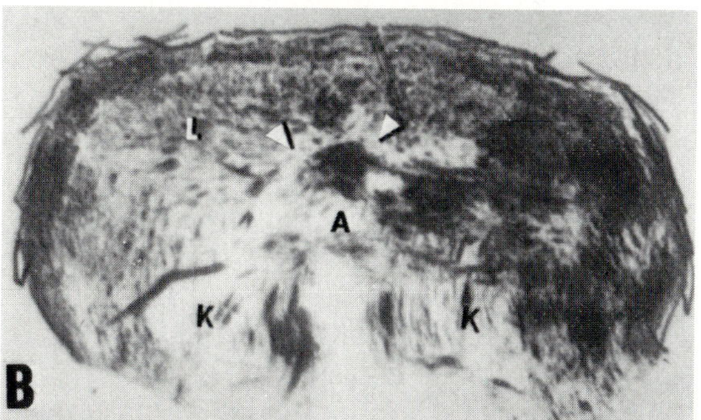

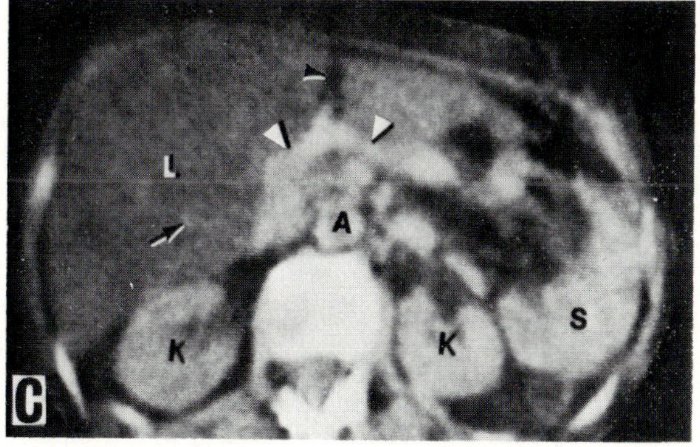

FIG. 15—Fatty liver. (A) Right longitudinal B-scan. The liver is enlarged, and echoes are diffusely increased. The penetration of sound is not decreased. (B) Transverse B-scan. The liver is much more echogenic than the pancreas (white arrowheads), which is the reverse of normal. (C) CT scan corresponding to (B). The liver has a much lower density than the pancreas. The small vessels (arrow) are more clearly seen than is usually the case. Black arrowhead indicates fat in the region of the falciform ligament.

DIFFUSE PARENCHYMAL DISEASES

Neither ultrasonography nor CT relies on hepatic function to obtain an image, nor do they reflect the status of hepatic function. Therefore, generally speaking, they are not sensitive to the changes resulting from diffuse hepatocellular diseases. Radionuclide scanning with ^{99m}Tc sulfur colloid, however, may detect such disease when the phagocytic activity of Kupffer cells is altered before gross changes in the parenchyma have occurred. When radionuclide scans show multiple filling defects suggestive of either multiple metastases to a cirrhotic liver or nodular regeneration from cirrhosis, a negative sonograph or CT may indicate that the filling defects in the radionuclide scan are caused by nodular regeneration.[4,8]

Early cirrhosis is not detectable by sonography or CT. The sonograph in more advanced cirrhosis shows increased internal echoes. The penetration of the ultrasound is decreased, and therefore the echoes decrease in the deeper portions of liver (Fig. 14A). By CT, the density of the cirrhotic liver is the same as that in the normal liver. CT may show a small liver or a liver with a nodular contour in advanced cirrhosis. The regenerated nodules have the same echo pattern or density as the adjacent hepatic parenchyma. Ascites can be easily recognized by sonography and CT.

The echoes in the liver in hepatitis and in fatty liver are diffusely increased, similar to those in cirrhosis. The penetration of the ultrasound is little affected, however. A diffuse increase in echoes has also been observed in sarcoidosis.[4] Hunter's syndrome (or gargoylism) shows multiple, highly echogenic streaks or flecks of echoes scattered in the liver in addition to diffusely increased echoes[4] that are somewhat similar to those found in ascending cholangitis.

CT features are characteristic for the well-developed fatty liver and for hemochromatosis. In the fatty liver, the density of the hepatic parenchyma is decreased and, in severe instances, may become less than that of water. The vessels stand out in contrast to the lucent parenchyma and become easier to recognize (Fig. 15). In hemochromatoses, the density of the parenchyma increases, in contrast to that in the fatty liver.

REFERENCES

1. Holm HH, Smith EH, Bartrum RJ: The relationship of computed tomography and ultrasonography in diagnosis of abdominal disease. J Clin Ultrasound 5:230–237, 1977
2. Harell GS, Marshall WH, Braiman RS, Seppi EJ: Early experience with the Varian six second body scanner in the diagnosis of hepatobiliary tract disease. Radiology 123:355–360, 1977
3. Yeh HC, Wolf BS: Ultrasonography and computerized tomography in the diagnosis of homogeneous masses. Radiology 123:425–428, 1977
4. Taylor KJW: Atlas of Gray Scale Ultrasonography. New York, Churchill Livingstone, 1978, pp 22–97
5. Michels NA: Newer anatomy of the liver and its variant blood supply and collateral circulation. Am J Surg 112:337–347, 1966
6. Leopold GR, Asher WM: Fundamentals of Abdominal and Pelvic Ultrasonography. Philadelphia, WB Saunders, 1975, pp 15–48
7. Lee TG, Henderson SC, Erlich R: Ultrasound diagnosis of common bile duct dilatation. Radiology 124:793–797, 1977
8. Bryan PJ, Dinn WM, Grossman ZD et al: Correlation of CT, gray scale ultrasonography and radionuclide imaging of the liver in detecting space-occupying processes. Radiology 124:387–393, 1977
9. Alfidi RJ, Haaga JR, Havrilla TR, Pepe RG, Cook SA: Computed tomography of the liver. Am J Roentgenol 127:69–74, 1976
10. Levitt RG, Sagel SS, Stanley RJ, Jost RG: Accuracy of computed tomography of the liver and biliary tract. Radiology 124:123–128, 1977
11. Havrilla TR, Haaga JR, Alfidi RJ, Reich NE: Computed tomography and obstructive biliary diseases. Am J Roentgenol 128:765–768, 1977
12. Taylor KJW, Rosenfield AT: Gray scale ultrasound in the differential diagnosis of jaundice. Arch Surg 112:820–825, 1977
13. Malini S, Sabel J: Ultrasonography in obstructive jaundice. Radiology 123:429–433, 1977
14. Conrad MR, Landy MJ, Jefferson OJ: Sonographic "parallel channel" sign of biliary tree enlargement in mild to moderate obstructive jaundice. Am J Roentgenol 130:279–286, 1978
15. Weill F, Eisencher A, Zeltner F: Ultrasonic study of the normal and dilated biliary tree

the "shotgun" sign. Radiology 127:221–224, 1978

16. Stephens DH, Sheedy PF, Hattery RR, MacCarty RL: Computed tomography of the liver. Am J Roentgenol 128:579–590, 1977

17. King DL: Ultrasonography of echinococcal cyst. J Clin Ultrasound 1:64–67, 1973

18. Scherer U: Diagnostic accuracy of CT in echinococcosis of the liver. Presented at the International Symposium and Course on Computed Tomography, Miami Beach, Florida, March 19-24, 1978

19. Landay M, Harless W: Ultrasonic differentiation of right pleural effusion from subphrenic fluid on longitudinal scans of the right upper guadrant: Importance of recognizing the diaphragm. Radiology 123:155–158, 1977

20. Taylor KJW, Sullivan D, Rosenfield AT, Gottschalk A: Gray scale ultrasound and isotope scanning: Complementary techniques for imaging the liver. Am J Roentgenol 128:277–281, 1977

21. Scheible W, Gosink BB, Leopold GR: Gray scale echographic patterns of hepatic metastatic disease. Am J Roentgenol 129:983–987

22. Green B, Bree RL, Goldstein HM, Stanley C: Gray scale ultrasonographic evaluation of hepatic neoplasms: Patterns and correlations. Radiology 124:203–208, 1977

23. Taylor KJW: Tumor of liver (letter). J Clin Ultrasound 2:74–76, 1974

24. Stanley RJ, Sagel SS: Computed tomography of the liver and biliary tract. Edited by RN Berk and AR Clemett: Radiology of the Gallbladder and Bile Ducts. Philadelphia, WB Saunders, 1977, pp 352–375

25. MacCarty RL, Wolner HW, Stephen DH, Sheedy PF, Hattery RR: Retrospective comparison of radionuclide scan and CT of the liver and pancreas. Am J Roentgenol 129:23–28, 1977

26. Katragadda CS, Goldstein HM, Green B: Gray scale ultrasonography of calcified liver metastases. Am J Roentgenol 129:591–593, 1977

Chapter 30

Vitamin D in Chronic Liver Disease

By RICHARD G. LONG, M.D., M.R.C.P., *and*
DAME SHEILA SHERLOCK, M.D., F.R.C.P.

BONE DISEASE, resulting in fractures and bone pains, has been recognized as a complication of chronic liver disease for many years. Bright described steatorrhea as a complication of obstructive jaundice in 1836.[1] Seidel, in 1910, reported a woman who developed kyphosis after having a biliary fistula for 3 years; an autopsy showed multiple long bone fractures.[2] Both osteomalacia and osteoporosis are well documented in patients with chronic liver disease. Hyperparathyroidism is not evident but periosteal new bone formation has been observed in a wide spectrum of patients with chronic liver disease.

Osteomalacia is usually caused primarily by deficiency of vitamin D with a secondary lack of calcium and phosphate. It results in bone pains and fractures; the classical radiologic lesion is the Looser's zone or pseudofracture (Fig. 1).

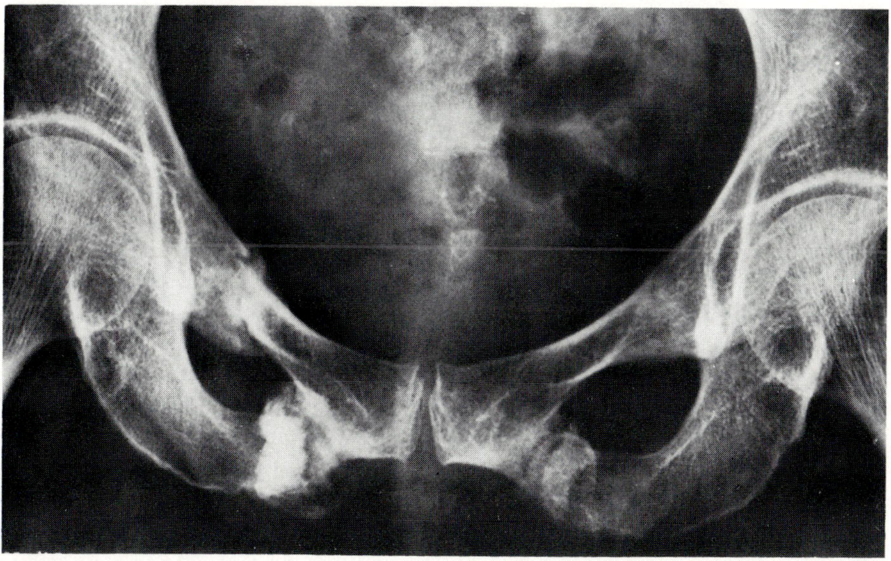

FIG. 1—Healing Looser's zones in the right inferior and superior pubic rami in a patient with chronic active hepatitis with cirrhosis. This radiograph was taken after treatment with 1,25-dihydroxycholecalciferol and calcium supplements. Bone biopsy before treatment confirmed osteomalacia.

From the Department of Medicine, Hammersmith Hospital and Royal Postgraduate Medical School, and the Department of Medicine, Royal Free Hospital School of Medicine, London, England.

Looser's zones are absent in many cases, however, and the diagnosis depends on showing increased osteoid tissue in histologic sections of bone, preferably along with a defect in the calcification front. Histologic osteomalacia is most common in long-standing cholestatic jaundice, particularly in primary biliary cirrhosis (PBC), and is well described.[3-6] It also occurs in chronic nonalcoholic and alcoholic liver disease.[3,6,7] The osteomalacia has been related to many factors, including vitamin D malabsorption, poor nutrition, and failure of synthesis of vitamin D_3 in the skin.

Osteoporosis is related to increasing age, gonadal hormone deficiency, immobilization, and chronic alcoholism. The role of calcium and vitamin D in its pathogenesis is controversial. Osteoporosis results in bone pain and fractures, particularly of the vertebral column. Multiple vertebral fractures (Fig. 2) in the absence of Looser's zones suggest the diagnosis of osteoporosis. The major histologic changes are a thin bone cortex and greatly reduced underlying trabecular bone. Histologic osteoporosis occurs in chronic biliary disease, especially when steroids have been given, and in alcoholic liver disease.[3,6] On rare occasions, we have also seen it in patients with cirrhosis resulting from chronic active hepatitis who have received long-term corticosteroid treatment. The exact cause of osteoporosis in patients with chronic liver disease remains obscure.

Many advances have been made recently in the biochemistry and physiology of vitamin D metabolism.[8-10] Abnormalities of vitamin D metabolism have been well recognized in patients with nutritional, renal, and anticonvulsant osteomalacia, but such abnormalities had been poorly documented in patients with chronic liver disease. It now appears that patients with chronic liver disease are commonly deficient in vitamin D. This deficiency presumably plays a role in the development of osteomalacia, and the observed histologic osteomalacia can be corrected by appropriate supplements.[5,11]

NORMAL BIOCHEMISTRY

Vitamin D metabolism is summarized in Fig. 3. There are two main forms of vitamin D, vitamin D_3 (cholecalciferol) and vitamin D_2 (ergocalciferol, calciferol). The molecular difference is small: the modified steroid nucleus is the same, but an additional methyl group and double bond are on the side chain of vitamin D_2 (Fig. 4). The metabolism of the two metabolites is thought to be identical, but in normal man the majority of circulating vitamin D is in the D_3 form, at least as reported in St. Louis and London.[12,13] Vitamin D_3 is synthesized in the skin from the action of ultraviolet light (wavelength, 280 nm) on 7-dehydrocholesterol. Vitamin D_2 is absorbed from the diet. In some countries, vitamin D_2 supplements have been put into foods such as margarine to prevent the development of dietary osteomalacia in susceptible people.

Both vitamin D_3 and D_2 are transported to the liver on a specific binding alpha-globulin, vitamin D binding protein, which is synthesized in the hepatocytes. Vitamin D 25-hydroxylation in man is thought to occur entirely in the liver, although in chicks 25-hydroxylase activity has been found in the intestine and the kidney.[14,15] In the rat, the vitamin D 25-hydroxylase enzyme has been

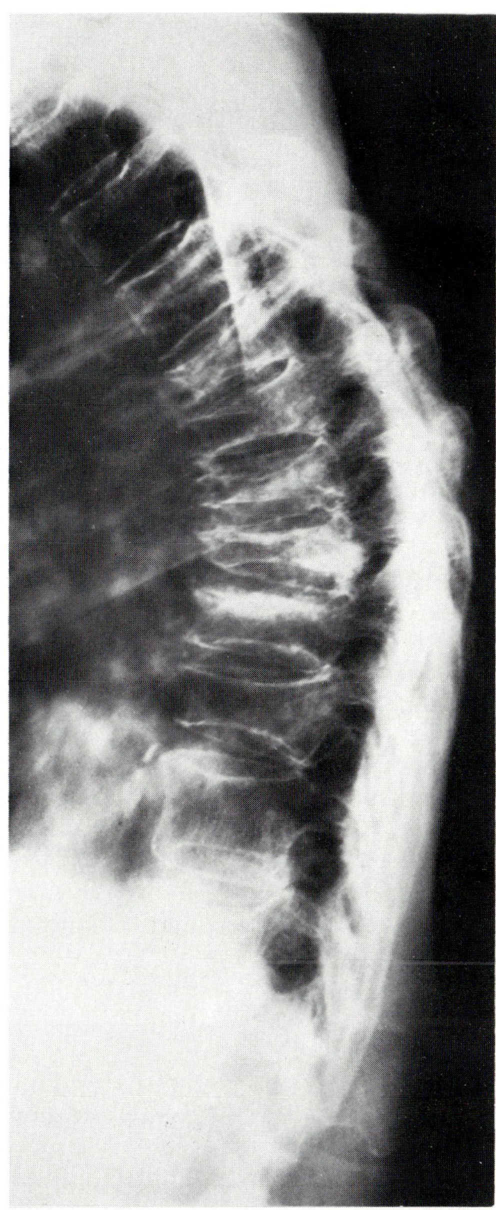

FIG. 2—Radiograph of a kyphotic spine with generalized loss of bone density and multiple vertebral collapse in a patient with PBC who had received long-term steroid therapy. Bone biopsy confirmed osteoporosis.

localized to the hepatocytic microsomal fraction.[16] The main circulating vitamin D metabolite in plasma is 25-hydroxyvitamin D [25-(OH)D].

Vitamin-D-binding globulin, the hepatocyte-synthesized protein, then transports 25-(OH)D to the kidney. Much of the 25-(OH)D in vitamin-D deficient persons is converted by a 1α-hydroxylase enzyme in the renal mitochondria to the most biologically active metabolite known, 1α,25-hydroxyvitamin D [1,25-(OH)$_2$D].[17] By contrast, in vitamin-D-replete persons, most of the 25-

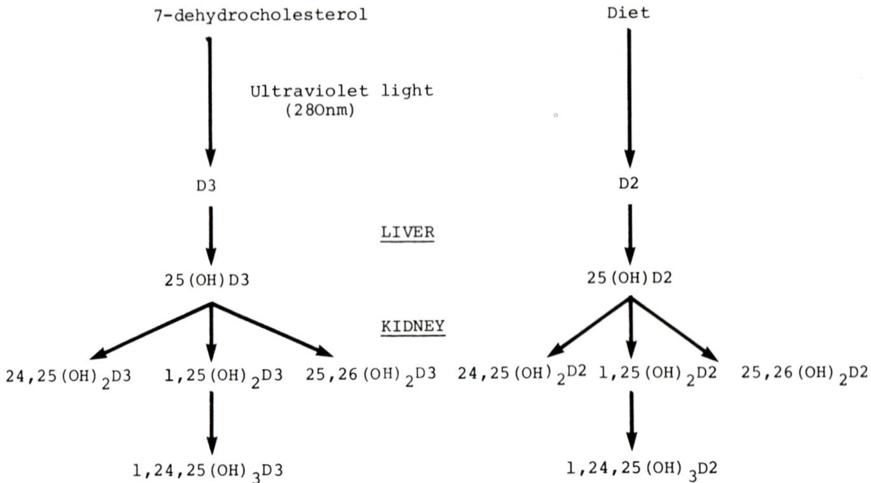

FIG. 3—Normal vitamin D metabolic pathway. Vitamin D_3 is formed in the skin. The 25-hydroxylation step of both vitamin D_2 and D_3 occurs in the liver; the addition of a second hydroxy step occurs predominantly in the kidney.

(OH)D is converted to 24,25-(OH)$_2$D and 25,26-(OH)$_2$D. The formation and role of 1,24,25-(OH)$_3$D are poorly understood. A small amount of 1-(OH)D may also be found and then metabolized in the liver to 1,25-(OH)$_2$D. Following injection of radiolabeled vitamin D, 25-(OH)D appears in the blood after about 4 hr, and the dihydroxy metabolites appear after 24 hr.

Other less polar metabolites are recognized. Many of these appear biologically inactive. The most important are probably the water-soluble forms. Vitamin D sulfate has been isolated in human breast milk, but its biologic activity is not established.[18] 1,25-(OH)$_2$D$_3$ glycosides have been found in South American plants[19,20] and are sometimes responsible for hypercalcemia in cattle; these glycosides may have a future therapeutic role.

NORMAL PHYSIOLOGY

The predominant action of 1,25-(OH)$_2$D is to stimulate calcium absorption from the gut, probably by stimulating the enterocyte to synthesize RNA and new proteins.[10] Calcium absorption is an active process against a concentration gradient; calcium-binding protein and intestinal alkaline phosphatase play a part.[21] Phosphorus follows as the accompanying anion. Vitamin D metabolites also act on bone primarily by calcium resorption. An effect on the kidney in promoting reabsorption of filtered calcium has been claimed.[22]

On the basis of bone reabsorption in tissue culture, 1,25-(OH)$_2$D has been found to be about 100 times more active than 25-(OH)D on a weight basis, and 25-(OH)D is more active than unhydroxylated vitamin D.[23] The exact effects of the different metabolites are poorly understood, but therapeutic roles have been claimed for 25-(OH)D[24] and 24,24(OH)$_2$D[25] in patients with chronic renal failure. Possibly, in normal man the different metabolites have different roles and work synergistically. The half-lives in the human body for vitamin D me-

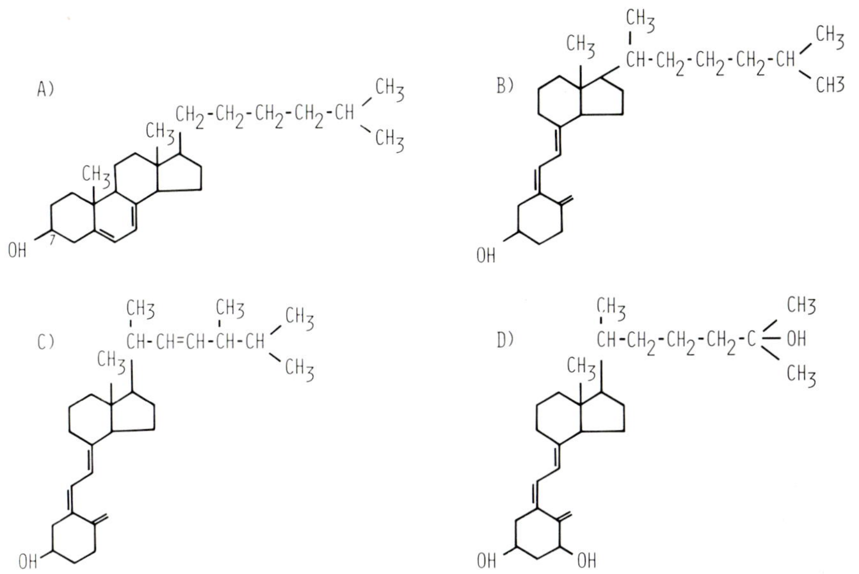

FIG. 4—Biochemical structure of (A) 7-dehydrocholesterol, (B) vitamin D_3 (cholecalciferol), (C) Vitamin D_2 (ergocalciferol), and (D) 1,25-dihydroxyvitamin D_3.

tabolites are approximately 1.5 days for 1,25-$(OH)_2D$, 3.5 days for 1-$(OH)D$, and 29.5 days for vitamin D_2.[26]

SERUM 25-(OH)D IN PATIENTS WITH HEPATOBILIARY DISEASE

Serum 25-(OH)D is the main form of circulating vitamin D and is the metabolite synthesized in the hepatocyte. It was also the first metabolite measured by a competitive protein-binding technique.[27] The standard methods measure both 25-$(OH)D_3$ and 25-$(OH)D_2$. The assay has now been performed in several series of patients with chronic liver disease. Recently developed assays for 1,25-$(OH)_2D$[28] and 24,25-$(OH)_2D$[29] have not been applied to patients with liver disease.

In England, allowing for seasonal change owing to variation in exposure to ultraviolet light, the normal range for 25(OH)D was found to be 9–44 ng/ml.[30] Normal persons were then compared with age-matched patients with chronic liver disease (Figs. 5 and 6). Nine patients with alcoholic hepatitis and 25 patients with alcoholic cirrhosis had mean ($\pm$ 1 SD) serum 25-(OH)D values of 9.8 $\pm$ 5.3 and 8.6 $\pm$ 4.9 ng/ml, respectively. Using the student's t-test, the results for both groups were significantly different ($p < 0.001$) from that of the control group, but there was no significant difference between the two groups. Reduced serum 25-(OH)D values have been described by others in patients with alcoholic liver disease.[31,32] The mean serum 25-(OH)D for the group of 6 patients with noncirrhotic chronic active hepatitis and the group of 26 patients with lupoid or cryptogenic cirrhosis were 10.6 $\pm$ 6.9 and 10.8 $\pm$ 8.0 ng/ml. The values were significantly less in both groups than those in the controls ($p < 0.01$) with no difference between the groups. The difference between the al-

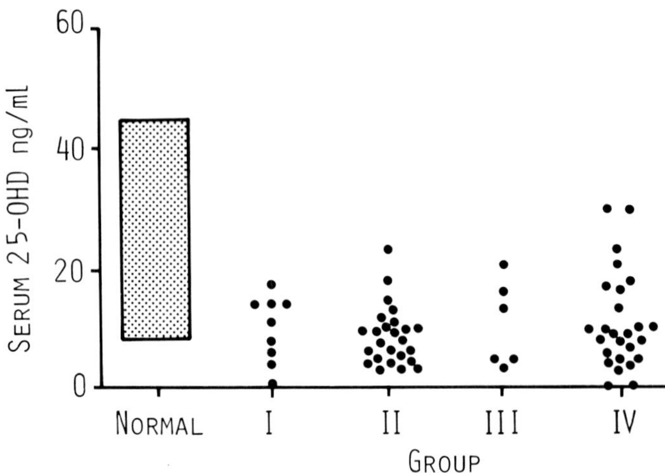

FIG. 5—Serum 25-(OH)D in parenchymal liver disease. Group I, alcoholic hepatitis without cirrhosis; group II, alcoholic cirrhosis; group III, chronic active hepatitis without cirrhosis; group IV, cryptogenic cirrhosis or cirrhosis secondary to chronic active hepatitis. (Reproduced by permission from Long RG, Skinner RK, Wills MR, et al: Serum-25-hydroxy-vitamin-D in untreated parenchymal and cholestatic liver disease. Lancet 2:650–652, 1976.)

coholic and the nonalcoholic cirrhotic patients was not significant. Five of the 6 with hepatocellular disease with values of serum 25-(OH)D greater than 20 ng/ml were anicteric patients who had had prolonged recent exposure to ultraviolet light in the form of bright sunshine. Some individuals with parenchymal liver disease did not fall into one of the above groups but had low 25-(OH)D values: acute fulminant viral hepatitis (1.3 ng/ml), Budd-Chiari syndrome (2.0 ng/ml), Dubin-Johnson syndrome (8.7 ng/ml), and an Asian girl with a portal vein thrombosis (2.2 ng/ml). One patient with Gilbert's disease had a normal serum 25-(OH)D (27.7 ng/ml).

Patients with cholestatic liver disease were also studied (Fig. 6). The mean ($\pm$ 1 SD) serum 25-(OH)D concentration for 7 patients with asymptomatic PBC (i.e., patients with PBC who have never had hepatobiliary symptoms[33]) was 22.3 $\pm$ 18.5 ng/ml, not significantly different from controls. The mean concentration for 11 patients with symptomatic PBC was 5.1 $\pm$ 3.8 ng/ml, which was significantly different from the values in the group of controls ($p < 0.001$) and the group of asymptomatic PBC patients ($p < 0.01$). Low serum 25-(OH)D concentrations have also been described in vitamin-D-untreated PBC by other workers.[4,27,31,34] The mean 25-(OH)D concentration for 5 patients with acute large bile duct obstruction resulting from either carcinoma or stones was 5.1 $\pm$ 4.8 ng/ml. In 11 patients with various forms of chronic cholestasis, the mean 25-(OH)D concentration was 6.4 $\pm$ 5.5 ng/ml. The results for the groups of 5 patients with acute and 11 patients with chronic cholestasis were significantly different from the controls ($p < 0.001$), but there was no difference between the groups. The serum 25-(OH)D concentration was 3.5 ng/ml in 1 patient with acute chlorpromazine cholestasis.

Simultaneous portal and peripheral or hepatic vein sampling was performed

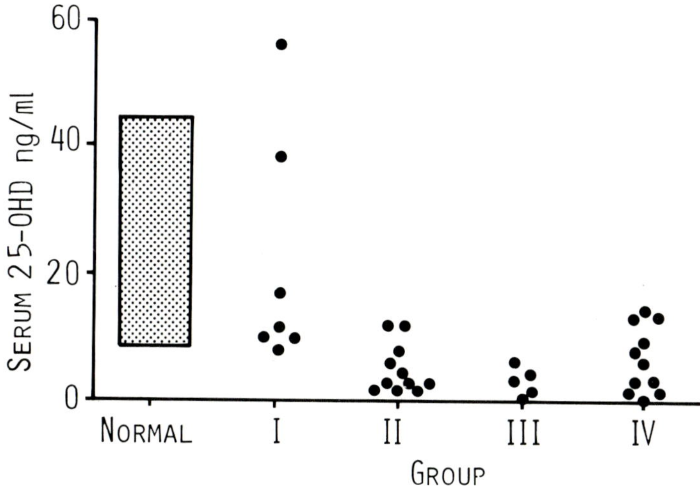

FIG. 6—Serum 25-(OH)D in cholestatic liver disease. Group I, asymptomatic PBC; group II, symptomatic PBC; group III, large bile duct obstruction secondary to carcinoma or gallstones; group IV, chronic cholestatic liver diseases. (Reproduced by permission from Long RG, Skinner RK, Wills MR, et al: Serum-25-hydroxy-vitamin-D in untreated parenchymal and cholestatic liver disease. Lancet 2:650–652, 1976.)

in cirrhotic patients undergoing percutaneous transhepatic sclerosis of varices.[35] The mean ± 1 SD serum 25-(OH)D in 5 cirrhotic patients was 8.8 ± 4.8 ng/ml in the portal vein and 8.5 ± 4.2 ng/ml in the peripheral vein. In 1 cirrhotic patient the hepatic vein serum 25-(OH)D was 9.1 ng/ml and the portal vein serum 25-(OH)D was 7.8 ng/ml. These data suggest that the serum 25-(OH)D concentration is not much greater in the peripheral and hepatic veins than it is in the portal vein.

The ability of patients with PBC to 25-hydroxylate vitamin D when substrate is provided was investigated in several series. The initial claim was that patients with PBC could not 25-hydroxylate vitamin D and that therefore 25-(OH)D$_3$ was the metabolite of choice for treating osteomalacia. This observation, however, was based on oral and subcutaneous administration of vitamin D to only 6 patients[36] and has not been supported in the great majority of patients by subsequent work.[4,7,31,34,37] When serum 25-(OH)D concentrations were measured in 27 PBC patients treated with regular monthly vitamin D$_2$ (100,000 IU in ethyl oleate), the concentrations were much higher ($p < 0.001$) than those in 11 comparable untreated patients (Fig. 7). Generally, the more advanced the histologic liver disease, the lower the serum 25-(OH)D concentrations. No significant rise in serum 25-(OH)D was seen after one injection over a 12-day period in 9 patients. Striking rises to the normal range were seen in 7 untreated PBC patients who were given regular monthly vitamin D$_2$ injections and were followed for 3 to 16 months. Other workers have also shown similar rises in serum 25-(OH)D values after unhydroxylated vitamin D injections and after the injection of radiolabeled unhydroxylated vitamin D. The conclusion, therefore, is that the great majority of PBC patients can 25-hydroxylate vitamin D if enough substrate is provided.

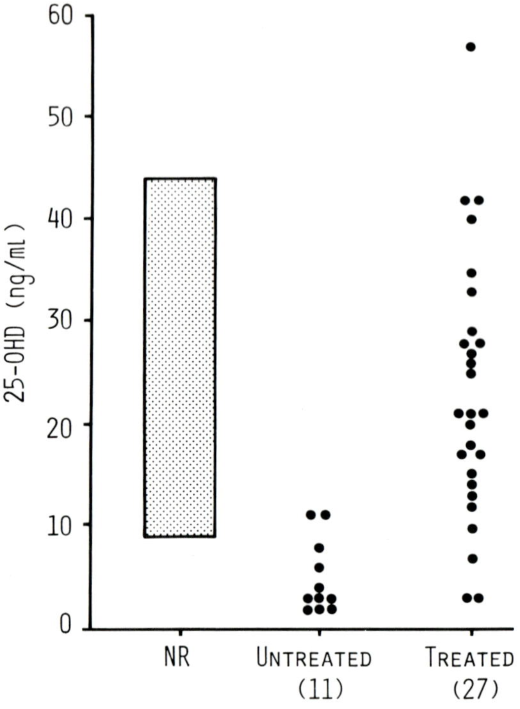

FIG. 7—Serum 25-(OH)D values in vitamin-D₂-treated and -untreated patients with PBC. The difference between the two groups of patients is highly significant (p <0.001). The patients treated with vitamin D_2 received 100,000 IU in ethyl oleate once monthly. (Reproduced by permission from Skinner RK, Long RG, Sherlock S, et al: Lancet 1:720–721, 1977.)

Changes in vitamin D 25-hydroxylation have also been observed in patients with alcoholic liver disease. Jung et al. found that serum 25-(OH)D concentrations were higher in anicteric alcoholic cirrhotic patients studied in the autumn than in the preceding spring.[38] When a large number of patients were studied serially, alcoholic patients with fatty liver disease, compensated cirrhosis, and severely decompensated cirrhosis could all form 25-(OH)D from vitamin D_3 substrate.[39] Therefore, vitamin D 25-hydroxylation appears to be adequate in the majority of patients with chronic cholestatic and hepatocellular liver disease if sufficient vitamin D substrate is provided to the liver.

FORMATION OF DIHYDROXYVITAMIN D

As in chronic renal disease, patients with chronic liver disease might possibly not be able to form dihydroxyvitamin D metabolites. A technique developed in Manchester to study the formation of certain biologically active vitamin D metabolites involves intravenous injection of vitamin D_3 labeled by ^{14}C in position 4 and ^{3}H in position 1.[40] Blood was taken at 6 and 12 hr and at 1, 2, 3, and 5 days after injection, centrifuged, and stored at −20°C. The serum was then extracted and chromatography performed using two Sephadex LH 20 columns. Both $1,25\text{-}(OH)_2D_3$ and $25,26\text{-}(OH)_2D_3$ elute from the columns in the same position. When hydroxylation in the 1α position occurs, however, ^3H is lost, the ratio of $^3H{:}^{14}C$ falls, and the amount of $1,25\text{-}(OH)_2D_3$ formed can be calculated. Thus the following radioactive metabolites can be assessed: D_3, $25\text{-}(OH)D_3$, $24,25\text{-}(OH_2D_3$, $1,25\text{-}(OH)_2D_3$, and $25,26\text{-}(OH)_2D_3$. Results can be expressed as the percentage of administered dose per liter of plasma.

Eight patients (7 PBC, 1 HB_sAg-negative chronic active hepatitis with cirrhosis) were studied at the Royal Free Hospital.[7] In 2 of the patients bone biopsies were performed which showed severe osteomalacia without osteoporosis. Four of the 8 patients studied were vitamin-D-replete and 4 were vitamin-D-deficient as assessed by serum 25-(OH)D concentrations at the start of the test. All 8 patients formed radiolabeled 25-(OH)D. Three of the 4 vitamin-D depleted patients formed radioactive $1,25\text{-}(OH)_2D_3$; 2 of the 3 patients forming this metabolite had osteomalacia. By contrast, all 4 of the vitamin-D replete patients formed $24,25\text{-}(OH)_2D_3$, and 1 also formed $1,25\text{-}(OH)_2D_3$. The results were quantitatively similar to those obtained in patients with normal liver function as performed by the Manchester group who established the technique. If sufficient vitamin D substrate is available, patients with chronic liver disease with or without osteomalacia seem to form monohydroxy- and dihydroxyvitamin D metabolites appropriately and in normal amounts.

CAUSES OF VITAMIN D SUBSTRATE DEFICIENCY

The ability to form mono- and dihydroxyvitamin D metabolites is relatively normal in patients with chronic liver disease, but vitamin D substrate may not be available. The possible causes of vitamin D deficiency in patients with chronic liver disease are numerous (Table 1), and different factors probably play varying roles in patients with different disease states.

The majority of circulating vitamin D is vitamin D_3, which is synthesized in the skin. Lack of exposure to sunlight is well accepted as causing vitamin D deficiency and osteomalacia. Patients with cirrhosis who are ill and confined to the house are not exposed to the sun. Ultraviolet light at the wavelength of 280 nm is required to convert 7-dehydrocholesterol to vitamin D_3. Bilirubin also has its maximum absorption of ultraviolet light at this wavelength. Con-

TABLE 1.—*Possible Causes for Lack of Vitamin D*

1. Skin
     Lack of sunlight
     ? Interference of bilirubin with ultraviolet light absorption
2. Poor nutrition
3. Malabsorption
     Exogenous vitamin D
     Endogenous vitamin D
     Exacerbated by cholestyramine
4. Increased urinary excretion
5. ?Lack of vitamin-D-binding protein
6. ? Enzyme induction

version to vitamin D_3 may be impeded by cutaneous jaundice, but to our knowledge, this hypothesis has not yet been tested.

Alcoholic patients are often malnourished.[41] Poor nutrition has also been demonstrated in patients with cryptogenic cirrhosis and chronic active hepatitis.[42] Patients with PBC may be deficient in vitamin C;[43] hypovitaminosis C is associated with osteoporosis. Accurate estimates of vitamin D intake have not been reported in cirrhotics, but dietary assessments on our patients have shown a tendency toward a low intake.

Malabsorption of vitamin D and 25-(OH)D has been demonstrated in patients with PBC, large bile duct obstruction, and cholestatic autoimmune hepatitis.[4,34,44,45] This malabsorption has been attributed to a lack of intraluminal bile acids. The absorption of vitamin D has been shown to correlate negatively with fecal fat excretion.[36] Cholestyramine may worsen the situation by increasing steatorrhea and vitamin D malabsorption.[4] In addition, vitamin D and some of its metabolites undergo an enterohepatic circulation. Arnaud et al. injected intravenous tritiated vitamin D_3 into normal controls and found that a mean of 17.1% of the dose reached the duodenum within 6 hr of administration and 35.5% of the dose after 24 hr. More than 85% of this secreted vitamin D was reabsorbed.[46] The amount of vitamin D secreted in the bile, its reabsorption, and the significance of an enterohepatic circulation remain to be assessed in patients with liver disease.

Increased radioactivity has been found in the urine of patients with PBC given intravenous radiolabeled vitamin D_3.[34] The radioactivity did not correspond on chromatography to known biologically active metabolites. As a result of this finding, urinary excretion has been suggested as a further source of loss of vitamin D. Alternatively, this excretion may be synonymous to bile acid sulfation in cholestasis and may represent biologically inactive metabolites which in healthy individuals are excreted via the bile.

Vitamin-D-binding protein (VDBG) is synthesized in the liver, has a molecular weight of 59,000, and binds circulating vitamin D metabolites in plasma. It is usually less than 5% saturated with vitamin D,[47] however. In a control group the mean ($\pm$ SEM) plasma VDBG was 27.6 $\pm$ 0.95 mg/dl, and in a total of 45 patients with chronic liver disease the mean plasma VDBG was 21.6 $\pm$ 0.9 mg/dl ($p < 0.01$). Similar mildly reduced plasma values were obtained in groups of patients with alcoholic cirrhosis or hepatitis (21.9 $\pm$ 1.4 mg/dl), chronic active hepatitis (22.8 $\pm$ 1.9 mg/dl), and PBC (20.3 $\pm$ 1.2 mg/dl). The mean plasma VDBG was 25.3 $\pm$ 5.6 mg/dl in 4 patients with extrahepatic biliary obstruction, a value not significantly lower than the control group.[48] Supplies of VDBG are therefore likely to be adequate for binding the vitamin in patients with chronic liver disease, and lack of circulating VDBG is unlikely to be clinically relevant.

Enzyme induction by drugs has been related to the formation of inactive metabolites and the development of osteomalacia in patients receiving long-term anticonvulsant therapy.[49] There is as yet no evidence for an increased metabolic turnover of vitamin D in patients with liver disease on enzyme-inducing drugs. Estrogens[50] and prolactin[51] have been shown to increase 25-(OH)D 1-hydroxylase activity. The possible increases of these circulating hormones in patients with chronic liver disease is controversial,[52] but, if confirmed, could be relevant to vitamin D metabolism in affected patients.

EFFECTS OF VITAMIN D

Clinical Observations

In the 1950s regular vitamin D supplements were reported to reduce bone symptoms.[3,53] Work with vitamin D_2 in patients with chronic cholestatic liver disease, however, showed improved plasma and urinary biochemical results and [47]Ca absorption but conferred little or no protection from bone pains and histologic bone disease.[6,54] Improvement of bone pain and myopathy has now been demonstrated with regular parenteral 1,25-$(OH)_2D_3$ in arachis oil in patients with biliary cirrhosis and proven histologic osteomalacia.[11]

Biochemical Findings

Regular parenteral vitamin D_2 therapy improves[47] Ca absorption in patients with PBC,[54] which may be defective in some jaundiced patients with parenchymal liver disease.[55] Although urinary calcium excretion in patients with osteomalacia resulting from chronic cholestatic and alcoholic liver disease is often reduced,[6] plasma total calcium and its ionized, complexed, and protein-bound fractions are usually in the normal range.[56] Likewise, plasma phosphorus concentrations tend to be in the low-normal range but are rarely subnormal in patients with chronic liver disease. Phosphorus malabsorption is common in patients with large bile duct obstruction and alcoholic liver disease[57] and can be corrected by 25-$(OH)D_3$ treatment.[58] In British patients, plasma magnesium deficiency is rare and does not appear to be associated with histologic osteomalacia.[6,56] We have failed to find significant correlation coefficients between serum 25-(OH)D and plasma calcium, phosphorus, and magnesium concentrations.

Bone Changes

Objective histologic evidence of healing of osteomalacia has only recently been described.[5,11] All 11 patients in these series have shown reduction in osteoid tissue on bone biopsy with either 25-$(OH)D_3$ or 1,25-$(OH)_2D_3$ treatment. An example of such healing is shown in Figs. 8A and 8B. The bone healing in the 4 patients studied at the Royal Free Hospital was not associated with large changes in biochemical variables, which also tended to be normal before 1,25-$(OH)_2D_3$ treatment (Table 2). The vitamin D_3 metabolites may have a direct healing effect on the demineralized bone. By contrast, vitamin D_2 appears not to heal or prevent osteomalacia in these patients.[6] Therefore, vitamin D_3 metabolites appear to reduce osteoid tissue, possibly by a direct action on bone, when vitamin D_2 does not. In view of the observation that the formation of mono- and dihydroxyvitamin D metabolites is relatively normal in these patients, we suggest that hepatic osteomalacia is sensitive to D_3 metabolites and resistant to D_2 metabolites, as has been proposed in chronic renal failure.[59]

Chapter 31

Alcoholic Hepatitis: Clinical, Morphologic, Pathogenic, and Therapeutic Aspects

By SAMUEL W. FRENCH, M.D., *and* EUGENE J. BURBIGE, M.D.

ALCOHOLIC HEPATITIS, a disease of growing importance, continues to elude precise clinical and pathologic definition. Its pathogenesis is poorly understood, and consequently, therapy is nonspecific and supportive. Many reviews on various aspects of these problems have appeared,[1,9] including one each in Volumes IV[10] and V[11] of this series. This progress report cites new leads and observations that signal hope that these problems can be solved.

CLINICAL DIAGNOSIS OF ALCOHOLIC HEPATITIS

At the 1975 meeting at the Fogarty International Center cosponsored by the International Association for the Study of Liver, the definition and the criteria for the diagnosis of alcoholic hepatitis were set forth.[12] The diagnosis of alcoholic hepatitis on a clinical basis remains difficult, however. The clinical criteria that were proposed include jaundice, abdominal distress, fever, leukocytosis, and the manifestations of portal hypertension, but all of these may be absent in the milder forms. Despite a vague set of rules, the clinician's job is not easy and is complicated by the fact that he or she must differentiate between fatty liver, alcoholic hepatitis, and alcoholic cirrhosis, as well as the nonalcoholic causes of hepatitis.

Frequently, there is little correlation between the duration of recognizable liver disease and the severity of the histologic lesion.[13,14] Furthermore, several reports[15-20] have documented hepatic abnormalities histologically in asymptomatic chronic alcoholics. The incidence of asymptomatic alcoholic hepatitis may be as high as 7% to 11% in a susceptible population. In addition to the problem of the asymptomatic patient, distinguishing clinically between alcoholic hepatitis, other forms of hepatitis and infection or surgical disease, such as acute abdomen or biliary obstruction, may be difficult.[21,22]

Investigation of a patient by searching for functional derangement resulting from parenchymal injury may not be helpful because the abnormalities are nonspecific for etiology. According to the criteria set forth, the SGOT level is slightly to moderately elevated and is characteristically higher than that of the SGPT. Frequently, there is hypoprothrombinemia and hypoalbuminemia and elevated activity of alkaline phosphatase. Although it is true that the only

From the Departments of Pathology and Medicine, Veterans Administration Hospital, Martinez, California, and the University of California-Davis, School of Medicine, Davis, California.

Supported by a Veterans Administration Support Grant and Grant #NIAAA 0229402.

biochemical abnormalities may be a slight increase in activities of SGOT, SGPT, or alkaline phosphatase, in some series the most frequent abnormality is direct-reacting bilirubin.[13,18] Again, all of these findings may be absent in the milder cases of alcoholic hepatitis. The discovery of biochemical abnormalities in alcoholic hepatitis is consistent with that diagnosis, but their absence is also consistent with it. The recent introduction of testing for glutamate dehydrogenase, an intramitochondrial enzyme, as a marker of hepatocellular necrosis may make the clinician's job easier. Measurement of glutamate dehydrogenase activities in a study of 100 alcoholics allowed clear discrimination between subjects with and without hepatitis and detection of cases of alcoholic hepatitis that were clinically silent.[23] Glutamate dehydrogenase activity may also be elevated in patients with right-sided heart failure and centrolobular necrosis, however.

In addition to the criteria already discussed, there must be a history of acute and chronic alcoholism in the absence of intestinal bypass surgery, primary biliary cirrhosis, and Wilson's disease. Although the absence of these entities may be determined clinically with some certainty, the level of an individual's alcohol intake may be difficult to ascertain accurately.[14,24] Although some studies suggest that a daily consumption of 80–160 g of ethanol is necessary to produce hepatic lesions,[24] the severity of the histologic lesions correlates poorly with either the duration of drinking or the amount of alcohol consumed.[13]

The definitive indication of alcoholic hepatitis remains a histologic diagnosis.[25] To quote Isselbacher, "I am reluctant to make a diagnosis on the basis of a single laboratory test, and I think that liver biopsy is more valuable in the diagnosis of alcoholic liver disease."

MORPHOLOGIC AND PATHOGENIC CORRELATES: CLINICAL AND EXPERIMENTAL

The morphologic features of alcoholic hepatitis are worth reviewing in order to understand the evolution of the current concepts of the disease. Many features first described in the older literature furnish clues regarding the pathogenesis of alcoholic hepatitis when correlated with newer experimental findings. For instance, when Mallory[26] first called attention to alcoholic hepatitis, he emphasized that the hyaline change affected the cells located near the portal tracts. This observation was based on a study of cirrhosis. Edmondson et al.,[27] however, made the important observation that alcoholic hyaline (Figs. 1 and 2) was located in the centrolobular hepatocytes (zone 3 of Rappaport) in the precirrhotic stage of the disease at a time when the periportal spaces showed no increase in connective tissue. They called this sclerosing hyaline necrosis because of the associated increase in centrolobular collagen and concomitant death of the liver cells. This concept was further amplified by Gerber and Popper,[28] who noted in acute alcoholic hepatitis that fibrosis first occurred in the centrolobular region. Later in the course of the disease, however, they noted that centrolobular-portal tract connections developed. These connections consisted of inflammatory reaction, fibrosis, and hepatocellular necrosis.

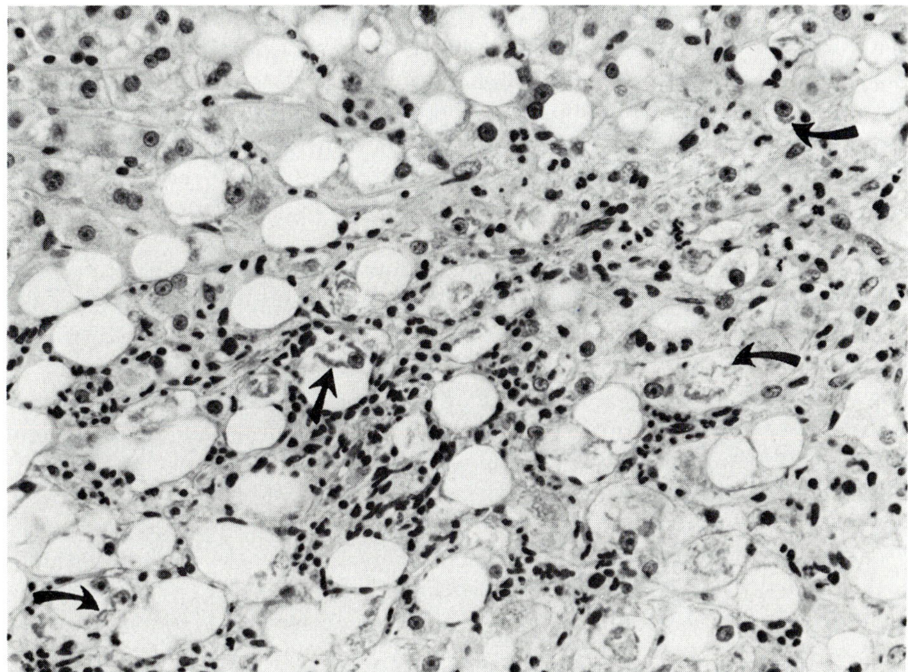

FIG. 1—Central hyaline necrosis. Note the prominent fatty change, hepatocellular swelling with rounded cellular contours, and mixed mononuclear and polymorphonuclear infiltrate. Alcoholic hyaline is present in many liver cells (arrows). Mallory bodies were numerous on electron-microscopic examination of this liver. (Hemotoxylin and eosin stain, ($\times$ 260).

At this point, alcoholic hyaline was also found in the peripheral part of the lobule (zone 1 of Rappaport). As a result of this "bridging" process, cirrhosis develops. Clinical studies have recently shown that, although acute alcoholic hepatitis may be reversible, sclerosing hyaline necrosis is an obligatory step in the natural evolution of alcoholic liver disease into cirrhosis.[29]

Centrolobular Location of Initial Injury

The recognition that alcoholic hepatitis starts in the centrolobular zone is helpful in the interpretation of experimental observations which indicate that this zone is the target of ethanol-induced liver injury. First, experimental liver lesions induced in baboons by chronic ethanol ingestion are located in the centrolobular zone.[30] This observation makes it possible to conclude that the baboon model reproduces the alcoholic liver disease experienced in man. This animal model now provides the opportunity to study its pathogenesis, which was not possible before.

Second, chronic ethanol feeding followed by 16-hr ethanol withdrawal causes an increase in the rate of oxygen consumption by the liver in rats.[31] Theoretically, this leads to an increase in the rate of the extraction of oxygen from the sinusoidal blood, which in turn leads to the reduction in the oxygen delivered to the centrolobular liver cells. Consequently, the centrolobular hepatocytes are more likely to undergo necrosis during hypoxic episodes.[31] A slight but statistically significant drop in the oxygen content of hepatic venous blood Po_2 occurs in the baboon model during the early phase of ethanol withdrawal (12-hr fast).[32] This observation provides a pathogenic mechanism for the degeneration and necrosis observed in the centrolobular zone in alcoholic hepatitis. Although this hypothesis remains to be proved, it provides the rationale for further investigation as well as for a therapeutic trial with propylthiouracil.[33]

Third, experimental chronic ethanol feeding induces an increased permeability of the mitochondrial membrane to phenazine methosulfate in the centrolobular hepatocytes in the rat.[34] A similar change has been observed in 3 alcoholic patients with fatty liver.[35] The significance of this change in man was not appreciated at the time it was reported (see Fig. 10 of that report[35]). This would indicate mitochondrial injury localized to the zone where injury is first detected in alcoholic hepatitis. Although no other studies indicate that liver mitochondrial injury caused by chronic ethanol ingestion is localized to the centrolobular hepatocytes, chronic ethanol ingestion does increase mitochondrial permeability in chronic alcoholics.[36] The serum activity of the intramitochondrial enzyme glutamate dehydrogenase is increased in 47% of chronic alcoholics.[36] The elevated serum glutamate dehydrogenase activity correlates well with the presence of alcoholic hepatitis.[23] Glutamate dehydrogenase activity is concentrated in the liver as compared to other organs. It is highest in the centrolobular hepatocytes, where alcoholic liver injury produces its major effects.[23] Viable isolated hepatocytes derived from the livers of chronic ethanol-fed rats leak mitochondrial glutamate dehydrogenase into the incubation medium.[37] Taken together the evidence indicates that chronic ethanol ingestion causes an increase in permeability of mitochondria to enzyme protein demonstrable in vivo and in vitro. This change may be centrolobular in distribution.

Fourth, the fact that the central hyaline necrosis lesion, indistinguishable from that seen in alcoholic hepatitis, also occurs in morbid obesity after jejunoileal bypass[38-40] (see Chapter 32) suggests that malnutrition plays a role in the pathogenesis of alcoholic hepatitis. This hepatitic lesion does not result from alcohol produced by fermentation in the intestinal lumen.[41] Since the pericellular fibrosis was noted prior to the bypass in some cases,[40] the role played by the bypass is to accentuate the sclerotic process by an undetermined mechanism.

Swelling of Hepatocytes

Swelling of hepatocytes is characteristic of alcoholic hepatitis.[2,4,42,43] Mallory[26] first noted this change associated with the development of alcoholic hyaline, and Hall and Morgan[44] postulated that it was caused by hydropic degeneration which leads to disintegration of the cell. Subsequently, others[45] described swelling of hepatocytes, and some[27,46] stressed that the swollen balloonlike appearance of hepatocytes was due to hydropic degeneration in sclerosing hyaline necrosis, usually preceding the formation of alcoholic hyaline. The formation of the balloon cells in subacute alcoholic hepatitis was regarded

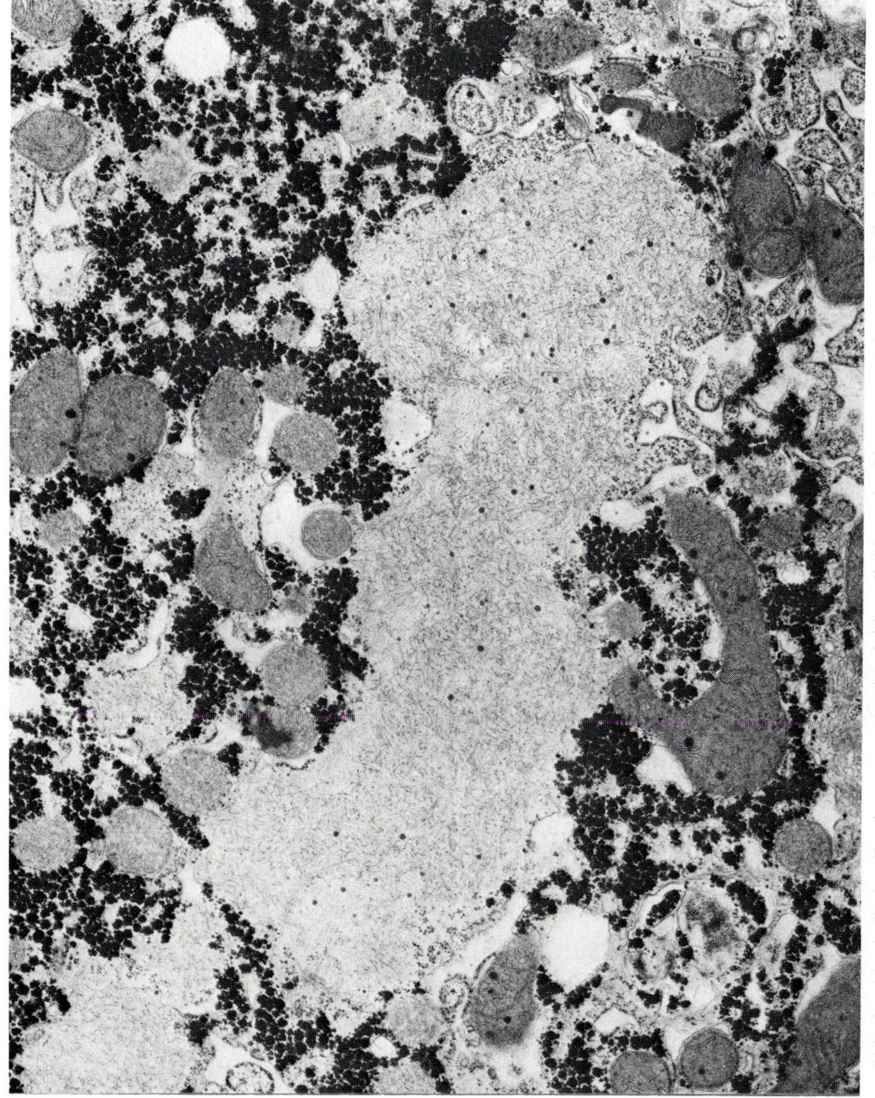

FIG. 2—Alcoholic hyaline in an apparently viable cell. Note the filamentous character indicative of a type II Mallory body. The hyaline is juxtaposed to glycogen, rough endoplasmic reticulum, and mitochondria. Electron micrograph (× 18,240).

as the primary reaction of hepatocytes to alcoholic injury.[47] The balloon cells often contain alcoholic hyaline[2] (Fig. 1). Cells appearing to undergo hydropic degeneration corresponded to cells that contained hyaline on electron microscopy.[48] Many other changes in the cytoplasm could account for the "hydropic" change, however, such as multiple small fat globules[4,48,49] and proliferation of smooth endoplasmic reticulum.[50] The latter, however, was not characteristic of alcoholic hepatitis.[50]

The mitochondrial changes seen in alcoholic hepatitis[51-55] are unlikely to be causally related to the cellular swelling because cellular integrity does not appear to be compromised in hepatocytes containing these mitochondrial alterations. The mitochondrial changes do not correlate with the severity of the hepatitis.[56,57] More recent evidence supports a new concept of alcohol-induced liver injury to explain the balloonlike swelling of hepatocytes in alcoholic hepatitis.[4] According to this hypothesis, hepatocellular swelling develops from accumulation of hepatocytic lipid and protein that normally would have been secreted into the plasma. Theoretically, the retention of export proteins in individual hepatocytes results from the failure of the microtubule-dependent secretory apparatus of the cell. The microtubular failure hypothesis was put forward when it was realized that alcoholic hyaline filaments could represent intermediate filaments. Alcoholic hyaline accumulation was proposed to be a response to the antimicrotubular action of ethanol in the same way that antimicrotubular agents induced alcoholic hyaline formation.[58] Retention of export proteins by the liver was demonstrated in the chronic ethanol-fed rat model.[59] The ethanol-induced hepatomegaly resulted in part from an increase in protein that accumulated primarily in the soluble fraction of the cell cytosol. Albumin and transferrin concentrations, both export proteins, increased in the liver of the ethanol-fed rats. The colchicine binding protein tubulin decreased, suggesting that retention of the export proteins in the cell was due to a decrease in functioning microtubules necessary for secretion. Retention of these export proteins could account for the hepatocytic swelling (balloon cell).[4,59]

Both acute and chronic exposure to ethanol interferes with the microtubular-dependent secretory functions of hepatocytes. Acutely, ethanol impedes the secretion of lipoproteins and serum proteins by hepatocytes, as does colchicine[60-63] and other antimicrotubular agents. Acute ethanol feeding causes lipoprotein globules to increase in the Golgi zone.[64] The latter is accentuated by colchicine.[64,65] This probably accounts for the inhibition of triglyceride release by the liver[66] and the reduction of serum very low density lipoproteins (VLDL) levels[67] after acute ethanol administration (see Chapter 13). This property of ethanol is exploited by biologists to increase the yield of the Golgi fractions isolated from hepatocytes because the Golgi apparatus retains VLDL after acute ethanol treatment.[68,69] Similar effects may be operative in ethanol inhibition of bile secretion,[70] since the microtubular-Golgi system is supposedly involved in the transport of bile acids and lecithin.[71]

Chronic ethanol ingestion inhibits the rate of secretion of liver albumin and transferrin[59,72] despite enhanced synthesis of liver protein and prealbumin.[72] The increase in retained protein, together with increased hepatic lipids, may account for the increase in cell size and hepatomegaly observed.[59,72] In this experimental model, the concentration of total serum albumin or transferrin was not reduced.[72] Polymerized tubulin was significantly reduced,[72] indicating that chronic ethanol ingestion interferes with microtubular assembly just as other antimicrotubular drugs do.

Any hypothesis to explain the balloonlike swelling of hepatocytes seen in alcoholic hepatitis must take into account the following observations: (1) The swelling is observed only after years of alcohol abuse in man and 9 months of high ethanol ingestion in baboons.[30] (2) The swelling is characteristically centrolobular.[46] (3) The swelling involves single or small groups of hepatocytes. (4) The swelling commonly accompanies alcoholic hyaline and the accumulation of numerous small lipid droplets. (5) An acidophilic body type of necrosis, granulocytic infiltrate (satellitosis), and fibrosis often coexist with the hepatocytic swelling.[9,42,43] Obviously, no single factor such as direct inhibition of protein secretion by ethanol could account for this constellation of factors.

Mice fed the antimicrotubulin agent griseofulvin for several months developed many of the features observed in alcoholic hepatitis described above. Balloon cells develop that often contain "alcoholic" hyaline.[4,73,74] The time interval for induction of "alcoholic" hyaline formation is several months. Fibrosis and granulocytic infiltrate occur but are less conspicuous than that observed in man.[73,74] Hyaline-containing hydropic hepatocytes first appear in the centrolobular location.[73] Structures resembling Councilman bodies and derived from necrotic liver cells develop.[73] "Alcoholic" hyaline and hepatocellular swelling are slowly reversible after griseofulvin withdrawal.[73] The griseofulvin-induced hepatitis thus bears sufficient similarity to alcoholic hepatitis, and they probably have at least one pathogenic factor in common, i.e., an antimicrotubulin effect. The reason for the prolonged induction period before the hepatitis becomes manifest remains unknown.

"Alcoholic" Hyaline (Mallory Bodies)

New insights into the nature of Mallory bodies has furnished some clues regarding the pathogenesis of alcoholic hepatitis. As indicated above the similarity of the Mallory body filaments to intermediate filaments suggests that they accumulate as a result of the antimicrotubulin action of ethanol.[4,58,75-77] Microtubules have been found in hepatocytes bearing Mallory bodies in alcoholic hepatitis.[78] Certainly, the fact that administration of the antimicrotubulin agent griseofulvin[73,74] and griseofulvin followed by colchicine[75] induce Mallory bodies supports this conclusion that Mallory bodies result from antimicrotubular effects. This conclusion, however, requires that the human and mouse Mallory bodies be the same. They appear identical on light and electron microscopy.[4,73,74] Additionally, the two types of Mallory bodies bind peroxidase-antiperoxidase[76,77] and cross-react with rat antihuman Mallory body antibody.[77] Cross-reactivity has also been observed using a guinea pig antihuman Mallory body antibody.[79]

Mallory bodies selectively bind immunoglobulins nonspecifically.[77-80] They share this property with intermediate filaments.[81] An anti-Mallory-body antibody raised in guinea pigs also bound intermediate filaments in PtK2 cells.[79] Mallory bodies, in an isolated fraction, also bind fluorescein-concanavalin A to a variable degree, and this binding was blocked by α-methylmannoside, indicating the presence of carbohydrate.[82] This property is shared by microtubules.[83] Purified Mallory bodies contain variable amounts of neutral sugar but no sialic acid.[82] Mallory bodies contain glycoprotein,[84] but this or carbohydrates may possibly be artifactually absorbed, since Mallory bodies have an affinity for immunoglobulins, thereby providing the explanation for the binding of IgA to Mallory bodies.[85]

The propensity of Mallory bodies to bind carbohydrates may have functional significance in that it could explain how Mallory bodies activate lymphocytes to secrete lymphokines in vitro. Purified hyaline alone had no chemotaxic, fibrogenic, or cytotoxic potential, but when added to serum, it was strongly chemotactic.[11] The chemotaxis and fibrogenesis may be phenomena associated with Mallory bodies in alcoholic hepatitis provoked by immunoglobulin and complement that become bound to Mallory bodies when the latter are exuded from dead liver cells. By contrast, specific antibodies to Mallory bodies have been reported in the serum of patients with alcoholic hepatitis, as well as immune complexes in the liver of these patients.[86] The presence of immune complexes in the liver could account for the chemotaxis by Mallory bodies observed in alcoholic hepatitis.

New insight into the significance of Mallory body formation has been gained through tissue culture experiments.[87] Mallory bodies produced by hepatocytes in tissue culture were not associated with hepatocellular degenerative changes. The hepatocytes did not become necrotic, indicating that hyaline formation did not result from cell injury or lead to cell death. Like the Mallory bodies observed in alcoholic hepatitis and after griseofulvin feeding, the diethylnitrosamine-induced Mallory body formation in tissue culture required several months to become manifest.[87] This suggests that a two-step process is involved in Mallory body formation analogous to the experimental induction of neoplasia, i.e., an initiating event (diethylnitrosamine) and a promoting event[88] (cell replication in tissue culture). This suggests the possibility that alcoholic hyaline may represent a epigenetic expression that has preneoplastic significance. Hepatocellular carcinomas containing Mallory bodies develop more frequently in alcoholic cirrhosis than in cirrhosis of any other etiology.[89]

A parallel can be drawn between the advent of Mallory body formation in alcoholic hepatitis and the appearance of fetoprotein in the liver and serum during liver regeneration[90-93] and in hepatocellular carcinoma.[94-100] Both appear to be gene derepression phenomena (activated fetal gene that is suppressed at the adult state.[101]) Like alpha-fetoprotein,[102] intermediate filaments (tonofilaments) are present in abundance in hepatocytes on the ninth and tenth days of gestation in the mouse fetus.[103] If Mallory bodies are intermediate filaments, as is suspected, then their appearance in hepatocytes in alcoholic hepatitis and cirrhosis may represent the expression of a gene normally repressed in the adult. The analogy to alpha-fetoprotein is further strengthened by the appearance of alpha-fetoprotein in the serum during alcoholic hepatitis when Mallory bodies were found in hepatocytes.[104,105] Another condition where alpha-fetoprotein occurs in the serum with high frequency (45%) is Indian childhood cirrhosis,[106] a condition that resembles alcoholic hepatitis in that Mallory bodies are present and the disease has a chronic course. Using immunofluorescent identification, alpha-fetoprotein-positive hepatocytes were found in 9 of 18 cases of alcoholic hepatitis.[107] This was not observed in controls or in cases of nonalcoholic hepatitis or cirrhosis. This establishes that the gene derepression phenomenon does indeed commonly occur in alcoholic hepatitis.

The prognostic significance of Mallory bodies in patients with alcoholic hepatitis who are undergoing portacaval anastomosis for portal hypertension is controversial. Even though Mallory bodies do not appear to affect the long-term survival rate in patients with alcoholic hepatitis,[7] many authors have observed that Mallory bodies correlated with a high postoperative death rate after portacaval anastomosis.[108,109] By contrast, others[110] did not observe a difference in survival when Mallory bodies were present. The percentage of hepatocytes that contain alcoholic hyaline may be critical. The postoperative death rate was significantly higher if hyaline was found in more than 10% of the hepatocytes in needle-biopsy specimens obtained preoperatively.[111] The correlation was better with this finding than with the Child's classification. Postponement of the shunt procedure was advocated if the 10% figure was exceeded. Possibly, the portacaval anastomosis is not the critical factor, since the same poor prognosis was observed when only open liver biopsy was performed without portacaval anastomosis.[112]

Lymphocytic Infiltration

There has been an increasing emphasis in the literature on the importance of the lymphocytic infiltrates observed in the liver in alcoholic hepatitis. Lymphocyte-mediated liver damage may play a role in the pathogenesis of alcoholic liver disease.[5,11] Autoimmune mechanisms have been held responsible for the progression of alcoholic hepatitis to cirrhosis in the absence of continued alcohol abuse.[11] Lymphocytic infiltrates in alcoholic liver disease sometimes resemble those of chronic active hepatitis,[42] and chronic alcohol ingestion may be one of the causes of chronic active hepatitis.[113] The resemblance is so close that pathologists diagnose chronic active hepatitis in alcoholics. Indeed, the diagnosis of chronic active hepatitis may be impossible to rule out in these cases.[17,114-116] The number of years of alcohol abuse is not different in cases of chronic hepatitis and alcoholic hepatitis in asymptomatic chronic alcoholics.[114] When features of chronic active hepatitis occur in chronic alcoholics without coexisting features of alcoholic hepatitis, such as Mallory body formation, the treatment and the prognosis may be quite different than in alcoholic hepatitis.[114,117]

Chronic lymphocytic infiltrates are often observed in livers of patients with alcoholic liver disease,[4,42,117-119] and more frequently in more advanced disease.[4] Lymphocytic infiltrates were found in 87% of patients with fatty liver and Mallory bodies and in 27% of patients with fatty liver without Mallory bodies.[120] This association of Mallory bodies with lymphocytic infiltrate supports the concept that Mallory bodies act as a neoantigen[121] but does not mean that the lymphocytic infiltrate is in the same location as the Mallory bodies. Lymphocytes and plasma cells may be observed in centrolobular locations, however[4] (Fig. 1). More often, the lymphocytes are located at the limiting plate (Figs. 3 and 4) (piecemeal necrosis), or within the parenchyma (Fig. 5) in direct contact with the plasma membranes of hepatocytes, or within hepa-

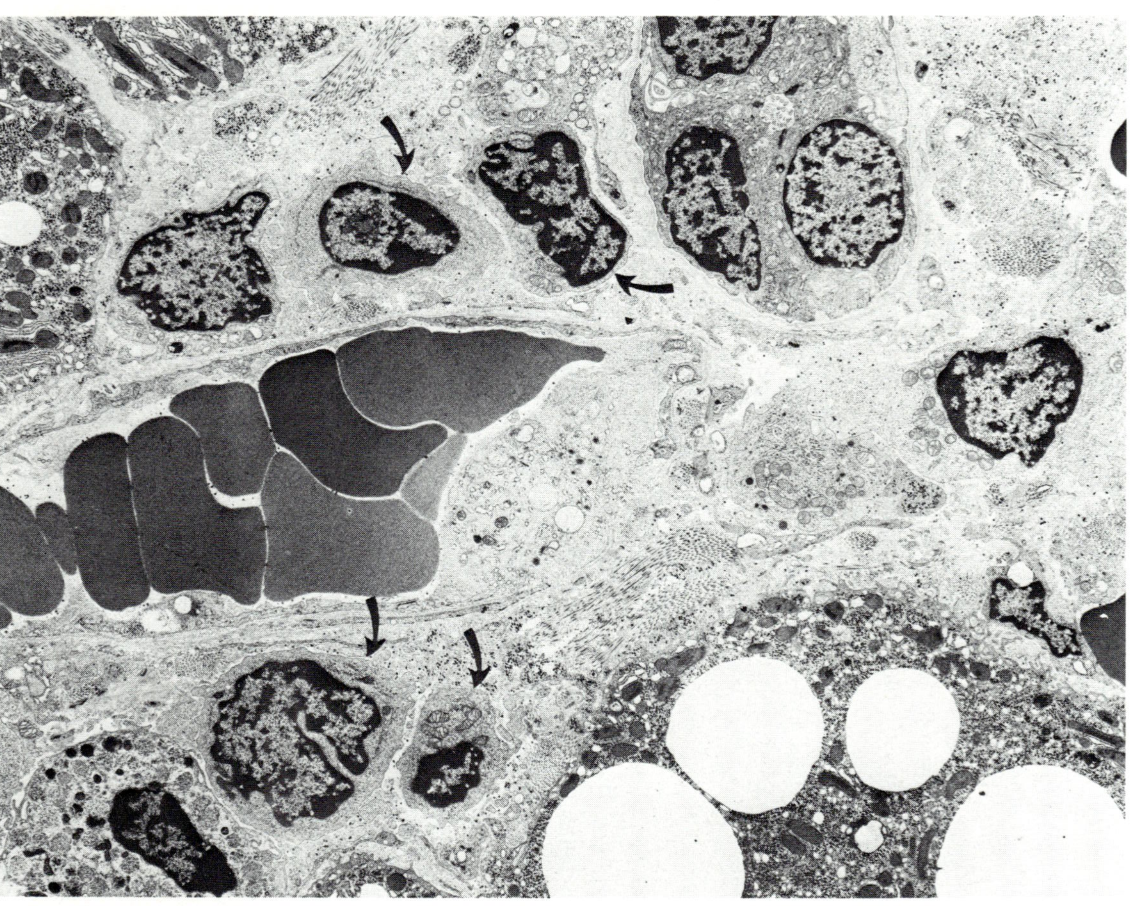

FIG. 3—Mononuclear infiltrate at the limiting plate in a patient with alcoholic hepatitis. Note the hepatocytes at the upper left and lower right and the cholangiole at the upper right. Lymphocytes are numerous in the portal connective tissue and around the sinusoid as it passes into the hepatic parenchyma to the left (arrows). Electron micrograph ($\times$ 3640).

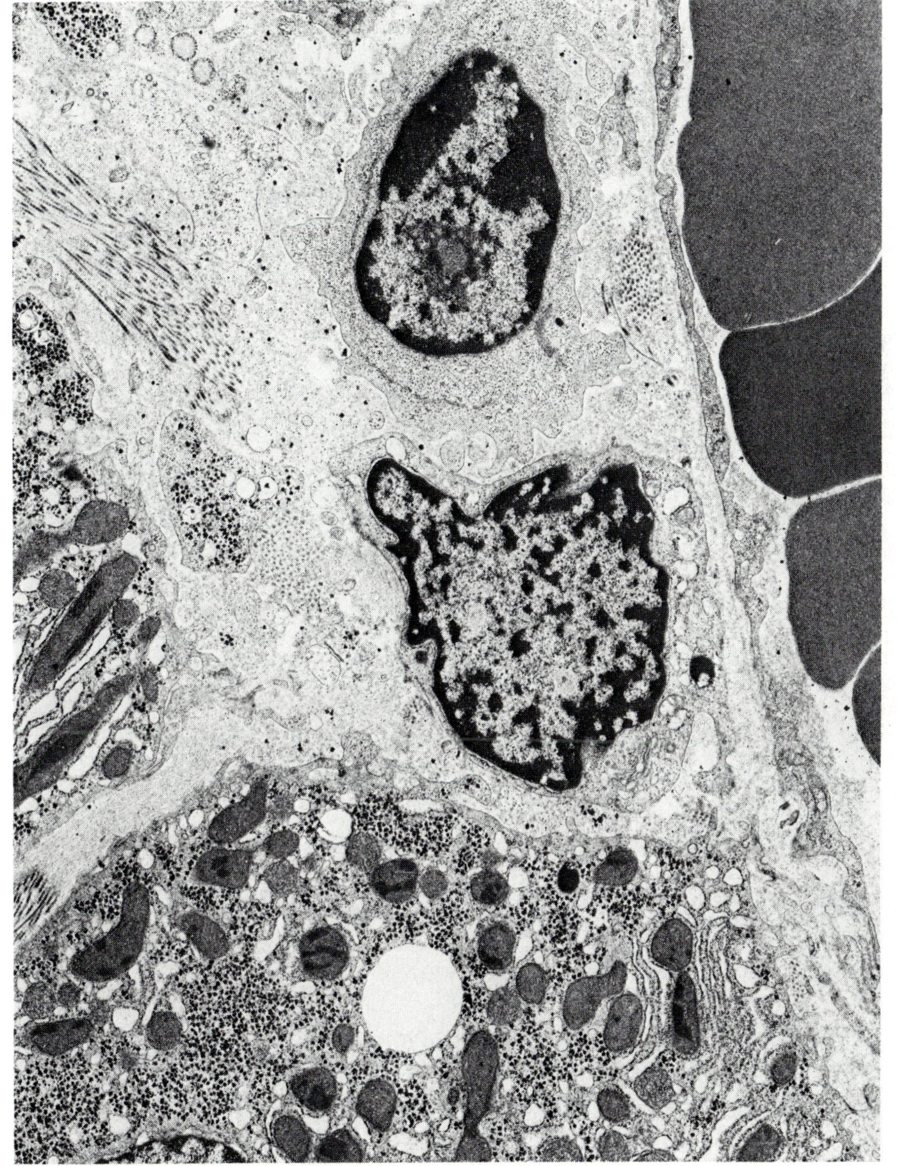

FIG. 4.—Higher magnification of Fig. 3 showing how portal lymphocytes closely approach hepatocytes at the point of sinusoidal penetration of the plate. Note the paracrystallin deposits in the liver cell mitochondria. Electron micrograph (× 7840).

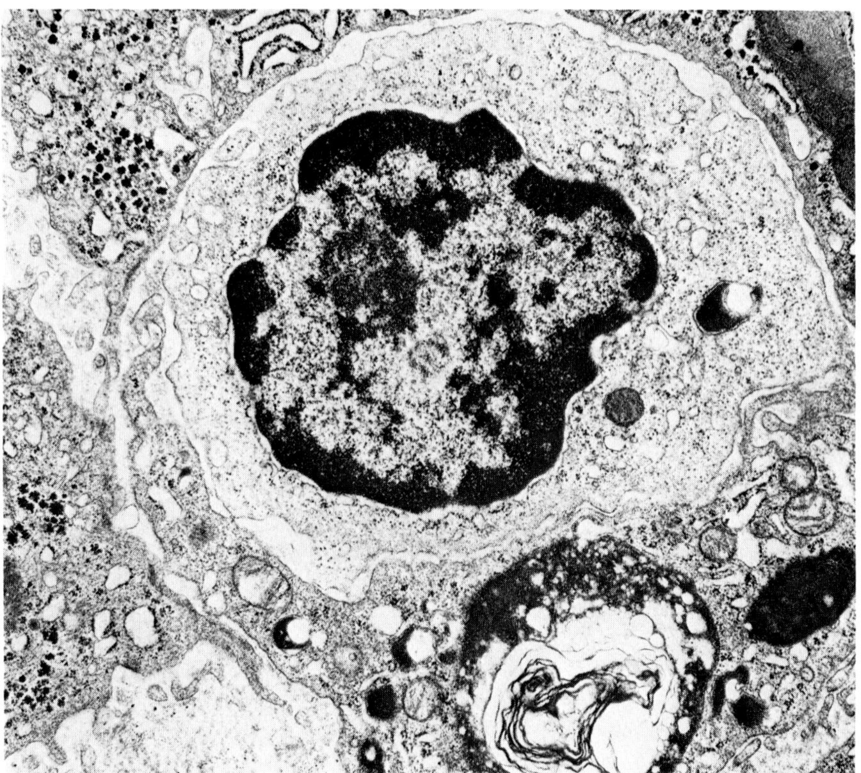

FIG. 5—Lymphocyte located in the space of Disse between a hepatocyte above and a Kupffer cell below. The lymphocyte has abundant free ribosomes and a paucity of organelles. Plasma membrane contact points between the lymphocyte and liver cell are not seen here, but these have been observed in alcoholic hepatitis. Electron micrograph ($\times$ 17,640).

tocytes.[4] This infiltration of the liver by lymphocytes in alcoholic hepatitis has not received as much emphasis in the literature as has infiltration by segmented leukocytes (Fig. 6).

The histologic features of the lymphocytic infiltrates suggest a cytotoxic role of lymphocytes similar to that in chronic active liver disease[122] or in orthotopic liver homograft rejection,[123] although the changes seen in alcoholic hepatitis are usually much less pronounced than those in chronic active hepatitis. The results from three studies using different methods indicate that T lymphocytes increase in the liver in alcoholic hepatitis.[107,124,125] Since T lymphocytes tend to be low in the peripheral blood in these patients,[107,124,126-128] sequestration of T lymphocytes in the liver has been postulated,[107,127,129] possibly resulting from antigen-antibody binding of the liver cell and lymphocyte plasma membranes. Such lymphocyte-hepatocyte binding could lead to hepatocellular destruction. Lymphocytes with cytotoxic potential adhere to target cells in vitro,[130] and those taken from the blood of patients with alcoholic hepatitis[131] and from baboons fed ethanol chronically[132] exhibit cytotoxic effects on hepatocytes in vitro. Chronic ethanol ingestion probably leads to sensitization of lymphocytes to a liver cell antigen.[11,124,86,133] Lymphocyte-hepatocyte interaction may lead

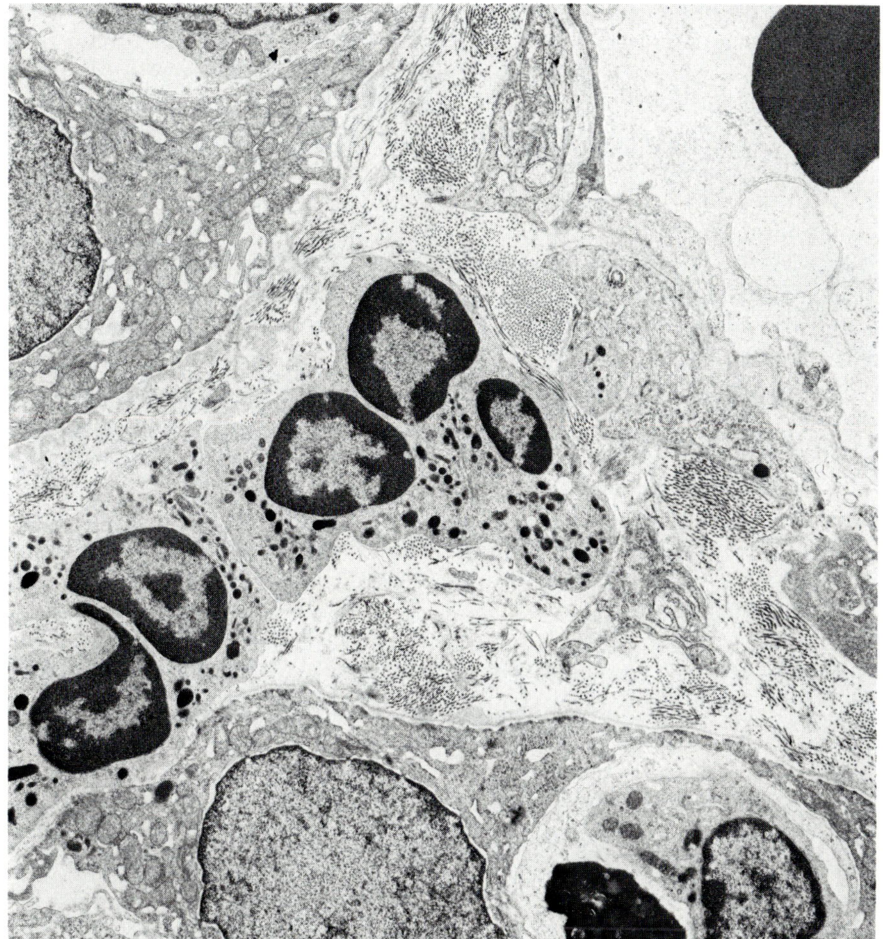

FIG. 6—Polymorphonuclear leukocytes in portal tract connective tissue between the two cholangioles. This acute cholangiolitis is commonly seen in alcoholic hepatitis as well as in other conditions. Electron micrograph ($\times$ 7000).

to hepatocellular death and perpetuation of the hepatitis process. This cytotoxicity could be mediated by either ''activated'' T cells or antibody assisted K lymphocytes.[124,134]

Hepatic Fibrosis

Mallory postulated that fibrosis results from the acute inflammatory exudate-induced ''stretching'' of the connective tissue.[26] Proliferation of fibroblasts, then, results from ''mechanical'' injury. Increase in glycosaminoglycuronan-rich ground substance was said to lead to the progressive fibrosis in alcoholic hepatitis.[7,117] Pericentral venous sclerosis typical of alcoholic liver disease has been thought to precede the inflammatory stage of alcoholic liver injury[135] and was noted in the fatty liver stage in both alcoholic patients and baboons fed ethanol. Sequential biopsies in baboons showed that the pericentral sclerosis increased with progressive liver injury. The opposite conclusion followed observations on serial biopsies of several cases of alcoholic hepatitis that centrolobular fibrosis followed, rather than preceded, the neutrophilic exudate, necrosis, and Mallory body formation (central hyaline necrosis).[29] In some cases, centrolobular fibrosis was encountered after central hyaline necrosis disappeared, supporting the concept that sclerosing hyaline necrosis is an essential step in the evolution of alcoholic hepatic damage that progresses to cirrhosis. Resolution of this controversy awaits further data.

Some alcoholic patients may develop cirrhosis without going through an alcoholic hepatitis phase,[136] since ethanol can stimulate collagen synthesis in the absence of the lesion of alcoholic hepatitis.[8,137-139] The various mechanisms involved in hepatic scarring in alcoholic liver disease, as well as in other types of liver disease, have been adequately summarized.[140] Of special interest is the theory that hepatic fibrosis may occur in alcoholic hepatitis as a result of Mallory-body-activated secretion of a lymphokine that is released as a result of an autoimmune mechanism.[141] Although fibrosis is usually preceded by inflammation in diseases causing hepatic scarring, this is not the case in iron overload.[140] Increased collagen synthesis and turnover in the liver in alcoholic hepatitis has been demonstrated in vitro.[8,138,142] Ethanol in these cases directly stimulated collagen synthesis.[142] These data clearly establish a fibroblastic role in the scarring process of alcoholic hepatitis. Colchicine might better be given during episodes of alcoholic hepatitis where collagen synthesis and turnover are at their peak,[139,145] rather than during the cirrhotic stage, since the rate of synthesis does not appear to be increased in inactive cirrhotics.[139]

Colchicine may also stimulate collagenase production.[146] The factors involved in colchicine therapy of hepatic fibrosis have been adequately reviewed in an earlier volume of this series.[147]

Not all patients with alcoholic hepatitis develop cirrhosis.[7,135] Apparently, both sex[148] and genetic factors[149] play a role in this selection. Alcoholic hepatitis was encountered with or without cirrhosis in 29% of men and 47% of female alcoholics with liver disease.[148] In the same study, 55% of men and 71% of female alcoholics had cirrhosis with or without alcoholic hepatitis. Cirrhosis was associated with specific histocompatibility antigens in patients with alcoholic liver disease.[149] HL-A-B8 was more prevalent in patients with cirrhosis than in controls, whereas patients with fatty liver and minimal fibrosis had a normal prevalence of this antigen. HL-A-A28 was found to be absent in the cirrhotic patients (See Chapter 15). These findings lend weight to the supposition that genetic factors determine the susceptibility of alcoholics to develop hepatic scarring in response to chronic alcohol abuse.

TREATMENT OF ALCOHOLIC HEPATITIS

Despite recent advances in understanding the pathogenesis of ethanol-induced liver damage, the mainstay of treatment continues to be withdrawal of alcohol and supportive therapy.[150] Although rats given alcohol daily along with a nutritious diet may not develop hepatocellular necrosis,[151] baboons do develop liver injury when fed alcohol despite a nutritious diet.[152] Because chronic alcohol abuse is often associated with malnutrition, however, it is reasonable to treat deficiencies in patients with a nutritious diet and multivitamin replacement.

Several early trials suggested that steroids might be helpful in the treatment of alcoholic liver disease.[153-155] They might be helpful because of their known effect in decreasing hyperbilirubinemia[156] and in increasing serum albumin.[157] With the realization that alcoholic hepatitis is associated with abnormal immunologic reactions, including lymphocytotoxicity[130] and the presence of alcoholic hyaline antigen and antibody,[85] the use of corticosteroids would seem to have a stronger foundation.

Steroids in initial trials were of benefit only in patients with severe alcoholic hepatitis.[18] Because the group treated with steroids had a significant improvement in caloric intake, it was postulated that prednisolone increased survival indirectly by its ability to improve the appetite and sense of well-being. Later studies, however, comparing the effect of prednisolone therapy with a dietary regimen of at least 1,600 calories per day without prednisolone, did not show an increased survival with caloric supplementation alone.[158] Whether corticosteroids have a beneficial effect in acute alcoholic hepatitis and whether they increase or decrease morbidity and mortality remain extremely controversial.[153,159-167]

Another justification for the use of corticosteroids is their possible effect on fibrogenesis[168] by inhibition of proline hydroxylase, an enzyme necessary for the hydroxylation of proline in collagen. The administration of prednisolone for 1 month did not show any effect on the morphologic evolution of alcoholic liver disease, however.[169]

Since alcoholic hepatitis is thought to be a precursor of cirrhosis,[170-172] agents that inhibit collagen formation may potentially be useful in the treatment of alcoholic hepatitis. Penicillamine, a drug that prevents the cross-linking of collagen molecules, has been used in the treatment of primary biliary cirrhosis.[173-175] Colchicine inhibits microtubular protein assembly in fibroblasts, and thereby collagen formation, and may be useful in inhibiting or decreasing fibrogenesis.[144,176] A proline analogue, L-azetidine-2-carboxylic acid, decreases fibrogenesis in carbon tetrachloride-induced hepatic injury in rats.[177]

Chronic alcohol abuse may be associated clinically with what appears to be a hypermetabolic state.[178] Chronic ingestion of ethanol increases oxygen consumption in rats probably through increased hepatic sodium-potassium–dependent ATPase activity.[179] If ethanol is fed to rats and the oxygen tension in the environment is lowered to make the rats hypoxic, hepatocellular necrosis is induced.[31] Preliminary studies in patients with alcoholic hepatitis given propylthiouracil to counteract the hypermetabolic state have shown a beneficial effect, with a decrease in mortality and recovery of liver function.[33] The beneficial effect of propylthiouracil may not be due to its effect on the hypermetabolic state, since the hypermetabolic state of the liver induced by ethanol withdrawal is transient. Rather, propylthiouracil probably acts through the reduction of the liver's response to adrenergic agonists. Rats pretreated with propylthiouracil[180] or reserpine[181] are less susceptible to hepatic necrosis caused by carbon tetrachloride poisoning. The protective effect of both of these drugs could result from the reduction of adrenergic activity. With reserpine, catecholamine depletion would result, whereas with propylthiouracil, an adrenergic subsensitivity would be expected, since adrenergic receptor sensitivity is increased in hyperthyroidism and decreased in hypothyroidism.[182-186] Theoretically, reserpine should be as effective as propylthiouracil in the treatment of alcoholic hepatitis.

Whether any of the agents discussed are useful clinically remains to be proven. Effective treatment is not likely to be available until the pathogenesis of alcoholic hepatitis is better understood.

REFERENCES

1. Isselbacher KJ: Metabolic and hepatic effects of alcohol. N Engl J Med 296:612–616, 1977
2. Galambos JT: Alcoholic hepatitis. Edited by F Schaffner, S Sherlock, and CM Leevy: The Liver and Its Diseases. New York, Intercontinental Medical Book Corp, 1974, pp 255–267
3. Davidson CS: Treatment of alcoholic liver diseases. Edited by F Schaffner, S Sherlock, and CM Leevy: The Liver and Its Diseases. New York, Intercontinental Medical Book Corp, 1974, pp 268–282.
4. French SW, Sim JS, Franks KE, Burbige EJ, Denton T, Caldwell MG: Alcoholic hepatitis. Edited by MM Fisher and JG Rankin: Alcohol and the Liver. New York, Plenum Press, 1977, pp 261–286
5. Fox RA: Immune mechanisms in alcoholic liver disease. Edited by MM Fisher and JG Rankin: Alcohol and the Liver. New York, Plenum Press, 1977, pp 309–320
6. Isselbacher KJ, Feller ER: The natural history and management of alcoholic liver disease. Edited by MM Fisher and JG Rankin: Alcohol and the Liver. New York, Plenum Press, 1977, pp 349–361
7. Galambos JT: The course of alcoholic hepatitis. Edited by JM Khanna, Y Israel, and H Kalant: Alcoholic Liver Pathology. Toronto, Addiction Research Foundation of Ontario, 1975, pp 97–111
8. Mezey E, Potter JJ, Maddrey WC: Hepatic fibrogenesis in alcoholism. Edited by JM Khanna, Y Israel, and H Kalant: Alcoholic Liver Pathology. Toronto, Addiction Research Foundation of Ontario, 1975, pp 145–156
9. Lieber CS, Baraona E, Borowsky SA, Leo MA: Effect of ethanol on lipoprotein and protein export from the liver and its relationship to progressive alcoholic liver injury. Edited by H Popper, L Bianchi, and W Reutter: Membrane Alterations as Basis of Liver Injury. Lancaster, MTP Press, 1977, pp 327–341
10. Galambos JT: Alcoholic hepatitis: Its therapy and prognosis. Edited by H Popper and F Schaffner: Progress in Liver Diseases. Vol. IV. New York, Grune & Stratton,1973, pp 567–588
11. Leevy CM, Chen T, Luisada-Opper A, Kanagasundaram N, Zetterman R: Liver disease of the alcoholic: Role of immunologic abnormalities in pathogenesis, recognition and treatment. Edited by H Popper and F Schaffner: Progress in Liver Diseases. Vol. V. New York, Grune & Stratton, 1976, pp 516–530
12. Nomenclature, diagnostic criteria and diagnostic methodology for diseases of the liver and biliary tract. Fogarty International Center, Proceeding 22. Washington DC, US Government Printing Office, 1976
13. Lischner MW, Alexander JF, Galambos JT: Natural history of alcoholic hepatitis. I. The acute disease. Am J Dig Dis 16: 481–494, 1971
14. Alexander JF, Lischner MW, Galambos JT: Natural history of alcoholic hepatitis. II. The long-term prognosis. Am J Gastroenterol 56:515–525, 1971
15. Ugarte G, Iturriaga H, Isurrza I: Some effects of ethanol on normal and pathologic livers. Edited by H Popper and F Schaffner: Progress in Liver Diseases. Vol. IV. New York, Grune & Stratton, 1970, pp 355–350
16. Green JR: Subclinical acute liver disease of the alcoholic. Aust Ann Med 14:111–124, 1965
17. Bruguera M, Bordas JM, Rodes J: Asymptomatic liver disease in alcoholics. Arch Pathol Lab Med 101:644–647, 1977

18. Helman RA, Temko MH, Nye SW, Fallon HJ: Alcoholic hepatitis: Natural history and evaluation of prednisolone therapy. Ann Intern Med 74:311–321, 1971

19. Beckett AG, Livingstone AU, Hill KR: Acute alcoholic hepatitis. Br Med J 2: 1113–1119, 1961

20. Green JR: Subclinical acute liver disease of the alcoholic. Aust Ann Med 14:111–124, 1965

21. Phillips GB, Davidson CS: Liver disease of the chronic alcoholic simulating extrahepatic biliary obstruction. Gastroenterology 33:236–244, 1957

22. Mikkelsen WP, Turrile FL, Kern WH: Acute hyaline necrosis of the liver: A surgical trap. Am J Surg 116:266–272, 1968

23. Van Waes LV, Lieber CS: Glutamate dehydrogenase: A reliable marker of liver cell necrosis in the alcoholic. Br Med J 2: 1508–1510, 1977

24. Turner TB, Mezey E, Kimball AW: Measurement of alcohol-related effects in man: Chronic effects in relation to levels of alcohol consumption. Part A. Johns Hopkins Med J 141:235–248, 1977

25. Isselbacher KJ: Metabolic and hepatic effects of alcohol. N Engl J Med 296:612–616, 1977

26. Mallory FB: Cirrhosis of the liver. Five different types of lesions from which it may arise. Bull Johns Hopkins Hosp 22:69–74, 1911

27. Edmondson HA, Perers RL, Telfer BR, Kuzma OT: Sclerosing hyaline necrosis of the liver in the chronic alcoholic. Ann Intern Med 59:646–673, 1963

28. Gerber MA, Popper H: Relation between central canals and portal tracts in alcoholic hepatitis. Hum Pathol 3:199–207, 1972

29. Karasawa T, Chedid A: Sclerosing hyaline necrosis in noncirrhotic chronic alcoholic hepatitis. Am J Clin Pathol 66:802–809, 1976

30. Lieber CS, DeCarli LM, Rubin E: Sequential production of fatty liver, hepatitis and cirrhosis in subhuman primates fed ethanol with adequate diets. Proc Natl Acad Sci USA 72:437–441, 1975

31. Israel Y, Kalant H, Orrego H, Khanna, JM, Videla L, Phillips JM: Experimental alcohol-induced hepatic necrosis: Suppression by propylthiouracil. Proc Natl Acad Sci USA 72:1137–1141, 1975

32. Shaw P, Heller EA, Friedman HS, Baraona E, Lieber CS: Increased hepatic oxygenation following ethanol administration in the baboon. Proc Soc Exp Biol Med 156: 509–513, 1977

33. Orrego H, Kalant H, Israel Y, Medline A, Rankin J, Findlay J, Deschenes J, Kreaden D, Armstrong A, Kapur B: Effect of propylthiouracil in the treatment of alcoholic liver disease (abstract). Gastroenterology, 73:1237, 1978

34. French SW: Succinic dehydrogenase: Histochemical "shift" in hepatic lobular distribution induced by ethanol. Lab Invest 13:1051–1056, 1964

35. French SW: Liver dehydrogenase activity in chronic alcoholism. Arch Pathol 69: 303–313, 1960

36. Konttinen A, Härtel G, Louhija A: Multiple serum enzyme analyses in chronic alcoholics. Acta Med Scand 188:256–264, 1970

37. Remmer H, Albrecht D, Kappus H: Lipid peroxidation in isolated hepatocytes from rats ingesting ethanol chronically. Naunyn-Schmiedebergs Arch Pharmacol 298: 107–113, 1977

38. Peters RL, Gay T, Reynolds TB: Post-jejunoileal bypass hepatic disease. Am J Clin Pathol 63:318–331, 1975

39. Peters RL: Patterns of hepatic morphology in jejunoileal bypass patients. Am J Clin Nutr 30:53–57, 1977

40. Marubbio AT Jr, Buchwald H, Schwartz MZ, Varco R: Hepatic lesions of central pericellular fibrosis in morbid obesity and after jejunoileal bypass. Am J Clin Pathol 66:684–691, 1976

41. Mezey E, Imbembo Al, Potter JJ, Rent KC, Lombardo R, Holt PR: Endogenous ethanol production and hepatic disease following jejunoileal bypass for morbid obesity. Am J Clin Nutr 28:1277–1283, 1975

42. Brunt PW, Kew MC, Scheuer PJ, Sherlock S, Studies in alcoholic liver disease in Britain. 1. Clinical and pathological patterns related to natural history. Gut 15:52–58, 1974

43. Schaffner F, Popper H: Alcoholic hepatitis in the spectrum of ethanol-induced liver injury. Scand J Gastroenterol [Suppl] 7: 69–78, 1970

44. Hall EM, Morgan WA: Progressive alcoholic cirrhosis. Arch Pathol 27:672–690, 1939

45. Phillip GB, Davidson CS: Acute hepatic insufficiency of the chronic alcoholic. Arch Intern Med 94:585–603, 1954

46. Edmondson HA, Peters RL, Frankel HH, Borowsky S: The early stage of liver injury in the alcoholic. Medicine 46:119–129, 1967

liams AO, Immunofluorescent localization of human α-fetoprotein in fetal and neonatal livers and cultured cells from hepatocellular carcinoma. Br J Cancer 25:343–349, 1971

100. Lehmann F-G, Lehmann D, Martini GA: α-Fetoprotein. Isolierung und kristallisation aus menschlichem plasma. Clin Chim Acta 33:197–206, 1971

101. Ruoslahti E, Seppälä M: Studies of carcinofetal proteins. III. Development of a radioimmunoassay for α-fetoprotein. Demonstration of α-fetoprotein in serum of healthy human adults. Int J Cancer 8:374–383, 1971

102. Peyrol S, Grimaud J-A, Pirson Y, Cayvialle J-A, Touillon C, Lambert R: Ultrastructural immunoenzymatic study of α-fetoprotein-producing cells in the human fetal liver. J Histochem Cytochem 25:432–438, 1977

103. Sugisaki T, Sakaguchi T: Intracytoplasmic tonofilaments: A desmosome-like structure in the mouse fetal liver cell. J. Ultrastruct Res 59:178–184, 1977

104. Miller AI, Moral MD, Schiff ER: Presence of serum α-fetoprotein in alcoholic hepatitis. Gastroenterology 68:381–383, 1975

105. Meshkinpour H, Wepsic HT, Schmalhorst WR: Alpha-1 fetoprotein and alcoholic hepatitis. Am J Dig Dis 19:709–713, 1974

106. Nayak NC, Ramalingaswami V: Childhood cirrhosis. Edited by FF Becker: The Liver. Normal and Abnormal Functions, Part B. New York, Marcel Dekker, 1975, pp 851–883

107. Husby G, Strickland RG, Caldwell JL, Williams RC Jr: Localization of T and B cells and alpha fetoprotein in hepatic biopsies from patients with liver disease. J Clin Invest 56:1198–1209, 1975

108. Kern WH, Mikkelsen WP, Turrill FL: The significance of hyaline necrosis in liver biopsies. Surg Gynecol Obstet 129:749–754, 1969

109. Mikkelsen WP, Therapeutic portacaval shunt. Arch Surg 108:302–305, 1974

110. Rouselot LM, Burchell AR, Panke WF, Lepone M, Medline A, Popper H: Prognostic value of liver biopsy in the electively shunted patient (abstract). Gastroenterology 64:165, 1973

111. Lang AP, Patel S, Langer B, Stone R, Phillips MJ: Preoperative liver biopsy and the prognosis of portosystemic shunt surgery (abstract). Lab Invest 38:353, 1978

112. Greenwood SM, Leffler CT, Minkowitz S: The increased mortality rate of open liver biopsy in alcoholic hepatitis. Surg Gynecol Obstet 134:600–604, 1972

113. Sherlock S: Chronic hepatitis. Gut 15:581–597, 1974

114. Goldberg SJ, Mendenhall CL, Connell AM, Chedid-A: "Nonalcoholic" chronic hepatitis in the alcoholic. Gastroenterology 72:598–604, 1977

115. Galambos JT: Chronic active hepatitis and ethanol-A form of drug hepatitis (abstract). Gastroenterology 68:1075, 1975

116. Goldberg S, Mendenhall CL, Connell A: Chronic active liver disease (CALD) in association with chronic alcoholism (CA) (abstract). Gastroenterology 68:1080, 1970

117. Galambos JT: Natural history of alcoholic hepatitis: III. Histological changes. Gastroenterology 63:1026–1035, 1972

118. Christoffersen P, Nielsen K: Histological changes in human liver biopsies from chronic alcoholics. Acta Pathol Microbiol Scand [Sect A], 80:557–565, 1972

119. Schaffner F, Loebel A, Weiner HA, Barka T: Hepatocellular cytoplasmic changes in acute alcoholic hepatitis. JAMA 183:343–346, 1963

120. Christoffersen P, Juhl E: Mallory bodies in liver biopsies with fatty changes but no cirrhosis. Acta Pathol Microbiol Scand [Sect A] 79:201–207, 1971

121. Sorrell MF, Leevy CM: Lymphocyte transformation and alcoholic liver injury. Gastroenterology 63:1020–1025, 1972

122. Kawanishi H: Morphologic association of lymphocytes with hepatocytes in chronic liver disease. Arch Pathol Lab Med 101:286–290, 1977

123. Cossel L, Mahnke PF, Schwarzer R: "Killer" lymphocytes in action? Light and electron microscopical findings in orthotopic liver homografts. Virchows Arch [Pathol Anat Histol] 364:179–190, 1974

124. Sanchez-Tapias J, Thomas HC, Sherlock S: Lymphocyte populations in liver biopsy specimens from patients with chronic liver disease. Gut 18:472–475, 1977

125. French SW, Burbige E, Luehrs D, Tarder G, Denton T, Harkin C, Bourke E: Percent T and B cells in the liver in alcoholic hepatitis (abstract). Am J Pathol 86:20, 1977

126. Lundy L, Raaf JH, Deakins S, Wanebo HJ, Jacobs DA, Lee T, Jacobwitz D, Spear C, Oettgen HF: The acute and chronic effects of alcohol on the human immune system. Surg Gynecol Obstet 141:212–218, 1975

127. Bernstein IM, Webster KH, Williams RC

Jr, Strickland RG: Reduction in circulating T lymphocytes in alcoholic liver disease. Lancet 2:488, 1974

128. Berenyi MR, Strars B, Avila L: T rosettes in alcoholic cirrhosis of the liver. JAMA 232:44–46, 1975

129. Wybran J, Goraerts A, Fudenberg HH: Alcoholic liver disease and the immune system. JAMA 232:57–58, 1975

130. Zagury D, Bernard J, Thierness N: Isolation and characterization of individual functionally reactive cytotoxic T lymphocytes: Conjugation, killing and recycling at the single cell level. Eur J Immunol 5:818–822, 1975

131. Kakumu S, Leevy CM: Lymphocyte cytotoxicity in alcoholic hepatitis. Gastroenterology 72:594–597, 1977

132. Paronetto F, Lieber CS: Cytotoxicity of lymphocytes in experimental alcoholic liver injury in the baboon. Proc Soc Exp Biol Med 153:495–497, 1976

133. Zetterman RK, Luisada-Opper A, Leevy CM: Alcoholic hepatitis cell-mediated immunological response to alcoholic hyaline. Gastroenterology 70:382–384, 1976

134. Wojciech KP: Cytodestructive mechanisms provoked by lymphocytes. Am J Med 61:1–8, 1976

135. Van Waes L, Lieber CS: Prognostic significance of pericentral venous sclerosis in alcoholic fatty liver (abstract). Fed Proc 36:332 1977

136. Popper H: The pathogenesis of alcoholic cirrhosis. Edited by MM Fisher and JG Rankin: Alcohol and the Liver. New York, Plenum Press, 1976, pp 289–307

137. Patrick RS: Alcohol as a stimulus to hepatic fibrogenesis. J Alcoholism 8:13, 1973

138. Feinman L, Lieber CS: Hepatic collagen metabolism: Effect of alcohol consumption in rats and baboons. Science 176:795–796, 1972

139. Mezey E, Potter JJ, Maddrey WC: Hepatic collagen proline hydroxylase activity in alcoholic liver disease. Clin Chim Acta 68:313–320, 1976

140. Popper H, Kent G: Fibrosis in chronic liver disease. Clin Gastroenterol 4:315–332, 1975

141. Zetterman R, Chen T, Leevy CM: Alcoholic hyaline and hepatic fibrosis. Clin Res 22:559A, 1974

142. Chen TSN, Leevy CM: Collagen biosynthesis in liver disease of the alcoholic. J Lab Clin Med 85:103–112, 1975

143. Ehrlich HP, Ross R, Bronstein P: Effects of antimicrotubular agents on the secretion of collagen. J Cell Biol 62:390–405, 1974

144. Kershenobich D, Uribe M, Suarez GI, Rojkind M: Treatment of cirrhosis with Colchicine: A randomized trial. Gastroenterology 70:A-128/986, 1976

145. Harris ED, Krane SM: Effects of Colchicine on collagenase in cultures of rheumatoid synovium. Arthritis Rheum 41:669–684, 1971

146. Mata JM, Villarreal E, Kershenobich D, Rojkind M: Serum free-proline in patients with chronic liver disease. Gastroenterology 68:1265–1269, 1975

147. Rojkin M, Kershenobich D: Hepatic fibrosis. Edited by H Popper and F Schaffner: Progress in Liver Diseases. Vol. V. New York, Grune & Stratton, 1976, pp 294–310

148. Morgan MY, Sherlock S: Sex-related differences among 100 patients with alcoholic liver disease. Br Med J 1:939–941, 1977

149. Bailey RJ, Krasner N, Eddleston ALWF, Williams R, Tee DEH, Doniach D, Kennedy LA, Batchelor JR: Histocompatibility antigens, autoantibodies and immunoglobulins in alcoholic liver disease. Br Med J 2:727–729, 1976

150. Gabuzda GJ: Nutrition and liver disease. Med Clin North Am 54:1455–1472, 1970

151. Patek AJ, Bowry SC, Sabesin SM: Minimal hepatic changes in rats fed alcohol and a high casein diet. Arch Pathol Lab Med 100:12–24, 1976

152. Rubin E, Lieber CS: Fatty liver, alcoholic hepatitis and cirrhosis produced by alcohol in baboons. N Engl J Med 290:128–135, 1974

153. Wells R: Prednisolone and testosterone proprionate in cirrhosis of the liver. A controlled trial. Lancet 2:1416–1419, 1960

154. Cachera R, Darnis F: Effect de la cortisone dans les cirrhoses alcooliques due foire (étude clinique, brologique et histologique). Sem Hôp Paris 28:1085–1095, 1952

155. Zoeckler SJ: Cortisone in portal cirrhosis: A controlled study. Gastroenterology 26:878–886, 1954

156. Williams R, Billings BH: Action of steroid therapy in jaundice. Lancet 2:392–396, 1961

157. Cain GD, Mayer G, Jones EA: Augmentation of albumin but not fibrinogenesis synthesis by corticosteroids in patients with hepatocellular disease. J Clin Invest 49:2198–2204, 1970

158. Lesesne HR, Bozymiski EM, Fallon HJ:

Treatment of alcoholic hepatitis with encephalopathy. Comparison of prednisolone with caloric supplements. Gastroenterology 79:169–173, 1978

159. Porter HP, Simon FT, Pope CR, Volwiler W, Fenster LF: Corticosteroid therapy in severe alcoholic hepatitis. N Engl J Med 284:1350–1355, 1971

160. Campra JL, Hamlin EM, Kirshbaum RJ, Oliver M, Redeker AG, Reynolds TB: Prednisone therapy of acute alcoholic hepatitis. Report of a controlled trial. Ann Intern Med 79:625–631, 1973

161. Copenhagen Study Group for Liver Diseases: Sex, ascites and alcoholism in survival of patients with cirrhosis: Effect of prednisone. N Engl J Med 291:271–273, 1974

162. Schumaker JB, Resnick RH, Galambos JT, et al: Steroids in alcoholic hepatitis: Survival related to biopsy feasibility (abstract). Gastroenterology 66:778, 1974

163. Schlichting P, Juhl E, Poulsen H, et al: Alcoholic hepatitis superimposed on cirrhosis: Clinical significance and effect of long term prednisone treatment. Scand J Gastroenterol 11:305–312, 1976

164. Maddrey WC, Boitnott KJ, Bedine MS et al: Corticosteroid treatment of alcoholic liver disease: A controlled trial (abstract). Gastroenterology 72:1171, 1977

165. Blitzer BL, Mutchnick MG, Joshi PH, Phillips MM, Fessel JM, Conn HO: Adrenocorticosteroid therapy in alcoholic hepatitis. A prospective double-blind randomized study. Am J Dig Dis 22:477–484, 1977

166. Depew WT, Boyer TD, Omata M, Redeker AG, Reynolds TB: Double-blind controlled trial of corticosteroid therapy in severe, alcoholic hepatitis with encephalopathy (abstract). Clin Res 26:150A, 1978

167. Conn HO: Steroid treatment of alcoholic hepatitis. The yeas and the nays. Gastroenterology 74:319–320, 1978

168. Minim ME, Bowetta LA: Collagen synthesis and turnover in the growing rat under the influence of methyl-prednisone. Proc Soc Exp Biol Med 117:618–623, 1964

169. Boitnott JK, Maddrey WC: Histologic correlations in alcoholic liver disease (abstract). Lab Invest 34:3–4, 1976

170. Leevy CM: Hard liquor and cirrhosis. Alcoholic cirrhosis and other toxic hepatopathies. Edited by A Engel and T Larsson: Skandia International Symposium. Stockholm, Nordiska Bakhandelns Forlag, 1970, pp 283–295

171. Lieber CS: Alcoholic fatty liver: Its pathogenesis and precursor role for hepatitis and cirrhosis. Panminerva Med 18:346–358, 1976

172. Edmonson HA, Peters RL, Hill KR: Acute alcoholic hepatitis. Br Med J 2:1113–1119, 1961

173. Deering TB, Dickson ER, Fleming CR, Geall MG, McCall JT, Baggenstoss AH: Effect of D-pencillamine or copper retention in patients with primary biliary cirrhosis. Gastroenterology 82:1208–1212, 1977

174. Jain S, McGee JOD, Scheuer PJ: A controlled trial of D-penicillamine in primary biliary cirrhosis and chronic active hepatitis (abstract). Digestion 14:523, 1976

175. Long RG, Scheuer PJ, Sherlock S: Presentation and course of asymptomatic primary biliary cirrhosis. Gastroenterology 72:1204–1207, 1977

176. Feldman G, Maurice M, Sapn C, Benhamon JP: Inhibition by colchicine of fibrinogen translocation in hepatocytes. J Cell Biol 67:237–243, 1975

177. Rojkind M: Inhibition of liver fibrosis by L-azetidine-s-carboxylic acid in rats treated with carbon tetrachloride. J Clin Invest 52:2451–2456, 1973

178. Israel Y, Videla L, Bernstein J: Liver hypermetabolic state after chronic ethanol consumption, hormonal interrelations and pathogenic implications. Fed Proc 34:2052–2059, 1975

179. Bernstein J, Videla L, Israel Y: Metabolic alterations produced by the liver by chronic ethanol administration: Change related to energetic parameters of the cell. Biochem J 134:515–521, 1973

180. Orrego H, Carmichael FT, Phillips MJ, Kalant H, Khanna J, Israel Y: Protection by propylthiouracil against carbon tetrachloride-induced liver damage. Proc Natl Acad Sci USA 71:821–827, 1976

181. Clower BR, Douglas BH, Carrier O Jr: Protection by reserpine of carbon tetrachloride-induced hepatic necrosis. Eur J Pharmacol 2:276–280, 1968

182. Emlen W, Segal DW, Mandell AJ: Thyroid state: Effects on pre- and postsynaptic central noradrenergic mechanisms. Science 175:79–81, 1972

183. Hartley EJ, McNeill JH: The effect of calcium on cardiac phosphorylase activation,

contractile force and cyclic AMP in euthyroid and hyperthyroid rat hearts. Can J Physiol Pharmacol 54:590–595, 1976

184. Engström G, Svensson TH, Waldeck B: Thyroxine and brain catecholamines: Increased transmitter synthesis and increased receptor sensitivity. Brain Res 77:471–483, 1974

185. Engström G, Strömbom U, Svensson TH, Waldeck B: Brain monoamine synthesis and receptor sensitivity after single or repeated administration of thyroxine. J Neural Transm 37:1–10, 1975

186. Karlberg BE, Hendriksson KG, Andersson RGG: Cyclic adenosine 3′, 5′-monophosphate concentration in plasma, adipose tissue and skeletal muscle in normal subjects and in patients with hyper- and hypothyroidism. J Clin Endocrinol Metab 39:96–101, 1974

Chapter 32

Hepatic Morphologic Changes After Jejunoileal Bypass

By ROBERT L. PETERS, M.D.

SURGICAL SHORTENING of the gastrointestinal system for the treatment of the morbidly obese patient apparently had its genesis as a result of the experimental work of Kremen et al.[1] and clinical observations of several alert surgeons.[2-4] Payne and associates in 1963 reported a series of patients upon whom jejunocolic bypass (JCB) had been performed as the "last resort" treatment of morbid obesity.[5] Subsequently, however, the seriousness of electrolyte problems, hematologic disorders, steatorrhea, hypoproteinemia, and intussusception were often profound, and the recognition of several cases of fatal acute liver disease[6-8] resulted in modification of the procedure, culminating in the jejunoileal bypass (JIB). The JIB operation, initially consisting of anastomosing the proximal 14 inches of jejunum to the terminal 4 inches of ileum, has undergone several minor modifications but all have resulted in quantitatively and qualitatively similar residual absorptive surfaces. The JIB operation evolved when two of Payne's JCB patients responded well after revision of the original JCB operation to the less severe JIB.[5] As might be anticipated, electrolyte and other disturbances were less pronounced, although weight loss was less profound. Reports of hepatic diseases associated with JIB were slow to appear; however, in 1969 Wills reported the development of cirrhosis in 1 of 50 JIB patients and several instances of fatty liver. Since all patients did not receive follow-up biopsies[9] and the ultimate outcome of the single patient considered to have cirrhosis was unstated, the significance of Wills' findings was uncertain. The histologic pattern of the liver of 4 of 25 JIB patients "deteriorated"; in a series reported a year later, 3 of the 4 were the "complete failures" of the group.[10] It is uncertain what the ultimate outcomes of the patients were. Whereas hepatic fatty change became severe in the first year after JIB, most patients seemed to improve after the first year. Furthermore, some patients who were considered to have "early cirrhosis" at original surgery did not appear to have progression of their liver disease. Review of the photomicrographs of supposedly cirrhotic lesions makes clear that the term "cirrhosis" was used quite loosely, both for the lesions so designated at the time of bypass and for those so classified at follow-up.

The first well-documented fatal case of cirrhosis following JIB was described in 1972.[11] The report was followed by several that indicated that fatal liver disease or liver disease of sufficient severity to require reestablishment of gut continuity may follow JIB surgery for obesity.[12-19]

From the University of Southern California, School of Medicine, Los Angeles, California.

Funded in part by John Wesley Attending Staff #6001.

From January 1973 to March 1978, 20 liver biopsies or segments of liver taken at autopsy representing post-JIB patients with serious liver disease, either terminating fatally or requiring reestablishment of gut continuity, were submitted to the pathology department of the University of Southern California Liver Unit (USC-Liver Unit); 9 were fatal cases. These patients represent a numerator extracted from a completely unknown denominator of obese patients subjected to JIB. In addition, the slides of the pre- and post-JIB liver biopsy series previously reported by Kern et al.[20] have been reviewed.

LIVER IN MORBID OBESITY, PREBYPASS

The liver of the hyperobese patient prior to bypass is not usually normal; between 60% and 84% have a fatty liver.[19-25] According to Salmon et al.[22] the fatty change is "severe" in 8.5% and "moderate" in 27.7%, but Kern et al. found that 34% had fat in more than half the hepatocytes.[9] The cause of the fatty liver is unclear, but the finding is consistent with the impression that the proportion of protein to the total caloric intake must be critical to prevent fat accumulation in hepatocytes. The distribution of the fat in the prebypass liver is inconstant. Some patients have irregular involvement from lobule to lobule, about 75% have diffuse involvement, most of the remaining have perivenular deposition, a few have periportal fatty change usually in an irregular fashion, and some have spotty, poorly defined foci of fatty change (Fig. 1).

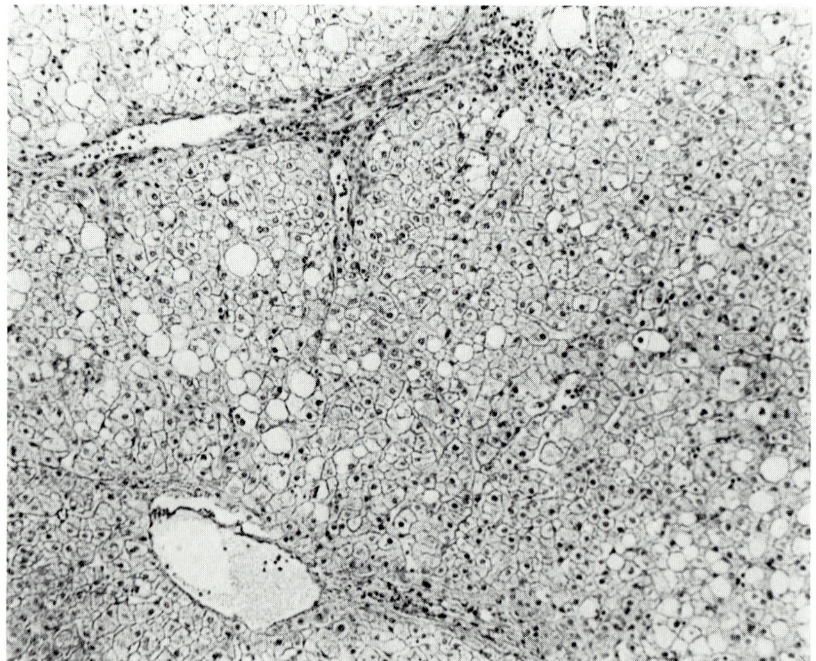

FIG. 1—Fairly scanty irregularly distributed foci of hepatocellular fat in the prebypass liver. Note also that the hepatocytes are large and watery, the pattern of the plates is poorly defined (72-11509, hemotoxylin and eosin stain, × 75).

In addition to the fat, minimal perivenular intrasinusoidal collagen[12] has been reported in up to 8.6% of livers of morbidly obese patients.[24] Kern et al.[25] reported that of 151 patients upon whom JIB was later performed, 3 had cirrhosis and 3 had portal fibrosis,[9] all in the absence of alcoholism. No relationship has been recognized between the amount of prebypass hepatic lipid and the development of post-JIB serious liver disease. Similarly the cases reported to have fibrosis or cirrhosis before bypass have not developed progressive disease.

The hepatocytes not containing fat in livers of many obese patients are large, polyhedral, and hydropic. Sometimes the arrangement of the liver cell plates is difficult to identify (Fig. 1). Similar nonspecific hydropic hepatocytic changes are often seen in livers of diabetics, as well as in many other patients, but the occurrence is somewhat greater in the morbidly obese.

Although mention has been made of portal lymphoid hyperplasia, this rather nonspecific response is no more common than in nonobese patients.

CHANGES OCCURRING AFTER BYPASS

Fatty Liver

The most consistent hepatic pattern in the post-JIB period is fatty liver. The maximal hepatic fat content was attained during the first 5 months, decreasing thereafter until about 3 years after bypass when the incidence of fatty change and amount of fat deposited were similar to that found preoperatively.[22] Over 95% of patients have fatty liver in the first 5 months after JIB. Apparently the increased mobilization of depot fat is partly responsible for the accumulation of lipid in the liver, and yet the morbidly obese individual who loses weight by fasting deposits very little fat in his liver. An excess in total body fat is apparently necessary for the accumulation of hepatic fat in JIB patients. JIB performed on normal rats results in little hepatic fatty change, but JIB performed on a "fat rat" is associated with a severely fatty liver.[26]

During the period of fat accumulation in the liver, serum amino acid levels, including essential amino acids, drop precipitously. The low serum amino acid and high hepatic lipid combination are characteristic of protein deficiency states such as kwashiorkor.[14] With passage of time and diminution of hepatic lipid, serum amino acids regain normal levels.

Postbypass Asymptomatic Hepatocytic Degeneration and Sinusoidal Collagenosis

Patients with fatty liver who are dying as a result of hepatic failure, whether the failure follows JIB or alcoholism, have changes beyond simple fatty change. Degenerative change in the fatty hepatocytes is invariably present when there is hepatic failure at the fatty stage of liver disease. Patients with neither symptoms nor laboratory changes suggesting liver disease may have alarming changes of hepatocytes that include a foamy degenerative appearance of perivenular hepatocytes, with breakdown of cell membranes and with cytoplasmic condensation. Thin, nearly inconspicuous collagen fibers may be deposited in perivenular spaces of Disse[27] (Fig. 2). The hepatocellular changes

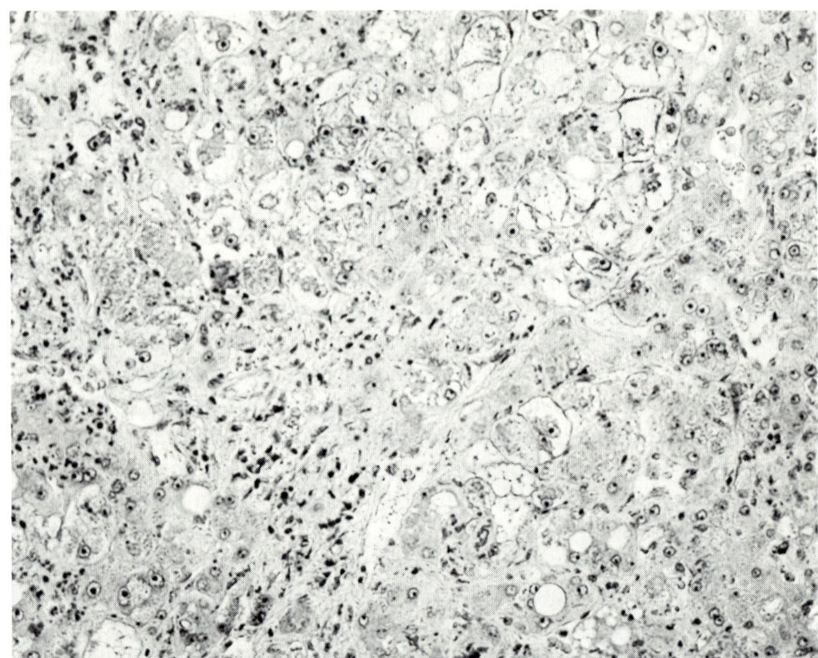

FIG. 4—Alcoholic hyaline necrosis, neutrophils in intrasinusoidal collagen in JIB patient at time of death, 9 months post-JIB, despite surgical reconstruction at 6 months (JWS365-73 H&E, × 125).

disorder despite abstinence from alcohol before and/or after JIB. Alcoholic hyaline has not usually been found in patients who recover but may be found in many patients who progress further into hepatic failure and death. If alcoholic hyaline necrosis is severe, there may be a heavy infiltration of neutrophils (Fig. 4). The similarity of these pathologic changes to those of patients with alcoholic liver disease is striking.[11,24,27,28,30] Alcoholic hyaline, however, does not occur in every patient who dies in hepatic failure from JIB any more than it does in all patients who die from alcoholic liver disease. Similarly, the hepatic neutrophilic infiltrate described in some patients dying after JIB[16] and in some patients dying of acute alcoholic liver disease[30] is only found in a minority of such patients. The most consistent feature found in livers of patients dying of either acute alcoholic liver disease or acute JIB hepatic disorder is the degenerative appearance of perivenular hepatocytes with fine vesiculation and disappearance of the cell membrane and the delicate deposition of fine collagen fibers in spaces of Disse and perivenular sinusoids.[16,24,27,30] The onset of these changes may be quite sudden, developing in a 2 month period even 8 months after JIB (Fig. 5A and B).

Tenuous Hepatic Reserve

A little-recognized facet of post-JIB liver disease may be the tendency for necrosis and hepatic failure to develop in the post-JIB patient when an ostensibly nonhepatic stress has occurred. Similarly, acute hepatic failure may apparently be precipitated in the alcoholic patient as a result of surgery, pneu-

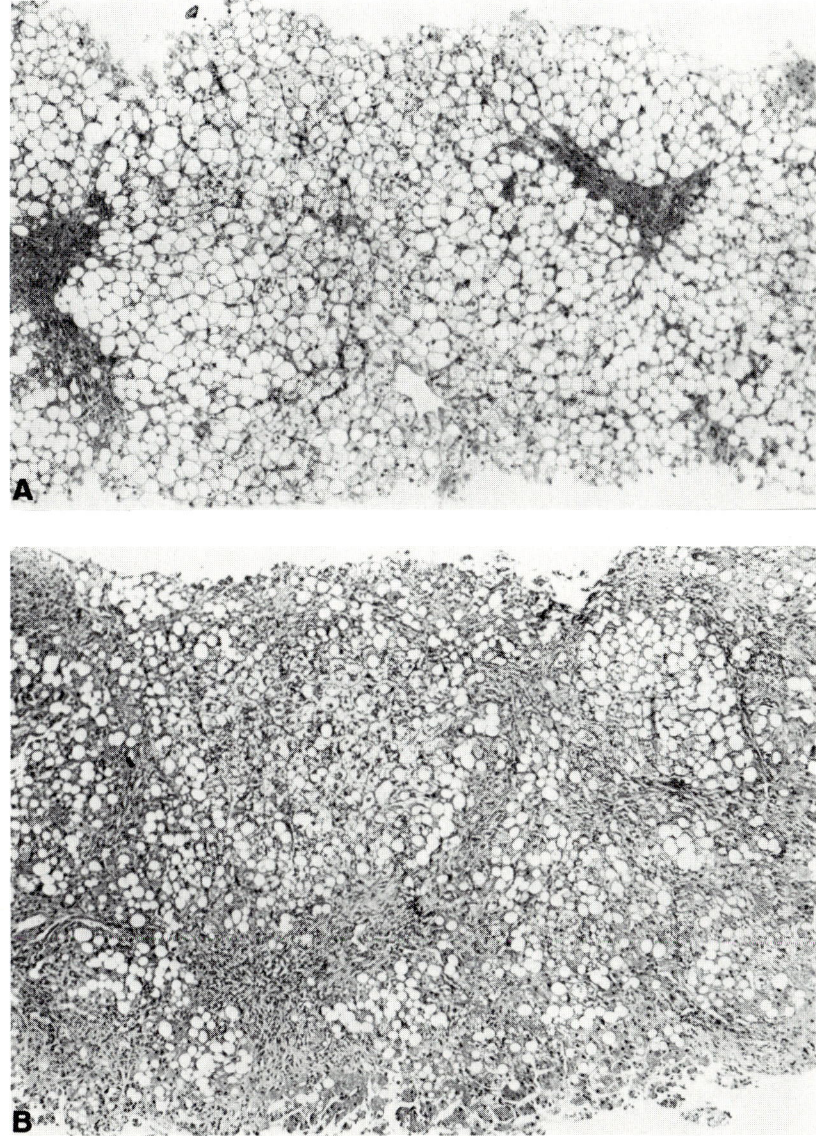

FIG. 5—(A) JIB patient 7 months after operation. Note intact lobular architecture (LUS416-78, 3121-76 H&E, × 37). (B) Two months later (9 months postoperatively) the liver has early cirrhotic changes (LUS416-76, 5019-76, H&E, × 37).

monia, or other traumatic events. One post-JIB patient developed hepatic failure and died in hepatic coma following a perforated colon. Although a biopsy taken 8 days before death (Fig. 6A) showed a small amount of fat and little else, at autopsy there was alcoholic hyaline in the perivenular areas with only minimal collagen deposition in the space of Disse (Fig. 6B and C).[27] There has been too little cumulative experience with the post-JIB patient regarding their ability to withstand stress.

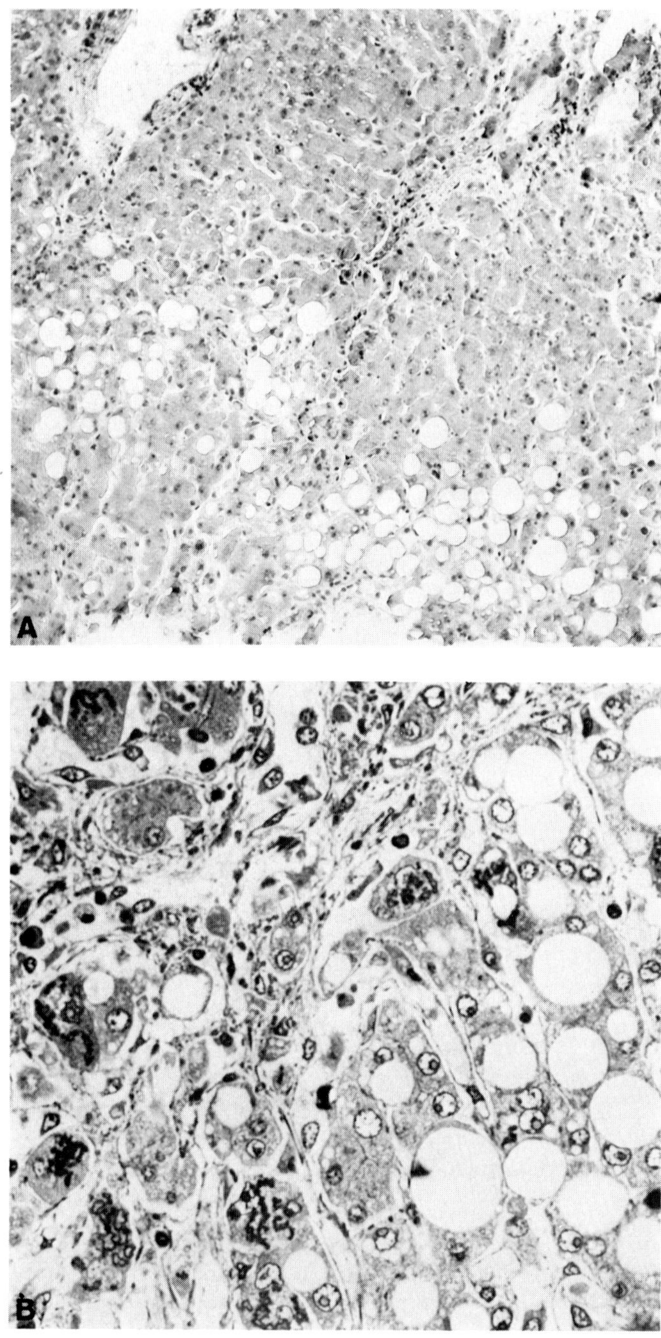

FIG. 6—(A) Liver of JIB patient who entered hospital with perforated colon 2 years post-JIB. There is only a small amount of fat (JWS3766-75 H&E, × 75). (B) Same patient as (A) 8 days later at autopsy. Note the alcoholic hyaline and sinusoidal collagen (JWS3766-75 araldite at 2 μ, H&E, × 240). (C) Higher power of (B) shows the fine character of collagen (long arrow) and the alcoholic hyaline (short arrow) (JWS3766-75 araldite at 2 μ, H&E, × 500).

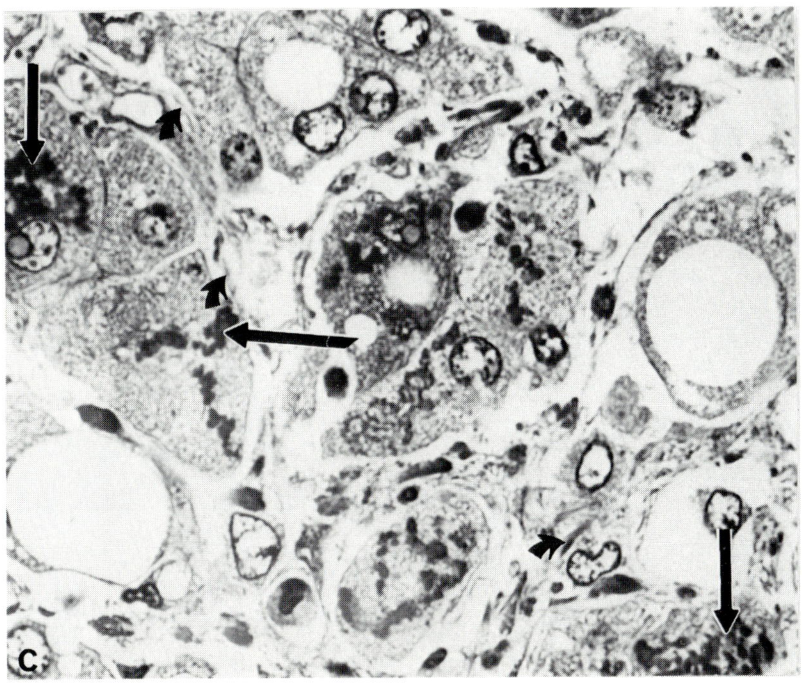

Insidious Cirrhosis

There has been considerable concern over the few cases of cirrhosis discovered accidentally in patients who have had JIB surgery more than a year earlier but who developed no signs of liver disease. The cirrhosis in such patients has usually been fatty, with small, poorly defined nodules and thin, arachnoid, fibrous septa (Fig. 7). The cirrhosis has been identified in patients from whom liver biopsies were taken purely for follow-up purposes. Three such patients have been studied at the USC Liver Unit, and 2 have been reported.[27] Marubbio et al. reported 3 such patients found among 88 studied at 2 years post-JIB,[24] and Salmon et al. reported 1 patient who developed cirrhosis not recognized until a routine follow-up biopsy was taken nearly 6 years after JIB.[22] The percentage of post-JIB patients who have had annual biopsies subsequent to the first postoperative year is unclear, however. Since most of the patients are asymptomatic with respect to liver disease, a true incidence would require biopsy, peritoneoscopy, or wedged hepatic vein pressure. One patient developed acute hepatic failure, without prior symptoms of liver disease, 2½ years after JIB and was found to have advanced cirrhosis at autopsy[31] (Fig. 8). The possibility that many other JIB patients may develop the manifestations of their cirrhosis many years after the event is a real one and the extent of the problem is unknown.

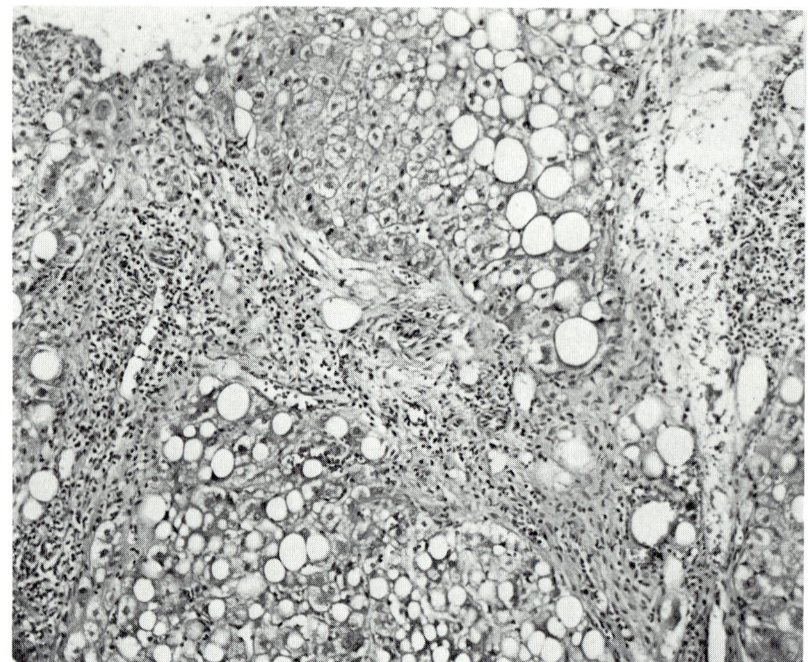

FIG. 7—Cirrhosis found incidentally in post-JIB patients 24 months after bypass surgery (JWS4327-75 H&E, × 75).

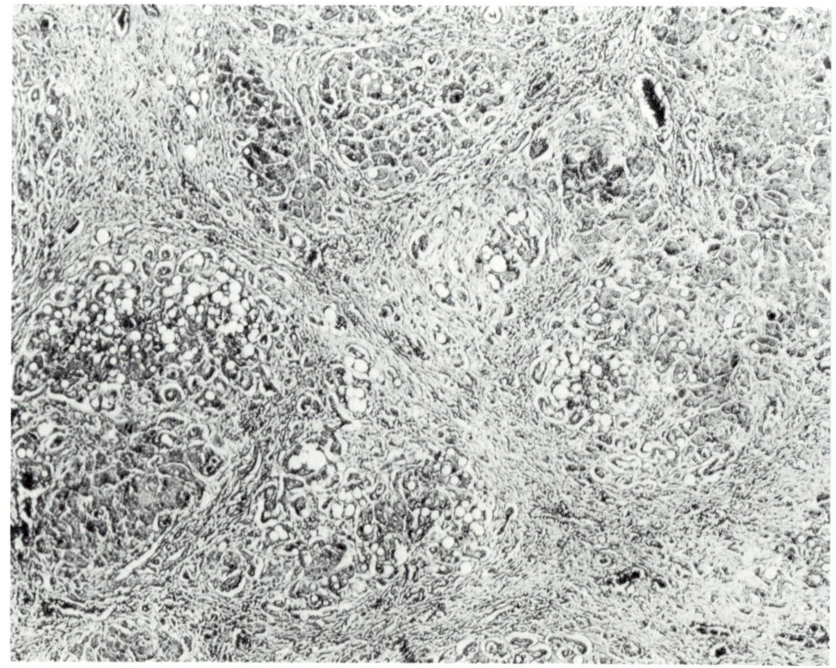

FIG. 8—Advanced cirrhosis at autopsy of patient who had JIB 22 months earlier but only terminal signs of liver disease. Note the invasive character of collagen (LUS1664-77, H&E, × 37).

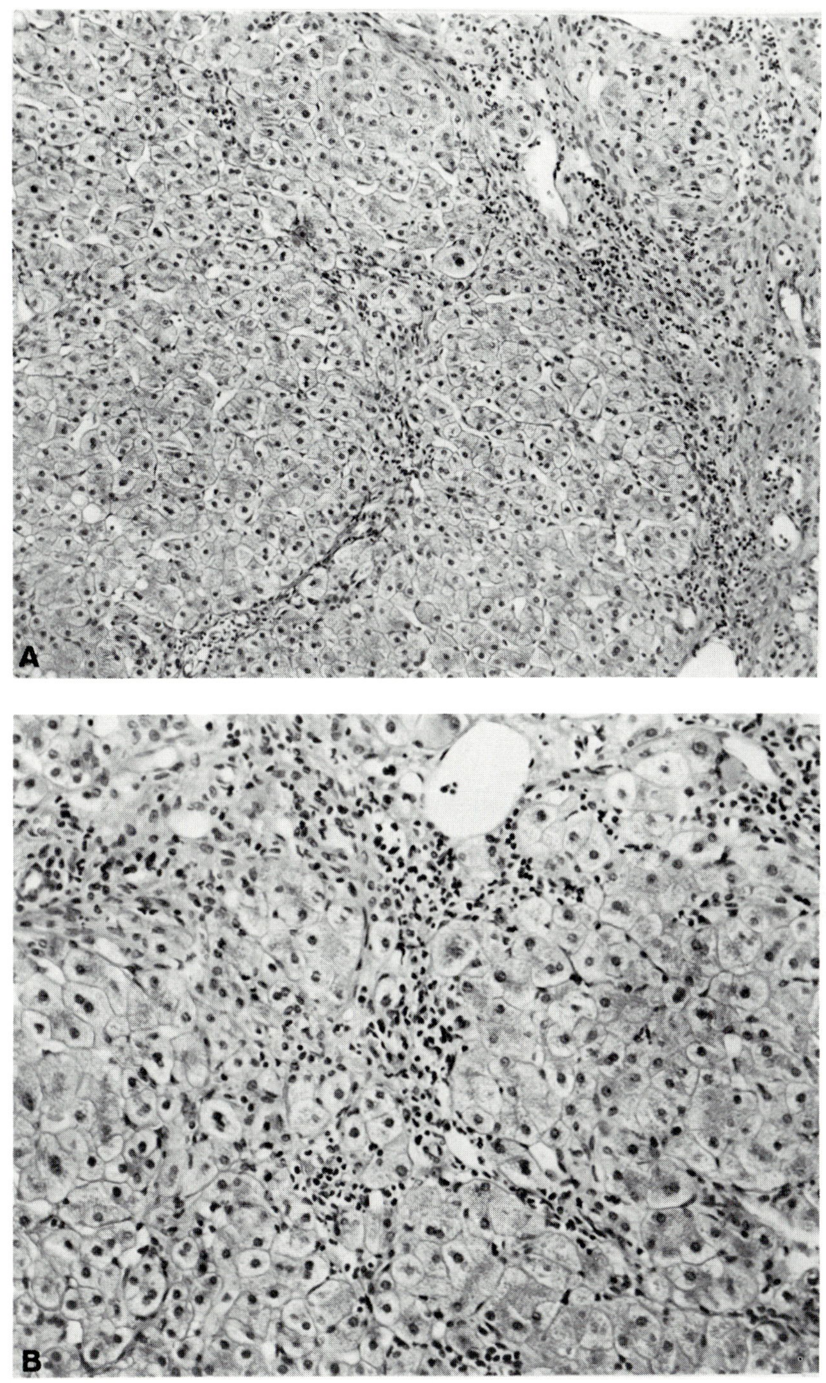

FIG. 9—(A) Cirrhosis with chronic active hepatitis (70-21976 H&E, × 76). (B) Note clusters of lymphocytes within parenchyma (70-21976 H&E, × 125).

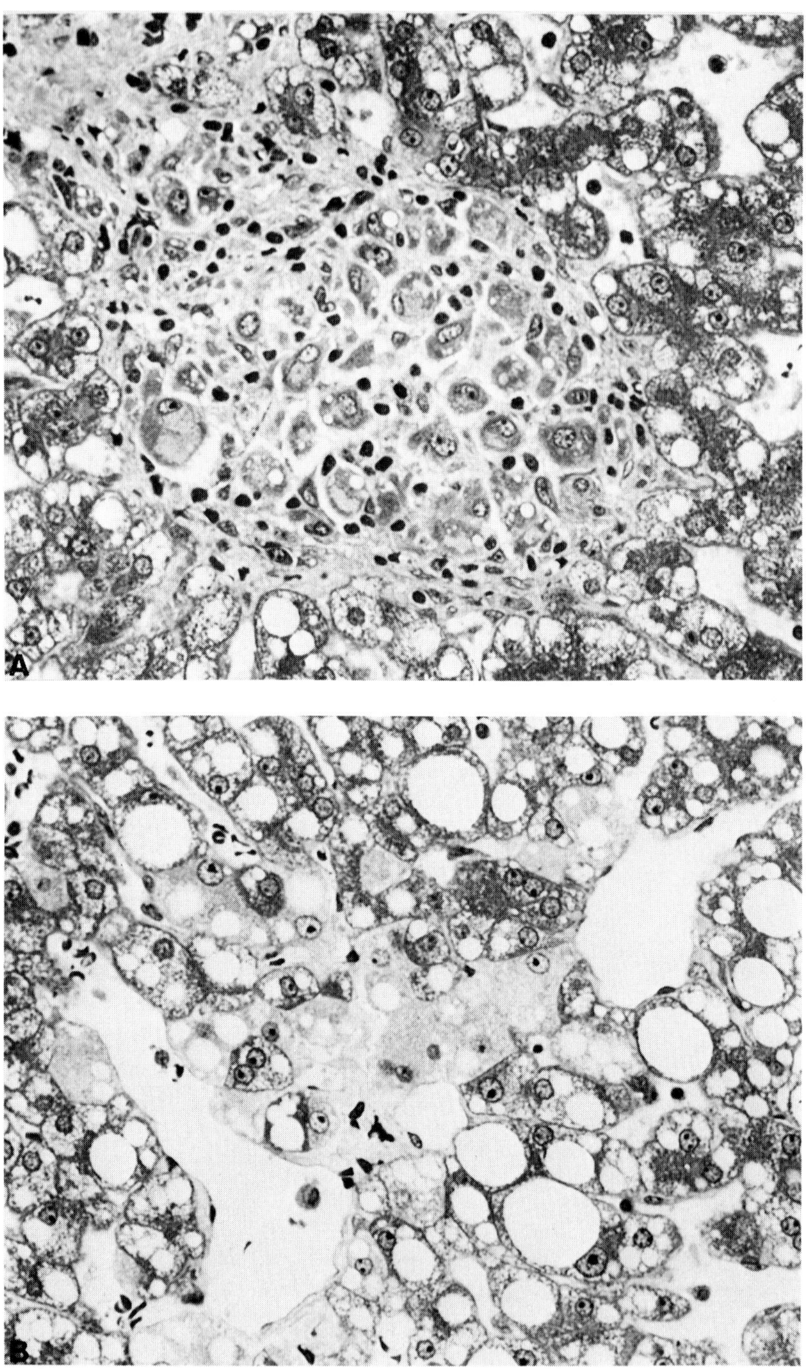

FIG. 10—(A) Granulomas, nontuberculous type, near terminal hepatic vein. Granulomas were not found in biopsy taken at time of bypass (LUS725-78 methacrylate at 2 μ, H&E, × 240). (B) Foamy sinusoidal histiocytes apparently antedating granuloma formation (Methacrylate, 2 μ × 250).

ADDITIONAL HEPATIC CHANGES

Chronic Active Hepatitis

At the USC Liver Unit, 1 patient was admitted for vitamin deficiency and ascites 15 months after a JIB, at which time her liver had been said to be normal. At reconstruction surgery, she had a portal vein pressure of 15 mm Hg above inferior vena caval pressure. A biopsy of liver showed cirrhosis with chronic active hepatitis (Fig. 9A and B). HB_sAg, smooth muscle antibodies, and lupus erythmatosus preparations were negative. Whereas this could be coincidental chronic active hepatitis, perhaps related to non-A, non-B hepatitis the patient's ascites did nonetheless subside with reestablishment of gut continuity.

Granulomas

Tuberculosis was first described in post-JIB patients by Wills.[9] Several other reports have appeared.[19,32-37] Whether the increased numbers of granulomas that seem to be found in liver biopsies from JIB patients are a result of tuberculosis is not clear. Some are histologically unlike tuberculosis (Fig. 10A and B). The granulomatous foci occur in patients without symptoms or changes of JIB liver disease. Halverson et al. report that 7% of JIB patients develop noncaseating granulomas.[19]

STATUS OF JEJUNOILEAL BYPASS PATIENTS

Unfortunately, the JIB is not the panacea for the treatment of obesity. Certain complications may develop, of which serious liver disease is the most important, perhaps leading to the patient's death. The hepatic lesion closely mimics alcoholic liver disease and could serve as a model for the study of this disease.

Although newer surgical procedures may negate the need for the JIB treatment of obesity, the clinician should consider liver biopsies at regular intervals, probably every 6 months, in JIB patients in order to avoid the development of insidious cirrhosis.

REFERENCES

1. Kremen AN, Linner JH, Nelson CH: Experimental evaluation of the nutritional importance of the proximal and distal small intestine. Ann Surg 140:439–498, 1954
2. Booth CC: The metabolic effects of intestinal resection in man. Postgrad Med J 37:725–739, 1961
3. Meyers HW: Acute superior mesenteric artery thrombosis: Recovery following extensive resection of small and large intestine. Arch Surg 53:298–303, 1946
4. Weckesser EC, Chinn AB, Scott MW, Prince JW: Extensive resection of small intestine. Am J Surg 78:706–714, 1949
5. Payne JH, DeWind LT, Commons RR: Metabolic observations in patients with jejunocolic shunts. Am J Surg 106:273–289, 1963
6. Bondary GF, Pisesky W: Complications of small intestinal short-circuiting for obesity. Arch Surg 94:707–716, 1967
7. Maxwell JG, Richards RC, Albo D: Fatty

degeneration of the liver after intestinal bypass for obesity. Am J Surg 116:648–652, 1968

8. Drenick EJ, Simmons F, Murphy JF: Effect on hepatic morphology of treatment of obesity by fasting, reducing diets and small bowel bypass. N Engl J Med 282:829–834, 1970

9. Wills GE: Jejuno-ileostomy for obesity: J Med Assoc Ga 58:436–461, 1969

10. Thompson RN, Meyerowitz BR: Liver changes after jejunoileal shunting for massive obesity. Surg Forum 21:366–367, 1970

11. McGill DB, Humphreys SR, Baggentoss AH, Dickson ER: Cirrhosis and death after jejunoileal shunt. Gastroenterology 63:872–877, 1972

12. Payne JH, DeWind L, Schwab CE, Kern WH: Surgical treatment of morbid obesity. Arch Surg 106:432–437, 1973

13. Brown RG, O'Leary JP, Woodward ER: Hepatic effects of jejunoileal bypass for morbid obesity. Am J Surg 127:53–58, 1974

14. Moxley RT, Pozefsky T, Lockwood DH: Protein nutrition and liver disease after jejunoileal bypass for morbid obesity. N Engl J Med 290:921–926, 1974

15. Mangle JC, Hoy W, Kim Y, Chopek M: Cirrhosis and death after jejunoileal shunt for obesity. Dig Dis 19:759–765, 1974

16. Peters RL, Gay T and Reynolds TB: Postjejunal bypass hepatic disease. Its similarity to alcoholic hepatic disease. Am J Clin Pathol 63:318–331, 1975

17. Spin FP, Weisman RE: Death from hepatic failure after jejunoileal anastomosis. Am J Surg 130:88–91, 1975

18. Jewel WR, Hermreck AS, Hardin CA: Complications of jejunoileal bypass for morbid obesity. Arch Surg 110:1039–1042, 1975

19. Halverson JD, Wise L, Wazna MF, Ballinger WF: Jejunoileal bypass for morbid obesity. A critical appraisal. Am J Med 64:461–475, 1978

20. Kern WH, Payne JH and DeWind L: Hepatic changes after small-intestinal bypass for morbid obesity. Am J Clin Pathol 61:763–768, 1974

21. Dean RH, Scott HW, Shull HJ, Gluck FW: Morbid obesity: Problems associated with operative management. Am J Clin Nutr 30:90–97, 1977

22. Salmon PA, Reedyk L: Fatty metamorphosis in patients with jejunoileal bypass. Surg Gynecol Obstet 141:75–84, 1975

23. Shibata HR, MacKenzie JR, Huang S-N: Morphological changes of the liver following small intestinal bypass for obesity. Arch Surg 103:229–257, 1971

24. Marubbio AT, Buchwald H, Schwartz MZ, Varco R: Hepatic lesions of central pericellular fibrosis in morbid obesity and after jejunoileal bypass. Am J Clin Pathol 66:684–691, 1976

25. Kern WH, Heger AH, Payne JH, DeWind LT: Fatty metamorphosis of the liver in morbid obesity. Arch Pathol 96:342–346, 1973

26. Madura JA, Csicsko JF, Cooney DR, Grossfeld JL: The "fat-rat" and new experimental jejunoileal bypass mode. J Pediatr Surg 10:349–352, 1975

27. Peters RL: Patterns of hepatic morphology in jejunoileal bypass patients. Am J Clin Nutr 30:53–57, 1977

28. Edmondson HA, Peters RL, Frankel HH, Borowsky S: The early stage of liver injury in the alcoholic. Medicine 46:119, 1967

29. Iber F and Cooper M: Jejunoileal bypass for the treatment of massive obesity. Prevalence, morbidity, and short and long term consequences. Am J Clin Nutr 30:4–15, 1977.

30. Edmondson HA, Peters RL, Reynolds TB, Kuzma OT: Sclerosing hyaline necrosis of the liver in the chronic alcoholic: A recognizable clinical syndrome. Ann Intern Med 59:646, 1963

31. Gay T, Peters RL: Death from hepatic failure as a late complication of jejunoileal bypass. (submitted)

32. Bray GA, Barry RE, Benefield JR, Castenuovo-Tedesco R, Drenick EJ, Passaro E: Intestinal bypass operations as a treatment for obesity. Ann Intern Med 85:97–109, 1976

33. Bruce RM, Wise L: Tuberculosis after jejunoileal bypass for obesity. Ann Intern Med 87:574–576, 1977

34. Wills CE: Tuberculosis after jejunoileal bypass. JAMA 235:1425, 1976

35. Pickleman JR, Evans LS, Kane JM, Freear KRS: Tuberculosis after jejunoileal bypass for obesity. JAMA 234:744, 1975

36. Wasson KR, Harris JO: The treatment of tuberculosis in the presence of malabsorption syndromes. Ann Intern Med 86:115–116, 1977

37. Batterskill JH: Tuberculosis after intestinal bypass surgery for obesity (letter). Chest 70:318, 1976

Chapter 33

Drug-induced Chronic Hepatitis
and Cirrhosis

By WILLIS C. MADDREY, M.D., *and* JOHN K. BOITNOTT, M.D.

HEPATIC INJURY OF many types may result from commonly used and generally well-tolerated therapeutic agents.[1-3] In this review we discuss those forms of drug-induced hepatic damage that closely mimic chronic hepatitis and cirrhosis of other etiologies, as well as those agents that produce a chronic cholestatic illness resembling primary biliary cirrhosis. While the most frequently recognized drug-induced hepatic reactions are asymptomatic increases in serum activities of aminotransferases detected on routine clinical laboratory screening, occasionally therapeutic drugs produce a symptomatic acute illness indistinguishable from viral hepatitis. Furthermore, several widely employed drugs, including methyldopa and isoniazid (INH), have produced the clinical and histologic patterns of chronic active hepatitis (CAH), which may progress as long as the drug is given and result in cirrhosis.[3-12]

Final proof of an association between a drug and liver injury can only be established by epidemiologic studies and rechallenge in an individual patient. The implication of a drug as the cause of a chronic liver disease has been particularly difficult. Individual drugs, however, often do have quite characteristic and reproducible patterns of liver damage as regards both the type of damage found and the duration of the presymptomatic interval. Recognition of these characteristic reaction patterns is often useful in diagnosis.

Drug reactions involving the liver may result from hepatotoxicity from the drug itself or from one of its metabolites (toxic reactions) or from the development of a sensitization reaction to the drug or a drug product (sensitivity or idiosyncratic reactions). Whereas previously the distinction between presumed toxic and sensitization reactions appeared clear, careful studies of several drugs have revealed that with some agents, idiosyncratic liver damage may also involve production of toxic intermediates (e.g., isoniazid-induced damage).[13] Genetically related differences in drug metabolism, such as in the increased production of toxic intermediates by patients who are rapid acetylators of isoniazid, may influence the occurrence of an adverse reaction.[13]

The type and extent of hepatic damage may also be affected by the dose, duration of administration, and patterns of usage of the drug. Some poorly defined influences on drug-induced hepatic injury include the age and sex of the patient and the role of associated drugs. Drug-induced liver injury is unusual in children, and for many drugs the incidence and severity of reactions

From the Departments of Medicine and Pathology, The Johns Hopkins University School of Medicine and The Johns Hopkins Hospital, Baltimore, Maryland.

are increased in women.[3,10,12] The effects of drugs in combination in the production or retarding of liver damage may account for part of the apparent increase in drug-induced liver injury. For example, the apparent decrease in the incidence of isoniazid hepatotoxicity in patients receiving INH and PAS, as compared to liver injury from INH alone, may reflect PAS blockage of isoniazid metabolism to acetylhydrazine and other toxic intermediates. The increased incidence of hepatic injury in patients receiving INH plus rifampin may result from rifampin induction and acceleration of INH metabolism to toxic intermediates.[13] Whether patients with underlying liver disease have an increased likelihood of developing drug-induced liver damage is unknown.

INCREASED SERUM AMINOTRANSFERASES: FOCAL HEPATITIS AND CHRONIC PERSISTENT HEPATITIS

The most frequently recognized hepatic reaction to therapeutic drugs is the asymptomatic elevation of serum aminotransferase activities detected on routine screening examinations while a patient is receiving a new drug or drug combination. Almost every therapeutic agent used has been suspect in the production of abnormal aminotransferase activity. For example, approximately 10% of patients receiving INH demonstrate an asymptomatic rise in the activity of serum aminotransferases.[14] These individuals do have minimal nonspecific focal hepatitis on liver biopsy often associated with both portal and intralobular inflammation. These elevated aminotransferase activities often return to normal despite continued administration of the INH.

The discovery of an elevated aminotransferase activity in a patient receiving a drug is an indication for consideration of whether the drug might be causing the injury and whether a liver biopsy should be performed. Clinical and laboratory evidences of liver disease may be deceptively misleading as an accurate reflection of severity in a patient with drug-induced liver injury.[3,10,12] In patients with isoniazid-induced liver injury, we found no instances of progression of minimal asymptomatic (< two- to threefold) elevated activities of aminotransferases alone to more severe damage, but the potential for such progression must be considered in an individual patient.[10] Such progression of damage in clinically asymptomatic patients has been observed with other drugs (e.g., methotrexate).[15,16]

ACUTE HEPATITIS WITH BRIDGING HEPATIC NECROSIS

The incidence of bridging necrosis is apparently increased in patients with drug-induced acute hepatitis.[3,9] Bridging necrosis is a histologic marker of aggressive disease in patients with acute viral hepatitis with a significant incidence of subsequent chronic hepatitis or cirrhosis.[17]

In their classical paper, Boyer and Klatskin presented 52 patients with acute, presumably viral hepatitis and liver biopsy evidence of bridging and multilobular necrosis.[17] Ten progressed to coma and death from massive hepatic necrosis. Twelve additional patients continued with chronic abnormalities of liver function, and in all 7 who were subsequently biopsied, postnecrotic cirrhosis was found. Of 28 patients who apparently recovered clinically and biochemically, 19 had a subsequent biopsy, with 9 having postnecrotic cirrhosis. Therefore, in patients with acute hepatitis and bridging necrosis, approximately one-half either died or had evidence of significant residual disease.

Follow-up information in 43 of 57 patients with bridging and multilobular necrosis occurring during acute hepatitis showed that 1 died with massive hepatic necrosis, and 8 developed clinical and histologic evidence of chronic active liver disease.[8] Seven of these 57 patients had a probable drug etiology for the hepatitis. The drugs involved were halothane (3 patients), methyldopa (2), isoniazid (1), and propylthiouracil (1). The follow-up information of the drug-related patients was not specifically reported.

To further evaluate the contribution of drug-induced hepatitis to bridging hepatic necrosis, we evaluated 42 consecutive patients with this finding on initial liver biopsy.[9] All 42 patients had their liver biopsy performed within 3 months of the onset of clinical illness. In 18 of the patients (43%), a drug was probably responsible for their hepatitis. Ten patients had HB_sAg-positive acute hepatitis; 14 had neither presumed drug-induced disease nor proved HB_sAg-positive hepatitis. The majority (89%) of the 18 patients in the drug-induced group were over 40 years of age at diagnosis, and 80% were female. Drugs were implicated on the basis of the temporal relation of the appearance of hepatitis to the administration of drug in all and from inadvertent rechallenge in 3. The drugs implicated were methyldopa in 8, isoniazid in 7; halothane in 3, and oxyphenisatin in 1. Of these 18 patients, 16 recovered completely without clinical evidence of chronic liver disease. One patient with isoniazid hepatitis died within a month of onset. Another patient, a 68-year-old female, had been continued on oxyphenisatin after an initial finding of bridging necrosis on liver biopsy and had progressed to an active postnecrotic cirrhosis. This postnecrotic cirrhosis had developed despite corticosteroid therapy. Upon identification of oxyphenisatin as the probable cause of her disease and withdrawal of the drug, she recovered with no further evidence of active liver disease. Therefore, we conclude from this study that the prognosis for bridging hepatic necrosis in a patient with drug-induced injury is excellent and does not have the same implication as bridging found in patients with viral illness.

In another study, none of 3 patients with halothane hepatitis with extensive bridging necrosis on initial liver biopsy had any evidence of residual disease on follow-up liver biopsy.[18] The suggestion was that the hepatic necrosis associated with halothane hypersensitivity is self-limited, and in patients who survive the initial illness, postnecrotic cirrhosis does not develop. However, instances of recurrent exposures to halothane with bouts of hepatitis and development of postnecrotic cirrhosis are known.[19] That a single exposure to halothane with resultant hepatitis led to cirrhosis is not established.

CHRONIC ACTIVE HEPATITIS: CONTRIBUTION OF DRUGS TO ETIOLOGY

The contribution of drug-induced injury to the overall pool of CAH has been examined in four series of patients. A probable drug etiology was reported for 14 of 21 consecutive patients who met histologic criteria of CAH.[5] The drugs implicated were oxyphenisatin in 9 and methyldopa in 5. The patients with drug-induced chronic hepatitis were similar clinically, biochemically, and histologically to those for whom no specific etiology was apparent. No CAH associated with hepatitis B antigen was in this series. Five of 12 female patients over the age of 30 with CAH had a history of prolonged ingestion of oxyphenisatin.[6] Two of these had a positive rechallenge with the drug. A history of prolonged ingestion of oxyphenisatin-containing laxatives[7] was elicited in 41 of 85 Danish patients with CAH. Of these, 19 were challenged with the drug and 8 had increases of serum bilirubin and/or aminotransferase activities, indicating a drug etiology. A series of 46 patients with histologically verified CAH was reported, in whom 13 had an apparently drug-induced hepatitis.[20] Oxyphenisatin was implicated in 8, sulfonamides in 2, nitrofurantoin in 2, and phenylbutazone in 1. All of these 13 patients had taken the apparent inciting drugs for several months to years before the onset of symptoms.

CAH from oxyphenisatin most closely resembles idiopathic CAH, with several patients having developed hyperglobulinemia and positive lupus erythematosus (LE) cell preparations.[4,21-23] In one series, 7 patients developed clinical and liver biopsy findings compatible with CAH while they were taking oxyphenisatin-containing laxatives;[4] six of them were women. The LE cell test was positive in 2 and suggestively positive in a third patient. Two others had antinuclear antibody, and 3 patients had smooth muscle antibody, further increasing the similarity of these patients to those with CAH of unknown etiology (so-called lupoid hepatitis).

COURSE OF DRUG-INDUCED CAH UPON DRUG WITHDRAWAL

Six of the 7 patients with oxyphenisatin-induced CAH in the series of Reynolds had complete clinical and biochemical remission once oxyphenisatin administration was discontinued.[4] In only 1 patient (case 3) was there any evidence of continuing damage. This patient had moderate increases in serum aminotransferase activities 6 months after withdrawal of the drug but was otherwise greatly improved. Follow-up liver biopsy in 2 patients showed considerable improvement, with no bridging necrosis or diffuse fibrosis. In three drug rechallenges with small doses of oxyphenisatin, activity of serum aminotransferases abruptly increased, further establishing the drug etiology of the liver disease. During follow-up the positive LE cell test disappeared in both patients in whom definite LE cells had been seen while on the drug.

Six cases of liver disease were reported after prolonged ingestion of oxyphenisatin.[21] Active cirrhosis was found in 2 of these patients who were husband and wife. All patients clinically improved after drug withdrawal. Results of tests of liver function returned to normal in 4 patients except for minimal increases in aminotransaminase activities in 3. One patient was clinically well but results of tests of liver function were not reported, and the sixth patient had been followed for less than 2 months. In another series, all 14 patients with drug-induced chronic hepatitis had clinical and biochemical improvement after withdrawal that was judged significantly greater than changes in patients with disease of unknown etiology.[5] In another series, only 1 of 5 patients with a history of regular oxyphenisatin ingestion did not improve clinically after discontinuation of the drug.[6] This patient also did not respond to a rechallenge with oxyphenisatin, suggesting that the disease may not have been related to the drug.

One patient was reported in whom an apparent halothane-induced liver injury did not subside, but CAH developed.[24] Multilobular necrosis was seen on a liver biopsy on the 14th postoperative day, and there was evidence of continuing cell necrosis and fibrosis on a second biopsy performed 3 months later at a time when the patient was on prednisone therapy. Other similar instances of ongoing hepatitis after halothane had not been reported. Likewise, we know of no instances of continued activity of CAH following identification and removal of isoniazid as the inducing agent. In our study of 14 patients with isoniazid, bridging and/or multilobular necrosis was found on liver biopsy in 8.[10] There was no clinical or biochemical evidence of continuing disease in any of these patients.

The issue of whether drug-induced CAH leads to progressive liver damage after drug withdrawal is unclear in patients with methyldopa-induced disease. There are suggestions that methyldopa may lead to CAH and postnecrotic cirrhosis, but these cases are not well documented. In our study of 6 patients with methyldopa-induced hepatitis, we had 4 of 5 surviving patients who had bridging and/or multilobular necrosis on liver biopsy.[12] None of these had clinical or laboratory evidence of continued CAH following drug withdrawal.

Two of a series of 20 patients with methyldopa-induced liver had clinical and histologic features of CAH.[11] One of these improved rapidly upon drug withdrawal, clearing his jaundice over the next 2 months, and the serum albumin increased to normal over the following year. Repeat liver biopsy 5 months after the onset of jaundice revealed an inactive postnecrotic cirrhosis. A second patient, who had typical changes of CAH with bridging necrosis on liver biopsy, also subsequently recovered.

A patient was reported who developed hepatitis 12 weeks after initiation of methyldopa therapy.[25,26] She recovered clinically after drug withdrawal and was well within 6 weeks. After 4 to 5 months, however, the drug was reintroduced, and severe hepatitis leading to her death developed 9 weeks later. At postmortem examination, there was submassive hepatic necrosis.

Another patient was reported who developed hepatitis 12 weeks after beginning methyldopa therapy.[27] An initial liver biopsy revealed large areas of hepatocellular necrosis and collapse, compatible with CAH. Serum aminotransferase activities fell after discontinuation of the drug. There was subsequent development of hepatic encephalopathy, however, and she died 4 months later despite corticosteroid therapy. At postmortem examination the liver was small and showed postnecrotic cirrhosis. Remaining hepatocytes revealed small droplet fat accumulation but no evidence of ongoing hepatitis.

A patient was reported who developed biopsy evidence of submassive hepatic necrosis after 10 weeks of methyldopa therapy.[18] In addition, this patient developed a positive LE cell reaction and a direct reacting Coombs reaction. This patient subsequently had a positive rechallenge to methyldopa administration. On follow-up evaluation, there was evidence of chronic liver disease with postnecrotic cirrhosis.

In a patient who developed hepatitis on several occasions while receiving sulfonamides, the drug etiology of her liver disease was proven by one deliberate positive rechallenge with the sulfonamide. A liver biopsy performed during the late resolving phase of her second bout of hepatitis was interpreted as showing changes resembling CAH. Her symptoms and liver function abnormalities resolved each time after drug withdrawal, and two subsequent liver biopsies have shown only minimal fibrosis. Two patients were described with presumed sulfonamide-induced liver injury leading to chronic hepatitis and cirrhosis.[1]

Several reports of a possible association between the administration of nitrofurantoin and hepatitis with clinical and histologic features of CAH are available.[31-33] All patients in whom follow-up information has been presented have had complete clinical recovery after discontinuation of the drug. Three of 4 patients with histologic evidence of CAH while receiving long-term nitrofurantoin were thought to have early cirrhosis on initial liver biopsy.[31] Two of these patients showed residual disease on follow-up liver biopsies despite clinical recovery.

A patient who received nitrofurantoin for recurrent urinary tract infections over several years developed evidence of hepatitis, with a liver biopsy revealing hepatocellular necrosis and portal fibrosis.[33] In addition, she developed antinuclear antibodies, increased gamma globulins, and smooth muscle antibodies. Upon drug withdrawal she rapidly improved clinically, and her laboratory studies (including gamma globulin) returned to normal. A follow-up liver biopsy 1 year after drug withdrawal revealed only minimal residual fibrosis.

One patient developed hepatitis with histologic features of CAH while on propylthiouracil.[34] He recovered rapidly and completely upon drug withdrawal. One patient with presumed propylthiouracil-induced hepatic injury had bridging necrosis on liver biopsy[35] but recovered clinically. We have encountered 2 patients who developed hepatitis with bridging necrosis while on propylthiouracil and both completely recovered clinically upon drug withdrawal.

A patient with aspirin-induced hepatotoxicity had a liver biopsy thought to be consistent with CAH.[36] The patient's liver function abnormalities returned to normal within a week of drug withdrawal. We have not seen any instances in which aspirin-induced hepatotoxicity could be confused with CAH histologically.

Chronic active hepatitis-like disease in patients receiving dantrolene has been reported.[37] One patient had two liver biopsies performed 2 years apart. The first biopsy done 5 months after initiation of drug therapy showed a pattern of CAH. A second biopsy 2 years later, while the patient was still on dantrolene, showed active cirrhosis. The patient died 3 months later and had cirrhosis at autopsy.

CHOLESTATIC DRUG REACTIONS

Drug-induced diseases that present predominantly as cholestatic reaction are characteristically found with phenothiazines and 17-alpha substituted testosterone derivatives.[1,38] Often such patients have evidence of both cholestasis and hepatitis. Drug-induced injury resulting from oral contraceptives is a further example of a mixed reaction. Whereas many patients with oral-contraceptive-induced liver disease present with a predominantly cholestatic picture, we have found evidence of hepatocellular necrosis in all in whom liver biopsies have been performed.

Several reports suggest that drug-induced cholestatic reactions may progress to primary biliary cirrhosis with continued liver damage despite drug withdrawal. The majority of such instances of chronic cholestasis have resulted from phenothiazine reactions, but tolbutamide, methyltestosterone, and organic arsenicals have also been implicated.[38-50] One patient died of bleeding esophageal varices 76 months after the onset of phenothiazine-induced cholestasis.[43] A second patient was jaundiced 46 months after onset of cholestasis. In six instances of chronic disease induced by phenothiazines, 2 patients had a late recovery (10 and 16 months) but 4 remained symptomatic 14, 15, 22, and 36 months after onset.[38] A patient with presumed phenothiazine-induced biliary cirrhosis died of bleeding esophageal varices 5 years after onset.[39]

While a clinical and histologic resemblance to primary biliary cirrhosis has been commented upon in some reports, no cases with the classical bile duct lesion of primary biliary cirrhosis have been described. Histologic changes interpreted as characteristic of CAH were reported in a 59-year-old man 8 months after an overdose of chlorpromazine.[51] Whether the histologic pattern in this case differed significantly from that seen in other reported cases of chronic or slowly resolving liver disease attributable to phenothiazines is not clear.

FUTURE PROGRESS

Several therapeutic drugs can produce typical CAH clinically and histologically. Recognition of the drug etiology is essential in these cases, since the prognosis is generally excellent upon drug withdrawal. Future progress in this area will depend upon better understanding of the pathogenesis of the injury and the development of specific tests for identifying drug-induced injury. A major area of concern is the possible role of drug-induced injury in aggravating an underlying liver disease. Until specific methods of testing are available for drug-induced injury, progress in this area will be limited.

REFERENCES

1. Klatskin G: Toxic and drug-induced hepatitis. Edited by L. Schiff: Diseases of the Liver (ed 4). Philadelphia, JB Lippincott, 1975, pp 604–710

2. Zimmerman HJ: Liver injury induced by chemicals and drugs. Edited by HL Bockus: Gastroenterology (ed 3). Vol III. Philadelphia, WB Saunders, 1976, pp 229–341

3. Maddrey WC, Boitnott JK: Drug-induced chronic liver disease. Gastroenterology 72:1348–1353, 1977

4. Reynolds TB, Peters RL, Yamada S: Chronic active and lupoid hepatitis caused by a laxative, oxyphenisatin. N Engl J Med 285:813–820, 1971

5. Goldstein GB, Lam KC, Mistilis SP: Drug-induced active chronic hepatitis. Am J Dig Dis 18:177–184, 1973

6. Cooksley WGE, Cowen AE, Powell LW: The incidence of oxyphenisatin ingestion in active chronic hepatitis: A prospective controlled study of 29 patients. Aust NZ J Med 3:124–128, 1973

7. Dietrichson O, Juhl E, Nielsen JO, Oxlund JJ, Christoffersen P: The incidence of oxyphenisatin-induced liver damage in chronic

non-alcoholic liver disease. A controlled investigation. Scand J Gastroenterol 9: 473–478, 1974

8. Ware AJ, Eigenbrodt EH, Combes B: Prognostic significance of subacute hepatic necrosis in acute hepatitis. Gastroenterology 68: 519–524, 1975

9. Spitz RD, Keren DJ, Boitnott JK, Maddrey WC: Bridging hepatic necrosis: Etiology and prognosis. Am J Dig Dis (in press)

10. Maddrey WC, Boitnott JK: Isoniazid hepatitis. Ann Intern Med 79:1–12, 1973

11. Toghill PJ, Smith PG, Benton P, Brown, RC, Matthews HL: Methyldopa liver damage. Br Med J 3:545–548, 1974

12. Maddrey WC, Boitnott JK: Severe hepatitis from methyldopa. Gastroenterology 68:351–360, 1975

13. Mitchell JR, Zimmerman HJ, Ishak KG, Thorgeirsson UP, Timbrell JA, Snodgrass WR, Nelson SD: Isoniazid liver injury: Clinical spectrum, pathology, and probable pathogenesis. Ann Intern Med 84:181–192, 1976

14. Scharer L, Smith JP: Serum transaminase elevations and other hepatic abnormalities in patients receiving isoniazid. Ann Intern Med 71:1113–1120, 1969

15. Dahl MGC, Gregory MM, Scheuer PJ: Liver damage due to methotrexate in patients with psoriasis. Br Med J 1:625–630, 1971

16. Weinstein G, Roenigk H, Maibach H, Cosmides J, Halprin K, Millard M: Psoriasis-liver-methotrexate interactions. Arch Dermatol 108:36–42, 1973

17. Boyer JL, Klatskin G: Pattern of necrosis in acute viral hepatitis. Prognostic value of bridging (subacute hepatic necrosis). N Engl J Med 283:1063–1071, 1970

18. Miller DJ, Dwyer J, Klatskin G: Follow-up of halothane hepatitis: Benign resolution of a severe lesion. Ann Intern Med, 89:212–215 1978

19. Klatskin G, Kimberg DV: Recurrent hepatitis attributable to halothane sensitization in an anesthetist. N Engl J Med 280;515–522, 1969

20. Lindberg J, Lindholm A, Lundin P, Iwarson S: Trigger factors and HL-A antigens in chronic active hepatitis. Br Med J 4:77–79, 1975

21. Willing RL, Hecker R: Oxyphenisatin and liver damage. Med J Aust 1:1179–1182, 1971

22. Reynolds JDH, Wilber RD: Chronic active hepatitis associated with oxyphenisatin. Am J Gastroenterol 57:566–570, 1972

23. Gjone E, Blomhoff JP, Ritland S, Elgio K. Husby G: Laxative-induced chronic liver disease. Scand J Gastroenterol 7:395–402, 1972

24. Thomas FB: Chronic agressive hepatitis induced by halothane. Ann Intern Med 81:487–489, 1974

25. Rehman OU, Keith TA, Gall EA; Methyldopa-induced submassive hepatic necrosis. JAMA 224:1390–1392, 1973

26. Hoyumpa AM Jr, Connell AM: Methyldopa hepatitis: report of three cases. Am J Dig Dis 18:213–222, 1973

27. Thomas E, Bhuta S, Rosenthal WS: Methyldopa-induced liver injury. Arch Pathol Lab Med 100:132–135, 1976

28. Schweitzer IL, Peters RL: Acute submassive hepatic necrosis due to methyldopa: a case demonstrating possible initiation of chronic liver disease. Gastroenterology 66:1203–1211, 1974

29. Rodman JS, Deutsch DJ, Gutman SI: Methyldopa hepatitis: a report of six cases and review of the literature. Am J Med 60:941–948, 1976

30. Tonder M, Nordoy A, Elgio K: Sulfonamide-induced chronic liver disease. Scand J Gastroenterol 9:93–96, 1974

31. Klemola H, Penttila O, Runeberg L, Tallquist G: Anicteric liver damage during nitrofurantoin medication. Scand J Gastroenterol 10:501–505, 1975

32. Stromberg A, Wengle B: Chronic active hepatitis induced by nitrofurantoin. Br Med J 3:174–175, 1976

33. Fagrell B, Strandberg I, Wengle B: A nitrofurantoin-induced disorder simulating chronic active hepatitis. Acta Med Scand 199:237–239, 1976

34. Fedotin MS, Lefer LG: Liver disease caused by propylthiouracil. Arch Intern Med 135: 319–321, 1975

35. Mihas AA, Holley P, Koff RS, Hirschowitz BI: Fulminant hepatitis and lymphocyte sensitization due to propylthiouracil. Gastroenterology 70:770-774, 1976

36. Seaman WE, Ishak WG, Plotz PH: Aspirin-induced hepatotoxicity in patients with systemic lupus erythematosus. Ann Intern Med 80:1–8, 1974

37. Utili R, Boitnott JK, Zimmerman HJ: Dantrolene-associated hepatic injury: incidence and character. Gastroenterology 72:510–516, 1977

38. Ishak KG, Irey NS: Hepatic injury associated with the phenothiazines. Arch Pathol 93:283–304, 1972

39. Myers JD, Olson RE, Lewis JH, Moran TJ: Xanthomatous biliary cirrhosis following chlorpromazine, with observations indicating overproduction of cholesterol, hyperprothrombinemia, and the development of portal hypertension. Trans Assoc Am Physicians 70:243–261, 1957

40. Beattie AS, Farris JM, Frempter GR: Hepatohypercholesterolemic cirrhosis: Report of a case implicating chlorpromazine as the etiologic agent. Calif Med 91:154–155, 1959

41. Kohn NN, Myerson RM: Xanthomatous biliary cirrhosis following chlorpromazine. Am J Med 31:665–670, 1961

42. Read AE, Harrison DV, Sherlock S: Chronic chlorpromazine jaundice. Am J Med 31:249–258, 1961

43. Walker CO, Combes B: Biliary cirrhosis induced by chlorpromazine. Gastroenterology 51:631–640, 1966

44. Norredam K: Chlorpromazine jaundice of long duration. Acta Med Scand 174:163–170, 1963

45. Levine RA, Briggs GW, Lowell DM: Chronic chlorpromazine cholangiolitic hepatitis. Gastroenterology 50:665–670, 1966

46. Bolton BH: Prolonged chlorpromazine jaundice. Am J Gastroenterol 48:497–503, 1967

47. Stolzer BL, Miller G, White WA, Morris Z: Postarsenical obstructive jaundice complicated by xanthomatosis and diabetes mellitus. Am J Med 9:124–132, 1950

48. Haubrich WS, Sancetta SM: Spontaneous recovery from hepatobiliary disease with xanthomatosis. Gastroenterology 26:658–665, 1954

49. Gregory DH, Zaki GF, Sarcosi GA, Carey JB: Chronic cholestasis following prolonged tolbutamide administration. Arch Pathol 84:194–201, 1967

50. Glober GA, Wilkerson JA: Biliary cirrhosis following the administration of methyltestosterone. JAMA 204:170–173, 1968

51. Russell RI, Allan JG, Patrick R: Active chronic hepatitis after chlorpromazine ingestion. Br Med J 1:655–656, 1973

Chapter 34

Environmental Hepatic Injury in Man

By HANS POPPER, M.D., Ph.D., MICHAEL A. GERBER, M.D., FENTON SCHAFFNER, M.D., *and* IRVING J. SELIKOFF, M.D.

THE RECENT YEARS have seen a rapid increase in the hazards to man and his surroundings from environmental factors. The liver plays a foremost role in this timely subject for two reasons: (1) It is the main site for the transformation of many environmental agents that become active only after this transformation. Moreover, hepatic transformation is a model for the study of biotransformation in other organs. (2) The liver may be the site of injury from environmental agents, with biotransformation representing a localizing factor. The recent observations of substantiated environmental hepatic injury, such as that from vinyl chloride, and the uncertainty about hepatic injury from other agents stimulated a review and evaluation of the available data to cover (1) the difficulties in establishing evidence of human hepatic injury, (2) the potential hazards to the liver, including tendency to carcinoma formation, from environmental agents by altering hepatic metabolism without creating hepatic disease, and (3) the acceptable evidence of such injuries from environmental agents, to be listed specifically.

ENVIRONMENTAL AGENTS

Environmental agents are difficult to define. In a restricted sense, they are the result of pollution. They include agents that are either manufactured directly or are by-products of industrial activities, in which case, their presence can easily be overlooked. Most industrial hazards are mixtures of various agents, and employees who are exposed to these mixtures, as well as their immediate families, may be at risk. Others may also be affected, since the surrounding area may be polluted, particularly as result of industrial accidents.

Environmental agents may be substances used in food processing, either for preservation or for coloring, or they may be contaminants of the food or water supply, or even ingredients of food. They may be derived from chemicals used in agriculture, particularly pesticides, which find their way into the human food chain, either directly by consumption of contaminated food or secondarily from animals or even plants incidentally exposed.

Drug-induced injuries can be considered an environmental hazard. However,

From the Stratton Laboratory for the Study of Liver Diseases, the Departments of Pathology and Medicine, and the Environmental Sciences Laboratory, Mount Sinai School of Medicine of the City University of New York, New York, New York.

Supported in part by National Institute of Occupational Safety and Health Contract No. 210-75-0044 and by National Institutes of Health, NIEHS Grant No. 2 P30 ES00928 06.

605

they are usually discussed independently as an important source of hepatic disease. Alcoholic and viral hepatic injuries can similarly be considered environmental hazards, but both are separately considered in hepatology. In a broad sense, any nongenetic factor can be thought of as environmental.

With the exception of accidents and suicidal or homicidal exposures, environmental injuries in man are characterized by long-term continuous or intermittent exposures to low doses of these agents, which are often hidden from recognition. A problem arises in the evaluation of conventional intoxication caused by homicidal or suicidal attempts or by negligence. Such incidents are well known and often reviewed. Although some are environmental, most are not referred to here, where the emphasis is mainly on hidden or unexpected etiologic factors that may be a preventable hazard to the liver. The characteristics of environmental injuries, namely long-term exposures to low doses, create particular difficulties in establishment of the injury. Therefore, problems of establishment are discussed first.

PROBLEMS IN EVALUATION OF ENVIRONMENTAL HEPATIC INJURIES

Evaluation in Man

Environmental injuries have a clearly identifiable clinical and morphologic picture only in few instances. This is best exemplified by the consequences of exposure to vinyl chloride, where both the early changes and the eventually developing tumor, namely hepatic angiosarcoma (see p. 624), are sufficiently rare in the general population to raise an index of suspicion, particularly when they occur in a relatively small work force. Usually, however, toxic hepatitis, cirrhosis, and hepatocellular carcinoma are found with sufficient frequency in the population at large so as to interfere with establishing a causal association with a newly suspected environmental agent.

Clinical Features

Clinical manifestations are of little diagnostic value, since in milder injury, they are nonspecific, such as fatigability and malaise. Acute severe hepatic injuries rarely occur as result of environmental exposure, with the exception of accidents. Manifestations of chronic liver injury, including portal hypertension, are even more nonspecific as to etiology. An attempt, however, has been made to describe the symptom complex as an entity in man.[1]

Laboratory Features

Abnormalities in results of laboratory examinations of single individuals are also of little help, since a demonstrated hepatic injury may be the result of an independent liver disease, most frequently of alcoholic or viral hepatitic origin and often detected in the absence of significant clinical manifestations. Better information has been sought by epidemiologic surveys of larger population groups. They have been carried out in industrial surveillance and in population groups accidentally exposed to environmental agents. The incidence of abnormalities, however, is not significantly different from that in similar population groups not exposed (Table 1), with the exception of gamma glutamyl transpeptidase activity,[2] the results of which deserve special consideration. This justifies the conclusion that application of the conventional liver function tests is of limited value, if any, in the detection of such abnormalities. Utilization of more sensitive and also more specific tests for hepatic abnormalities, specifically of liver function and functional capacity, may be more revealing. For instance, clearance of dyes such as indocyanine green, response of the bile acid level to bile acid loads,[3-5] or tests for biotransformation of drugs have been repeatedly recommended and sporadically used, but no test for practical use, particularly in surveys, is available to prove or definitely exclude environmentally induced injury to population groups. Standardization of available tests, with better delineation of the range of abnormalities, may provide this information.

Morphologic Features

Morphologic studies of biopsy or autopsy specimens appear more reliable, although they also present difficulties in practical application, particularly in evaluation of the results obtained. Liver biopsy is a useful procedure despite its invasive character. However, sinusoidal dilatation in established environmental injury, such as following exposure to sex steroids, arsenics and vinyl chloride,[6-10] raises the danger of peritoneal hemorrhage. This danger is reduced if liver biopsy is obtained by the transjugular approach, which requires even more invasive procedures.[11] The interpretation offers difficulties, however, because of the possibility of alterations, particularly of alcoholic and viral hepatitic origin mentioned above. Preexposure biopsies for comparison are, of course, unavailable, for technical and ethical reasons. Liver biopsy thus will render interpretable results only if either a specific lesion is noted or the same, though nonspecific, lesion is seen in a higher incidence than would be expected in a random population. Examples of the former are focal hyperplasia of the hepatocytes with or without simultaneous proliferation of sinusoidal cells and reticulum framework and sinusoidal dilatation not related to lobular architecture.[10] Examples of the latter are steatosis; accumulation of hepatocytic pigment not explained by age or wasting; centrolobular necrosis often associated with many pigmented macrophages; diffuse alterations of the hepatocytes, such as hydropic swelling or irregular clumping of the cytoplasm, variations of hepatocytic nuclei, and accumulation of sinusoidal macrophages with PAS-positive diastase-resistant granules. Hepatocytic alterations may be associated with an inflammatory reaction and fibrosis.

Small and large droplet steatosis with occasional foci of necrosis or fibrosis, associated with conspicuous variations of hepatocytic nuclei, may be observed in persons exposed to fumes containing various solvents. These features may be accompanied by abnormalities of results of hepatic tests. This lesion is difficult to distinguish from alcoholic liver injury. Its disappearance together with that of the functional abnormalities after cessation of the exposure support the etiologic role of the exposure.

Both centrolobular necrosis and diffuse alterations of the hepatocytes with-

TABLE 1—*Prevalence of Abnormal Results of Hepatic Tests in Cohorts with Various Occupational and Environmental Exposures*

Cohort	Percentage of Abnormal Results of Hepatic Tests					
	Number	Bilirubin (>1.1 mg/dl)	Alk. Phos. (>86 IU/liter)	SGPT (>36 IU/liter)	SGOT (>50 IU/liter)	LDH (>225 IU/liter)
Painters	503	3.8	23.7	2.0	6.6	2.4
Vinyl chloride polymerization workers	1177	3.8	22.7	4.4	3.3	—
Styrene polymerization workers	471	3.2	5.9	4.0	3.4	—
Controls	286	7.3	8.7	—	2.1	—
			>95	>45	>40	>225
Michigan dairy farmers (polybrominated biphenyls)	614	—	11.1	11.1	10.7	6.8
Michigan chemical workers (polybrominated biphenyls)	55	—	25.5	10.9	9.1	7.3
Wisconsin dairy farmers	141	—	14.2	2.8	2.8	2.8
		>1.7	>50	>50	>50	>250
Capacitor manufacturing workers (polychlorinated biphenyls)	321	0	1.2	7.2	2.2	2.5

out other characteristic features are conventionally designated as toxic hepatitis. The inflammatory component is insignificant except for macrophages, and the degenerative changes of the hepatocytes, such as hydropic swelling, often associated with cytoplasmic clumping, as well as ground-glass hepatocytes produced by increased smooth endoplasmic reticulum[12] and nuclear alterations, are in the foreground. These are the morphologic features in toxic hepatitis, especially if steatosis is also seen. Cholestasis may be present. The differentiation from other forms of hepatitis, however, particularly that of viral origin, remains an unresolved problem.[13]

Histochemical analysis of human material has occasionally been applied, but standardized observations in man do not exist. Similarly, electron-microscopic studies have offered anecdotal observations of essentially nonspecific changes of organelles that defy reliable interpretation.

Even more difficulties exist in the interpretation of autopsy findings if nonspecific lesions are encountered. Centrolobular necrosis may be the result of an intoxication. More frequently, however, it is produced by terminal interference with hepatic circulation caused by cardiac failure or a lesion in another organ and does not necessarily indicate a hepatotoxic effect. Disagreement in nomenclature, as well as inadequate descriptions in the literature, interfere significantly with the evaluation of hepatic injury from environmental factors. The recognition of precancerous manifestations in the human liver with or without cirrhosis has made distinct progress. They are either dysplastic changes of single hepatocytes with enlargement and polyploidy of the nuclei, reported initially in association with hepatitis B[14] but also occurring without it, or focal accentuation of architectural features of regeneration with plates that are more than one cell thick, designated as adenomatoid changes.[15]

Extrapolation from Animals

Uncertainty in environmental hepatic injury in man encourages extrapolation from observations in domestic or wild animals following incidental exposure or experimentally controlled injuries.

Environmental Liver Injury in Animals

A series of toxic injuries has been reported in animals, particularly from plant poisons, such as senecio, causing cirrhosis in horses, swine, cattle, and sheep in Nebraska, Texas, Canada, South Africa, Australia, and New Zealand.[16] The hepatic alterations resemble veno-occlusive disease in man (see later). Mycotoxins, such as aflatoxins in contaminated food, have produced periportal and centrolobular hepatic necrosis in domestic animals and cirrhosis in some species.[17,18] Food poisoning, possibly from aflatoxin, resulting in toxic hepatitis has been reported in dogs coinciding with human intoxication in India.[19] Aflatoxin carcinoma is common in trout.[17] Veno-occlusive disease of the liver occurred in horses and other animals after accidental dioxin poisoning.[20,21] Cattle accidentally exposed to polybrominated biphenyls in Michigan showed hepatocytic injury associated with lymphocytic infiltration and scarring.[22] An epizootic of chick edema disease in Japan was shown to be due to contamination of chicken feed by polychlorinated biphenyls.[23,24]

Experimental Observations in Animals

Conclusions for human disease are conventionally drawn from study of hepatic alterations produced in experimental animals, utilizing biochemical as well as morphologic parameters that represent the basis of many decisions of regulatory agencies.

Biochemical Investigations

The toxicologic study of hepatic injuries has developed into a well-reviewed technology.[25-27] Nevertheless, the utilization of hepatic tests, including those measuring hepatic function, is not fully standardized. Although the significance of borderline abnormalities is unknown, these tests represent the most reliable techniques. Observations are more important in demonstrating acute lesions rather than chronic ones, since the latter are influenced to a great degree by individual variations. Chemical analysis of liver tissue is a valuable supplement, but the greatest difficulty in the extrapolation of results of animal observations lies in species variations, especially in metabolic transformation, and also in tissue distribution of toxic agents. Enzyme patterns in the liver vary with age, with the fetal and neonatal liver being different from the mature one. Developmental enzyme differentiation in man is similar to that in rats.[28] Study of the effect of environmental agents, particularly of chemical carcinogens, on cultures of hepatic cells may develop into a useful technique if it can be applied to cultured human adult hepatocytes.[29-33]

An important contribution of animal experimental studies is elucidation of the mechanism of hepatotoxic injury,[34] such as formation of free radicals, for instance in carbon tetrachloride intoxication, synthesis of epoxides, oxidative dealkylation, or *N*-oxidation. From precursors of lower bioactivity, all of these reactions produce an electrophile with greater ability to bind macromolecules. Thus, they develop increased carcinogenic, and possibly also necrogenic, potential. The relation between necrosis and covalent binding to protein is not established, however.[35] Another example of synthesis of potential hepatotoxins is formation of aldehydes from alcohols. Trapping of cofactors exemplified by ATP in ethionine intoxication and UTP in galactosamine intoxication is also injurious. Antitubulin action results in retention of protein secreted by the hepatocytes, producing hydropic swelling. This has been demonstrated following alcohol exposure[36] but is probably applicable to many other conditions. Finally, some environmental agents like hexachlorobenzene and lead, produce porphyria by destroying heme and stimulating synthesis of delta-aminolevulinic acid.

Morphologic Investigations

Toxicologic/morphologic studies are essential supplements to biochemical investigations. Extrapolation to man, however, is complicated by the same difficulties as biochemical studies in terms of interpretation and species variations. Light-microscopic hepatocellular necrosis, fibrosis, cirrhosis, and specific lesions such as vascular alterations, including sinusoidal dilatation, arteritis, and fibrosis, present few problems. Steatosis is harder to interpret, since it might be caused by independent nutritional factors including vomiting or inadequate food intake. Cholestasis can be recognized in many species, except in rats, by light microscopy. Histochemical demonstration of the reaction products of enzymes has been useful but is not standardized. The same holds true for electron-microscopic study, where adequate controls are not always available and the interpretation of changes is often difficult, even when time-consuming morphometry is applied.[37] Electron microscopy is, however, useful in demonstration of cholestasis in rodents. Nevertheless, the combined toxicologic/morphologic investigation remains the mainstay in the evaluation of environmental injuries, although relatively few observations in experimental animals have demonstrated counterparts in human lesions.

Three specific problems require consideration in the extrapolation of animal experimental data to man: acute hepatic necrosis, chronic liver injury, and hepatocellular tumors.

ACUTE HEPATIC NECROSIS

The pathogenesis of hepatocellular necrosis in general is not established, with the exception of anoxic injury, although rapid inhibition of energy supply need not result in morphological recognizable changes, for example, that following cyanide intoxication. Otherwise, a sequential process sets in, the terminal event of which is an alteration of cell membranes, possible resulting in irreversible calcium accumulation.[37a] Increase of microsomal transformation, by phenobarbital and other inducing agents, is a useful procedure to produce hepatic necrosis by otherwise nontoxic environmental and other agents;[38] inhibition of the transformation, for instance by low-protein diets, inhibits hepatocellular necrosis.[39] The action of environmental agents, many inducing the biotransformation system, may thus represent a potential hazard. Metabolic transformation includes not only formation of a bioactive metabolite but also its degradation. The lack of predictability of the metabolic process might explain special risks of population groups, such as children, malnourished persons, and pregnant and lactating women.

CHRONIC LIVER INJURY

The demonstration of acute hepatic injury and necrosis by large doses in acute experiments does not necessarily point to a danger in sustained administration of small doses. Even continued exposure to medium doses of toxic agents that initially cause hepatocellular injury may be tolerated for a long time, with disappearance of the original injury. This is explained by metabolic adaptation which permits the complete restitution of the liver in subsequent months even with continued exposure. The establishment of chronic liver injury in man by extrapolation from long-term animal experiments is thus difficult. Experiences with drugs, however, such as methyldopa, isoniazid, nitrofurantoin, and oxiphenisatin (see Chapter 33) point to the potential of environmental agents producing chronic hepatitis and cirrhosis.

HEPATOCELLULAR TUMORS

Many environmental agents produce proliferative lesions of the liver in experimental animals, proceeding in many instances to frank carcinoma.[39a] They include polychlorinated biphenyls, polybrominated biphenyls, organochlorine insecticides, nitroso compounds such as dimethyl and diethyl nitrosamines,[40] and agents used in food processing, such as Safrol and Ponceau-MX.[41,42] In rodents, a characteristic morphologic sequence has been established.[39a,43,44] It starts with the formation of hyperplastic areas in which the hepatocytes differ from the surrounding parenchyma by histochemical characteristics. These include increase in glycogen; loss of enzymes characteristic of the adult liver, such as glucose-6-phosphatase and 5′-nucleotidase; appearance of enzymes characteristic of the fetal liver, such as gamma glutamyl transpeptidase; and emergence of fetal proteins such as alpha-fetoprotein and of a preneoplastic antigen which may be an epoxide hydrase.[45,46] Eventually, neoplastic, previously called "hyperplastic," nodules form and exert pressure on the surrounding parenchyma. The cells show increased basophilia or ground-glass cytoplasm characterized by increased smooth endoplasmic reticulum. The lobular architecture becomes distorted; excess arteries and sinusoidal dilatation may be found, and the nodules may become grossly visible, even distorting the shape of the organ. Variations in cell populations, "nodules in nodules," develop, and carcinomatous transformation may set in. The application of these rodent nodules as predictive of carcinogenicity in man was initially challenged.[47] Subsequently, the same lesions were demonstrated as a result of administration of large doses of anabolic steroids to men and women[48-51] and, although in very low incidence, also in pregnant women and in those taking contraceptive drugs;[52-59] occasionally, these lesions also occurred without substantiated etiology. Moreover, a similar, but less well identified sequence has been produced in primates after administration of nitroso compounds and aflatoxin, although not after organochlorine pesticides.[60,61]

Cytologically the sequence has been explained by Farber[62] as the selection of individual hepatocytes which become tolerant to the carcinogenic agent and proliferate, especially when stimulated to do so, for instance, by partial hepatectomy. The nonselected hepatocytes are prevented from proliferating by the presence of inhibitory agents. These agents do not affect the selected hepatocytes, however, which eventually may become carcinomatous after multiple cell divisions.

The underlying metabolic process is explained by a carcinogenic chain, a multistep process consisting of initiation and promotion.[63] Most carcinogens are fat-soluble and, as such, are of low reactivity. In one or several metabolic steps in which mono-oxygenases of cytochrome P-450/P-448 variety are active, these carcinogens are transformed into electrophilic agents by hydroxylation, epoxide formation, and methylation.[35] The active agent may bind to macromolecules like DNA, which is of major importance in carcinogenesis.[63,64] This is recognized by the Ames test for mutagenicity with *Salmonella* species, although the mutagenic and carcinogenic compounds may not be identical. Moreover, subsequent events may account for additional differences.[63,64] The active agent is further metabolized by several processes that might either be enzymatic or nonenzymatic. They include action of a hydrase, binding to glutathione, and antioxidant action, as well as glucuronidation, all of which might result in a less active compound, often water-soluble and excreted by the cell or the body. The carcinogenic effect thus depends on amount and life span of the active agent.

Subsequent processes determining the carcinogenic effect include potential excision of the altered DNA by nucleases, which would terminate the carcinogenic event.[65,66] The tissue concentration of nucleases may be a crucial factor. For instance, single large doses of diethyl nitrosamine produce hepatocellular carcinoma presumably because they overwhelm the activity of the nucleases. By contrast, repeated small doses of the same agent lead to renal tumors, since the activities of the nucleases in the kidneys are lower than in the liver. Another factor is proliferation of hepatocytes, since DNA during synthesis in the s phase is more susceptible to binding.[63] In addition, cell division fixes the DNA change in the template. Agents favoring cell proliferation and division may nonspecifically increase carcinogenesis.[67,68] Hepatocytes with persisting alteration of DNA presumably represent the selected cell population previously referred to and permit the initiating process of relatively short duration to progress to the promoting sequence, requiring multiple cell divisions and a long period of time, presumably years, in man. These events in the carcinogenic chain explain the low susceptibility of the adult human liver to hepatocellular carcinoma, even to carcinogens that undergo biotransformation in the liver. This includes the most common human carcinogens, the polycyclic hydrocarbons, which do not produce hepatocellular carcinomas in any species. There is no convincing evidence that the nitroso compounds that produce carcinomas of the liver in many species, including subhuman primates, are hepatocarcinogenic in man. By contrast, this group of compounds is incriminated in human bronchogenic carcinoma. The protection is presumably broken in the case of established human carcinogens, which include aflatoxin.[69] The association with hepatitis B virus is more complex. Hepatitis B may cause incorporation of viral DNA into host genome or alternatively may change the biotransformation system in selected cells in which an excess amount of the surface antigen is found in the proliferated smooth endoplasmic reticulum.[70]

CONSEQUENCES FROM ALTERATIONS OF HEPATIC METABOLISM BY ENVIRONMENTAL AGENTS

The most important contribution of environmental factors to human hepatocarcinogenesis may be a modulation of the carcinogenic chain.[71] This includes increased formation and reduced degradation in the microsomal biotransformation system of the active electrophilic metabolite, alteration of the nucleases, and more importantly, stimulation of cell proliferation. While the mono-oxygenases have limited substrate specificity, their activity may be nonspecifically enhanced by a metabolic transformation of chemically unrelated substances if this metabolism is delayed and if the binding of the substances to the enzyme is prolonged.[72] This process results in an increase of the smooth endoplasmic reticulum, accompanied by increased activity of mono-oxygenases and their cofactors, but also an increase of other cell organelles with enlargement of the cells and often with cell division. This process is designated induction. Modulating agents have known enhancing effects in experimental chemical carcinogenesis, depending on the time of administration.[73,74] They also determine the extent of hepatocellular necrosis in human nonpredictable drug reactions.[75,76] Most aliphatic drugs are metabolized by cytochrome P-450, while the usually aromatic carcinogens are transformed by cytochrome P-448 in experimental animals. The inducing capacity may therefore differ, although some overlap exists; some agents, like polychlorinated biphenyl, induce both variants of the cytochrome.[77] Multiple variants of the mono-oxygenases exist. Biotransformation depends on a variety of other factors, including genetic predisposition, physical factors, and diet, both its protein and fat content.[78-84]

Increase of the smooth endoplasmic reticulum need not imply increased enzymatic activity, which may be reduced for most or selected enzymes, so-called hypertrophic hypoactive endoplasmic reticulum.[85] Butylated hydroxytoluene and phenobarbital in rats produce sustained liver enlargement and increased activities of various microsomal enzymes without producing nodular changes, and the cellular hypertrophy is reversible after 80 weeks of treatment.[86] By contrast, other agents, such as safrol, produce an initially similar enzyme induction, but nodules appear eventually and the elevated activity of the drug-metabolizing enzymes drops, although the liver remains enlarged and NADPH-cytochrome C reductase, cytochrome b-5, and microsomal protein remain elevated.[41] This therefore represents hypertrophic hypoactive endoplasmic reticulum[85] associated with histochemical and ultrastructural evidence of liver damage. These observations raise the possibility that subsequent hepatocellular injury and not induction by itself is predictive of formation of tumors in the liver.

A series of agents with proven capacity to produce hepatic tumors in some species are not mutagenic, and their chemical structure does not suggest formation of an active electrophilic metabolite.[87] This includes organochlorine pesticides and most sex steroids. Some of them are inducing. Moreover, many agents, such as polybrominated and polychlorinated biphenyls and dioxin, which produce hepatic tumors in experimental animals, are potent inducers primarily before tumors appear.[88-91] This raises the questions of whether these substances have an inducing potential in man and what the consequences of this induction are to man. Induction, which can be looked upon as a promotion, is readily reversible, in contrast to initiation of the carcinogenic chain. Induction therefore represents a target for preventive management.

Recognition of Induction in Man

The following procedures have been formulated to recognize induction:

1. Response to administration of drugs by determining their decay in blood or by measuring CO_2 excretion in breath tests.[92-94] This, however, has only been applied to agents metabolized by cytochrome P-450, but not by P-448.
2. Increased urinary excretion of total porphyrins in random samples, with creatinine concentrations as a reference point. By contrast with the reversal of the ratio of corproporphyrin to uroporphyrin in hepatic disease, this ratio is not altered.[95]
3. Altered steroid pattern in the urine, which requires a complex technology.
4. Elevated excretion of D-glucaric acid in the urine.[96-100] It has been demonstrated following phenobarbital administration in man, is reduced in liver injury, and may be useful in investigations in industrial workers.

5. Elevated serum activities of gamma glutamyl transpeptidase, but the evidence so far indicates that too many other processes influence this activity in man to make it a useful index of induction.[101-106]
6. Histologic visualization of increased smooth endoplasmic reticulum reflected light microscopically in ground-glass cells and electron microscopically by morphometry, which is not feasible in field studies.
7. Hepatomegaly in the absence of other alterations, determined by scanning.[107] This may develop into a useful method if quantitation can be accomplished.
8. Demonstration of induction of enzymes, for instance, of aryl hydroxylases in lymphocytes or skin samples, which may eventually become a practical method.
9. Increased clearance of dyes, such as sulfobromophthalein.[108]

Consequences of Induction in Man

Two epidemiologic studies of the incidence of hepatic and other tumors in epileptics on long-term therapy with phenobarbital and phenytoin have been conducted.[109,110] One study[110] showed an increased incidence in hepatic tumors that, however, was related to the use of thorium dioxide in these patients. There was a definite increase in brain tumors, which may be explained by the underlying disease. Long-term studies on larger human populations would be required to establish beneficial or harmful effects of induction in man.

A specific problem is the interaction with ethanol, which has a somewhat controversial inducing effect. Experimentally, it enhances the carbon tetrachloride liver injury.[111] Moreover, the vinyl chloride experimental lesion is aggravated by simultaneous administration of alcohol.[112] The postulated greater risk of the alcoholic or the malnourished person to environmental liver injury remains to be substantiated, however, if increased susceptibility in accidental intoxication is excluded.

DISEASE PATTERNS RELATED TO ENVIRONMENTAL FACTORS

The toxicologist is concerned with the question of the effect and dose of toxic agents in man and uses a classification as to the responsible agent. The hepatologist, by contrast, attempts to determine whether an observed clinical/pathologic entity may be the result of environmental exposure, often not an obvious one. Intoxications as a result of suicidal, homicidal, or negligence-induced events do not as a rule present a problem of diagnosis but rather of management. Therefore, in the subsequent listing of hepatic disease processes, the best-described intoxications are only recorded to prove the toxic potential of the agent in question.

Acute and Subacute Liver Injury

Acute Massive Hepatic Necrosis with Potentially Fatal Outcome

This condition follows accidental exposure to large doses of environmental agents, many of them in industry, or deliberate or accidental intake by mouth. The clinical manifestations are those of rapidly developing hepatic failure with jaundice, proceeding to coma. Recovery of a variable frequency usually occurs without a persisting hepatic deficit like chronic hepatitis, although postnecrotic scarring has been recorded at autopsy in some cases. The interval between effective exposure and appearance of manifestations is short, and children are at greater risk. The liver is almost never the only target organ, and associated manifestations, such as renal failure, central nervous dysfunction, or gastrointestinal symptoms from topical effects, are often in the foreground. At autopsy, massive hepatic necrosis, usually associated with severe steatosis, represents a typical picture, depending upon the duration of the disease. The environmental agents discussed below represent examples rather than a comprehensive enumeration.

PHOSPHORUS

The yellow form of phosphorus, rather than the red one, is poisonous, and intake results from ingestion of roach pastes, rat poisons, or "firecrackers."[113-115] Although most matches no longer contain phosphorus, in countries where they do, the risk continues. The classic term "acute yellow atrophy" was coined by Rokitansky for phosphorus intoxication in the middle of the last century.

CARBON TETRACHLORIDE

Carbon tetrachloride is the classic example of a hepatotoxic effect in view of the similarity of clinical and experimental experiences.[116,117] The greater susceptibility of alcoholics is well known[118] and is explained by increased absorption, preferential fat solubility, and activation of the microsomal biotransformation system, increasing the concentration of the active metabolite.[111,119] Renal failure is more important in the majority of human cases than hepatic failure. Rapid recovery from even severe hepatic lesions is well documented by biopsy observations in survivors.[120]

OTHER AGENTS

Occasionally, anesthesia and exposure in dry cleaning establishments to *trichlorethylene* has led to massive necrosis.[121] Sniffing of trichlorethylene and of toluene[122-125] has also been incriminated.

Tetrachloroethylene has been reported to cause toxic hepatitis.[126]

Industrial exposure to *dimethyl nitrosamine* resulted in severe liver injury after a variable duration.[127-129]

Trinitrotoluene produced massive necrosis in munitions workers.[130-132] Hepatic damage in these instances may be very much delayed,[133] however, and the question of a hypersensitivity reaction should be raised, in contrast to the other agents.

Tetrachloroethane caused massive hepatic necrosis after inhalation by aircraft factory workers.[133-137]

Chlorinated naphthalene used in insulation has led to massive necrosis associated with chloracne.[138-140] The reported cases in the older literature seem to have had a more delayed course.

Central necrosis rapidly following accidental intake of large doses of *DDT* has been reported.[141]

Lead poisoning in youngsters after intravenous injection is reported to have caused one case of massive necrosis.[142]

Aflatoxin has induced centrolobular necrosis in man.[143-145] An epidemic presumably of toxic hepatitis, with a high mortality, has been reported from northwest India.[146,147] Food poisoning, probably aflatoxin, was incriminated because of simultaneous disease in dogs. Acute aflatoxinosis has also been reported from other countries.[148]

Amanita phalloides intoxication may produce rapid hepatic necrosis with steatosis, for which the amanitin component is responsible rather than phalloidin.[149-151]

Herbal remedies are said to cause a rapidly developing, often fatal centrolobular necrosis in blacks in South Africa, occurring in all age groups but preferentially in children below 5 years of age.[152-154] Hypoglycemia is frequent, but jaundice is not regularly found.

Delayed Massive Hepatic Necrosis

In several of the intoxicants listed above, massive necrosis results after prolonged administration and thus might justify a distinction. The applicable drugs are trinitrotoluene, dimethyl nitrosamine, chlorinated naphthalene, and possibly also tetrachlorethane.

Moderate Acute Hepatic Injury Substantiated by Liver Biopsy

A survey of the literature reveals a limited number of environmental exposures in which the presence of significant liver injury is documented not only by laboratory findings but also by liver biopsy observations. Recovery is the rule. This includes findings after trichlorethylene intoxication, in which mainly fatty infiltration was noted;[155] acute cholestatic hepatitis after dinitrophenol[156] or chromium intoxication;[157] *Amanita phalloides* poisoning, where elevated serum aminotransferase activity was associated with centrolobular necrosis without inflammation;[150] and heat stroke, possibly considered environmental, in which centrolobular necrosis was associated with cholestasis.[158,159] Such milder lesions were also found in youngsters after lead poisoning.[142] The best-documented episode is Epping jaundice,[160,161] in which at least 84 persons ate bread made from flour accidentally contaminated with 4,4'-diaminodiphenylmethane. The clinical manifestations varied. Upper abdominal pain and jaundice sometimes lasted for months, as did abnormalities in results of hepatic tests. Liver biopsy specimens showed hepatocellular injury, portal inflammation, eosinophilic infiltration, and bile duct injury, as well as cholestasis. Thus, histologically, the differential diagnosis from viral hepatitis does not appear easy. A similar disease was caused by methylenedianiline.[162] Jamaican vomiting sickness, resulting from toxic hypoglycine in a local fruit, clinically and histologically resembles Reye's syndrome.[163]

Metabolic Effects of Environmental Agents on the Liver

Many environmental agents produce porphyria in man, either acute hepatic porphyria or porphyria cutanea tarda.[163a] Hypercholesterolemia or hypertriglyceridemia have also been described, but space does not permit discussion of these functional consequences.

Chronic Liver Disease

Abnormalities in the Results of Hepatic Tests

In view of the difficulty in individual cases of associating exposure to industrial agents with abnormalities of hepatic function and structure, field studies on large population groups, such as workers, have been applied. They require control groups without exposure for evaluation before a significant incidence of abnormalities can be assumed. Michigan dairy farmers were exposed to polybrominated biphenyls as result of an accidental contamination of animal feed with a fire retardant.[164] This resulted in chemical contamination of cattle and their milk. In 614 such farmers, compared with 141 Wisconsin dairy farmers not exposed, activities of alkaline phosphatase were elevated in 11.1%, as compared to 14.2% in the controls; SGPT in 11.1% as compared to 2.8%; SGOT in 10.7%, as compared to 2.8%; and LDH in 6.8%, as compared to 2.8% (Table 1). Bilirubin elevation, by contrast, was more frequent in the Wisconsin farmers, but none of the recorded elevations reached twice the upper limit of normal.[165] In 493 workers exposed to styrene, no significant alterations of similar, mainly enzyme-based test results were found, with the exception of gamma glutamyl transpeptidase, where the elevation depended on both level and duration of the exposure.[2] In a major German chemical factory, similar results were obtained on a very large material, but no distinct differences were found between the percentage of abnormalities in preemployment test results as compared to those in the exposed workers.[166] An effect of socioeconomic factors was suggested by the lower incidence of abnormalities in salaried employees, however. Similar studies are being conducted in other settings, such as one begun following the explosion in Sevoso in northern Italy, which resulted in pollution by dioxin-containing agents.[167] Abnormalities in the results of hepatic tests have been observed following prolonged exposure to fumes containing organic solvents or to other chemicals. Whether these abnormalities, usually not accompanied by disturbed health, are related to development of disabling liver diseases is not established, even if they are associated with nonspecific histologic alterations (see p. 607). Frequently the abnormalities disappear on termination of the exposure. Elevation of gamma glutamyl transpeptidase and hepatomegaly appeared to be the most sensitive indicators of an alteration. It is not established whether this reflects liver injury or induction, however (see before).

Partially Established Chronic Liver Injury

Sustained liver injury in man from a variety of environmental agents, mainly industrial, is often invoked, particularly in view of experimental evidence of liver damage by these agents, including oncogenicity. An attempt to collect hard data in man was barely successful, however. A 3-year study of the effects of *tetrachloroethane* on workers in a penicillin factory revealed hepatomegaly, urobilinogenuria, hyperbilirubinemia, and positive thymol coagulation tests, but two other studies were negative.[137] *Trichloroethylene* exposure resulted in hyperglobulinemia suggestive of liver damage, while several other studies showed no changes of laboratory tests of hepatic function.[168] There is no factual evidence available that would relate chronic liver disease in man or monkey to *organochlorine pesticide* exposure (DDT, Aldrin, Dieldrin, Chlordecone), although these agents stimulate hepatic drug and steroid metabolism.[169-173] Elevated DDT and Dieldrin concentrations in cirrhotic liver appear to be related to the lipid content in the liver.[174,175] An extensive clinical study of Yusho disease (poisoning caused by ingestion of rice oil contaminated with *polychlorinated biphenyls*) in Japan revealed no abnormalities of laboratory tests of hepatic function except for the results of Bromsulphalein test, which were abnormal in several cases.[176-179] Liver biopsies disclosed hypertrophy of smooth endoplasmic reticulum and mitochondrial changes[180] but no specific alterations.[181] No definite clinical evidence of hepatotoxicity was associated with *polybrominated biphenyl* exposure.[182] Hepatomegaly and liver tenderness were not prominent findings, although results of hepatic tests were abnormal in about 25% of those tested.[165] There is little evidence of liver disease as a result of exposure to *pentachlorophenol*[183] or *tetrachlorodibenzo-p-dioxin*.[184,185]

In workers exposed to *styrene*, indications of chronic liver injury are listed in various papers mainly from East European countries.[186,187] The evidence is not convincing, however. The National Institute for Occupational Safety and Health is conducting a number of studies to assess the effects of chemical exposures upon the digestive system. The liver may be involved by exposure to epichlorohydrin, ethylene dibromide, benzene, tri- and perchloroethylene, methylene chloride, and toluene diisocyanate, but detailed information is not available.[188]

In conclusion, while evidence exists for exposure of man to many environmental agents that are hepatotoxic in animals, chronic liver disease in man is not established for the bulk of them. The sequence exemplified following exposure to vinyl chloride (see p. 622) is the most glaring exception.

Cirrhosis

The large number of cases of cirrhosis without known etiology, designated as cryptogenic cirrhosis, raises the suspicion that some may be environmentally induced, as defined in the introduction, for instance, from industrial chemicals. A thorough literature search reveals little evidence in support of this assumption. In the few instances published, it is not clear whether the cirrhosis represents simple postnecrotic scarring, as seen after carbon tetrachloride,[189,190] trichlorethane, or chlorinated naphthalene[140] injury, or real cirrhosis. In the first identification of hepatotoxicity of dimethyl nitrosamine in industrial workers, the presence of cirrhosis is listed,[127] and the same holds true for another case.[128] Aflatoxin supposedly has produced cirrhosis in children.[191,192] There is evidence of cirrhosis formation following exposure to a few chemicals in which hypersensitivity rather than a direct toxic effect is incriminated, e.g., trinitrotoluene.[193] This agrees with experiences with medicinal drugs where only those associated with the morphologic picture of chronic active hepatitis and hypersensitivity (nonpredictable drug reaction) lead to cirrhosis (see Chapter 33). The chances for insidious transformation to cirrhosis from environmental chemicals are therefore low. Cirrhosis resulting from hepatic vein obstruction is discussed later, as is cirrhosis from arsenic or vinyl chloride.

Veno-occlusive Disease

Pyrrolizidine alkaloids in senecio, crotalaria, and heliotropium plants cause veno-occlusive disease of the liver,[194] as first reported after ingestion of contaminated bread.[195] Subsequently, it was described in malnourished children in Jamaica and other Caribbean areas, where bush tea is the vehicle.[196] Epidemics of this lesion were reported from India[197] and Afghanistan[198] in adults and also in 2 Mexican-American children in Arizona.[199] The same lesion in live stock is well known to veterinarians in South Africa and Australia.[200,201] (see before). The obstruction of medium-sized and small hepatic vein tributaries causes severe passive congestion of the liver, potentially progressing to cirrhosis, although portal tract structures are long preserved. Ascites is the most prominent symptom. Therapeutic radiation to the liver in excessive doses causes a similar obstruction of the hepatic vein tributaries progressing to fibrosis.[202-205] There is no evidence of similar effects of environmental radiation.

Granulomas

Exposure in the handling of beryllium may result after a long latent period in a granulomatous reaction of the liver,[206-209] usually associated with a clinically more significant pulmonary lesion. Beryllium granulomatosis has many features of sarcoidosis, sharing with it a specific diagnostic skin reaction. Exposure to copper in Bordeaux solution in Portugal also has caused hepatic granulomas.[210]

Hepatocellular Carcinoma

Epidemiologic observations suggest an environmental origin of hepatocellular cancer, reflected in the great geographical variations. The highest incidence has been recorded in the blacks of sub-Saharan Africa, particularly the Shangaans of Mozambique.[211] This is followed by many other African countries, East Asia and Oceania, Japan, and Southern Europe, with the lowest incidence in Central and Northern Europe and North America. In Western countries, however, pockets of higher incidence exist, for instance, in the Oriental population of the United States, although it is significantly lower in this group than in the Oriental countries of their ancestors.[212-214] The *Atlas of Cancer Mortality in the United States* indicates a higher incidence of cancer of biliary passages and the liver, unfortunately not separated from each other, in circumscribed areas where industrial plants, primarily petrochemical, aggregate.[215] Moreover, the common production of hepatocellular cancer in experimental animals by various chemicals, following the initial demonstration by Sasaki and Yoshida[216] in Japan, suggests a chemical environmental origin for hepatocellular carcinoma. Despite the abundance of chemical agents producing hepatocellular carcinoma in experimental animals, however, the documentation of these manifold agents having produced carcinoma in the human liver is far less convincing, indeed missing for most, in contrast to ample evidence in other organ sites.

The most common factors associated with hepatocellular carcinoma in man are alcohol abuse and hepatitis B virus infection. Both of these factors, despite their environmental nature, deserve specific consideration in a hepatologic text (for hepatitis B, see Chapter 35). The relation between alcoholic liver injury and hepatocellular carcinoma is not clear. The epidemiologic evidence is convincing in countries where the carrier rate of hepatitis B is low and where the majority of hepatocellular carcinomas is observed in alcoholics. Whether the incidence of hepatocellular carcinoma in a given area is related to the incidence of alcoholic cirrhosis is not established. Evidence suggests that the incidence rate of carcinoma in alcoholic cirrhosis has increased. To what degree this reflects variations in diagnosis and autopsy rate, age of population, or longer survival of alcoholics because of improved therapy is not established. Supposedly the rate is higher in reformed alcoholics.[217] Incidence rates of up to 15% cancer in alcoholics are quoted.[218] Carcinoma also develops in noncirrhotic livers of alcoholics, and the mechanism of alcohol-induced carcinogenesis remains problematic. Alcohol may alter the microsomal biotransformation system,[111] but a direct carcinogenic effect of alcohol is not excluded because of its mutagenic potential[219] and the liberation of free radicals.[220] Finally, the possibility that the cirrhotic liver is more susceptible to additional carcinogenic factors, e.g., ubiquitous ones, should be considered, suggesting that a cirrhotic process itself may be the basis of carcinomatous transformation.

MYCOTOXINS

The chemical possibly responsible for a significant portion of hepatocellular carcinomas in man is the mycotoxic agent aflatoxin,[17,221] the most potent hepatocarcinogenic substance per unit weight in animals. Significant species differences exist, the mouse being the least sensitive animal. The metabolic basis of the formation of the responsible ultimate carcinogen(s) is known. The epidemiologic basis of occurrence of aflatoxin in food contaminated with *Aspergillus flavus*, particularly in hot humid areas, is clearly delineated.[222] This includes the often-reviewed geographic association between aflatoxin exposure and incidence of hepatocellular cancer in Africa, particularly Uganda, Swaziland, Kenya, and Mozambique, and in Asia in Thailand and the Philippines.[17] Despite these many surveys, the evidence that aflatoxin is responsible for human hepatocellular carcinoma is still circumstantial, as it is for other human liver-related disorders, such as Reye's disease in Thailand.[148] The possibility has been raised that aflatoxin cooperates with hepatitis B antigens[223] in inducing hepatocellular carcinoma on the basis of experimental evidence of combined viral and chemical carcinogenesis.[224,225] The evidence for other myocotoxins, such as sterigmatocystin, producing hepatocellular carcinoma in man is far less convincing, as it also is for plant poisons carcinogenic in animals, such as cycasin.[226] As already pointed out, no convincing evidence was found in an extensive survey as to the ability of a large number of proven hepatocarcinogens in animals, including primates,[61] to produce hepatocellular carcinoma in man. This includes carbon tetrachloride,[227] the nitroso compounds, organochlorine pesticides, and polyhalogenated biphenyls.

The Sequence Exemplified by Exposure to
Vinyl Chloride, Arsenic, and Thorotrast

Environmental, predominantly industrial, exposure to vinyl chloride, inorganic arsenicals and probably inorganic copper, as well as agents in therapeutic use [thorium dioxide (Thorotrast) and arsenic], produce a characteristic morphologic sequence. This is characterized by focal hepatocytic hyperplasia combined with focal hyperplasia of sinusoidal cells, progressing potentially to angiosarcoma and exceptionally to hepatocellular carcinoma and possibly cirrhosis. The vinyl-chloride-induced lesion represents the prototype of this sequence, which guided the elucidation of the lesion induced by the other agents.[10]

Vinyl Chloride

The availability of follow-up biopsy specimens in man permitted the construction of the sequence,[9,10,228] correlated with and supplemented by light- and electron-microscopic observations in animals exposed to prolonged inhalation of vinyl chloride.[229,230] The correlation of the entire sequence in man and rodents is by far the most complete for any known hepatocarcinogen. Moreover, the experimental production of angiosarcoma preceded or coincided with the recognition of the relation between vinyl chloride and angiosarcoma in man and also assisted in setting allowable tolerance levels in the ambient air in factories. Furthermore, the rarity of hepatic angiosarcoma in man made the multiple occurrence in the relatively small work force of plants engaged in the polymerization of the gaseous monomer, vinyl chloride, to the widely used plastic polymer, polyvinyl chloride, a convincing argument for an etiologic relation. This was strengthened by the greater incidence in workers with the highest exposure, such as those cleaning the polymerization vats. Finally, the appreciation of various well-defined stages of "vinyl chloride disease" facilitated the search for clinical and biochemical tools to identify early and late stages and thus provide parameters of clinical recognition of a potentially reversible early stage and to take appropriate hygienic action. In the clinical recognition of the morphologically defined precursor stages, however, the least progress has been made. Nevertheless, the vinyl-chloride-induced sequential changes represent the best-studied and best-understood industrial hepatic lesion, indeed the prototype. They also provided the stimulus for this entire chapter, particularly since the experiences from the study of vinyl chloride disease may serve in the management of other industrial hepatic injuries that might appear.

CLINICAL INVESTIGATIONS

Nonspecific hepatic injury in vinyl chloride polymerization workers was described by Russian[231] and Roumanian scientists.[232] Several years later, with the first appreciation of angiosarcomas in vinyl chloride workers[233] and in rats exposed to vinyl chloride,[234] splenomegaly, laboratory evidence of liver injury, and hepatic fibrosis associated with portal hypertension were recognized in German workers who were examined because of a vinyl-chloride-induced skin lesion (osteoacrolysis).[235] This led rapidly to surveys of workers in such factories.[236,237] The abnormalities found by conventional biochemical tests did not differ significantly from control populations and did not match, in diagnostic significance, laparoscopy;[238] extensive physical methods, including scanning[239,240] and angiography;[241,242] and hemodynamic studies for portal hypertension.[243,244] It is not established, however, whether these physical methods, particularly angiography, detect the precursor stage or only the angiosarcoma, for which surgical excision offers no hope in view of its multicentric nature. Effective chemotherapy has not been established.

METABOLIC STUDIES

The metabolism of vinyl chloride has been extensively studied, particularly in the rat,[245-247] in which liver function impairment has also been noted.[248] Vinyl chloride ($ClCH=CH_2$) undergoes three metabolic transformations in the rat: (1) change to chlorethanol, becoming chloracetaldehyde with the help of alcohol dehydrogenase; (2) transformation of chlorethanol to chloracetic acid by a catalase; and (3) the most important for toxic effects, transformation by cytochrome P-448 to an epoxide, chloro-oxiran, which is capable of covalent binding to macromolecules[246] and alkylation.[249] Vinyl chloride itself is not bound to macromolecules.[250] The biologic fate of vinyl chloride explains its oncogenic potential, as well as the mutagenic activity of its metabolites.[251-253] As with any other epoxide formation, the presence of hydrases[254] and glutathione determines the final outcome. The important role of the biotransformation system is illustrated by the extensive hepatic necrosis produced by large doses of vinyl chloride in rats exposed to inducing chemicals. This is not found without induction.[38]

MORPHOLOGIC STUDIES

The earliest lesion in both man and rodents is focal hyperplasia of hepatocytes, with variation of nuclei and cytoplasm in neighboring cells.[229,255] This lesion seems to be associated with portal hypertension, as judged from serial biopsies obtained before the connection with vinyl chloride was known.[256] Subsequently, in a second stage, the hepatocytic hyperplasia is associated with hyperplasia of polymorphic sinusoidal cells and focal increase of the reticulum framework,[230] accompanied by numerous perisinusoidal fat-storing cells,[257] presumably precursors of fibroblasts. Electron microscopically, the hepatocytes show only insignificant lesions.[258] Light microscopy shows subtle intralobular fibrosis, not characteristic portal, and characteristic subcapsular fibrosis, the last being the basis for the diagnostic laparoscopic picture. This stage may be associated with portal hypertension, splenomegaly, sometimes with thrombocytopenia, and bleeding esophageal varices, manifestations considered characteristic of Banti's syndrome.[8,240,259] Whether this stage undergoes regression on discontinuation of exposure is not established. Progression may take place in three directions: one, into hepatocellular carcinoma, rare in man (reference 261 and some personal observations) but developing in rats exposed to inhalation of vinyl chloride at birth;[260] the other two pathways, more common in man and adult animals, lead to angiosarcoma (text Fig. 1). One pathway represents transformation of the endothelial cells in the mixed hyperplastic nodules to angiosarcoma cells associated with the disappearance of most other

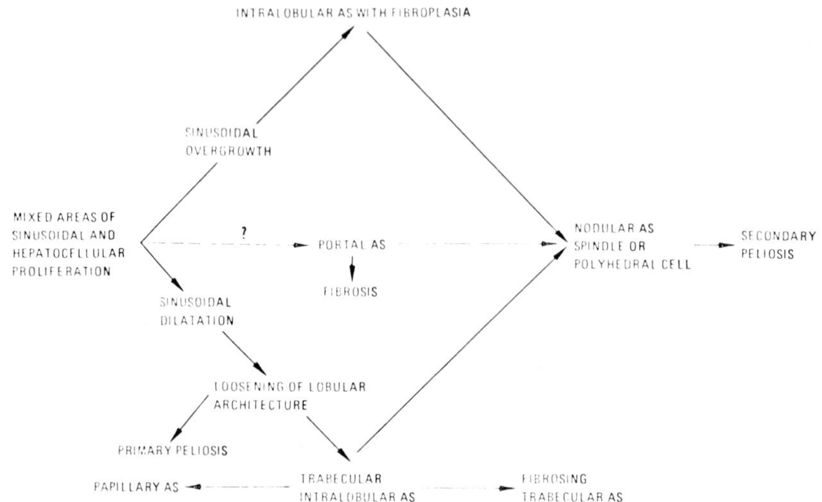

FIG. 1—Proposed schema of evolution of hepatic angiosarcoma (AS). (Reprinted from Ref. 10 with permission of the American Journal of Pathology.)

cells characteristic of inflammation. Significant parenchymal and subsequent portal fibrosis complicates this form of intralobular angiosarcoma in both man and animal. The third and most frequent pathway is initiated by dilatation of sinusoids without relation to lobular architecture which may progress to peliosis. Such sinusoidal dilatation is not diagnostic of the sequence, since it occurs in women on contraceptive drugs,[6] in men and women on anabolic steroids,[7,262] even without tumor formation, and after administration of chenodeoxycholate.[262a] The dilatation of the sinusoidal spaces leads to loosening of the architecture until trabecles, consisting of hepatocytic plates with multiple layers of hepatocytes covered by angiosarcoma cells, traverse the dilated blood spaces to produce the most characteristic picture of the trabecular form of angiosarcoma. Subsequent fibrosis in the core of these trabecles crowds the hepatocytes, and papillary structures or diffuse fibrosis develop. In all described forms of angiosarcoma, solid nodules of various sizes may develop, consisting of either spindle-shaped or polyhedral tumor cells. Extensive hemorrhage may lead to "secondary peliosis." Exceptionally, cirrhosis may develop.[263]

Study of a relatively large material of these tumors in man[264] revealed no significant differences between angiosarcoma related to vinyl chloride and that of unknown etiology, with the vinyl-chloride-induced tumor representing 11% to 20% of the studied material.[10,265,266] The similarity in all stages between vinyl-chloride-induced and idiopathic angiosarcoma suggests an environmental factor, so far not detected in the idiopathic group, possibly related to arsenic. Hepatic angiosarcoma is far more frequent in animals than in man. It occurs spontaneously in dogs and has been observed in rodents and primates after treatment with various chemicals, particularly those that also cause hepatocellular carcinoma.[267-270]

There are over 75 instances of vinyl-chloride-associated angiosarcomas in man.[271] By reducing the amount of vinyl chloride permissible in the air to less than 1 ppm, it is hoped that new cases will not be initiated, but in view of a probable induction period of up to 20 years, additional cases have to be expected. Apparently, 6,000 workers are engaged in the polymerization of vinyl chloride at one time. With turnover, we can assume that about 30,000 are at risk. One million workers have been engaged in processing of vinyl chloride and may have been exposed to up to 100 ppm. These smaller doses, and possibly inhalation of particulate material containing polyvinyl chloride may lengthen the induction period to 30 years.

Inorganic Arsenicals

The sequence just discussed has also been postulated in liver lesions induced by inorganic arsenicals on the basis of single biopsy and autopsy observations but without the benefit of confirmation in experimental animals. The hepatic changes in animals from chronic exposure to inorganic arsenicals are nonspecific. The human sequence has been observed after both medicinal and industrial exposure. Cases with portal hypertension, such as Banti's syndrome and angiosarcoma,[272,273] have been reported following prolonged administration of inorganic arsenic-containing medicinal agents. Excess arsenic in drinking water in India was associated with portal hypertension[274] and, predominantly, angiosarcoma, but also carcinoma, and supposedly, cirrhosis has followed exposure to arsenic-containing pesticides in vineyards in Germany.[275,276] Cirrhosis was slightly increased among smelter workers exposed to arsenic.[277] Study revealed the same mixed hyperplastic areas in the noninvolved liver of autopsy specimens of arsenic-induced angiosarcoma, as well as in idiopathic angiosarcoma.[10]

Thorotrast

Previously administered for radiologic demonstration, mainly of cerebral lesions, Thorotrast is associated with the same sequence of mixed hyperplastic nodules, sinusoidal dilatation, and angiosarcoma.[10] While this is a medicinal injury, it illustrates the potential of local radiation to produce the sequence, which has not been substantiated with other types of radiation. There are few reports of the precursor lesion[10,278] but many of angiosarcoma.[279,280,281] Thorotrast also produces carcinoma, however, mainly of the cholangiocarcinoma type[282,283] and possibly cirrhosis.[284] Malignant vascular tumors were produced by Thorotrast in rabbits.[285] Hepatocellular carcinoma has been reported following therapeutic hepatic irradiation in man.[286] Finally, the same sequence has been reported after exposure to *copper* in Bordeaux mixture in Portugal,[210] although it is not certain that arsenical admixture can be excluded.

THE PROBLEM OF THE ETIOLOGY
OF HEPATIC MALIGNANCIES

Most hepatocellular carcinomas are associated with three factors[287]: hepatitis B virus and alcohol abuse, for which no experimental models exist, and aflatoxin, which has ample experimental support. Other environmental or industry-related malignancies of the liver are better substantiated, and most have experimental counterparts. Their contribution to the total number of hepatic

malignancies in man is small, however. The best substantiated preferentially produce angiosarcoma. Other exogenous factors contribute very little to the number of hepatic malignancies, and the same holds also true for hepatocellular carcinoma associated with endogenous metabolic abnormalities, such as hemochromatosis, alpha-1-antitrypsin deficiency, and tyrosinemia. This contrasts to the many chemicals that have proven hepatocarcinogenic potential in animals but the effects of which in man are not established.[288]

OUTLOOK

The search for evidence of environmental hepatic lesions, stimulated by the vinyl chloride experience, detected a disappointingly small number of substantiated hepatic injuries of the chronic variety. It did not significantly enlarge the substantiated number of etiologic factors for cirrhosis and hepatic cancer appreciated long ago. This result of the literature search was predictable from careful study of available reviews,[287,289,290] but does not exclude the possibility that environmental factors may have been overlooked because of a weak, ill-defined, or incomplete data base. Thus, the meager results should not reduce vigilance particularly in view of the potential significance of metabolic alterations.

Table 2 provides a list of specific agents incriminated in environmental hepatic injury and the numbers of pages where they are discussed.

REFERENCES

1. Martini GA: Toxische hepatitis. Edited by L Wannagat: Toxische Leberschaeden. Stuttgart, Georg Thieme Verlag, 1976, pp 121–128

2. Lorimer WV, Lilis R, Nicholson WJ, Anderson H, FE Fischbein A, Daum S, Rom W, Rice C, Selikoff IJ: Clinical studies of styrene workers: Initial findings. Environ Health Perspect 17:171–181, 1976

3. Struthers JE Jr, Mehta SJ, Kay MD, Naylor JL: Relative concentrations of individual nonsulfated bile acids in the serum and bile of patients with cirrhosis. Am J Dig Dis [New Series] 22:861–865, 1977

4. Demers LM, Hepner GW: Levels of immunoreactive glycine-conjugated bile acids in health and hepatobiliary disease. Am J Clin Pathol 66:831–839, 1976

5. Stiehl L, Ast E, Czygan P, Fröhling W, Raedsch R, Stiel A, Kommerell B: Die Ser-

umgallensaeuren bei Patienten mit hepatobiliaeren Erkrankungen: Ein empfindlicher Indikator eines Leberparenchymschadens oder einer Cholestase. Inn Med 5:14–21, 1978

6. Winkler K, Poulsen H: Liver disease with periportal sinusoidal dilatation. A possible complication to contraceptive steroids. Scand J Gastroenterol 10:699–704, 1975

7. Bagheri SA, Boyer JL: Peliosis hepatis associated with androgenic anabolic steroid therapy. Ann Intern Med 81:610–618, 1974

8. Thomas LB, Popper H, Berk PD, Selikoff I, Falk H: Vinyl chloride induced liver disease. From idiopathic portal hypertension (Banti's syndrome) to angiosarcoma. N Engl J Med 292:17–22, 1975

9. Müller R, Bechtelsheimer H, Gedigk P, Marstelle JH, Lelbach WK: Das morphologische Bild der Leberschaedigung nach

59. Palmer PE, Christopherson WM, Wolfe HJ: Alpha$_1$-antitrypsin, protein marker in oral contraceptive-associated hepatic tumors. Am J Clin Pathol 68:736–739, 1977
60. Gopalan C, Tulpule PG, Krishnamurthi D: Induction of hepatic carcinoma with aflatoxin in the rhesus monkey. Food Cosmet Toxicol 10:519–521, 1972
61. Adamson RH, Correa P, Dalgard DW: Occurrence of a primary liver carcinoma in a rhesus monkey fed aflatoxin B$_1$. J Natl Cancer Inst 50:549–553, 1973
62. Farber E, Solt D, Cameron R, Laishes B, Ogawa K, Medline A: Newer insights into the pathogenesis of liver cancer. Am J Pathol 89:477–482, 1977
63. Berenblum I: Established principles and unresolved problems in carcinogenesis. J Natl Cancer Inst 60:723–726, 1978
64. Frei JV: Some mechanisms operative in carcinogenesis. A review. Chem Biol Interact 13:1–25, 1976
65. Kleihues P, Cooper K, Buecheler J: Involvement of DNA repair in the organ-specific carcinogenicity of alkylating agents. Edited by H Remmer, HM Bolt, P Bannasch, and H Popper: Primary Liver Tumors. Lancaster, MTP Press, 1978, pp 319–326
66. Craddock VM, Henderson AR: De novo repair replication of DNA in liver of carcinogen-treated animals. Cancer Res 36:2135–2143, 1978
67. Schulte-Hermann R: Induction of liver growth and tumor promotion by drugs and environmental pollutants. Edited by H Remmer, HM Bolt, P Bannasch, and H Popper: Primary Liver Tumors. Lancaster, MTP Press, 1978, pp. 385–394
68. Craddock VM: Cell proliferation and induction of liver cancer. Edited H Remmer, HM Bolt, P Bannasch, and H Popper: Primary Liver Tumors. Lancaster, MTP Press, 1978, pp 377–383
69. Peers FG, Linsell AC: Dietary aflatoxins and liver cancer. A population based study in Kenya. Br J Cancer 27:473–484, 1973
70. Bianchi L: Personal communication
71. Remmer H, Bolt HM, Bannasch P, Popper H (eds): Primary Liver Tumors. Lancaster, MTP Press, 1978
72. Ioannides C, Parke DV: Mechanism of induction of hepatic microsomal drug metabolizing enzymes by a series of barbiturates. J Pharmacol Pharmaceut 27:739–746, 1975
73. Peraino C, Fry RJM, Staffeldt E, Christopher JP: Comparative enhancing effects of phenobarbital, amobarbital, diphenylhydantoin, and dichlorodiphenyltrichloroethane on 2-acetylaminofluorene-induced hepatic tumorigenesis in the rat. Cancer Res 35:2884–2890, 1975
74. Nishizumi M: Enhancement of diethylnitrosamine hepatocarcinogenesis in rats by exposure to polychlorinated biphenyls or phenobarbital. Cancer Lett 2:11–16, 1976
75. Von Schmidt-Wilcke HA, Wolfert W, Grundmann E: Halothan und Tuberkulostatica als hepatotoxische Arzneimittelkombination. Z Gastroenterol 15:504–511, 1977
76. Pessayre D, Bentata M, Degott C, Nouel O, Miguet J-P, Rueff B, Benhamou J-P: Isoniazid-rifampin fulminant hepatitis. A possible consequence of the enhancement of isoniazid hepatotoxicity by enzyme induction. Gastroenterology 72:284–289, 1977
77. Alvares AP, Bickers DR, Kappas A: Polychlorinated biphenyls: A new type of inducer of cytochrome P-448 in the liver. Proc Natl Acad Sci USA 70:1321–1325, 1973
78. Labadarios D, Dickerson JWT, Parke DV, Lucast EG, Obuwa GH: The effects of chronic drug administration on hepatic enzyme induction and folate metabolism. Br J Clin Pharmacol 5:167–173, 1978
79. Clayson DB: Nutrition and experimental carcinogenesis: A review. Cancer Res 35:3293–3300, 1975
80. Rogers AE, Sanchez O, Feinsod FM, Newberne PM: Dietary enhancement of nitrosamine carcinogenesis. Cancer Res 35:96–99, 1974
81. Pantuck EJ, Hsiao K-C, Conney AH, Garland WA, Kappas A, Anderson KE, Alvares AP: Effect of charcoal-broiled beef on phenacetin metabolism in man. Science 194:1055–1057, 1976
82. Wattenberg LW, Loub WD, Lam LK, Speier JL: Dietary constituents altering the responses to chemical carcinogens. Fed Proc 35:1327–1331, 1976
83. Campbell TC: Nutrition and drug-metabolizing enzymes. Clin Pharmacol Ther 22:699–706, 1977
84. Vesell ES, Passananti GT: Genetic and environmental factors affecting host response to drugs and other chemical compounds in our environment. Environ Health Perspect 20:159–182, 1977

85. Hutterer F, Klion FM, Wengraf A, Schaffner F, Popper H: Hepatocellular adaptation and injury. Structural and biochemical changes following dieldrin and methyl butter yellow. Lab Invest 20:455–464, 1969

86. Crampton RF, Grays TJB, Grasso P, Parke DV: Long-term studies on chemically induced liver enlargement in the rat. I. Sustained induction of microsomal enzymes with absence of liver damage on feeding phenobarbitone or butylated hydroxytoluene. Toxicology 7:289–306, 1977

87. Parke DV: The role of the endoplasmic reticulum in carcinogenesis. (in press)

88. Alvares AP, Kappas A: Induction of aryl hydrocarbon hydroxylase by polychlorinated biphenyls in the foeto-placental unit and neonatal livers during lactation. Fed Eur Biochem Soc Lett 50:172–174, 1975

89. Argus MF, Arcos JC, Hoch-Ligeti C: Studies on the carcinogenic activity of protein-denaturing agents. Hepatocarcinogenicity of dioxane. J Natl Cancer Inst 35:949–958, 1965

90. Woo Y-t, Argus MF, Arcos JC: Effect of mixed-function oxidase modifiers on metabolism and toxicity of the oncogen dioxane. Cancer Res 38:1621–1625, 1978

91. Hinton DE: Studies on the cellular toxicity of polychlorinated biphenyls (PBCs). I. Effect of PBCs on microsomal enzymes and on synthesis and turnover of microsomal and cytoplasmic lipids of rat liver - A morphological and biochemical study. Virchows Arch B [Zellpathol] 27:279–306, 1978

92. Hepner GW, Vesell ES: Assessment of aminopyrine metabolism in man by breath analysis after oral administration of ^{14}C-aminopyrine. Effects of phenobarbital, disulfiram and portal cirrhosis. N Engl J Med 291:1384–1388, 1974

93. Hepner GW, Vesell ES: Quantitative assessment of hepatic function by breath analysis after oral administration of [^{14}C]aminopyrine. Ann Intern Med 83:632–638, 1975

94. Audétat V, Preisig R, Bircher J: Der Aminopyrin-Atemtest unter akuter Äthanoleinwirkung. Schweiz Med Wochenschr 107:231–235, 1977

95. Strik JJTWA: personal communication

96. Hunter J, Maxwell JD, Stewart DA, Williams R: Urinary D-glucaric acid excretion and total liver content of cytochrome P-450 in guinea-pigs: Relationship during enzyme induction and following inhibition of protein synthesis. Biochem Pharmacol 22:743–747, 1973

97. Notten WRF, Henderson PT: Effect of disulfiram on the urinary D-glucaric acid excretion and activity of some enzymes involved in drug metabolism in guinea-pig. Arch Int Pharmacodyn Ther 2–5:199–208, 1973

98. Herzberg M, Fishel B, Wiener MH: Hepatic microsomal enzyme induction and its evaluation in a clinical laboratory. Israel J. Med Sci 13:471–476, 1977

99. Herzberg M, Tenenbaum E, Fishel B, Wiener MH: D-glucaric acid and gamma glutamyltransferase as indices of hepatic enzyme induction in pregnancy. Clin Chem 23:596–598, 1977

100. Carrella M, D'Arienzo A, Manzillo G, De Ritis F: An evaluation of urinary D-glucaric acid excretion during acute hepatitis in man. Dig Dis 23:18–22, 1978

101. Whitfield JB, Moss DW, Neale G, Orme M, Breckenridge A: Changes in plasma gamma-glutamyl transpeptidase activity associated with alterations in drug metabolism in man. Br Med J 1:316–318, 1973

102. Martin PJ, Martin JV, Goldberg DM: Gamma-glutamyl transpeptidase, triglycerides, and enzyme induction. Br Med J 1:17–18, 1975

103. Martin JV, Martin PJ: Enzyme induction as a possible cause of increased serum-triglycerides after oral contraceptives. Lancet 1:1107–1108, 1976

104. Bartels H, Hauck W, Vogel I: Aminopyrine—an effective modifier of liver and serum gamma glutamyl transpeptidase. J Pediatr 86:298–301, 1975

105. Teschke R, Brand A, Strohmeyer G: Induction of hepatic microsomal gamma-glutamyltransferase activity following chronic alcohol consumption. Biochem Biophys Res Commun 75:718–724, 1977

106. Oldigs HD, Bartels H: Cytochrom P-450 in der Leber und Gamma-glutamyltransferase in Leber und Serum Phenobarbital—und Phenytoin-behandelter Ratten. Klin Wochenschr 55:85, 1977

107. Jujii M, Wakisaka G, Yamamoto T: Determination of liver volume by use of a gamma camera connected with 1600 or 4096 channel analyser in diffuse liver diseases. Gut 17:289–294, 1976

108. Capron J-P, Erlinger S, Feldmann G: Increased sulfobromophthalein clearance in a patient receiving phenobarbital and other anticonvulsant drugs. Gastroenterology 69:756–760, 1975

109. McLean AEM: Personal communication

110. Clemmesen J, Hjalgrim-Jensen S: Is phenobarbital carcinogenic? A follow-up of 8078 epileptics. Ecotoxicol Environ Safety 1:457–470, 1978

111. Lieber CS: Pathogenesis and early diagnosis of alcoholic liver injury. N Engl J Med 298:888–893, 1978

112. Tamburro CH: personal communication

113. Ganote CE, Otis JB: Characteristic lesions of yellow phosphorus-induced liver damage. Lab Invest 21:207–213, 1969

114. Marin GA, Montoya CA, Sierra JL, Senior JR: Evaluation of corticosteroid and exchange-transfusion treatment of acute yellow-phosphorus intoxication. N Engl J Med 284:125–128, 1971

115. Salfelder K, Doehnert HR, Doehnert G, Sauerteig E, De Liscano TR, Fabrega, SE: Fatal phosphorus poisoning; A study of forty-five autopsy cases. Beitr Pathol 147:321–340, 1972

116. Stewart RD, Boetthner EA, Southsorth RR, Cerney JC: Acute carbon tetrachloride intoxication. JAMA 183:994–997, 1963

117. Kennaugh RC: CCl₄ overdosage: A case report. S Afr Med J 49:635–636, 1975

118. Moon HD: The pathology of fatal carbon tetrachloride poisoning with special reference to the histogenesis of the hepatic and renal lesions. Am J Pathol 26:1041–1057, 1950

119. Rao SK, Recknagel RO: Early incorporation of carbon-labeled carbon tetrachloride into rat liver particulate lipids and proteins. Exp Mol Pathol 10:219–228, 1969

120. Dume T, Schroder E, Wetzels E: Clinical features and treatment of carbon tetrachloride poisoning. Dtsch Med Wochenschr 94:1646–1651, 1969

121. Joron GE, Cameron DG, Halpenny GW: Massive necrosis of the liver due to trichlorethylene. Can Med Assoc J 73:890–891, 1955

122. Baerg RD, Kimberg DV: Centrilobular hepatic necrosis and acute renal failure in "solvent sniffers." Ann Intern Med 73:713–720, 1970

123. Litt IF, Cohen MI: "Danger . . . vapor harmful." Spot-remover sniffing. N Engl J Med 281:543–544, 1969

124. James WRL: Fatal addiction to trichlorethylene. Br J Indust Med 20:47–49, 1963

125. O'Bien ET, Yeoman WB, Hobby JAE: Hepatorenal damage from toluene in a "glue sniffer." Br Med J 2:29–30, 1971

126. NIOSH: Tetrachloroethylene (perchloroethylene). Current Intelligence Bulletin 20. DHEW (NIOSH) Publication No. 78–112, 1978

127. Barnes JM, Magee PN: Some toxic properties of dimethylnitrosamine. Br J Indust Med 11:167–170, 1954

128. Freund HA: Clinical manifestations and studies in parenchymatous hepatitis. Ann Intern Med 10:1144–1155, 1937

129. Magee PN: Toxic liver injury. The metabolism of dimethylnitrosamine. Biochem J 64:676–682, 1956

130. Himsworth HP, Glynn LE: Toxipathic and trophopathic hepatitis. Lancet 1:457–461, 1944

131. Stewart MJ: Toxic jaundice in munition workers and troops. Br Med J 1:156–159, 1917

132. Stewart MJ: Atrophy of the liver. Br Med J 2:584–587, 1920

133. Willcox WH, Spilsbury BH, Legge TM: An outbreak of toxic jaundice of a new type amongst aeroplane workers—its clinical and toxicological aspect. Trans Med Soc London 38:129–1256, 1915

134. Coyer HA: Tetrachloroethane poisoning—seven cases. Ind Med 13:230–233, 1944

135. Wilson RH, Brumley DR: Health hazards—in the use of tetrachloroethane. Ind Med 13:233–234, 1944

136. Gurney R: Useful procedures in early diagnosis of liver damage following exposure to the chlorinated hydrocarbons. NY J Med 47:2566–2568, 1947

137. NIOSH: Criteria for a recommended standard occupational exposure to 1,1,2,2 tetrachloroethane. DHEW (NIOSH) Publication No. 77–121, 1976

138. Flinn FB, Jarvik NE: Liver lesions caused by chlorinated napthalene. Am J Hyg 27:19–25, 1938

139. Greenburg L, Mayers MR, Smith RA: The systemic effects resulting from exposure to certain chlorinated hydrocarbons. J Indust Hygiene Toxicol 21:29–38, 1939

140. Strauss N: Hepato-toxic effects following occupational exposure to Halowax (chlorinated hydrocarbons). Rev Gastroenterol 11:381–389, 1944

141. Smith NJ: Death following accidental

ingestion of DDT; experimental studies. JAMA 136:469–471, 1948

142. Beattie AD, Mullin P, Baxter R, Moore MR: Acute lead poisoning—an unusual cause of hepatitis. Gut 18:A968, 1977

143. Sereck-Hanssen A: Aflatoxin-induced fatal hepatitis? Arch Environ Health 20:729–731, 1970

144. Emmrich P, Toussaint W, Jungst BK, Neidhardt M, Straub E: Akute gelbe Leberdystrophie infolge von mit Mycotoxinen verunreinigter Xylitloesung. Fortschr Med 89:190–194, 1971

145. Campbell TC, Hayes JR: The role of aflatoxin in its toxic lesion. Toxicol Appl Pharmacol 35:199–222, 1976

146. Krichnamachari KAVR, Bhat RV, Nagajaran V, Tilak TBG: Investigations into an outbreak of hepatitis in parts of Western India. Indian J Med Res 63:1036–1049, 1975

147. Tandon BN, Krishnamurthy L, Koshy A, Tandon HD, Ramalingaswami V, Bhandari JR, Mathur MM, Mathur PD: Study of an epidemic of jaundice, presumably due to toxic hepatitis in Northwest India. Gastroenterology 72:488–494, 1977

148. Bourgeois CH, Shank RC, Grossman RA, Johnson DO, Wooding WL, Chandavimol P: Acute aflatoxin B_1 toxicity in the Macaque and its similarities to Reye's syndrome. Lab Invest 24:206–216, 1971

149. Panner BJ, Hanss RJ: Hepatic injury in mushroom poisoning. Electron microscopic observations on two nonfatal cases. Arch Pathol 87:35–45, 1969

150. Wepler W, Opitz K: Histologic changes in the liver biopsy in *Amanita phalloides* intoxication. Hum Pathol 3:249–254, 1972

151. Matthes KJ, Leber HW, Etesham-Schahabi S, Gerhardt H, Wizemann V: Amanitaphalloides-Intoxikation. Verlaufsbeobachtungen an 5 Faellen von schwerer Knollenblaetterpilzvergiftung. Med Welt 29:823–827, 1978

152. Mokhobo KP: Herb use and necrodegenerative hepatitis. S Afr Med J 50:1096–1099, 1976

153. Mokhobo KP: Acute necrodegenerative hepatitis. S Afr Med J 48:833–834, 1974

154. Wainwright J, Schonland MM: Toxic hepatitis in black patients in Natal. S Afr Med J 51:571–73, 1977

155. Smith GF: Trichlorethylene: a review. J Indust Med 23:249–269, 1966

156. Sidel N: Dinitrophenol poisoning causing jaundice: report of a case. JAMA 103:254, 1934

157. Pascale LR, Waldstein SS, Englering G, Dubin A, Szanto PB: Chromium intoxication with special reference to hepatic injury. JAMA 149:1385–1389, 1952

158. Bianchi L, Ohnacker H, Beck K, Zimmerli-Ning M: Liver damage in heat stroke and its regression. Hum Pathol 3:237–248, 1972

159. Kew MC, Minick OT, Bahu RM, Stein RJ, Kent G: Ultrastructural changes in the liver in heat stroke. Am J Pathol 90:609–618, 1978

160. Kopelman H, Robertson MH, Sanders PG, Ash I: The Epping jaundice. Br Med J 1:514–516, 1966

161. Kopelman H, Scheuer PJ, Williams R: The liver lesion of the Epping jaundice. Q J Med 35:553–567, 1966

162. McGill DB, Motto JD: An industrial outbreak of toxic hepatitis due to methylenedianiline. N Engl J Med 291:278–282, 1974

163. Tanaka K, Kean EA, Johnson B: Jamaican vomiting sickness. Biochemical investigation of two cases. N Engl J Med 295:461–467, 1976

163a. Doss M: Pathobiochemie der Porphyrien. Med Klin 72:1501–1518, 1977

164. Humphrey HEB, Hauner NS, Budd ML: Polybrominated biphenyls (PBB). Edited by DD Hemphill: Trace Substances in Environmental Health. Columbia, University of Missouri Press, 1975, pp 56–63

165. Selikoff IJ: personal communication

166. Steinborn J, Schmitz, T, Thiess AM: Recognition and interpretation of liver impairments in the chemical industry. Proceedings of the V Medichem Congress, San Francisco, 5th-9th September 1977 (in press)

167. NIEHS/IARC: Coordination of epidemiological studies on the long-term hazards of chlorinated dibenzodioxins/chlorinated dibenzofurans. IARC Internal Technical Report No. 78/001. Lyon, International Agency for Research on Cancer, 1978

168. NIOSH: Criteria for a recommended standard occupational exposure to trichloroethylene. HSM 73-11025, 1973

169. Deichmann WB, MacDonald WE: Organochlorine pesticides and liver cancer deaths in the United States, 1930–1972. Ecotoxicol Environ Safety 1:89–110, 1977

170. Wright AS, Donninger C, Greenland RD, Stemmer KL, Zavon MR: The effects of prolonged ingestion of dieldrin on the livers of male rhesus monkeys. Ecotoxicol Environ Safety 1:477–502, 1978
171. Taylor JR, Selhorst JB, Houff SA: Kepone intoxication in man. Neurology (Minneap) (in press)
172. Cohn WJ, Boylan JJ, Blanke RV, Fariss MW, Howell JR, Guzelian PS: Treatment of chlordecone (Kepone) toxicity with cholestyramine. Results of a controlled clinical trial. N Engl M Med 298:243–248, 1978
173. Kaminky LS, Piper LJ, McMartin DN, Fasco MJ: Induction of hepatic microsomal cytochrome P-450 by mirex and Kepone. Toxicol Appl Pharmacol 43:327–338, 1978
174. Radomski JL, Deichmann WB, Clizer EE, Rey A: Pesticide concentrations in the liver, brain and adipose tissue of terminal hospital patients. Food Cosmet Toxicol 6:209–220, 1968
175. Oloffs PC, Hardwick DF, Szeto SY, Moerman DG: DDT, dieldrin, and heptachlor epoxide in humans with liver cirrhosis. Clin Biochem 7:297–306, 1974
176. Kuratsune M: An abstract of results of laboratory examinations of patients with Yusho and of animal experiments. Environ Health Perspect 1:129–136, 1972
177. Kuratsune M, Yoshimura T, Matsuzaka J, Yamaguchi A: Epidemiologic study on Yusho, a poisoning caused by ingestion of rice oil contaminated with a commercial brand of polychlorinated biphenyls. Environ Health Perspect 1:119–128, 1972
178. Okumara M: Course of serum enzyme change in PCB poisoning. Fukuoka Acta Med 63:396–400, 1972
179. Hirayama C, Okumura M, Magai J, Masuda Y: Hypobilirubinemia in patients with polychlorinated biphenyl poisoniong. Clin Chim Acta 55:98–100, 1974
180. Hirayama C, Irisa T, Yamamoto T: Fine structural changes of the liver in a patient with chlorobiphenyl intoxication. Fukuoka Acta Med 60:455–461, 1969
181. Umeda G, Nakajima H, Yatsuki K: Some problems on health effects of polychlorinated biphenyls. Ecotoxicol Environ Safety 1:437–446, 1978
182. Kay K: Polybrominated biphenyls (PBB) environmental contamination in Michigan, 1973–1976. Environ Res 13:74–93, 1977
183. Dougherty RC: Human exposure to pentachlorophenol. Edited by KR Rao: Pentachlorophenol. New York, Plenum Press, 1978, pp 351–361
184. Ton That T: Pathologic humaine et animale de la dioxine. Rev Med (Paris) (in press)
185. Hay WM: Tetrachlorodibenzo-p-dioxin release at Seveso. Disasters 1:289–308, 1977
186. Zlobina NS: The toxicity of low concentrations of styrene vapors. Gig Sanit 28:29–35, 1963
187. Troshin IM, Sechenov IM: Some morbidity features of workers coming into contact with styrene. Gig Tr Prof Zabol 7:17–20, 1962
188. Bridbord K: Presentation to the National Commission on Digestive Diseases on the NIOSH role in digestive disease research. Department of Health, Education, and Welfare Center for Disease Control, National Institute for Occupational Safety and Health, Office of Extramural Coordination and Special Projects, March 3, 1978
189. Poindexter CA, Green CH: Toxic cirrhosis of the liver. JAMA 102:2015 1934
190. McDermott WV, Hardy HL: Cirrhosis of the liver following chronic exposure to carbon tetrachloride. J Occup Med 5:249–251, 1963
191. Robinson P: Infantile cirrhosis of the liver in India. With special reference to probable aflatoxin etiology. Clin Pediatr (Phila) 6:57–62, 1967
192. Amla I, Kamla CS, Gopalakrishna GS, Jayaraj AP, Sreenivasamurthy V, Parpia HAB: Cirrhosis in children from peanut meal contaminated by aflatoxin. Am J Clin Nutr 24:609–614, 1971
193. Wilcox WW: Toxic jaundice. Lancet 2:1–6, 1931
194. Bras G: Aspects of hepatic vascular diseases. Edited by EA Gall and FK Mostofi: The Liver. Baltimore, Williams & Wilkins, 1973, pp 406–430
195. Selzer G, and Parker RGF: Senecio poisoning exhibiting as Chiari's syndrome; report on 12 cases. Am J Pathol 27:885–907, 1951
196. Stuart KL, Bras G: Veno-occlusive disease of the liver. Q J Med 26:291–315, 1957
197. Tandon BN, Tandon HD, Tandon RK, Narndranathan M, Joshi YK: An epidemic of veno-occlusive disease of liver in central India. Lancet 2:271–272, 1976

198. Mohabbat O, Younos MS, Merzad AA, Srivastava RN, Sedig GG, Aram GN: An outbreak of hepatic veno-occlusive disease in north-western Afghanistan. Lancet 2:269–271, 1976

199. Stillman AE, Huxtable R, Consroe P, Kohnen P, Smith S: Hepatic veno-occlusive disease due to pyrrolizidine (Senecio) poisoning in Arizona. Gastroenterology 73:349–352, 1977

200. Bull LG, Culvenor CCJ, Dick AT: The Pyrrolizidine Alkaloids. Amsterdam, North-Holland, 1968, pp 1–293

201. McLean EK: The toxic actions of pyrrolizidine (Senecio) alkaloids. Pharmacol Rev 22:429–483, 1970

202. Reed GB, Cox AJ: The human liver after radiation injury. Am J Pathol 48:597–611, 1966

203. Lansing AM, Davis WM, Brizel HE: Radiation hepatitis. Arch Surg 96:878–882, 1968

204. Samuels LD, Grosfeld JL, Kartha M: Radiation hepatitis in children. J Pediat 78:68–73, 1971

205. Lewin K, Millis RR: Human radiation hepatitis. A morphologic study with emphasis on the late changes. Arch Pathol 96:21–26, 1973

206. Chesner C: Chronic pulmonary granulomatosis in residents of a community near a beryllium plant; three autopsied cases. Ann Intern Med 32:1028, 1950

207. DeNardi JM, Van Ordstrand HS, Carmody M: Chronic pulmonary granulomatosis; report of 10 cases. Am J Med 7:345–355, 1949

208. DeNardi JM, Van Ordstrand HS, Curtis GH, Zielinski J: Berylliosis: Summary and survey of all clinical types observed in a twelve-year period. Arch Indust Hyg 8:1–24, 1953

209. Van Ordstrand HS: Current concepts of beryllium poisoning. Ann Intern Med 35:1203–1217, 1951

210. Pimentel JC, Menezes P: Liver disease in vineyard sprayers. Gastroenterology 72:275–283, 1977

211. Prates MD, Torres FO: A cancer study in Lourenco Marques, Portuguese East Africa. J Natl Cancer Inst 35:729–757, 1965

212. MacDonald RA: Primary carcinoma of the liver; a clinicopathologic study of one hundred eight cases. Arch Intern Med 99:266–279, 1957

213. Steiner PE: Cancer of the liver and cirrhosis in Trans-Saharan Africa and the United States of America. Cancer 13:1085–1166, 1960

214. Peters RL, Afroudakis AP, Tatter D: The changing incidence of association of hepatitis B with hepatocellular carcinoma in California. Am J Clin Pathol 68:1–7, 1977

215. Mason TJ, McKay FW, Hoover R, Blot WJ, Fraumeni JF Jr: Atlas of Cancer Mortality for U.S. Counties: 1950–1969. DHEW Publication No. (NIH) 75–780. US Department of Health, Education and Welfare

216. Sasaki T, Yoshida T: Experimentelle Erzeugung des Lebercarcinoms durch Fuetterung mit o-amidoazotoluol. Virchows Arch [Pathol Anat Physiol] 295:175–200, 1935

217. Lee F: Cirrhosis and hepatoma in alcoholics. Gut 7:77–85, 1966

218. Martini GA: The role of alcohol in the etiology of cancer of the liver. Dtsch Med Wochenschr (in press)

219. Obe G, Herha J: Chromosomal damage in chronic alcohol users. Humangenetik 29:191–200, 1975

220. Gordon ER: Pyridine nucleotides and ethanol. Edited by MM Fisher and JG Rankin: Alcohol and the Liver. New York, Plenum Press, 1977, pp 63–78

221. Butler WH: Aflatoxicosis in laboratory animals. Edited by LA Goldblatt: Aflatoxin: Scientific Background, Control and Implications. New York, Academic Press, 1969, pp 223–236

222. Shank RC: Epidemiology of aflatoxin carcinogenesis. Edited by HF Kraybill and MA Mehlman: Environmental Cancer. Vol. 3. Washington, Hemisphere Publishing Corporation, 1977, pp 291–318

223. Larouze B, London WT, Saimot G, Werner BG, Lustbader ED, Payet M, Blumberg BS: Host responses to hepatitis-B infection in patients with primary hepatic carcinoma and their families. A case/control study in Senegal, West Africa. Lancet 2:534–538, 1976

224. Casto BC, Pieczynski J, Janosko N, Dipaolo JA: Significance of treatment interval and DNA repair in the enhancement of viral transformation by chemical carcinogens and mutagens. Chem Biol Interact 13:105–125, 1976

225. Huberman E: Viral antigen induction and mutability of different genetic loci by metabolically activated carcinogenic polycyclic hydrocarbons in cultured mammalian cells. Edited by HH Hiatt, JD Watson,

and JA Winsten: Origins of Human Cancer. Book C, Human Risk Assessment. Cold Spring Harbor Conferences on Cell Proliferation, Vol. 4. Cold Spring Harbor, Cold Spring Harbor Laboratory, 1977, pp 1521–1535

226. Lacqueur GL: Oncogenicity of cycads and its implications. Edited by HF Kraybill and MA Mehlman: Environmental Cancer. Vol. 3. Washington, Hemisphere Publishing Corporation, 1977, pp 231–262

227. Tracey JP, Sherlock P: Hepatoma following carbon tetrachloride poisoning. NY State J Med 68:2202–2204, 1968

228. Thomas LB, Popper H, Berk PD, Selikoff I, Falk H: Vinyl-chloride-induced liver disease. From idiopathic portal hypertension (Banti's syndrome) to angiosarcoma. N Engl J Med 292:17–22, 1975

229. Popper H, Selikoff IJ, Maltoni C, Squire RA, Thomas LB: Comparison of neoplastic hepatic lesions in man and experimental animals. Edited by HH Hiatt, JD Watson, and JA Winsten: Origins of Human Cancer. Book C, Human Risk Assessment. Cold Spring Harbor Conferences on Cell Proliferation, Vol. 4. Cold Spring Harbor, Cold Spring Harbor Laboratory, 1977, pp 1359–1382

230. Popper H, Thomas LB, Schaffner F, Maltoni C, Selikoff IJ: Interaction between sinusoidal cells and hepatocytes in human and experimental angiosarcoma induced by environmental factors. Edited by E Wisse and DL Knook: Kupffer Cells and Other Liver Sinusoidal Cells. Amsterdam, Elsevier/North Holland Biomedical Press, 1977, pp 173–181

231. Pushin GA: O porashenii petscheni i sheltschnyich putei u rabotschich zanjatyich w proizqodstwe nekatoriyich widow plastmass. Sov Med 28:132–138, 1974

232. Suciu I, Drejman I, Valaskai M: Étude des maladies dues au chlorure de vinyle. Med Lav 58:261–271, 1967

233. Creech JL Jr, Johnson MN: Angiosarcoma of liver in the manufacture of polyvinyl chloride. J Occup Med 16:150–151, 1974

234. Maltoni C, Lefemine G: Carcinogenicity bioassays of vinyl chloride. 1. Research plan and early results. Environ Res 7:378–405, 1974

235. Marsteller HJ, Lelbach WK, Müller R, Jühe S, Lange CE, Rohner HG, Veltman G: Chronisch-toxische Leberschaeden bei Arbeitern in der PVC-Produktion. Dtsch Med Wochenschr 98:2311–2314, 1973

236. Lilis R, Anderson H, Nicholson WJ, Daum S, Fischbein AS, Selikoff IJ: Prevalence of disease among vinyl chloride and polyvinyl chloride workers. Ann NY Acad Sci 246:22–41, 1975

237. Mákk L, Creech JL, Whelan JG, Johnson MN: Liver damage and angiosarcoma in vinyl chloride workers. A systematic detection program. JAMA 230:64–68, 1974

238. Marsteller HJ, Lelbach WK, Müller R, Gedigk P, Lange CE: Klinische und laparoskopische Aspekte der Leberschaeden bei Chemiearbeitern in der Vinylchlorid-Polymerisation. Leber Magen Darm 5:196–202, 1975

239. Biersack HJ, Lange CE, Ebinger H, Marsteller HJ, Lelbach WK, Veltman G, Winkler C: Sequenzszintigraphische Untersuchungen von Leber und Milz by Patienten mit Vinylchlorid-Krankheit. Dtsch Med Wochenschr 100:615–617, 1975

240. Gutacker HW, Lelbach WK (eds): Leberschaeden durch Vinylchlorid-Krankheit. Baden-Baden, Verlag Gerhard Witzstrock, 1977

241. Whelan JG, Creech JL, Tamburro CH: Angiographic and radionuclide characteristics of hepatic angiosarcoma found in vinyl chloride workers. Radiology 118:549–557, 1976

242. Biersack HJ, San Luis T Jr, Lange CE, Thelen M, Veltmann G, Winkler C: Scintigraphy of liver and spleen in vinyl chloride workers. Acta Hepatogastroenterol (Stuttg) 24:357–361, 1977

243. Blendis LM, Smith PM, Lawrie BW, Stephens MR, Evans WD: Haemodynamic studies in vinyl chloride monomer workers with portal hypertension. Gut 18:400–401, 1977

244. Blendis LM, Smith PM, Lawrie BW, Stephens MR, Evans WD: Portal hypertension in vinyl chloride monomer workers. A hemodynamic study. Gastroenterology 75:206–211, 1978

245. Watanabe PG, McGowan GR, Gehring PJ: Fate of [^{14}C] vinyl chloride after single oral administration in rats. Toxicol Appl Pharmacol 36:339–352, 1976

246. Bolt HM, Laib RJ, Kappus H, Buchter A: Pharmacokinetics of vinyl chloride in the rat. Toxicology 7:179–188, 1977

247. Gehring PJ, Watanabe PG, Park CN: Resolution of dose-response toxicity data for

chemicals requiring metabolic activation: Example—vinyl chloride. Toxicol Appl Pharmacol 44:581–591, 1978

248. Watanabe PG, Hefner RE Jr, Gehring PJ: Vinyl chloride-induced depression of hepatic non-protein, sulfhydryl content and effects on bromosulphalein (BSP) clearance in rats. Toxicology 6:1–8, 1976

249. Osterman-Golkar S, Hultmark D, Segerbäck D, Calleman CJ, Göthe R, Ehrenberg L, Wachtmeister CA: Alkylation of DNA and proteins in mice exposed to vinyl chloride. Biochem Biophys Res Commun 76:259–266, 1977

250. Watanabe PG, Zempel JA, Pegg DG, Gehring PJ: Hepatic macromolecular binding following exposure to vinyl chloride. Toxicol Appl Pharmacol 44:571–579, 1978

251. Greim H, Bonse G, Radwan Z, Reichert D, Henschler D: Mutagenicity in vitro and potential carcinogenicity of chlorinated ethylenes as a function of metabolic oxirane formation. Biochem Pharmacol 24:2013–2017, 1975

252. McCann J, Simmon V, Streitwieser D, Ames BN: Mutagenicity of chloroacetaldehyde, a possible metabolic product of 1,2-dichloroethane (ethylene dichloride), chloroethanol (ethyl chlorohydrin), vinyl chloride, and cyclophosphamide. Proc Natl Acad Sci USA 72:3190–3193, 1975

253. Loprieno N, Barale R, Baroncelli S, Bartsch H, Bronzetti G, Cammellini A, Corsi C, Frezza D, Nieri R, Leporini C, Rosellini D, Rossi AM: Induction of gene mutations and gene conversions by vinyl chloride metabolites in yeast. Cancer Res 37:251–257, 1977

254. Walker CH, Bentley P, Oesch F: Phylogenetic distribution of epoxide hydratase in different vertebrate species, strains and tissues measured using three substrates. Biochim Biophys Acta 539:427–434, 1978

255. Popper H, Thomas LB: Alterations of liver and spleen among workers exposed to vinyl chloride. Ann NY Acad Sci 246:172–194, 1975

256. Bianchi L, Popper H: Multiple-biopsy observations of the sequence from precursor stage to angiosarcoma in vinyl chloride worker. (in preparation)

257. Triche T, Nanba K, Ishak K, Wolkoff A, Berk PD: Hepatic ultrastructural changes in vinyl-chloride (VC) workers. Clin Res 23:259A, 1975

258. Schattenberg P-J, Totovic V, Gedigk P, Marsteller HJ: Die Ultrastruktur der Leberschaedigung bei der chronischen Vinylchlorid-Intoxikation. Virchows Arch [Pathol Anat] 373:233–247, 1977

259. Smith PM, Crossley IR, Williams DMJ: Portal hypertension in vinyl-chloride production workers. Lancet 2:602–604, 1976

260. Maltoni C: Predictive value of carcinogenesis bioassays. Ann NY Acad Sci 271:431–447, 1976

261. Gokel JM, Liebezeit E, Eder M: Hemangiosarcoma and hepatocellular carcinoma of the liver following vinyl chloride exposure: A report of two cases. Virchows Arch [Pathol Anat] 372:195–203, 1976

262. Nadell J, Kosek K: Peliosis hepatis. Twelve cases associated with oral androgen therapy. Arch Pathol Lab Med 101:405–410, 1977

262a. Levy VG, Bouma ME, Lageron A, Darnis F, Infante R: Hepatic sinusoidal dilatation after chenodeoxycholic-acid therapy. Lancet 1:206, 1978

263. Smith PM, Williams DMJ: Vinyl chloride and cirrhosis. Digestion 10:321–322, 1974

264. Ishak KG: Mesenchymal tumors of the liver. Edited by K Okuda and RL Peters: Hepatocellular Carcinoma. New York, John Wiley & Sons, 1976, pp 286–298

265. Baxter PJ, Anthony PP, MacSween RNM, Scheuer PJ: Angiosarcoma of the liver in Great Britain, 1963–73. Br Med J 2:919–921, 1977

266. Brady J, Liberatore F, Harper P, Greenwald P, Burnett W, Davies JNP, Bishop M, Polan A, Vianna N: Angiosarcoma of the liver: An epidemiologic survey. J Natl Cancer Inst 59:1383–1385, 1977

267. Stewart HL: Hemangiosarcoma (malignant hemangioendothelioma). Edited by FF Becker: Cancer. Vol. 4. New York, Plenum Publishing Co, 1975, pp 303–374

268. Herrold KM: Histogenesis of malignant liver tumors induced by dimethylnitrosamine: An experimental study in Syrian hamsters. J Natl Cancer Inst 39:1099–1111, 1967

269. Andervont H: Induction of hemangioendotheliomas and sarcomas in mice with o-aminoazotoluene. J Natl Cancer Inst 10:927–941, 1950

270. Narisawa T, Wong C-Q, Weisburger JH: Azoxymethane-induced liver hemangiosarcomas in inbred strain-2 guinea pigs. J Natl Cancer Inst 56:653–654, 1976

271. Spirtas R, Kamisnki R: Angiosarcoma of the liver in vinyl chloride/polyvinyl chloride workers. J Occup Med 20:427–429, 1978

272. Regelson W, Kim U, Ospina J, Holland JF: Hemangioendothelial sarcoma of liver from chronic arsenic intoxication by Fowler's solution. Cancer 21:514–522, 1968

273. Lander JJ, Stanley RJ, Sumner HW, Boswell DC, Aach RD: Angiosarcoma of the liver associated with Fowler's solution (potassium arsenite). Gastroenterology 68:1582–1586, 1975

274. Datta DV: Arsenic and non-cirrhotic portal hypertension. Lancet 1:433, 1976

275. Denk R, Holzmann H, Lange HJ, Greve D: Ueber Arsenspaetschaden bei obduzierten Moselwinzern. Med Welt 20:557–567, 1969

276. Luechtrath H: Cirrhosis of the liver in chronic arsenical poisoning of vintners. Ger Med Mon 2:127–128, 1972

277. Axelson O, Dahlgren E, Jansson C-D, Rehnlund SO: Arsenic exposure and mortality: A case-referent study from a Swedish copper smelter. Br J Indust Med 35:8–15, 1978

278. da Silva Horta J: Late effects of thorotrast on the liver and spleen, and their efferent lymph nodes. Ann NY Acad Sci 145:676–699, 1967

279. da Silva Horta J: Late lesions in man caused by colloidal thorium dioxide (thorotrast): A new case of sarcoma of the liver twenty-two years after the injection. Arch Pathol 62:403–418, 1956

280. Dahlgren S: Thorotrast tumours: A review of the literature and report of two cases. Acta Pathol Microbiol Scand 53:147–161, 1961

281. Telles NC, Thomas LB, Popper H, Ishak K, Falk H: Evolution of thorotrast-induced hepatic angiosarcomas. Environ Res (in press)

282. Smoron GL, Battifora HA: Thorotrast-induced hepatoma. Cancer 30:1252–1259, 1972

283. Johnson PK, Babb RR: Cholangiocarcinoma in a patient previously given Thorotrast. Dig Dis 20:384–390, 1975

284. Mori T, Maruyama T, Hatakeyama S, Miyaji T, Tsuya A, Takahashi S: Thorotrast injury in Japan. Statistical study on autopsy cases and follow-up study on 147 cases. J Jpn Med Radiol Soc 35:439–452, 1975

285. Swarm RL, Miller E, Michelitch HJ: Malignant vascular tumors in rabbits injected intravenously with colloidal thorium dioxide. Pathol Microbiol (Basel) 25:27–44, 1962

286. Moore TA, Ferrante WA, Crownon TD: Hepatoma occurring two decades after hepatic irradiation. Gastroenterology 71:128–132, 1976

287. Higginson J: Chronic toxicology—An epidemiologist's approach to the problem of carcinogenesis. Edited by WJ Hayes Jr: Essays in Toxicology. Vol. 7. New York, Academic Press, 1976, pp 29–71

288. Farber E: On the pathogenesis of experimental hepatocellular carcinoma. Edited by K Okuda and RL Peters: Hepatocellular Carcinoma. New York, John Wiley & Sons, 1976, pp 3–22

289. Steinborn J: Toxische Leberschaeden durch berufliche Exposition. Edited by L Wannagat: Toxische Leberschaeden. Stuttgart, Georg Thieme Verlag, 1976, pp 3–22

290. Higginson J: The role of the pathologist in environmental medicine and public health. Am J Pathol 86:459–484, 1977

Chapter 35

Hepatocellular Carcinoma: A Review of the Recent Studies and Developments

By KUNIO OKUDA, M.D., *and* TOSHIRO NAKASHIMA, M.D.

HEPATOCELLULAR CARCINOMA (HCC) has been an inoperable tumor with no means for early detection. It may no longer be so, thanks to recent studies demonstrating its close relation to hepatitis B virus (HBV) infection. This chapter summarizes several recent developments of importance.

HEPATITIS B VIRUS AND HEPATOCARCINOGENESIS

Although early reports carried conflicting data, the surface antigen (HB$_s$Ag) is frequently positive in HCC in countries where the incidence of HB$_s$Ag carriers is high, and HCC occurs frequently in livers with nonalcoholic macronodular cirrhosis. The rate of positivity for HB$_s$Ag varies with the test procedure, particularly when the level of antigenemia is low, as in HCC.[1-3] The rate is about 50% by radioimmunoassay in Japan, where frequency of HB$_s$ antigenemia is about 2%;[1,3] about 80% of patients with HCC are positive by the micro-Ouchterlony method in Taiwan, where more than 10% of the general population has antigenemia.[4] These serologic parameters for HBV infection are perhaps highest in some areas of Africa.[5-7]

Anti-HB$_s$ is relatively infrequent in HCC patients,[1,8] but the reported figures vary,[5,9,10] and whether or not a low incidence of antibody indicates an immunodeficient state has not clearly been demonstrated. Simons et al.,[10] using a radioelectrocomplexing technique, demonstrated that the rates of both HB$_s$ antigenemia and immune complexemia were higher in HCC patients than in control blood donors. They suggested that immune complexemia frequently reflects an inability to produce high avidity anti-HB$_s$ and that the immune deficiency might have a primary genetic basis or might be secondary to the immunodepressive effects of concurrent viral or parasitic infections. Antibody to the core (HB$_c$) antigen is a sensitive indicator of persistent viral replication[11] and more definitely so if its titer is high.[12] Anti-HB$_c$ is more frequently positive than is HB$_s$Ag in HCC patients, and their titers are usually high.[13,14] If tests for HB$_s$Ag, anti-HB$_s$, and anti-HB$_c$ are considered together, nearly all HCC patients are positive in Africa and Southeast Asia.[15] These figures are slightly lower among Japanese with HCC.[13] HB$_e$ antigen is seldom positive in HCC patients with HB$_s$ antigenemia, and hence anti-HB$_e$ is more frequently positive.[16]

From the First Department of Medicine, Chiba University School of Medicine, Chiba, and First Department of Pathology, Kurume University School of Medicine, Kurume, Japan.

Studies on familial clustering of HB$_s$Ag-positive HCC, cirrhosis, and chronic hepatitis suggest maternal transmission as the main route of infection.[17] Maternal transmission is almost inevitable when the mother is positive for HB$_e$Ag,[18] and efforts are currently made to prevent such transmission in order to reduce the number of carriers and thereby the number of HCC cases in the long run. Infants who have acquired HB$_s$Ag during the paranatal period become chronic carriers.[19] Some of them may develop chronic liver disease and eventually HCC. Sakuma et al.[20] followed 341 adult asymptomatic carriers in Tokyo for a period of up to 3½ years; 3 of them developed HCC and died. Epidemiologic data seem to suggest that a correlation exists between the frequency of HB$_s$Ag carriers and the incidence of HCC.

A case/control study on 28 HCC patients and matched controls and their families in Senegal, West Africa, revealed that nearly all patients and controls had some evidence of HBV infection and that the cases were more frequently positive for anti-HB$_c$ and less frequently for anti-HB$_s$.[21] Most of the mothers of the cases were HB$_s$Ag carriers, suggesting that HCC patients had been infected by maternal transmission. None of the fathers of the cases had anti-HB$_s$, and the sibs had low titers of anti-HB$_s$, as compared with the sibs of the controls. These latter findings strongly suggested an environmental factor which affected the immunologic response of all family members to HBV infection.

The intracellular localization of HB$_s$Ag and HB$_c$Ag demonstrable by immunohistologic techniques is still puzzling. Bianchi (see Chapter 20), who analyzed the distribution of these antigens in relation to histological types, proposed four patterns of differing prognostic implications.[22] One unrefutable pattern is the "elimination" type in which no HB$_s$Ag is demonstrated in hepatocytes at the height of acute hepatitis. A liver bearing HCC perhaps falls in his "non- or low-grade infective HB$_s$-predominance" type. Using the Shikata (orcein) stain and immunoperoxidase technique, the distribution of HB$_s$Ag is seen to be random in a cirrhotic liver, and the size of the sample makes a difference in the rate of positivity.[23,24] In our study of 160 livers with HCC, a cross section of the entire liver was examined. Orcein stain was positive in 39 (24.4%), and most were also seropositive. Areas with positive cells were irregularly distributed with no consistent relation to tumors (Fig. 1). In the hepatocyte, orcein-positive material (HB$_s$Ag) was seen either diffusely, or in an inclusion-body-like deposit (Fig. 2), or in a mixture of both. While the inclusion-body-type cells were sparsely seen, diffuse-type cells were more densely distributed, in clear contrast to areas of negative cells, suggesting slow infection of regenerating cells. Positive cells were seen in tumor areas in only 2 (1.25%), but the possibility of nontumorous hepatocytes left among infiltrating tumor cells could not entirely be dismissed (Fig. 3).

Hepatocarcinogenesis has long been postulated to be a result of cell regeneration and the malignant transformation that ensues. Anthony and associates[9] demonstrated in Ugandan patients with cirrhosis that hepatocellular swelling and dysplasia, i.e., cellular enlargement, nuclear pleomorphism, and multinucleation occurring in groups, were closely associated with the presence of HB$_s$Ag. They further investigated the frequency of such changes in relation to

HCC and found dysplasia in 64.5% of 124 patients with HCC in contrast to an incidence of 1% in the controls.[25] Dysplasia was regarded as a precancerous change, and HBV was postulated to induce malignant changes in liver cells, which then fuse with normal liver cells to form large, abnormal, dysplastic cells.[26] Similar changes called adenomatous paraplastic changes, and ground-glass-like alterations of hepatocytes were also described in the same lesion.[27]

More recently, Popper[28] studied livers bearing HCC and found eosinophilic ground-glass appearance in Shikata-positive cells, often with hyperplastic features proceeding to focal dysplasia. Shikata-positive cells were in diffusely hyperplastic portions of regenerative nodules of cirrhotic livers. He hypothesized that the centricellular deposition of HB_sAg, which prevents an immunologic attack on these hepatocytes in the carrier stage, predisposes them to malignant transformation. To explain the observed sparsity of the c component or virion in nuclei and excessive synthesis of the s component, Popper offered an alternative theory that alteration of increased smooth endoplasmic reticulum as the site of microsomal biotransformation renders these cells more susceptible to additional carcinogens, owing to excessive formation or reduced degradation of a biologically active metabolite. Localization of alpha-fetoprotein (AFP) was demonstrated in dysplastic cells in human biopsies.[29] However, whether survivors long after resection had dysplasia at the time of surgery, or whether dysplastic changes persist for years without malignant transformation remains to be investigated.

Another piece of evidence for the oncogenic property of HBV comes from a recent study in which HB_sAg-positive patients with chronic liver disease developed HCC earlier during the follow-up than did antigen-negative patients.[30]

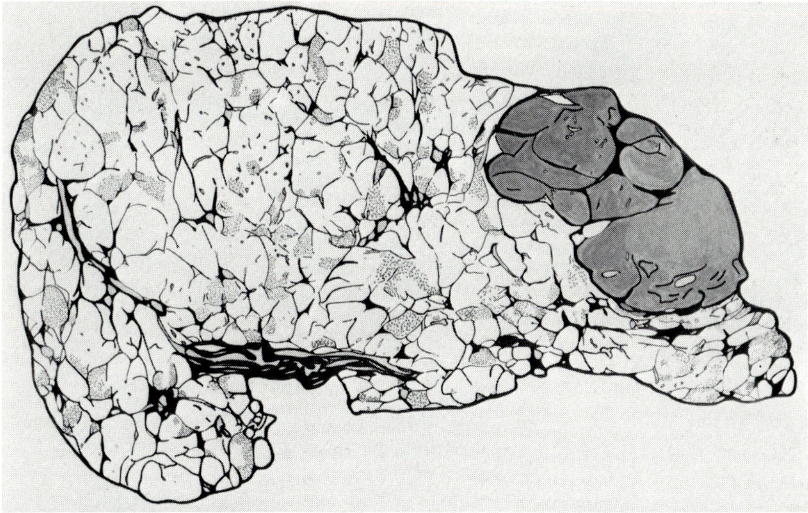

FIG. 1—Orcein (HB_sAg)-positive cells are irregularly distributed with no consistent relation to tumor as demonstrated in this drawing of a large cross section of the liver (composite map made from 15 large tissue sections). Areas of positive cells are indicated by dots, and tumor is located in lightly shaded area.

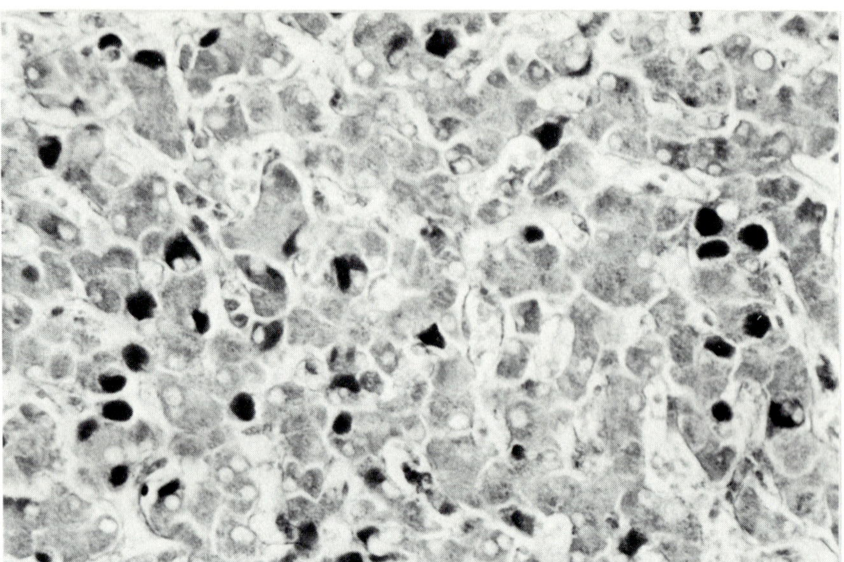

FIG. 2—Inclusion-body-like deposits of orcein-positive material in the hepatocytes. They are sparsely distributed with more negative cells ($\times$ 350).

Despite these observations, the problem still remains as to whether HBV is, in fact, an oncogenic virus, or whether HBV induces a chronic immunologic derangement leading to an immunodeficiency state, which in turn expedites carcinogenesis. Demonstration of HBV genome in the DNA of HCC would provide more direct evidence for the first possibility.

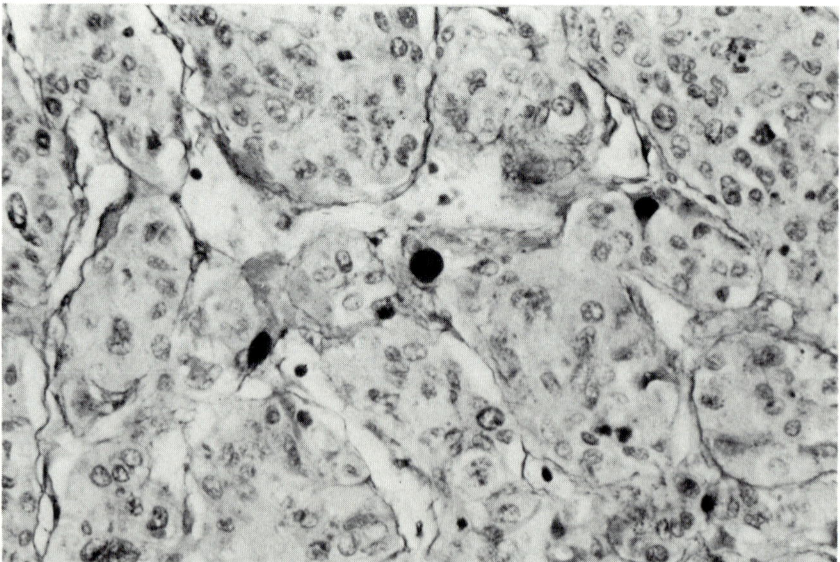

FIG. 3—Inclusion-body-like deposits of Hb$_s$Ag (orcein stain) in tumor tissue. They are located in the periphery of a trabecular tumor cell cord, and the possibility cannot be denied that they represent hepatocytes that remain in tumor tissue and are about to vanish ($\times$ 400).

DIAGNOSIS AND EARLY DETECTION

Diagnosis of advanced HCC only requires differentiation from metastatic cancers. Recently, computed tomography and ultrasonography have joined the diagnostic armamentarium for localized hepatic lesions, and their reliability is being assessed and compared (see Chapter 29). Gray-scale ultrasonography seems to be just as reliable as liver scanning.[31-33] Computed tomography perhaps has similar diagnostic value,[34-36] but its cost is much greater. Theoretically, HCC that has a tissue density similar to that of liver parenchyma, would not be discerned on the film. By contrast, one having a greater density, such as sclerosing HCC,[27] or one having a firm capsule[37] may be delineated. Enhancement by some hepatophilic contrast medium may assist in the detection of low-density tumors.

When tests for AFP first became available, it was thought that they would detect early HCC. Although serum AFP levels above several micrograms per milliliter, or detectable by immunodiffusion techniques are highly diagnostic, some HCCs demonstrate low AFP or negative tests. AFP is often mildly elevated in various liver diseases, making interpretation difficult.[3,38,39] In 1975, we first documented the progressive changes of AFP in the range below 1,000 ng/ml in 5 patients who had relatively small HCCs, and, in fact, hepatic resection was possible in 2 of them.[40] Similar observations have since been made on sporadic cases.[41] The serum AFP level and its changes correlate with the clinical course, especially with therapeutic effects,[40-42] and even with gross anatomic types.[43]

Systematic investigations on diagnostic procedures for small HCCs are under way, particularly in Japan, where nearly 40% of cirrhotic livers harbor HCC at autopsy,[23,44] and clinical follow-up of patients with cirrhosis eventually demonstrates HCC in a similar proportion. A group of 19 male patients was described who had clinical acute hepatitis and subsequently died from HCC.[45] The interval from acute hepatitis to the diagnosis of HCC ranged from 6 to 20 years, averaging 12.8 years. More recently, clinical follow-up of 31 patients with an initial diagnosis of cirrhosis or chronic hepatitis was reported, in whom HCC was found after 1 to 14 years.[30] Those with antigenemia developed HCC after an interval of 48 months on the average, as compared with a 74-month interval for the negative patients, and the difference was statistically significant. Similar studies demonstrated that in patients who have a small growing HCC, serum AFP remains mildly abnormal for some time and then rises steeply.[46] In most of the latter cases, however, in which monitoring of AFP helped in the diagnosis of HCC, the tumor was already 3–5 cm in diameter. Thus, only HCC with a high AFP-producing capacity seems detectable before it reaches such sizes. Obviously, AFP alone is not sufficient for early detection, and more specific and sensitive tests for HCC are needed. To that end, immunologic methods utilizing tumor-specific antigens have to be developed. Whether the leukocyte adherence inhibition test[47] suits the same purpose requires confirmation. Carcinoembryonic antigen (CEA) is elevated in metastatic hepatocarcinoma to a greater extent and more frequently than in primary hepatocarcinoma.[48,49] Although CEA by itself is not diagnostic for HCC, if both AFP and CEA were measured, it can differentiate between primary and secondary hepatic tumors. Other carcino-fetal proteins such as ferritins,[50] isoenzymes,[51,52] and other cancer-specific substances[53] have been demonstrated in sera of HCC patients, but none has been shown to be of value in early diagnosis.

Another approach to the detection of resectable HCC is to understand the clinical and pathologic properties of minute HCC. Many of the primary tumors among 16 autopsied and 4 resected livers bearing one to several small HCCs, were well differentiated and encapsulated, especially in the autopsy material, suggesting a slow expanding growth.[54] The growth pattern changed later in some cases, and the accompanying cirrhosis was advanced. Serum AFP was usually low, and a positive test for HB_sAg was infrequent in the autopsied patients. These HB_sAg-negative livers having a small HCC and HB_sAg-negative patients who developed HCC during the follow-up in Kubo's series[30] may represent one type of cirrhosis-associated HCC that is different from the more common HCC that is closely associated with HB_sAg-positive cirrhosis. Whether the nonalcoholic, chronic liver disease in these HB_sAg-negative cases represents a non-A, non-B virus hepatitis, and whether this virus is less carcinogenic than HBV remain to be determined.

The best policy for the detection of small HCC is to follow patients with chronic liver disease regularly, with radioimmunoassay of AFP at short intervals. When AFP starts to rise, it must be followed more closely. If it rises continuously and steeply for several months or if it reaches a level far above 1,000 ng/ml, celiac angiography and other diagnostic procedures should be carried out.

For the detection of small HCC, selective celiac or hepatic arteriography is often, if not always, helpful. Angiographic demonstration of small HCC depends on its vascularity, which also depends on the histologic type, and an HCC as small as 1 cm may be detected.[3,55] Liver scintiscan is less sensitive in this respect, although several carcinophilic and other radionuclides have been used as an adjunct to radiocolloid.[56-59] Furthermore, certain angiographic characteristics of HCC, such as arterioportal anastomoses, assist in the diagnosis.[60,61] Small hypervascular HCCs were found by preoperative celiac angiography done for bleeding varices and could be excised in 2 patients.[62]

MANAGEMENT OF HEPATOCELLULAR CARCINOMA

The response rate to systemic chemotherapy generally is low, irrespective of the agent if used singly. Currently available agents such as 5-fluorouracil (5-FU), cyclophosphamide, vinblastine, and mitomycin C have been disappointing,[42,63-67] but favorable responses have also been observed by some investigators,[68] and occasional remarkable responses have been recorded.[65,69] One of the problems is the lack of methods for predicting the response. Ftoraful [FT-207 or N_1-(2'-furanidyl)-5-fluorouracil], a compound developed by the Russians and metabolically related to 5-FU,[70] has recently been preferred to 5-FU in systemic chemotherapy in Eastern European countries and in Japan. It can be given orally and intravenously as well as rectally. Several reports advocate the use of adriamycin, but the rate of response varies considerably among the investigators.[71,72] Combination chemotherapy seems somewhat superior in rate of response,[42,65,73] but it is usually partial.

Intra-arterial delivery of a single dose (one-shot) of chemotherapeutic agents, combined with systemic administration, has been a popular procedure in Japan.[74] This type of treatment ensures a high drug concentration locally and is based on the facts that HCC has mainly an arterial blood supply[75] and that nontumorous hepatocytes are relatively tolerant to high doses of chemotherapeutic agents. Intra-arterial infusion chemotherapy, using a continuous infusion pump, has been attempted by several investigators. Catheterization of the gastroepiploic or gastroduodenal artery at laparotomy has been more popular than the percutaneous procedure, which is less effective in catheterizing the intended artery, although it circumvents surgical operation.[76] This procedure, using either 5-FU or methotrexate, prolongs survival considerably in some patients with tumor regression, relief of pain, and decline in serum AFP[66,74] but often must be terminated because of complications such as peptic ulceration[77,78] and infection,[74] and the overall results are not necessarily satisfactory. Unfortunately, well-controlled studies comparing the efficacy of these therapies are lacking.

Radiation therapy, particularly orthovoltage radiotherapy, has been regarded as almost useless.[67] Excellent results, however, have been reported in nonresectable cases in which hepatic artery ligation was combined with supervoltage radiotherapy (2,500–3,000 rads) and BCG immunotherapy.[73] The assessment of the effect of radiotherapy alone is difficult, however. Internal radiation using radioactive particles or colloids delivered intra-arterially has been attempted in combination with chemotherapy, but the results were not impressive.[79]

There is good evidence, particularly based on the serologic studies of HBV infection, that patients with HCC have defective immune responses.[10,21] A patient with HCC has been described who developed lung metastasis after hepatic resection and in whom continuous immunization using BCG mixed with autologous tumor cells inactivated by irradiation suppressed further tumor growth.[80] An animal experiment using tumor-specific immunoglobulin conjugated with chlorambucil yielded promising results[81] and suggests a novel approach for the future.

Surgical management of HCC includes resection, dearterialization, and perhaps portal vein ligation.[82] In 1955, Lin developed a technique called the ''finger fracture'' method in which blunt fingers are used to fracture away liver tissue to expose and ligate large vessels, thereby shortening operating time and minimizing bleeding. With the conventional technique, profuse bleeding is inevitable during the isolation of blood vessels. Lin further improved his technique in such a way that he now uses a crush clamp instead of fingers, while bleeding is prevented by a large hepatic clamp applied around the liver near the separating line.[83,84] A technique for lobectomy was developed with complete vascular isolation and cold perfusion.[85] By this technique, the liver is completely mobilized except for major vascular attachments and the external bile ducts. The inflow and outflow vessels are clamped, and then the liver is cold-perfused. This method was used in 33 patients, with only 2 deaths. More recently, H.

Hasegawa in Japan (personal communication) developed a technique that permits resection of more than 80% of the liver. The main features include the use of a huge amount of fresh human plasma postoperatively to prevent deficiency of short-lived essential plasma proteins and development of hepatic failure and the postoperative management of fluid-electrolyte imbalance. He also performed cavography and hepatic venography simultaneously with a balloon catheter and used a stereo-viewer for hepatic arteriograms and venograms in order to orient vessels with regard to depth. Only 1 death occurred in 40 cases of hepatic resections, including 23 trisegmentectomies or extended hemihepatectomies; 6 patients had cirrhosis, and trisegmentectomy was carried out in 2 with an uneventful postoperative course. Early reports stressed the inevitability of splanchnic bed pooling of blood following major hepatic resection, but this contention has been refuted.[86] Angiography is of particular importance for the selection of patients for surgical treatment,[87,88] and tumor growth in the portal vein, which contraindicates resection and dearterialization,[89] can be detected by celiac arteriography.[90] Tumor growth in the hepatic vein and extension into the inferior vena cava can also be diagnosed angiographically.[91] Dearterialization alone is generally inadequate and should be combined with other forms of chemotherapy.[92,93] Whether liver transplantation is indicated for unresectable HCC has not been determined.[94,95] The results have been generally poor for hepatic malignancies[96] and are comparable with those of hepatic resection. Reports from Taiwan[83] and Japan[97] record several postresection survivals of more than 10 years.

The efficacy of therapeutic regimens can only be compared if the patients are in a similar disease stage. Although a proposal for staging was made,[98] in actuality it is not easy because of the variable growth pattern of tumor and the state of the nontumorous parenchyma. Some HCC grows very slowly, and survival after detection can be as long as 5 years without treatment.[37] Survival even varies with the serology for HBV.[99] For the assessment of tumor regression, AFP may be more quantitative than the size assessment by scanning or palpation;[42,64,100] sometimes, however, AFP rises despite progressive diminution of tumor size, representing perhaps a clonal change with respect to sensitivity to chemotherapy,[74] or it may decrease in spite of tumor recurrence.[101]

REFERENCES

1. Nishioka K, Hirayama T, Sekine T, Okochi K, Mayumi M, Sung JL, Liu CH, Lin TM: Australia antigen and hepatocellular carcinoma. Gann Monogr Cancer Res 14:167–175, 1973

2. Simons MJ, Yap EH, Yu M, Shanmugaratnam K: Australia antigen in Singapore Chinese patients with hepatocellular carcinoma and comparison groups: Influence of technique sensitivity on differential frequencies. Int J Cancer 10:320–325, 1972

3. Okuda K: Clinical aspects of hepatocellular carcinoma—analysis of 134 cases. Edited by K Okuda and RL Peters: Hepatocellular Carcinoma. New York, John Wiley & Sons, 1976, pp 387–436

4. Tong MJ, Sun SC, Schaeffer BT, Chang NK, Lo KJ, Peters RL: Hepatitis-associated antigen and antibody in hepatocellular carcinoma in Taiwan. Ann Intern Med 75:687–691, 1971

5. Vogel CL, Anthony PP, Sadikali F, Barker LF, Peterson MR: Hepatitis-associated antigen and antibody in hepatocellular carci-

noma: Results of a continuing study. J Natl Cancer Inst 48:1583–1588, 1972

6. Macnab GM, Urbanowicz JM, Geddes EW, Kew MC: Hepatitis-B surface antigen and antibody in Bantu patients with primary hepatocellular cancer. Br J Cancer 33:544–548, 1976

7. Prince AM, Szmuness W, Michon J, Demaille J, Diebolt G, Linhard J. Quenum C, Sankale M: A case/control study of the association between primary liver cancer and heptitis B infection in Senegal. Int J Cancer 16:374–383, 1975

8. Anand S, Malavia AN: H.A.A. in primary liver-cell carcinoma. Lancet 2:1032–1033, 1971

9. Anthony PP, Vogel CL, Sadikali F, Barker LF, Peterson MR: Hepatitis-associated antigen and antibody in Uganda: Correlation of serological testing with histopathology. Br Med J 1:403–406, 1972

10. Simons MJ, Yu M, Shanmugaratnam K: Immunodeficiency to hepatitis B virus infection and genetic susceptibility to development of hepatocellular carcinoma. Ann NY Acad Sci 259:181–195, 1975

11. Hoofnagle JH, Gerety RJ, Ni LY, Barker LF: Antibody to hepatitis B core antigen. A sensitive indicator of hepatitis B virus replication. N Engl J Med 290:1336–1340, 1974

12. Kojima M, Kazumichi U, Takahashi Y, Yoshizawa H, Tsuda F, Itoh Y, Miyakawa Y, Mayumi M: Correlation between titer of antibody to hepatitis B core antigen and presence of viral antigens in the liver. Gastroenterology 73:664–667, 1977

13. Kubo Y, Okuda K, Hashimoto M, Nagasaki Y, Ebata H, Nakajima Y, Musha H, Sakuma K, Ohtake H: Antibody to hepatitis B core antigen in patients with hepatocellular carcinoma. Gastroenterology 72:1217–1220, 1977

14. Furuta S, Nagata A, Kiyosawa K, Akahane Y, Koike Y, Sahara T, Oda M, Mayumi M, Tsuda F: Anti-HBc titer in relation to the etiological role of hepatitis B virus in primary hepatocellular carcinoma. Acta Hepatogastroenterol 24:306, 1977

15. Maupas P, Werner B, Larouze B, Millman I, London WT, O'Connell A, Blumberg BS: Antibody to hepatitis-B core antigen in patients with primary hepatic carcinoma. Lancet 2:9–11, 1975

16. Eleftheriou N, Thomas HC, Heathcote J, Sherlock S: Incidence and clinical significance of e-antigen and antibody in acute and chronic liver disease. Lancet 2:1171–1173, 1975

17. Ohbayashi A: Genetic and familial aspects of liver cirrhosis and hepatocellular carcinoma. Edited by K Okuda and RL Peters: Hepatocellular Carcinoma. New York, John Wiley & Sons, 1976, pp 43–51

18. Okada K, Kamiyama I, Inomata M, Imai M, Miyakawa Y, Mayumi M: e Antigen and anti-e in the serum of asymptomatic carrier mothers as indicators of positive and negative transmission of hepatitis B virus to their infants. N Engl J Med 294:746–749, 1976

19. Merrill DA, Dubois RS, Kohler PF: Neonatal onset of the hepatitis-associated-antigen carrier state. N Engl J Med 287:1280–1282, 1972

20. Sakuma K, Ohtake H, Okuda K, Mayumi M: Prognosis of asymptomatic HBsAg carriers in adults. A prelim Hepatitis Sci Memo H-1310. Buffalo, Calspan, 1977

21. Larouze B, London WT, Saimot G, Werner BG, Lustbader ED, Payet M, Blumberg BS: Host responses to hepatitis B infection in patients with primary hepatic carcinoma and their families. A case/control study in Senegal, West Africa. Lancet 2:534–538, 1976

22. Bianchi L, Gudat F: Hepatitis B: Immunpathologie der verschiedenen Verlaufsformen. Schweiz Med Wochenschr 107: 929–935, 1977

23. Shikata T: Primary liver carcinoma and liver cirrhosis. Edited by K Okuda and RL Peters: Hepatocellular Carcinoma. New York, John Wiley & Sons, 1976, pp 53–72

24. Nayak NC, Dhar A, Sachdeva R, Mittal A, Seth HN, Sudarsanam D, Reddy B, Wagholikar UL, Reddy CRRM: Association of human hepatocellular carcinoma and cirrhosis with hepatitis B virus surface and core antigens in the liver. Int J Cancer 20:643–654, 1977

25. Anthony PP, Vogel CL, Barker LF: Liver cell dysplasia: a premalignant condition. J Clin Pathol 26:217–223, 1973

26. Anthony PP: Precursor lesions for liver cancer in human. Cancer Res 36:2570–2583, 1976

27. Peters RL: Pathology of hepatocellular carcinoma. Edited by K Okuda and RL Peters:

Hepatocellular Carcinoma. New York, John Wiley & Sons, 1976, pp 107–168

28. Popper H: Cytoplasmic HBsAg in liver tissue outside of hepatocellular carcinoma. Hepatitis Sci Memo H-1306. Buffalo, Calspan, 1977

29. Okita K, Kodama T, Harada T, Noda K, Fukumoto Y, Takenami T, Shigeta K, Mizuta M, Takemoto T: Early lesions and development of primary hepatocellular carcinoma in man—association with hepatitis B viral infection. Gastroenterol Jpn 12:51–57, 1977

30. Kubo Y, Okuda K, Musha H. Nakashima T: Detection of hepatocellular carcinoma during a clinical follow-up of chronic liver disease. Observations in 31 patients. Gastroenterology 74:578–582, 1978

31. Vicary FR: Ultrasound and gastroenterology. Technical considerations. Gut 18:386–397, 1977

32. Gilby ED, Taylor KJW: Ultrasound monitoring of hepatic metastases during chemotherapy. Br Med J 1:371–373, 1975

33. Green B, Bree RL, Goldstein HM, Stanley C: Gray scale ultrasound evaluation of hepatic neoplasms: Patterns and correlations. Radiology 124:203–208, 1977

34. Alfidi RJ, Haaga JR, Havrilla TR, Pepe RG, Cook SA: Computed tomography of the liver. Am J Roentgenol 127:69–74, 1976

35. Levitt RG, Sagel SS, Stanley RJ, Jost RG: Accuracy of computed tomography of the liver and biliary tract. Radiology 124:123–128, 1977

36. Stephens D, Sheedy PF, II, Hattery RR, MacCarty RL: Computed tomography of the liver. Am J Roentgenol 128:579–590, 1977

37. Okuda K, Musha H, Nakajima Y, Kubo Y, Shimokawa Y, Nagasaki Y, Sawa Y, Jinnouchi S, Kaneko T, Obata H, Hisamitsu T, Motoike Y, Okazaki N, Kojiro M, Sakamoto K, Nakashima T: Clinicopathological features of encapsulated hepatocellular carcinoma. A study of 26 cases. Cancer 40:1240–1245, 1977

38. Lehman FG: Early detection of hepatoma: prospective study in liver cirrhosis using passive hemagglutination and the radioimmunoassay. Ann NY Acad Sci 259:196–210, 1975

39. Kew MC: Alpha-fetoprotein in primary liver cancer and other diseases. Gut 15:814–821, 1974

40. Okuda K, Kotoda K, Obata H, Hayashi N, Hisamitsu T, Tamiya M, Kubo Y, Yakush-iji F, Nagata E, Jinnouchi S, Shimokawa Y: Clinical observations during a relatively early stage of hepatocellular carcinoma, with special reference to serum α-fetoprotein levels. Gastroenterology 69:226–234, 1975

41. Niermeijer P, Gips CH, Marrink J. Que GS: Early detection of hepatoma in cirrhosis by serial quantitation of alpha-1-foetoprotein in serum. Neth J Med 19:15–18, 1976

42. Matsumoto Y, Suzuki T, Ono H, Nakase A, Honjo I: Evaluation of hepatoma chemotherapy by α-fetoprotein determination. Am J Surg 132:325–328, 1976

43. Okuda K, Kubo Y, Obata H: Serum α-fetoprotein in the relatively early stages of hepatocellular carcinoma and its relationship to gross anatomical types. Ann NY Acad Sci 259:248–252, 1975

44. Miyaji T: Association of hepatocellular carcinoma with cirrhosis among autopsy cases in Japan during 14 years from 1958 to 1971. Gann Monogr Cancer Res 18:129–149, 1976

45. Ohta Y: Viral hepatitis and hepatocellular carcinoma. Edited by K Okuda and RL Peters: Hepatocellular Carcinoma. New York, John Wiley & Sons, 1976, pp 73–82

46. Obata H, Hayashi N, Okuda K, Nishioka K: Continuous monitoring of HBsAg and alpha-fetoprotein in patients with cirrhosis and detection of hepatocellular carcinoma in early stage. Hepatitis Sci Memo H-881. Buffalo, Calspan, 1975

47. Halliday WJ, Maluish AE, Little JH, Davis NC: Leukocyte adherence inhibition and specific immunoreactivity in malignant melanoma. Int J Cancer 16:645–658, 1975

48. Loewenstein MS, Zamcheck N: Carcinoembryonic antigen and the liver. Gastroenterology 72:161–166, 1977

49. McCartney WH, Hoffer PB: Carcinoembryonic antigen assay in hepatic metastases detection. An adjunct to liver scanning. JAMA 236:1023–1027, 1976

50. Alpert E, Coston RL: Carcino-foetal human liver ferritins. Nature 242:194–196, 1973

51. Higashino K, Ohtani R, Kudo S, Hashimotsume M, Hada T, Kang K-Y, Ohkochi T, Takahashi Y, Yamamura Y: Hepatocellular carcinoma and a variant alkaline phosphatase. Ann Intern Med 82:74–78, 1975

52. Tsuo MG, McCoy MG, Lo KW: An isoenzyme of 5'-nucleotide phosphodiesterase and α-fetoprotein in human hepatic cancer patient sera. Cancer Res 34:2459–2463, 1974

53. Okazaki N, Araki E: Eicosatrienoic acid ω9 in serum lipids of patients with hepatocellular carcinoma. Clin Chim Acta 53:11–21, 1974

54. Okuda K, Nakashima T, Obata H, Kubo Y: Clinicopathological studies of minute hepatocellular carcinoma. Analysis of 20 cases, including 4 with hepatic resection. Gastroenterology 73:109–115, 1977

55. Nakashima T, Sakamoto K, Okuda K: A minute hepatocellular carcinoma found in a liver with clonorchis sinensis infection. Report of two cases. Cancer 39:1306–1311, 1977

56. Suzuki T, Matsumoto Y, Manabe T, Honjo I, Hamamoto K, Torizuka K: Serum alpha-fetoprotein and 67Ga citrate uptake in hepatoma. Am J Roentgenol 120:627–633, 1974

57. Kew MC, Geddes EW, Levin J: False-negative 75Se-seleno methionine scans in primary liver cancer. J Nucl Med 15:234–236, 1974

58. Levin J, Kew MC: Gallium-67-citrate scanning in primary cancer of the liver:diagnostic value in the presence of cirrhosis and relation to alpha-fetoprotein. J Nucl Med 17:369–373, 1976

59. Burraggi GL, Oaurini R, Rodari A, Bombardieri E: Double-tracer scintigraphy with 67Ga-citrate and 99mTc-sulfar colloid in the diagnosis of hepatic tumors. J Nucl Med 17:369–373, 1976

60. Kido C, Sasaki T, Kaneko M: Angiography of primary liver cancer. Am J Roentgenol 113:70–81, 1971

61. Okuda K, Musha H, Yamasaki T, Jinnouchi S, Nagasaki Y, Kubo Y, Shimokawa Y, Nakayama T, Kojiro M, Sakamoto K, Nakashima T: Angiographic demonstration of intrahepatic arterio-portal anastomoses in hepatocellular carcinoma. Radiology 122:53–58, 1977

62. Kobayashi M, Inokuchi K, Nagasue N, Saku M, Iwaki A: Successful treatment of early cancer of the liver and portal hypertension in patients presenting with bleeding oesophageal varices. Br J Surg 64:542–544, 1977

63. Link JS, Bateman JR, Paroly WS, Durkin WJ, Peters RL: 5-fluorouracil in hepatocellular carcinoma. Report of twenty-one cases. Cancer 39:1936–1939, 1977

64. McIntire KR, Vogel CL, Primack A, Waldmann TA, Kyalwazi SK: Effect of surgical and chemotherapeutic treatment on alpha-fetoprotein levels in patients with hepatocellular carcinoma. Cancer 37:677–683, 1976

65. Okazaki N: Systemic chemotherapy of hepatocellular carcinoma. Edited by K Okuda and RL Peters: Hepatocellular Carcinoma. New York, John Wiley & Sons, 1976, pp 469–475

66. Al-Sarraf M, Go TS, Kithier K, Vaitkevicius VK: Primary liver cancer: A review of the clinical features, blood groups, serum enzymes, therapy, and survival of 65 cases. Cancer 33:574–582, 1974

67. Geddes EW, Falkson G: Malignant hepatoma in the Bantu. Cancer 25:1271–1278, 1970

68. Kennedy PS, Lahane DE, Smith FE, Lane M: Oral fluorouracil therapy of hepatoma. Cancer 39:1930–1935, 1977

69. Ramirez G, Ansfield FJ, Curreri AR: Hepatoma: long-term survival with disseminated tumor treated with 5-fluorouracil. Am J Surg 120:400–403, 1970

70. Smart CR, Townsend LB, Rusho WJ, Eyre HJ, Quagliana JM, Wilson ML, Edwards CB, Manning SJ: Phase I study of Ftoraful, an analog of 5-fluorouracil. Cancer 36:103–106, 1975

71. Olweny CLM, Toya T, Katongole-Mbidde E, Mugerwa J, Kyalwazi SK, Cohen H: Treatment of hepatocellular carcinoma with adriamycin. Preliminary communication. Cancer 36:1250–1257, 1975

72. Vogel CL, Bayley AC, Brooker RJ, Anthony PP, Ziegler JL: A phase II study of adriamycin (NSC 123127) in patients with hepatocellular carcinoma from Zambia and the United States. Cancer 39:1923–1929, 1977

73. Balasegaram M: Management of primary liver cell carcinoma. Am J Surg 130:33–37, 1975

74. Kubo Y, Shimokawa Y: Arterial injection chemotherapy. Edited by K Okuda and RL Peters: Hepatocellular Carcinoma. New York, John Wiley & Sons, 1976, pp 477–490

75. Nakashima T: Vascular changes and hemodynamics in hepatocellular carcinoma. Edited by K Okuda and RL Peters: Hepatocellular Carcinoma. New York, John Wiley & Sons, 1976, pp 169–203

76. Massey WH, Fletcher WS, Kudkins MP, Dennis DL: Hepatic artery infusion for metastatic malignancy using percutaneously placed catheter. Am J Surg 121:160–164, 1971

77. Cady B: Hepatic arterial patency and complications after catheterization for infusion chemotherapy. Ann Surg 178:156–161, 1973

78. Lange M, Falkson G, Geddes E: Intra-ar

terial chemotherapy in the treatment of primary liver cancer. S Afr J Surg 12:245–249, 1974

79. Ariel IL, Pack GT: Treatment of inoperable cancer of the liver by intra-arterial radioactive isotopes and chemotherapy. Cancer 20:793–804, 1967

80. Hahn E, Hehmann F-G, Ferlemann J, Ax W, Hamelmann H, Hort W, Havemann K: Immuntherapie eines metastasierten primären Leberzellkarzinoms mit autologen Tumorzellen und BCG. Verh Dtsch Ges Inn Med 83:1205–1208, 1977

81. Smith GV, Grogan JB, Stribling J, Lockard J: Immunochemotherapy of hepatoma in rats. Am J Surg 129:146–155, 1975

82. Honjo I, Suzuki T, Ozawa K, Takasan H, Kitamura O, Ishikawa T: Ligation of a branch of the portal vein for carcinoma of the liver. Am J Surg 130:296–302, 1975

83. Lin TY: Results in 107 hepatic lobectomies with a preliminary report on the use of a clamp to reduce blood loss. Ann Surg 177:413–421, 1973

84. Lin TY: A simplified technique for hepatic resection: the crush method. Ann Surg 180:285–290, 1974

85. Fortner JQ, Shiu MH, Kinne DW, Castro EB, Watson RC, Hawland WS, Beattie EJ: Major hepatic resection using vascular isolation and hypothermia perfusion. Ann Surg 180:644–652, 1974

86. Buerk CA, Putnam CW, Starzl TE: Major hepatic resection and portal pressure. Surg Gynecol Obstet 144:853–854, 1977

87. Gammill SL, Takahashi M, Jingu K, Stumpe W, Font R: A comparison of scan and angiograms in selecting patients with hepatomas for hepatic lobectomy. Am J Roentgenol 123:522–530, 1975

88. Nagasue N, Inokuchi K, Kobayashi M, Ogawa Y, Saku M, Yukaya H: Angiographic evaluation of hepatoma for surgical treatment. Surgery 143:184–190, 1976

89. Shiu MH, Fortner JG: Current management of hepatic tumors. Surg Gynecol Obstet 140:781–788, 1975

90. Okuda K, Musha H, Yoshida T, Kanda Y, Yamazaki T, Jinnouchi S, Moriyama M, Kawaguchi S, Kubo Y, Shimokawa Y, Kojiro M, Kuratomi S, Sakamoto K, Nakashima T: Demonstration of growing casts of hepatocellular carcinoma in the portal vein by celiac angiography: The thread and streaks sign. Radiology 117:303–309, 1975

91. Okuda K, Jinnouchi S, Nagasaki Y, Kuwahara S, Kaneko T, Kubo Y, Shimokawa Y, Nakajima Y, Takasha M, Musha H, Kudo T, Sakamoto K, Kojiro M, Nakashima T: Angiographic demonstration of growth of hepatocellular carcinoma in the hepatic vein and inferior vena cava. Radiology 124:33–36, 1977

92. Nagasue N, Inokuchi K, Kobayashi M, Ogawa Y, Iwaki A, Yukaya H: Hepatic dearterialization for nonresectable primary and secondary tumors of the liver. Cancer 38:2593–2603, 1976

93. Almersjö O, Bengmark S, Hafström L, Leissner H: Results of liver dearterialization combined with regional infusion of 5-fluorouracil. Acta Chir Scand 142:131–138, 1976

94. Starzl TE, Brettschneider LB, Putnam CW: Transplantation of the liver. Edited by H Popper and F Schaffner: Progress in Liver Diseases. Vol. III. New York, Grune & Stratton, 1970, pp 495–542

95. William R, Smith MGM: Liver transplantation: A clinical and immunological appraisal. Edited by H Popper and F Schaffner: Progress in Liver Diseases. Vol. IV. New York, Grune & Stratton, 1972, pp 433–446

96. Starzl TE, Porter KA, Putnam CW, Schroter GPJ, Halgrimson CG, Weil III R, Hoescher M, Reid HAS: Orthotopic liver transplantation in ninety-three patients. Surg Gynecol Obstet 142:487–505

97. Honjo I, Mizumoto R: Primary carcinoma of the liver. Am J Surg 128:31–36, 1974

98. Primack A, Vogel CL, Kyalwazi SK, Ziegler JL, Simon R, Anthony PP: A staging system for hepatocellular carcinoma: prognostic factors in Ugandan patients. Cancer 35:1357-1364

99. Fisher RL, Scheuer PJ, Sherlock S: Primary liver cell carcinoma in the presence or absence of hepatitis B antigen. Cancer 38:901–905, 1976

100. Nagasue N, Inokuchi K, Kobayashi M, Saku M: Serum alpha-fetoprotein levels after hepatic artery ligation and postoperative chemotherapy. Cancer 40:615–618, 1977

101. Esterhay RJ, Shapiro HM, Sutherland JC, McIntire KR, Wiernik PH: Serum alpha fetoprotein concentration and tumor growth dissociation in a patient with ovarian teratocarcinoma. Cancer 31:835–839, 1973

Index

Ouabain
  and hepatic DNA synthesis, 127
  and synthesis of α_1-fetoprotein and albumin,
    132
Oxidase reactions, mixed function, microsomal
    enzymes in, 264, 275-276
Oxygen consumption, cerebral, in hepatic coma,
    334
Oxyphenisatin, liver damage from 597, 598

Pancreas
  endoscopic retrograde
    cholangiopancreatography,   510-512
  and hepatic regeneration, 143
Pancreatitis, and cholestasis, 505-506
Parenchymal cells. *See* Hepatocytes
Penicillamine, in primary biliary cirrhosis, 498,
    571
Pentachlorophenol, liver damage from, 619
Periarteritis nodosa, hepatitis B immune
    complexes in, 401-403
Peroxidase activity, in Kupffer cells, 162-164
Peroxisomes of hepatocytes, 95-99
  abnormalities of, 97-99
  inclusions in, 99
  matrix consistency changes in, 99
  normal, 95-97
  number of, changes in, 97-98
  shape of, changes in, 98
  size of, changes in, 98
Phalloidin, 465
  affecting actin filaments, 115
Phenothiazines, liver damage from 489, 600, 601
Phenylalanine
  brain levels in hepatic encephalopathy, 330
  injections of lethal doses, 335
Phosophorus, liver damage from, 616
Pit cells, 158
PIVKA effect, in liver disease, 304, 308
Platelets
  endotoxin interaction with, 314
  transfusions of, 310
  uptake of octopamine and NE in hepatic
    encephalopathy, 337
Polymyxin B antiendotoxin effect of, 320, 321
Porphyria, microsomal enzymes in, 271-274
Portacaval shunt
  clinical evaluation of, 146-147
  hepatic changes from, 135-136
  and prognostic significance of Mallory bodies,
    565
Portal blood hepatotrophic factors, 135-147
  clinical implications of, 146-147
  and effects of Eck's fistula, 135-136, 140-141
  and effects of insulin, 138-139
  experimental studies

  with intestinal venous blood, 137-139
  with pancreaticoduodenal venous effluent,
    137-139
  with splanchnic venous blood, 136-137
  with systemic venous blood, 136-137
  and hepatic lipid synthesis, 139
  and regeneration, 142-146
Potassium, transport in cells, 58
Pregnancy, liver disease in
  and mitochondria of hepatocytes, 89
  and peroxisomes of hepatocytes, 98
Profilin, properties of, 106
Propylthiouracil
  in alcoholic hepatitis, 571-572
  liver damage from 597, 600
Prostaglandins, receptors for, on hepatic cell
    surface, 57
Proteases, at cell surface, 179
Protein
  in brain, in hepatic coma, 333
  cell-surface, 177-179
  deprivation of, and microsomal enzyme
    activity, 275
  hepatic-binding, 61-63, 68-70
  liver-specific, 408-409
  microtubule-associated, 111-112
  secretion after ethanol ingestion, 562
  synthesis in hepatocytes, 11-12, 25-31
    in diseases, 34-37
    experimental modification of, 31-34
    localization of, 25-31
Pruritus
  in cholestasis, 236
  in primary biliary cirrhosis, 495
Psychometric testing, in hepatic encephalopathy,
    333

Receptors in hepatic cell surfaces, 43-70, 113-114
  and carrier-mediated transport, 58-60
  for catecholamines, 57
  for glucagon, 54-56
  for glycoproteins, 61-63
  for growth-promoting hormones, 57
  for hormones, 51-58
  and immunologic phenomena, 64-70, 414
  for insulin, 51-54
  for lactogenic hormones, 57
  and ligand-receptor interactions, 47-50
  for lipoproteins, 63-64
  methods of study, 45-47
  for prostaglandins, 57
  for secretin, 56
  for transferrin-bound iron, 60-61
  for triiodothyronine and thyroxine, 57
  for vasoactive intestinal polypeptide, 56
Reflux esophagitis, bile acid metabolism in, 234